THEORETICAL IMMUNOLOGY

IMMUNOLOGY SERIES

Edited by NOEL ROSE

Professor and Chairman
Department of Immunology and Microbiology
Wayne State University
Detroit, Michigan

1. Mechanisms in Allergy: Reagin-Mediated Hypersensitivity
   Edited by Lawrence Goodfriend, Alec Sehon, and Robert P. Orange
2. Immunopathology: Methods and Techniques
   Edited by Theodore P. Zacharia and Sidney S. Breese, Jr.
3. Immunity and Cancer in Man: An Introduction
   Edited by Arnold E. Reif
4. *Bordetella pertussis:* Immunological and Other Biological Activities
   J. J. Munoz and R. K. Bergman
5. The Lymphocyte: Structure and Function, Parts I and II
   Edited by John J. Marchalonis
6. Immunology of Receptors
   Edited by B. Cinader
7. Immediate Hypersensitivity: Modern Concepts and Developments
   Edited by Michael K. Bach
8. Theoretical Immunology
   Edited by George I. Bell, Alan S. Perelson, and George H. Pimbley, Jr.

Other Volumes in Preparation

THEORETICAL IMMUNOLOGY

Edited by

George I. Bell
Alan S. Perelson
George H. Pimbley, Jr.

Theoretical Division
University of California
Los Alamos Scientific Laboratory
Los Alamos, New Mexico

MARCEL DEKKER, INC. New York and Basel

Library of Congress Cataloging in Publication Data

Main entry under title:

Theoretical immunology.

(Immunology series ; 8)
Includes indexes.
1. Immunology--Mathematical models. I. Bell, George I., 1926- II. Perelson, Alan S., 1947- III. Pimbley, George H., Jr. IV. Series.
QR182.2.M36T48 574.2'9 77-26655
ISBN 0-8247-6618-0

MARCEL DEKKER, INC.
270 Madison Avenue, New York, New York 10016

Current printing (last digit):
10 9 8 7 6 5 4 3 2 1

PRINTED IN THE UNITED STATES OF AMERICA

PREFACE

During the past two decades, immunology has moved a long way from its origins among the healing arts toward becoming one of the biological sciences. Two factors have been critical in facilitating this progress. The first was the development of the clonal selection theory, which, now amply confirmed by experiment, has furnished at least a working outline of the operation of the immune system. The second has been the development of quantitative experimental techniques for studying the molecules and the cells of the immune system and their interactions.

Immunology now has a solid conceptual basis, and a vast amount of hard data has been accumulated; yet important uncertainties remain. Many of these are concerned with the mechanisms which govern the initiation and regulation of immune responses. Understanding these mechanisms would have important clinical implications especially for those conditions for which immune responses may be ineffective, such as cancer, or self-destructive, as in autoimmune diseases.

Under these circumstances it is natural that many scientists, trained in the physical sciences or mathematics, have become interested in immunology and in what they might be able to contribute to further progress. During the past few years we have encountered many theoretically inclined scientists who would like to become more involved, perhaps in collaboration with immunologists, in the modeling and analysis of immunological assays, experiments, or theories. We believe that this is a healthy trend which should be encouraged. It may, however, be difficult for a physical scientist to learn enough immunology to make an informed choice of problems on which to work. While some have been fortunate in finding sympathetic collaborators, and have been able to bridge the communication gap, many more are discouraged from trying.

In order to promote the interaction between immunologists and physical or mathematical scientists we have assembled the papers in this book. The contributions contained herein are of two types. Some are by immunologists and describe various theoretical problems which might be appropriate subjects for mathematical modeling and analysis. Others portray the current state of modeling of some important problems in immunology. We hope that the juxtaposition of these two kinds of contributions will prove stimulating, both to theoretically inclined immunologists and to mathematicians and physical scientists who may be seeking to contribute to immunology.

Those with no previous exposure to immunology and without knowledge of some of the basic facts of immunology may find portions of this book difficult to understand. We recommend that such readers consult a textbook of immunology such as I. Roitt, *Essential Immunology* (2nd ed., Blackwell, Oxford, 1974), H. Eisen, *Immunology* (2nd ed., Harper and Row, New York, 1974), or M. J. Hobart and I. McConnell, *The Immune System: A Course on the Molecular and Cellular Basis of Immunity* (Blackwell, Oxford, 1975). These books are listed in order of increasing sophistication.

This book is an introduction to theoretical immunology and provides a summary of work to date in many problem areas. The book begins with an historical introduction which is followed by two papers with a philosophical emphasis (Burnet and Cunningham). Examples by Goldstein and Nossal follow on the analysis of assays, after which there are papers by DeLisi, Ault and Unanue, Perelson, and Inman on the interactions of antigens with antibodies and with lymphocytes and the resulting cell behaviors. Interactions among B cells, T cells, and macrophages, and the architecture of the immune system are next considered by Feldmann, Dutton and Swain, and Bell. Following this, several models of cell population dynamics are developed. Those of Bruni, Giovenco, Koch and Strom, of Waltman, and of Mohler, Barton, and Hsu are primarily models of the lymphocyte proliferation and differentiation that occur following antigen injection, while those of Aris, Pimbley, and Lefever and Garay are concerned with the competition between replicating antigen and cells of the immune system. The models of Richter, Hoffman, and Adam are distinguished by the fact that they assume that lymphocytes recognize each other's idiotopes, forming a network of interacting cells.

We are delighted to acknowledge the expert typing and other assistance of Mrs. Mary Plehn in preparing the final camera-ready copy of each manuscript.

George I. Bell
Alan S. Perelson
George H. Pimbley, Jr.

CONTRIBUTORS

Gerold Adam, Fachbereich Biologie, Universität Konstanz, Konstanz, Federal Republic of Germany

Rutherford Aris, Department of Chemical Engineering and Materials Science, University of Minnesota, Minneapolis, Minnesota

Kenneth A. Ault, Department of Pathology, Harvard Medical School, Boston, Massachusetts

Claude F. Barton, Department of Electrical and Computer Engineering, Oregon State University, Corvallis, Oregon

George I. Bell, Theoretical Division, University of California, Los Alamos Scientific Laboratory, Los Alamos, New Mexico

Carlo Bruni, Istituto di Automatica, University of Rome, Rome, Italy

F. M. Burnet, Department of Microbiology, University of Melbourne, Parkville, Victoria, Australia

A. J. Cunningham,* Department of Microbiology, John Curtin School of Medical Research, Australian National University, Canberra, Australia

Charles DeLisi, Laboratory of Theoretical Biology, National Cancer Institute, National Institutes of Health, Bethesda, Maryland

Richard W. Dutton, Department of Biology, University of California at San Diego, La Jolla, California

Marc Feldmann, ICRF Tumour Immunology Unit, Department of Zoology, University College, London, England

Ricardo Garay, Chimie Physique II, Faculté des Sciences, Université Libre de Bruxelles, Brussels, Belgium

Maria Adelaide Giovenco, Centro Studi Sistemi, Controllo e Calcolo Automatici, C.N.R., Rome, Italy

Byron Goldstein, Theoretical Division, University of California, Los Alamos Scientific Laboratory, Los Alamos, New Mexico

**Present affiliation*: Division of Biological Research, Ontario Cancer Institute, Toronto, Ontario, Canada

Geoffrey W. Hoffmann, Basel Institute for Immunology, Basel, Switzerland.

Chin-Shung Hsu, Department of Electrical and Computer Engineering, Oregon State University, Corvallis, Oregon

John K. Inman, Laboratory of Immunology, National Institute of Allergy and Infectious Diseases, National Institutes of Health, Bethesda, Maryland

Giorgio Koch,[*] Istituto di Automatica, University of Rome, Rome, Italy

René Lefever, Chimie Physique II, Faculté des Sciences, Université Libre de Bruxelles, Brussels, Belgium

R. R. Mohler, Department of Electrical and Computer Engineering, Oregon State University, Corvallis, Oregon

Ralph Nossal, Physical Sciences Laboratory, Division of Computer Research and Technology, National Institutes of Health, Bethesda, Maryland

Alan S. Perelson, Theoretical Division, University of California, Los Alamos Scientific Laboratory, Los Alamos, New Mexico

George H. Pimbley, Jr.,[†] Theoretical Division, University of California, Los Alamos Scientific Laboratory, Los Alamos, New Mexico

Peter H. Richter,[††] Department of Biochemical Kinetics, Max-Planck-Institut für Biophysikalische Chemie, Göttingen-Nikolausberg, Federal Republic of Germany

Roberto Strom, Istituto di Chimica Biologica, University of Rome, Rome, Italy

Susan L. Swain, Department of Biology, University of California at San Diego, La Jolla, California

Emil R. Unanue, Department of Pathology, Harvard Medical School, Boston, Massachusetts

Paul Waltman, Department of Mathematics, The University of Iowa, Iowa City, Iowa

---

[*] *Present affiliation:* Istituto di Matematica, University of Lecce, Lecce, Italy

[†] *Present affiliation:* National Science Foundation, Washington, D.C.

[††] *Present affiliation:* Department of Theoretical Chemistry, Massachusetts Institute of Technology, Cambridge, Massachusetts

CONTENTS

Part I

HISTORICAL SURVEY

Chapter 1

AN HISTORICAL INTRODUCTION TO THEORETICAL IMMUNOLOGY

George I. Bell and Alan S. Perelson

Theoretical Division
University of California
Los Alamos Scientific Laboratory
Los Alamos, New Mexico

Two types of theories in immunology are reviewed. First, some of the major nonmathematical theories which have traditionally furnished the framework for immunological thought and controversy are outlined. It is pointed out that although there is now a dominant theoretical model, namely the clonal selection theory, many important questions remain unresolved. These involve such key issues as the origin of antibody diversity, mechanisms of self-nonself discrimination, and the regulation of expression of genetic information. Second, theories having a significant mathematical content are described. Some have made possible the quantitative understanding of immunological assays or procedures, including complement-mediated lysis, antigen-antibody precipitation, and the Jerne hemolytic plaque assay. Others have helped to elucidate the interactions between antigens and cells, which may be important in triggering immune responses. Finally, several attempts to model the cell kinetics in an immune response are described. An extensive list of references to immunological theories is included.

I. INTRODUCTION

So rich is the phenomenology of immunology that theoretical frameworks are almost always required for understanding of immunological data. An example may be taken from the beginnings of immunology. The phenomenon of immunity to smallpox was known in ancient societies and even exploited by dangerous immunization procedures (Langer, 1976). Around 1800 Jenner developed sucessful immunization techniques against smallpox, but this discovery of vaccination had little impact on the treatment or understanding of any other disease for nearly 100 years. As pointed out by Ehrlich (1900), "that Jenner's discovery remained so isolated was due essentially to the fact that the theoretical conceptions of the cause and nature of infectious diseases made no advance during the subsequent decades." That is, not until the germ theory of disease became accepted was there any basis for understanding the response of the organism.

As immunology has developed during this century, the field has been dominated by various theoretical controversies, for example, (a) instructive vs. selective theories of antibody formation, (b) germ-line vs. somatic mutation origin of antibody diversity, and (c) one specific signal vs. one nonspecific signal vs. two-signal models of lymphocyte activation. The theories have been almost entirely conceptual or nonmathematical in nature. This volume is, however, at least partially dedicated to the proposition that mathematical analysis can make an important contribution to immunology. In this chapter we will first briefly review some of the major nonmathematical theories which have played important roles in immunology and second, efforts to formulate and solve mathematical models of immunological assays, phenomena, and systems.

II. MAJOR NONMATHEMATICAL THEORIES

A. Instructive vs. Selective Theories of Antibody Formation

An animal which has survived a first exposure to an antigen, such as a pathogenic virus or bacterium, is commonly far better able to cope with a subsequent exposure. It has acquired immunity or an immunological memory. A most important challenge to early immunologists was to provide a satisfactory theory for this development of immunity. Such theories may be broadly categorized as selective or instructive. In a selective theory, the antigen is postulated to selectively stimulate the production of those preexisting antibodies which are complementary to and bind to the antigen, while in an instructive theory, the antigen is viewed as instructing the animal how to make complementary antibody where none existed before.

An early and influential selective model was formulated by Ehrlich (1900), who postulated that every responding cell has a diversity of surface receptors (in modern terminology) which are complementary to possible antigens. Contact with an antigen was then assumed to stimulate the cell to synthesize those particular receptors, complementary to the antigen, in great excess and to release them as circulating antibodies. As noted by Burnet in Chap. 3, Ehrlich's model was largely abandoned as immunologists began in the 1920s to obtain increasing evidence of the great diversity of antibody molecules that could be produced in response to synthetic compounds. The preexistence of such diversity, particularly on a single cell, became difficult to understand. Although Ehrlich's model is no longer believed to be correct, the existence of diversity prior to antigen stimulation is now generally accepted. It is also interesting to note that Szilard (1960) developed a model for the operation of selection at the subcellular level according to concepts of molecular biology. Szilard had been considering the induction and repression of enzyme synthesis in bacteria and constructed his model along analogous lines. Contrary to Ehrlich, he postulated that the antigen enters the lymphocyte where it binds to receptors that also serve as enzymes in mediating the formation of molecules which repress the synthesis of antibodies complementary to stimulating antigen. The antigen thereby serves to derepress the synthesis of complementary antibody molecules in an irreversible manner. Szilards' model was developed, however, after the clonal selection theory and had little influence on immunology.

During the 1930s many immunologists believed that antigen must instruct the antibody forming mechanism to somehow produce complementary antibodies. Pauling (1940) presented a particularly clear instructive model. He postulated that all antibodies have the same amino acid sequence but that the three-dimensional conformation of their ends was determined during synthesis by direct contact with the antigen serving as a template. Moreover, he assumed that their conformation would be stable once the molecule was separated from the antigen. While this model could explain a virtually infinite repertoire of antibody conformations, it offered little insight into the nature of immunological memory. Furthermore, it has been found that the conformations of antibody molecules, like those of other proteins, are determined by their amino acid sequences.

Selective theories of antibody formation were revived by Jerne (1955), who assumed that a diverse population of natural antibodies arises during development, even in the absence of antigen. Antigen then selectively combines with complementary circulating antibodies. It was further assumed that the antigen-antibody complexes, on being taken up by phagocytic cells of the immune system, somehow stimulate the further and more abundant production of antibodies of the same specificity in either the phagocyte or other cells. The vigor of a response would depend on the concentration of circulating antibodies and could thus be enhanced by prior exposure to antigen.

It remained for Burnet (1957) (and also Talmage, 1957) to make the key assumption that each responsive cell makes and expresses on its surface only a single type of antibody molecule, and that the *selective event* is the stimulation by antigen of those *cells* making complementary antibodies, resulting in proliferation of the cells and secretion of the antibodies. This clonal selection theory, which was given definitive form by Burnet (1959), is briefly brought up to date by Burnet in this volume, and is generally accepted as a valid outline of the functioning of the immune system. Many details of the outline remain controversial, and some of these are worth special attention.

B. The Origin of Antibody Diversity: Somatic Mutation vs. Germ Line, Self vs. Nonself Discrimination

The diversity of antibody molecules arises from the variability of their amino acid sequences. As the structure of antibody molecules became understood during the 1960s and as amino acid sequences were measured, some aspects of this variability became clear. First of all, it was found that antibody molecules are composed of light and heavy polypeptide chains containing somewhat more than 200 and 400 amino acids, respectively (Fig. 1).

Moreover, a high degree of variability was found in the 100 or so amino acids at the amino terminal end of each chain. Wu and Kabat (1970) further analyzed sequence variability and showed that it was confined to three or four hypervariable regions which have now been found on both light and heavy chains. It is now known that an antigen binding site on an antibody molecule is formed from the variable regions of both heavy and light chains and that amino acids in the hypervariable regions are particularly available for establishing bonds with an antigen. This structure of antibody molecules quantitatively eases the diversity problem since, for example, from 10^3 light chain sequences and 10^3 heavy chains, it would in principle be possible to assemble 10^6 different antibody molecules. But this does not *solve* the diversity problem.

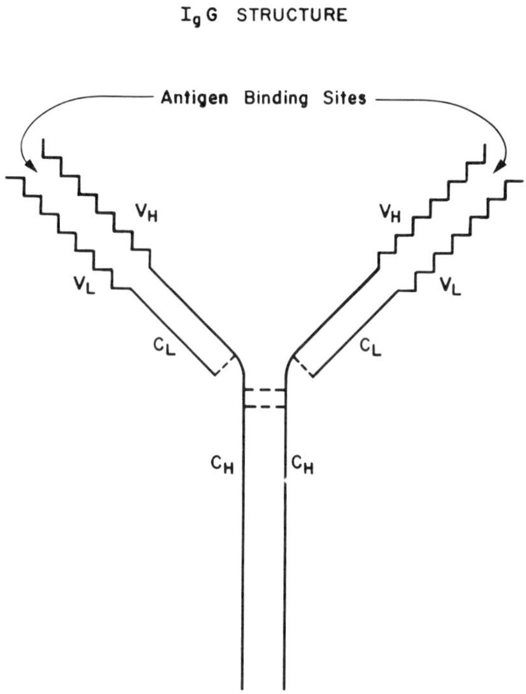

FIG. 1. Each of the four polypeptide chains in this antibody molecule is indicated by a solid line, two light and two heavy. The straight portions depict the constant regions (C_L and C_H) wherein the amino acid sequences are more or less invariant for antibodies of a given class, while the zigzag portions depict the variable regions (V_L and V_H) in which the amino acid sequences are highly variable. V_L and V_H regions combine to form the two antigen binding sites.

Two extreme theoretical positions may be distinguished for explaining the generation of antibody diversity. In the germ-line theory it is postulated that there are DNA sequences in the germ line for each of the amino acid sequences which may appear in the variable portions of light or heavy chains. These "genes" are presumed to have arisen through evolution and natural selection of the species. The alternative theory, somatic mutation, postulates that variability is generated by a process of somatic mutation (or some other randomization process) during ontogeny and/or differentiation of the lymphocytes. In either case it must be explained why an animal does not make antibodies against self components.

In his clonal selection theory, Burnet (1957, 1959) assumed that diversity was generated by random processes such as somatic mutation during perinatal life, so that shortly after birth the animal would have a fixed repertoire of antibody combining sites. Moreover, he postulated the death of any lymphocyte which recognized a self (or foreign) antigen during this sensitive time of diversity generation. In a particularly clear elaboration of Burnet's clonal selection theory, Lederberg (1959) favored the possibility that somatic mutation may generate new clones throughout the life of an animal, and it is only required that each clone pass through a sensitive stage during which contact with self antigen will eliminate it. In either case, self-reactive clones would not be found in normal mature animals.

In 1971, Jerne argued that the elimination of self-reactive clones could furnish a powerful negative selection mechanism favoring diversity in cells which could recognize *slightly different from self* antigens. Such antigens, for example on virally infected host cells, might otherwise be particularly hard to detect and therefore dangerous. Jerne (1971) postulated that a significant fraction of the germ-line genes code for variable regions on antibody molecules which recognize self antigens, and that these self-recognizing clones proliferate and mutate within such primary lymphoid organs as the thymus. After considerable proliferation, the nonmutant, self-reactive cells would be killed by contact with self antigen, and only the mutants would survive. Further consideration of the ways in which self antigens, in particular those on antibody molecules themselves (idiotypes), may affect the generation of diversity and the regulation of immune responses, led Jerne to propose his network theory (Jerne, 1973, 1974, 1976) which is considered in this volume by Adam (Chap. 21), by Hoffman (Chap. 21), and by Richter (Chap. 19).

It has been argued by the proponents of somatic mutation theory, from Burnet on, that unusually high mutation rates (e.g., $> 10^{-7}$ per base-pair per cell division) are not required for generation of diversity. The possibility that diversity is generated by recombination between germ-line genes has been proposed (Edelman and Gally, 1967; Smithies, 1967). Some attractive features of this hypothesis will be considered in Section II.C. Recombination among only a few genes is not supported by sequence data; many genes would be required. Baltimore (1974) has called attention to the enzyme terminal deoxynucleotidyl transferase, as a possible mechanism for enhancing mutation rates in certain DNA segments. This enzyme is found preferentially in the thymus and adds deoxyribonucleotides at random to the ends of DNA primers.

The germ-line theory of antibody diversity was encouraged by the finding that antibody binding sites were formed from two separate polypeptide chains. Thus a rather modest investment of DNA would suffice in coding for all of the required variability.* In addition, the amino acid sequences could be grouped into families (e.g., Hood and Talmage, 1970) which might represent germ-line genes. More convincing evidence has come from repeated findings of the same sequence in independent myelomas induced in inbred mice (e.g., Cohn et al., 1974). Such sequences are generally agreed to represent germ-line genes, but few such genes have been reliably identified by this method.

Amino acid sequence data do not suffice for a clean solution to the germ- line vs. somatic mutation controversy, since much the same sequence patterns could be expected to result whether mutation

---

*For example, consider 2×10^3 polypeptide chains, half heavy and half light, and thus having an average of about 330 amino acids per chain. These would be coded by 2×10^6 nucleotide pairs having an aggregate molecular weight of 1.3×10^9. This is approximately equal to 10^{-3} of the DNA content of a mammalian cell. These chains could in principle be used for assembling 10^6 distinct antibody molecules, which is a rough median estimate of the required diversity (e.g., Cohn et al., 1974; Jerne, 1971; Klinman and Press, 1975; see also Inman, Chap. 9).

and selection occur during lymphocyte differentiation or during species evolution. Cohn (1968) has argued forcefully for a strong role for somatic mutation in enabling an animal to cope with the unexpected. He has advanced the model (Cohn et al., 1974) that variability in the hypervariable or complementarity-determining regions of immunoglobulin (Ig) chains results from somatic mutation, whereas variability elsewhere in the variable regions (in framework regions) defines germ-line genes. This method of counting implied somewhat over 100 germ-line genes for light chains alone. Further clarification is to be expected from current studies of the hybridization of DNA with homogeneous mRNA coding for a particular variable chain. The results (e.g., Tonegawa, 1976; Honjo et al., 1976) appear to indicate that a substantial and perhaps crucial role remains for somatic variation, in that the number of germ-line genes is much less than the number of different sequences which have been identified.

In analyzing the possible evolution of families of immunoglobulin genes, Hood and others (1975; Smith, 1976) have indicated a variety of ways in which such evolution may differ from that of individual genes, as studied, for example, in bacteria. For example, the number of copies of a gene and the number of DNA sequences in a family may be expanded or contracted as a result of homologous but unequal crossing-over between sister chromatids. Smith (1973), Black and Gibson (1974), Ohta (1976, 1977), and Perelson and Bell (1977), have studied the evolution of multigene families by unequal crossing-over. Since repeated DNA sequences are common in eukaryotic DNA, the careful study of the immunoglobulin gene family may reveal some general principles of eukaryotic evolution.

We have thus seen that although the original somatic mutation theory of Burnet and Lederberg has been modified and enriched by subsequent data and theory, it appears to retain considerable validity. It remains to reconsider the problem of self-nonself discrimination.

First of all, it should be noted that self-nonself discrimination cannot be coded in the germ line. It must be learned. This is because, except in the unnatural case of highly inbred strains, each parent of an animal is capable of responding to and rejecting the other parent's antigens, in particular the histocompatability antigens. Therefore, each parent contains the genetic information which is required for rejecting the other parent's antigens. Since the offspring will derive genetic information and express antigens from each parent, it must have the information for making antibodies against self antigens and somehow learn not to do so.

During the 1960s immunologists found that exposure of an animal to an antigen could render the animal either specifically unresponsive (tolerant), or immune, depending on the details of antigen presentation (e.g., Mitchison, 1964). This suggested that mature lymphocytes could be either stimulated or paralyzed by contact with antigen. On this basis, Bretscher and Cohn (1970) devised a theory in which self-reactive cells would usually be paralyzed, while nonself-reactive cells would be stimulated, by exposure to complementary foreign antigens. According to the theory, contact of antigen with a lymphocyte always delivers a paralytic signal to the cell, and for stimulation or induction a second signal is required. This second signal must also be antigen-specific and was assumed to be due to a second cell or to a diffusable factor derived from a second antigen recognizing cell. In the model, antigen reactive cells are assumed to be generated continuously during an animal's life, and the distinction between self and nonself antigens arises from the requirement that the former always be present (at least during the generation of responsive cells) while the latter appear at some first time. To see how this distinction leads to paralysis of self antigens and responsiveness of foreign antigens, consider first the self antigen case. As cells are generated with receptors for self antigens, they will appear one (or possibly two) at a time and they will encounter antigen's, one by one, without any helper factors or cells to give a second signal. They will thus all be paralyzed. A foreign antigen is, however, absent for some duration, during which helper cells and factors may accumulate to some extent. When, therefore, the antigen is introduced and encounters a responsive cell, there will already be present sufficient helper cells and/or factors to result in a strong second signal and induction. See Bretscher (1972) for a discussion of some quantitative aspects of the theory.

This two-signal hypothesis remains controversial, and we are a long way from being able to define necessary and sufficient conditions for either lymphocyte activation or paralysis (see e.g., Möller, 1975). Nevertheless, it is impressive that the model did predict a requirement for helper cells before the cooperation between T cells and B cells was known. More recently, Bretscher (1974) has generalized the theory to account for control of cell-mediated and humoral immunity, the IgM to IgG switch, and possibly suppressor T cells. In part the modifications are based upon a general hypothesis, namely, that when an animal is first confronted with a threatening antigen, it should respond in the most effective way possible, that is, by using the cell-mediated immune system. If the animal obtains evidence that its defense is going to be successful, it should then switch to IgM and IgG responses successively, in order to minimize possible damage to itself. This later model requires more factors than the original one, but the factors do not approach in number those identified by Feldmann in Chap. 10.

C. Regulation of the Expression of Genetic Information. Translocons

The light and heavy polypeptide chains of an antibody molecule are composed of both variable and constant regions. The constant regions are responsible for the functioning of the antibody once it has bound antigen. In particular, the constant parts of the heavy chain govern the binding to cells or to complement.

It appears that each immunoglobulin chain is specified by two separate genes, a V gene and a C gene (Gally and Edelman, 1972), which is a striking departure from the one gene-one polypeptide rule. Gally and Edelman (1970) proposed that when a particular V gene (out of many choices) is to be expressed, it must be excised from its initial position in the DNA and spliced-in adjacent to the corresponding C gene. This process, or more generally, any process in which the genome is reorganized so that two genes not originally functionally related become so organized, was called translocation, and the family of V and C genes within which translocation is permitted is called a translocon. Three unlinked translocons were identified, namely, those coding for two kinds of light chains (called κ and λ light chains) and for heavy chains. Nucleic acid hybridization studies have recently provided evidence for the joining of V and C genes during the differentiation of lymphocytes (Hozumi and Tonegawa, 1976).

Gally and Edelman (1970) also pointed out that if the several V genes are adjacent and if the excision process does not precisely remove one V gene but perhaps, say, the first third of one V gene and the last two-thirds of the adjacent V gene, then diversity will be generated by somatic recombination.

Recent studies of the conversion of a response from IgM to IgG production (reviewed by Hood et al., 1975) suggest that this represents expression of a new C gene for the heavy chain, namely one coding for a γ as opposed to a μ chain, while the translocated V genes remain invariant. This may imply another form of translocation, either of the V or C_μ gene.

III. MATHEMATICAL THEORIES

Although the majority of theories in immunology have been nonmathematical, there are a variety of quantitative questions whose solutions require mathematical analysis and mathematically formulated models. To obtain quantitative, and not merely qualitative, information about immune phenomena, theoretical models have been made of many of the assays and experimental methods commonly employed in immunology. Without attempting to be exhaustive we shall review some of the major theoretical efforts in this direction in Section III.A.

In order for the cells of the immune system to detect antigen there must be some interaction between antigen and receptors on the cell's surface. Models of such interactions, which may help elucidate the nature of the signal antigen gives a cell, are reviewed in Section III.B.

As discussed by Burnet and by Cunningham in Chap. 2, a number of immune phenomena may not be amenable to analysis by a purely reductionist approach. Thus only looking at the molecules or single cells may not be sufficient to allow one to understand many immune phenomena. The regulation and control of the immune system, while clearly utilizing molecules and cells, also seems to involve the interaction of various cell populations. In fact, the very notion of clonal selection is a population level idea. In Section III.C a number of population level models will be discussed with emphasis on the types of phenomena each class of model can address.

A. Models of Assays and Experimental Procedures

1. *Complement*

One of the earliest applications of mathematics to immunology was in the development of theories to explain the biological action of complement. Complement was discovered between 1880 and 1890 in studies by Nuttall, Buchner, and others of the capacity of blood serum to kill certain microorganisms. The ability of antibody, which had been discovered somewhat earlier, to kill bacteria (in vitro) was found to depend upon the presence of another serum constituent called "alexin" (protective substance) or *complement*, to indicate that the agent helped antibody perform its protection function.

Leschly (1914) showed that plots of percent hemolysis of sensitized red cells vs. the quantity of complement added have a sigmoid shape. Thus small amounts of complement are without lytic effect, but as the amount of complement increases, lysis begins, then increases sharply, and finally approaches completion. Von Krough (1916) showed the if one plots the logarithm of the quantity of complement used, log x, vs. log[y/1 - y)], where y is the fraction of cells that have been lysed, then a straight line with slope 1/n is obtained, that is,

$$\log x = \log K + \left(\frac{1}{n}\right) \log \frac{y}{1 - y} \tag{1}$$

or

$$x = K\left(\frac{y}{1 - y}\right)^{1/n} \tag{2}$$

where K is a constant.

As a possible explanation for the sigmoidal shape of the hemolysis curve, Brooks (1919) pointed out that red cells may vary in their susceptibility to lysis, with some cells requiring more complement than others. Implicit in this interpretation is the notion that lysis results from accumulation of damage, with some cells requiring more damaged sites than others before lysing.

The cumulative damage concept was further analyzed by Alberty and Baldwin (1951). They pointed out that it is not necessary to assume differences in the susceptibilities of red cells to lysis if one supposes that lytic action is a multiple-hit phenomenon involving cumulative damage. Probability effects alone could explain the sigmoid curve. Alberty and Baldwin assumed that all red cells were identical, that each contained m substrate regions at which antibody and complement could act, and that a cell does not lyse until a certain critical number, r, of these substrate regions have reacted. The fraction of cells lysed, y, may then be calculated from the binomial distribution as

$$y = \sum_{i=r}^{m} \binom{m}{i} p^{i}(1 - p)^{m-i} \tag{3}$$

where $\binom{m}{i} = \frac{m!}{i!(m - i)!}$ is the binomial coefficient, i is the number of reacted substrate regions on any one cell, and p is the fraction of the total number of substrate regions in the entire cell population which has reacted. Assuming that the extent of reaction p is proportional to the amount of complement added, Alberty and Baldwin found that their theory agreed with experimental titration data and the von Krough equation, if r had a value of about 10, assuming that the total number of substrate regions is 49 or greater. They also introduced heterogeneity of the red cell population into their theory by allowing r to vary from cell to cell. However, they showed that the shape of the dose response curve was not very sensitive to heterogeneity if the number of reactions involved was small ($r \leq 10$).

Even though the Alberty-Baldwin theory suffered from some oversimplifications, their results appeared reasonable, and the underlying concept of cumulative damage was firmly established at the time (Mayer, 1961). However, from experiments in which the total number of red cells was varied, Mayer and his colleagues noticed some discrepancies with the Alberty and Baldwin theory. For example, at the usual cell concentration of 6.7×10^6 cells/ml the value of $1/n$ in the von Krough equation is about 0.2, which corresponds to $r = 10$ in the Alberty-Baldwin theory. However, if 2×10^9 cells/ml are used, $1/n \approx 0.43$, and a value of $r = 2$ is needed to fit the data. To explain this shift in r it would be necessary to make the unreasonable assumption of a corresponding change in lytic susceptibility as the red cell density is increased. Mayer (1961), recognizing the multicomponent nature of the complement, then formulated a one-hit theory in which a single, but random, critical event is all that is needed to force a red cell on the pathway to lysis. We now know that the critical event is the binding of one IgM or a pair of IgG molecules in close proximity, followed by the binding of all the complement components on the red cell surface. By the one-hit theory, the proportion of cells with k lytic lesions per cell is given by the Poisson distribution, i.e.,

$$P(k) = \frac{\ell^k \exp(-\ell)}{k!} \tag{4}$$

where ℓ is the average number of lytic lesions per cell. A variety of observations have now confirmed the Mayer one-hit theory (Mayer, 1972, 1973). For example, Eq. (4) predicts that the average number of lytic lesions per cell, ℓ, can be calculated by examining the unlysed cells, i.e.,

$$P(0) = \exp(-\ell)$$

and hence

$$\ell = -\ln P(0) = -\ln(1 - y) \tag{5}$$

where, as before, y is the fraction of cells lysed. The number of lesions per cell as seen by electron microscopy has been determined by Humphrey and Dourmashkin, and for the most part seems to agree with the one-hit theory. In some instances the number of lesions far exceeded the predicted value; it is presumed that clusters of lesions were formed by enzymatic showers after the binding of one molecule each of C1, C4, and C2 (Humphrey and Dourmashkin, 1969).

For a more detailed summary of one-hit theory see Rapp and Borsos (1970). A kinetic theory of complement-mediated hemolysis has recently been proposed by Pruitt et al. (1974). From the historical perspective that we are adopting here, both the multi-hit and single-hit theories of complement action are mathematical theories that were formulated to explain experimental data and which were used to predict the outcome of future experiments.

2. *The Quantitative Precipitin Reaction*

After a foreign protein, an antigen, is injected into an animal, new substances, antibodies, usually appear in the blood serum of the animal. Historically, these substances have been characterized by their property of reacting with the antigen injected. When the antigen-antibody interaction results in the formation of a precipitate it is called a *precipitin reaction*. When the antigen is an invading microorganism, say a bacterium, the antibodies found in the serum may react with antigenic determinants on the bacterial surface causing the bacteria to clump together. This special case of the precipitin reaction is called an *agglutination reaction*. Not all antigens will form an insoluble precipate. We know that complexes formed by antibodies and small univalent ligands are soluble, while macromolecular multivalent antigens frequently form insoluble complexes.

In a typical precipitin reaction, such as those performed by Heidelberger and Kendall (1935), an antiserum is prepared by immunizing an animal, such as a horse or rabbit, with a multivalent antigen such as type S III pneumococcal polysaccharide. When purified S III is added to the antiserum a precipitate appears. The protein in the precipitate is essentially all antibody; trace amounts of complement may also be precipitated. As the amount of antigen added to the antisera is increased, the amount of antibody precipitated increases up to a maximum and then progressively decreases, as shown in Fig. 2. The rising portion of the curve is called the region of antibody excess; the falling portion of the curve is known as the region of antigen excess, or inhibition zone, while the region of maximum precipitation is called the equivalence zone. A more complete discussion can be found in Eisen (1973) or Day (1972).

Ehrlich proposed that immune reactions such as the precipitin reaction involved the chemical combination of antigen and antibody in stoichiometric proportions in a reaction that was analogous to the almost complete neutralization reaction that occurs between a strong acid and a strong base. Arrhenius and Madsen suggested that the precipitin reaction might be more similar to the reaction between weak acids and weak bases, in which a reverssible equilibrium is reached according to the mass action law of Guldberg and Waage. This purely chemical view of antigen-antibody reactions was opposed by Bordet who felt chemical reactions with their fixed stoichiometry

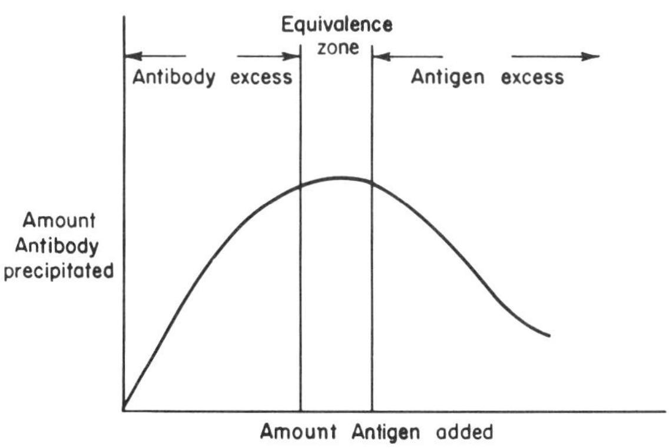

FIG. 2. Precipitin curve for a system containing one antigen and the corresponding antibodies.

could not explain the equivalence and inhibition zones of the precipitin curve, that is, as more antigen is added it should react with more antibody and give greater amounts of precipitate. Thus, Bordet held that antigen-antibody reactions were more like adsorption phenomena found in colloidal systems. When two colloids of opposite electrical charge are mixed in suitable proportions they may be precipitated, but an excess of either may prevent precipitation. As Bechhold and von Krough pointed out, the adsorption theory failed to account for the specificity of antigen-antibody reactions. Thus hybrid theories which suggested that adsorption might bring the antigen and antibody together with secondary chemical processes occurring in the colloidal complex were proposed. (For a more detailed historical account see Wells, 1925.) At the time these theories were proposed little was known about the chemical nature of antigens and antibodies, and precise analytical methods were not available.

The first quantitative studies of the precipitin reaction yielding accurate data were performed by Heidelberger and coworkers in the 1920s and 1930s (for a review see Heidelberger, 1939). Besides doing careful measurements of the amount of antibody and antigen in a precipitate, Heidelberger and Kendall (1935) attempted to model their results with mass-action equations. First, they found that up to the equivalence zone, the course of the reaction could be expressed by the empirical equation

$$A = aS - bS^2 \qquad (6)$$

where A and S are the amounts of antibody and antigen, respectively precipitated, and a and b were constants for a given experiment. Next they showed that this equation could result from a sequence of competing reversible bimolecular reactions in which antigen and antibody would first form a complex

$$S + A \rightleftharpoons SA$$

which then could react, say in the region of antibody excess, either with antibody or itself

$$AS + A \rightleftharpoons ASA$$
$$AS + AS \rightleftharpoons ASAS$$

followed by subsequent reactions in which free antibody or complexes would join to already formed complexes, until particles large enough to settle from solution were formed. The final precipitate would then consist of antibody molecules held together by varying proportions of antigen molecules. A similar lattice view of precipitation was also presented by Marrack (1934); however, Heidelberger and Kendall (1935) developed a mathematical theory of precipitation based on this reaction scheme which fit their empirical observations. A similar theory was developed by Pauling et al. (1942). Kendall (1942) extended the theory and explicitly considered reactions between antibodies of valence one or two and multivalent antigens. He also treated the case in which there were two different types of antigenic determinants on the same antigen molecule or two groups with different reactivities on a bivalent antibody molecule. Morales et al. (1948) used statistical mechanics to derive relations between reactant concentrations and the dissociation constants describing the equilibrium of antigen-antibody complex formation. Goldberg (1952) applied methods pioneered by Flory (1941) and Stockmayer (1943) for describing condensation polymerization reactions in order to obtain the distribution of antigen-antibody aggregate sizes. The assumption in these theories that all antigen-antibody bonds were equivalent was dispensed with by Palmiter and Aladjem (1963) and Whittle (1965). Aladjem and Palmiter (1965) generalized Goldberg's treatment and considered aggregation phenomena in a system with bivalent antibodies having a spectrum of affinities. DeLisi (1974) treated similar reactions in which he also allowed certain types of competing intramolecular reactions. The range of antigen-antibody concentration ratios that give rise to precipitates can also be derived by using percolation theory (Bell, 1971a, DeLisi and Perelson, 1976). Perelson and DeLisi (1975) described the formation of antigen-antibody aggregates via graph theory. Palmiter and Aladjem (1968) established a relation between the behavior of precipitin curves in the regions of far antibody and antigen excess and the composition of insoluble antigen-antibody complexes. The statistical theory of branching or cascade processes has also been applied to the precipitin reaction (Watson, 1958; Gordon, 1962; Good, 1963).

The theory of the precipitin reaction is still not complete. Intramolecular rearrangements of antigen-antibody aggregates that cause ring or cycle formation with a concommitant stabilization of the aggregate have not been dealt with (Bell, 1977). If aggregates contain large cycles, there is a possibility of two aggregates becoming entangled or knotted, hence forming a larger hydrodynamic mass even though no covalent bonds have formed. Similar problems have been treated in polymerization theory by Frank-Kamenetskii et al. (1975). In the development of the theory, no assumptions have been made as to the cause of the insolubility of antigen-antibody aggregates, nor have assumptions been made about the kinetics of precipitation. It has always simply been assumed that antigen-antibody complexes are insoluble (Kendall, 1942), and hence, all one needs to do is compute the most probable size and composition of an aggregate without regard to its distribution between solution and solid phases. However, one knows that precipitation phenomena may involve complex nucleation events with nontrivial kinetics. Thus, problems remain in describing the kinetics of the precipitin reaction.

One further problem related to the agglutination reaction should be mentioned. A number of stochastic models have been devised to describe the attachment of antibodies to viruses and the subsequent loss of virial infectivity. References include Gani (1967a,b), Gani and Srivastava (1968), and Morgan (1971).

3. *The Jerne Hemolytic Plaque Assay*

Although the precipitin assay has proven very useful in detecting small amounts of antigen and specific antibody in antisera, other techniques were needed to detect and study cells that were secreting antibody. The Jerne hemolytic plaque-in-agar technique (Jerne and Nordin, 1963; Jerne et al., 1963) and its various modifications were designed to identify antibody secreting cells, but have also been used to obtain information regarding the rate of antibody secretion (Jones et al., 1976; Perelson and Goldstein, 1977). Additional experimental results such as the distribution of plaque radii as a function of time, and the extent to which plaque formation can be inhibited either by free hapten or antigen, are potentially relatable to the antibody affinity and the kinetic parameters characterizing antigen-antibody reactions (DeLisi and Goldstein, 1974; DeLisi, 1976a,b; see also Goldstein, Chap. 4). In order to obtain quantitative information of this type, a mathematical theory of plaque growth was developed by DeLisi and Bell (1974) and independently by Jerne (Jerne et al., 1974).

In a typical plaque experiment, lymphoid cells from the spleen of a mouse previously immunized with sheep red blood cells (RBC) or haptenated sheep RBC are mixed with the antigen (sheep RBC), plated in a thin layer of agar,* and incubated at 37°C for an hour or two. Complement is added either before incubation to the original cell mixture or poured over the plate after incubation. The complement causes RBC which have sufficient antibody bound to their surface to lyse. Clear areas of lysed RBC called *plaques* are seen surrounding antibody secreting cells.

Mathematical models of the plaque assay using diffusion-reaction equations have been constructed (DeLisi and Bell, 1974; DeLisi and Goldstein, 1975; DeLisi, 1975a,b,c; Goldstein and Perelson, 1976, 1977). The models have been idealized and assume that the antibody forming cell (AFC) secretes antibodies isotropically at a constant rate S. These antibodies are assumed to diffuse with constant diffusion coefficient D and to bind to sites on RBC distributed uniformly throughout the system. The size of the RBC and the AFC are assumed to be sufficiently small that a continuum model with a point source can be utilized. The free antibody concentration, at position r, $C(r, t)$, is assumed to obey an equation of the form

---

* Liquid layer techniques which do not use agar are also widely employed (Cunningham and Szenberg, 1968).

$$\frac{\partial C}{\partial t} = D\nabla^2 C - \frac{\partial C_b}{\partial t} + S\delta(r) \tag{7}$$

with the boundary condition $C(r, t) \to 0$ as $|r| \to \infty$ for all finite t, where C_b is the bound antibody concentration, $\delta(\cdot)$ is the Dirac delta function, and r is a position vector with origin at the AFC. Various models have been used for the binding of antibodies to RBC, which depend upon whether the antibody is IgG or IgM. For example, a reversible single-site binding model would yield

$$\frac{\partial C_b}{\partial t} = k_f C(\rho_0 - C_b) - k_r C_b \tag{8}$$

where ρ_0 is the total concentration of sites (epitopes) on RBC to which the antibody under discussion binds. Goldstein (Chap. 4) discusses the predictions of mathematical models of this type, their usefulness, and their limitations.

Diffusion-reaction equations of the form of Eqs. (7) and (8) have also been used to analyze the diffusion of antiserum from a circular well into a thin layer of gel containing red blood cells and complement (Goldstein et al., 1975; Goldstein and DeLisi, 1976).

Cunningham and Fordham (1974) and Cunningham and Pilarski (1974) have used a variant of the hemolytic plaque technique to show that antibody diversity can be generated after B cells have been stimulated to proliferate. In this modified plaque technique, the indicator layer of red cells is formed by mixing the immunizing red blood cells with some other type of erythrocyte. Antibody secreting cells are observed to form direct plaques of three distinct morphological classes: clear, cloudy, and sombrero. The clear plaques are formed by antibodies which lyse both types of red cells with equal or near-equal efficiency. Cloudy plaques are thought to occur when only one type of red cell is lysed. The sombreros, characterized by a clear central area surrounded by a cloudy brim, are assumed to arise from antibodies which lyse the two red cell types with unequal efficiency. Cunningham and Fordham (1974) found that the progeny of a single antibody forming lymphocyte gave rise to plaques of a different morphological class with an unexpectly high frequency ($\sim$ 3% per mitosis). Goldstein (1975a) and DeLisi and Bell (1976) constructed mathematical models of this modified plaque technique to ascertain the reliability of plaque morphology as a measure of antibody specificity, to determine the optimal experimental conditions for this technique, and to define precise criteria by which plaque morphologies should be distinguished.

4. *The Distribution of Antibody Affinities*

One use of the plaque assay is to determine antibody affinity, that is, the equilibrium constant for the binding of a single antibody site to a single antigenic determinant. For this purpose the inhibition of plaques by free hapten or antigen is measured; the validity of this assay depends on the details of the experimental procedure as described by DeLisi (1976b).

Since each lymphoid cell produces antibodies with a unique affinity, the distribution of affinities in an antiserum reflects the properties of the antibody secreting B-cell population. Considerable theoretical and experimental effort has been directed toward determining the affinity distribution of an antiserum.

Attempts to measure directly the affinity distribution by fractionation of an antiserum on the basis of affinity through the use of immunoabsorption techniques have so far not yielded accurate information (Kim et al., 1974). Indirect methods such as equilibrium dialysis (cf Eisen, 1973) and the Farr assay (Farr, 1958) measure the fraction of haptens that are bound by an antiserum as a function of total hapten concentration. On the basis of mass-action equations one can show that at equilibrium the number of haptens bound per antibody molecule, r, is given by

$$r(H) = \frac{vHK}{1 + KH} \tag{9}$$

for a homogeneous antiserum (cf Eisen, 1973); for a heterogeneous antiserum (cf Goldstein, 1977; Bruni et al., 1976)

$$r(H) = vH \int_0^{\infty} \frac{Kf(K)}{1 + KH} dK \tag{10}$$

where H is the free hapten concentration, K is the hapten-antibody binding site affinity, f(K) is the fraction of antibodies with affinity K, and v is the antibody valence (v = 2 for IgG and v = 10 for IgM). From experimental measurements of r at different values of H, one wishes to obtain f(K). Weblin and Siskind (1972) and Erwin and Aladjem (1976) have written Eq. (10) as a finite sum and then used computer curve-fitting techniques to determine a "best" f(K). Bruni et al. (1976) rewrite Eq. (10) as a Stieltjes transform

$$r\left(\frac{1}{y}\right) = v \int_0^{\infty} \frac{Kf(K)\ dK}{K + y} \tag{11}$$

where y = 1/H, and then compute the inverse Stieltjes transform of r(1/y). However, they must first determine an analytical expression for r from the experimental points. Unfortunately, the choice of the analytic form for r influences the type of f(K) curve obtained. For example, the form Bruni and his colleagues have chosen tends to yield bimodal affinity distributions. Many workers simply assume that f(K) is a Sips distribution (Sips, 1948). If ln r(H)/[v - r(H)] plotted against ln H yields a straight line, then f(K) is Sipsian. (The slope of a Sips plot is a measure of the heterogeneity of the antisera.) A number of experiments have yielded data which seem to have this property (Nisonoff and Pressman, 1958; Karush, 1962). However, from a theoretical viewpoint one can show that there are difficulties with the Sips distribution function for very large or very small values of H (Bruni et al., 1976; Goldstein, 1975b). Bowman and Aladjem (1963) have suggested an empirical method of determining the affinity heterogeneity. A plot of r/H versus r, a Scatchard plot (Scatchard, 1949), can be used to obtain the mean and variance of the affinity distribution as well as the valence of the antibody (cf Goldstein, 1975b); however, further theoretical work is needed in order to provide an adequate and rigorous description of the antibody affinity distribution (Goldstein, 1977).

B. Models of the Interaction Between Cells and Antigen

The recognition of a molecule as being antigenic, and the subsequent triggering of an immune response, are believed to involve the binding of antigen to cells bearing antigen-specific receptors. Since all cells which bind antigen are not stimulated to proliferate and secrete antibodies or otherwise respond, quantitative factors such as the rate of binding, total amount of antigen bound, and the amount of receptor-ligand lattice formation, as well as the presence of additional stimuli or signals, may determine the response pattern of a cell. Further, assays such as the hemolytic plaque assay and agglutination tests depend on the binding of molecules to cell surfaces. For these and other reasons, models of the binding of univalent and multivalent ligands to cell surfaces have been constructed.

Bell and DeLisi (1974) developed simple mathematical models for treating the kinetics of binding of multivalent antigens to cell receptors when the binding may be in competition with the nonspecific binding of antigen to cell surfaces and with the binding of hapten to the receptors. Their models, based on the mass-action description of reversible bimolecular reactions, were used to analyze experiments of Davie and Paul (1972) on the binding of antigen to immunocompetent cells. A later model of Bell's (1974) incorporated a two-step mechanism for the binding of multivalent antigens to cells. In this mechanism an antigen molecule is assumed to first bind to a single receptor site, and then either to dissociate or to form irreversibly a bond with another receptor molecule, thereby establishing a multivalent attachment. The binding of an antigen to both sites of the monomeric IgM or IgD cell receptor molecule, which has been termed monogamous bivalency, has been elegantly treated from an equilibrium statistical-mechanical viewpoint by Crothers and Metzger (1972). Earlier, Jacobson and Stockmayer (1950) considered intramolecular reactions in linear polycondensation systems. DeLisi (Chap. 8), DeLisi (1976a), and DeLisi and Perelson (1976) pursue some of the consequences of allowing both bimolecular and intramolecular binding reactions. Bell (1975b) has considered the types of signals that can be generated by the binding of multivalent antigens to lymphocytes. Using Bell's two-step mechanism for the binding of multivalent antigens to the cell surface and the Flory-Stockmayer-Goldberg theory of polymerization reactions, DeLisi and Perelson (1976) constructed a model for patch formation on lymphocyte membranes (see Perelson, Chap. 7). DeLisi and Thakur (1976) used Bell's model to investigate the thermodynamic and biological implications of requiring receptor cross-linking for B-cell activation.

More complicated and more realistic models of the binding of multivalent ligands to cells should be explored. If the multivalent ligand is a long, flexible, chain-like molecule, as is commonly the case with many T-independent antigens, "zipper" models in which there is an initial nucleation event, such as weak one-point binding, followed by progressive sequential binding of the remaining portion of the ligand, may prove valuable. Such models have been used to explain double-helix formation in nucleic acids (Applequist and Damle, 1965; Poland and Scheraga, 1970; Porschke and Eigen, 1971; Craig et al., 1971) and have been proposed to explain the binding of hormones to cellular receptors (Cuatrecasas and Hollenberg, 1976; Burgen et al., 1975). For large chainlike ligands the possibility of loop formation, in which two portions of the molecule bind to the surface leaving an intervening unattached loop unbound, and the possibility of the entanglement of several ligand chains before binding, may also need to be considered.

C. Population Level Models of the Immune Response

A number of investigators have constructed mathematical models of the humoral immune response. Hege and Cole (1966) constructed a simple model which attempted to relate the time dependent changes in the concentration of circulating antibody after immunization to the changes in the number of antibody forming cells as measured by the Jerne hemolytic plaque assay. Choosing different functional forms for the rate at which a single cell secretes antibody, they attempted to match experimental measurements of 19S serum antibody concentrations. Closest agreement between model and experiment was obtained when the antibody secretion rate was increasing rapidly (proportional to t^2) during the initial phase of the response, but was constant later.

Jilek and Sterzl (1970, 1971), Jilek and Ursínyová (1970a,b), and Jilek (1971a,b, 1973), developed stochastic models for the dynamics of the immune response based on the Sercarz and Coons (1962) X, Y, Z model of lymphocyte differentiation. Jilek's models were aimed at assessing the probability of an antigen encountering an immunocompetent cell, determining the mean number of memory cells and antibody forming cells as a function of time, and the number of memory cells after repeated immunizations. Groves et al. (1970) have also proposed a stochastic model for the initiation of the immune response, but base it on the interaction of two cell types.

Cohen (1970,1971) developed a model for the induction of antibody production and tolerance based on interactions between antigen and cell-bound antibody-like receptors. Cohen assumes that the binding of one antigen molecule to a single receptor (a singlet) is the signal for activation, while the binding of two antigen molecules to two adjacent receptors (a doublet) is the suppressive signal. If α is the fraction of sites on the cell surface which are bound, and δ is the fraction which take part in doublet formation, then Cohen assumes that $A = \alpha - \delta$ must be above some threshold, A_c, for activation of the cell. Using simple probability considerations, Cohen shows that the model can account for high and low zone tolerance, and the variations in antibody affinity observed during an immune response. The essential feature of Cohen's model is that the curve of A vs. α is zero at $\alpha = 0$ and $\alpha = 1$, and rises to a single maxima for intermediate values of α. Coupled with the threshold A_c, this predicts that some finite range of α leads to activation. More recent models, discussed below, which do not make the a priori assumptions that singlet formation is activating and doublet formation is suppressive, have similar properties and make similar predictions.

Bell (1970, 1971a) constructed a model that assumed that the interaction between antigen and cellular receptors is governed by the law of mass action, that such binding reactions are sufficiently rapid compared to the time course of the immune response that they may be considered at equilibrium, and that the probability that a target cell becomes activated depends on the fraction of receptor sites bound or cross-linked (Bell, 1975a). In order to obtain the possibility of producing tolerance to an antigen, Bell also assumed that most target cells are killed when nearly all their receptor sites are occupied. Bell then coupled this model for activation and tolerance with a population dynamic model incorporating the major features of the clonal selection hypothesis. The target cell population was broken up into discrete subpopulations each with a different affinity for antigen. Once a target cell was stimulated by antigen it became a proliferating cell which could secrete antibody and undergo further differentiation into a memory cell or plasma cell. Both plasma cells and proliferating cells secreted antibody of the same affinity as the target cells from which they were derived. This model was formulated mathematically by a system of ordinary differential equations which were then solved numerically on a digital computer. The parameters of the model were chosen to simulate the response of rabbits to the antigen 2,4-dinitrophenyl bovine gamma globulin. The model showed considerable agreement with experiments which determined the average antibody affinity as a function of time and antigen dose. There also was qualitative agreement between experiment and predictions of antibody concentration as a function of time, and primary antigen dose required to produce a given antibody concentration. Bell (1971b) also used his model to analyze experiments of Mitchison in which immunological paralysis was induced by repeated injections of high or low doses of antigen; low dose tolerance was found to result from exhaustion of the target and memory cell populations as they are stimulated to become terminal plasma cells with little intervening proliferation.

Bruni et al. (1975; see also, Chap. 13) have developed a model similar to Bell's in which the affinity of antibodies and cellular receptors is treated as a continuous variable, resulting in an integro-differential equation model. However, neither Bell's nor Bruni, Giovenco, Koch, and Strom's model include T cells. The article by Mohler, Barton, and Hsu (Chap. 14) develops a population level model which explicitly incorporates T cell-B cell interaction.

The population level models all make some assumptions about the mechanism of lymphocyte stimulation and the processes controlling the decision of a lymphocyte to proliferate or differentiate into a plasma cell or memory cell. Models have been constructed by a number of investigators which attempt to determine the correct description of these processes. For example, Waltman (Chap. 15) and Waltman and Butz (1977) develop a dynamical model based on treating lymphocyte stimulation and the decision of proliferating cells to differentiate into plasma cells as threshold phenomena. Merrill (1977) has developed a model of B-cell stimulation and the primary immune response which incorporated ideas from Thom's recently developed catastrophe theory (1975). Perelson et al. (1976, 1977) have utilized ideas from optimal control theory to determine the best pattern of B lymphocyte proliferation and differentiation so as to eliminate antigen in an optimal fashion.

Mathematical models of the control of the immune response have been developed along the lines of Jerne's network hypothesis (Chaps. 19 and 20).

The models discussed so far all assume that the antigen is nonself-replicating. Bell (1973) developed a predator-prey model which dealt with replicating antigens. Pimbley (1974a,b,c; see also Chap. 16) and Hsu and Kazarinoff (1977) have done an extensive mathematical analysis of Bell's original two-variable model and of a three-dimensional generalization. Threshold models of the humoral immune response to reproducing antigens have been developed by Dibrov et al. (1977) and Freedman and Gatica (1976). DeLisi and Rescigno (1977) and Rescigno and DeLisi (1977) have used predator-prey equations to model the interaction of the immune system with a growing tumor (antigen). Dubin (1976) uses a nonlinear birth-death process to model tumor growth with immunological feedback. Lefever and Garay (Chap. 17) also present a mathematical model of immune surveillance.

All of the models referred to in this section ignored the architecture of the immune system and have treated the antigen as a given source for stimulation of cell proliferation, differentiation, and antibody secretion, within a uniform volume. Evidently much remains to be done in devising more realistic models which take into account the many compartments of the immune system and the possible molecular and cellular events in each.

This survey is by no means complete. For example, from an historical viewpoint we have omitted important topics concerned with the analysis of antibody-hapten reactions by methods such as thermodynamics, chemical kinetics, Scatchard plots, and Sips plots, which yielded significant information about the specificity of antibodies, antibody affinity, and antibody valence before the structure of the antibody molecule was elucidated. [These methods are discussed in text books such as Day (1972), Eisen (1973), and Nisonoff et al. (1975).] However, we hope that our historical prelude coupled with this volume will provide a detailed introduction and selective bibliography of work in theoretical immunology.

REFERENCES

Aladjem, F. and Palmiter, M. T. (1965). The antigen-antibody reaction. V. A quantitative theory of antigen-antibody reactions which allows for heterogeneity of antibodies. *J. Theor. Biol.* *9:* 8-21.

Alberty, R. A. and Baldwin, R. L. A. (1951). A mathematical theory of immune hemolysis. *J. Immunol.* *66:* 725-735.

Applequist, J. and Damle, V. (1965). Thermodynamics of the helix-coil equilibrium in oligoadenylic acid from hypochromicity studies. *J. Am. Chem. Soc.* *87:* 1450-1458.

Baltimore, D. (1974). Is terminal deoxynucleotidyl transferase a somatic mutagen in lymphocytes? *Nature* *248:* 409-410.

Bell, G. I. (1970). Mathematical model of clonal selection and antibody production. *J. Theor. Biol.* *29:* 191-232.

Bell, G. I. (1971a). Mathematical model of clonal selection and antibody production, II. *J. Theor. Biol.* *33:* 339-378.

Bell, G. I. (1971b). Mathematical model of clonal selection and antibody production. III. The cellular basis of immunological paralysis. *J. Theor. Biol.* *33:* 379-398.

Bell, G. I. (1973). Predator-prey equations simulating an immune response. *Math. Biosciences* *16:* 291-314.

Bell, G. I. (1974). Model for the binding of multivalent antigen to cells. *Nature 248:* 430-431.

Bell, G. I. (1975a). B lymphocyte activation and lattice formation. *Transplant. Rev. 23:* 23-36.

Bell, G. I. (1975b). On the signals generated by the binding of multivalent antigens to lymphocytes. In *Proceedings of the First Los Alamos Life Sciences Symposium, Mammalian Cells: Proves and Problems*. USERDA Technical Information Center, Oak Ridge, Tennessee.

Bell, G. I. (1977). Some mathematical models in immunology, I. In *Lectures on Mathematics in the Life Sciences,* Vol. 9. Am. Math. Soc. Providence, Rhode Island.

Bell, G. I. and DeLisi, C. P. (1974). Antigen binding to receptors on immunocompetent cells. I. Simple models and interpretation of experiments. *Cell. Immunol. 10:* 415-431.

Black, J. A. and Gibson, D. (1974). Neutral evolution and immunoglobulin diversity. *Nature 250:* 327-328.

Bowman, J. D. and Aladjem, F. (1963). A method for the determination of heterogeneity of antibodies. *J. Theor. Biol. 4:* 242-253.

Bretscher, P. (1972). The control of humoral and associative antibody synthesis. *Transplant. Rev. 11:* 217-267.

Bretscher, P. (1974). On the control between cell mediated, IgM, and IgG immunity. *Cell. Immunol. 13:* 171-195.

Bretscher, P. and Cohn, M. (1970). A theory of self-nonself discrimination. *Science 169:* 1042-1049.

Brooks, S. C. A. (1919). A theory of the mechanism of disinfection, hemolysis and similar processes. *J. Gen. Physiol. 1:* 61-80.

Bruni, C., Germani, A., Koch, G., and Strom, R. (1976). Derivation of antibody distribution from experimental binding data. *J. Theor. Biol. 61:* 143-170.

Bruni, C., Giovenco, M. A., Koch, G., and Strom, R. (1975). A dynamical model of humoral immune response. *Math. Biosciences 27:* 191-211.

Burgen, A. S. V., Roberts, G. C. K., and Feeney, J. (1975). Binding of flexible ligands to macromolecules. *Nature 253:* 753-755.

Burnet, F. M. (1957). A modification of Jerne's theory antibody production using the concept of clonal selection. *Austr. J. Sci. 20:* 67-69.

Burnet, F. M. (1959). *The Clonal Selection Theory of Acquired Immunity,* Vanderbilt and Cambridge University Presses, Nashville, Tennessee, and London.

Cohen, S. (1970). A model for the mechanism of antibody induction and tolerance, with specific attention to the affinity characteristics of antibodies produced during the immune response. *J. Theor. Biol. 27:* 19-29.

Cohen, S. (1971). A quantitative model for the mechanism of antibody formation and tolerance. In *Morphological and Functional Aspects of Immunity, Adv. Exp. Med. Biol.*, vol. 12. (K. Lindahl-Kaessling, G. Alm, and M. G. Hanna, Jr., eds.). Plenum, New York, pp. 323-331.

Cohn, M. (1968). The molecular biology of expectation. In *Nucleic Acids in Immunology* (O. J. Prescia and W. Braun, eds.). Springer-Verlag, New York, pp. 671-715.

Cohn, M., Blomberg, B., Geckeler, W., Raschke, W., Riblet, R., and Weigert, M. (1974). First order considerations in analyzing the generator of diversity. In *The Immune System, Genes, Receptors, Signals* (E. E. Sercarz, A. R. Williamson, and C. F. Fox, eds.). Academic, New York, pp. 89-117.

Craig, M. E., Crothers, D. M., and Doty, P. M. (1971). Relaxation kinetics of dimer formation by self complementary oligonucleotides. *J. Molec. Biol. 62:* pp. 383-401.

Crothers, D. M. and Metzger, H. (1972). The influence of polyvalency on the binding properties of antibodies. *Immunochem. 9:* 341-357.

Cuatrecasas, P. and Hollenberg, M. D. (1976). Membrane receptors and hormone action. *Adv. Protein Chem. 30:* 251-451.

Cunningham, A. J. and Fordham, S. A. (1974). Antibody cell daughters can produce antibody of different specificities. *Nature 250:* 669-671.

Cunningham, A. J. and Pilarski, L. M. (1974). The generation of antibody diversity. II. Plaque morphology as a simple marker for antibody specificity at the single-cell level. *Eur. J. Immunol. 4:* 457-761.

Cunningham, A. J. and Szenberg, A. (1968). Further improvements on the plaque technique for detecting single antibody-forming cells. *Immunology 14:* 599-600.

Davie, J. M. and Paul, W. E. (1972). Receptors on immunocompetent cells. IV. Direct measurement of avidity of cell receptors and cooperative binding of multivalent ligands. *J. Exp. Med. 135:* 643-659.

Day, E. D. (1972). *Advanced Immunochemistry*, Williams and Wilkins, Baltimore.

DeLisi, C. (1974). A theory of precipitation and agglutination reactions in immunological systems. *J. Theor. Biol. 45:* 555-575.

DeLisi, C. (1975a). The kinetics of hemolytic plaque formation. III. Inhibition of plaques by antigen. *J. Theor. Biol. 51:* 337-345.

DeLisi, C. (1975b). The kinetics of hemolytic plaque formation. IV. IgM plaque inhibition. *J. Theor. Biol. 52:* 419-440.

DeLisi, C. (1975c). The kinetics of hemolytic plaque formation. V. The influence of geometry on plaque growth. *J. Math. Biol. 2:* 317-331.

DeLisi, C. (1976a). *Antigen Antibody Interactions, Lecture Notes in Biomathematics,* Vol. 8, Springer-Verlag, New York.

DeLisi, C. (1976b). Hemolytic plaque inhibition: the physical chemical limits on its use as an affinity assay. *J. Immunol. 117:* 2249-2257.

DeLisi, C. P. and Bell, G. I. (1974). The kinetics of hemolytic plaque formation. *Proc. Nat. Acad. Sci. (USA) 71:* 16-20.

DeLisi, C. and Bell, G. I. (1976). Plaque morphology as an antibody specificity marker: an analysis of the physical chemical foundations of the method. *Immunochem. 13:* 21-28.

DeLisi, C. and Goldstein, B. (1974). On the mechanism of hemolytic plaque inhibition. *Immunochem. 11:* 661-665.

DeLisi, C. and Goldstein, B. (1975). The kinetics of hemolytic plaque formation. II. Inhibition of plaques by hapten. *J. Theor. Biol. 51:* 313-335.

DeLisi, C. and Perelson, A. (1976). The kinetics of aggregation phenomena. I. Minimal models for patch formation on lymphocyte membranes. *J. Theor. Biol. 62:* 159-210.

DeLisi, C. and Rescigno, A. (1977). Immune surveillance and neoplasia. I. A minimal mathematical model. *Bull. Math. Biol. 39:* 201-221.

DeLisi, C. and Thakur, A. K. (1976). Antigen binding to receptors on immunocompetent cells. II. Thermodynamic and biological implications of the receptor cross-linking requirement for B cell activation. *Cell. Immunol. 28:* 416-426.

Dibrov, B. F., Livshits, M. A., and Volkenstein, M. V. (1977). Mathematical models of immune processes. *J. Theor. Biol. 65:* 609-631.

Dubin, N. (1976). *A Stochastic Model for Immunological Feedback in Carcinogenesis: Analysis and Approximations, Lecture Notes in Biomathematics,* Vol. 9. Springer-Verlag, New York.

Edelman, G. M. and Gally, G. M. (1967). Somatic recombination of duplicated genes: an hypothesis on the origin of antibody diversity. *Proc. Nat. Acad. Sci. (USA) 57:* 353-358.

Ehrlich, P. (1900). On immunity with special reference to cell life. *Proc. Roy. Soc. B 66:* 424-448.

Eisen, H. N. (1973). Immunology, In *Microbiology,* 2nd ed. (B. D. Davis, R. Dulbecco, H. N. Eisen, H. S. Ginsberg, and W. B. Wood, eds.). Harper and Row, New York, pp. 349-624.

Erwin, P. M. and Aladjem, F. (1976). The heterogeneity of antibodies with respect to equilibrium constants, calculation by a new method using delta functions, and the analysis of the results. *Immunochem. 13:* 873-883.

Farr, R. S. (1958). A quantitative immunochemical measure of the primary interaction between I*BSA and antibody. *J. Infect. Dis. 103:* 239-262.

Flory, P. J. (1941). Molecular size distributions in three-dimensional polymers. *J. Am. Chem. Soc. 63:* 3083-3100.

Frank-Kamenetskii, M. D., Lukashin, A. V., and Vologodskii, A. V. (1975). Statistical mechanics and topology of polymer chains. *Nature 258:* 398-402.

Freedman, H. I. and Gatica, J. A. (1976). A threshold model simulating humoral immune response to replicating antigens. *University of Iowa Technical Report IM76-5,* Iowa City.

Gally, J. A. and Edelman, G. M. (1970). Somatic translocation of antibody genes. *Nature 227:* 341-348.

Gally, J. A. and Edelman, G. M. (1972). The genetic control of immunoglobulin synthesis. *Ann. Rev. Genet. 6:* 1-46.

Gani, J. (1967a). Models for antibody attachment to virus and bacteriophage. *Proc. Fifth Berkeley Symp. on Math. Statist. and Prob. 4:* 537-547.

Gani, J. (1967b). A problem of virus populations: attachment and detachment of antibodies. *Math. Biosciences 1:* 545-554.

Gani, J. and Srivastava, R. C. (1968). A stochastic model for the attachment and detachment of antibodies to virus. *Math. Biosciences 3:* 307-321.

Goldberg, R. J. (1952). A theory of antibody-antigen reactions. I. Theory for reactions of multivalent antigen with bivalent and univalent antibody. *J. Am. Chem. Soc. 74:* 5715-5725.

Goldstein, B. (1975a). Effects of antibody emission rates on plaque morphology. *Nature 253:* 637-639.

Goldstein, B. (1975b). Theory of hapten binding to IgM: the question of repulsive interactions between binding sites. *Biophysical Chem. 3:* 363-367.

Goldstein, B. (1977). Some mathematical models in immunology, II. In *Lectures on Mathematics in the Life Sciences,* Vol. 9. Am. Math. Soc., Providence, Rhode Island.

Goldstein, B. and DeLisi, C. (1976). Immunodiffusion in gels containing erythrocyte antigen. II. Analysis of experiments involving the diffusion of antiserum from a circular well. *Immunochem. 13:* 39-43.

Goldstein, B., DeLisi, C., and Abate, J. (1975). Immunodiffusion in gels containing erythrocyte antigen. I. Theory for diffusion of antiserum from a circular well. *J. Theor. Biol. 52:* 317-334.

Goldstein, B. and Perelson, A. S. (1976). The electrophoretic plaque assay -- theory. *Biophysical Chem. 4:* 349-362.

Goldstein, B. and Perelson, A. S. (1977). The hemolytic plaque assay: theory for finite layers. *Biophysical Chem.* (in press)

Good, I. J. (1963). Cascade theory and the molecular weight averages of the sol fraction. *Proc. Roy. Soc. A 272:* 54-59.

Gordon, M. (1962). Good's theory of cascade processes applied to the statistics of polymer distributions. *Proc. Roy. Soc. A 268:* 240-259.

Groves, D. L., Lever, W. E., and Makinodan, T. (1970). A model for the interaction of cell types in the generation of hemolytic plaque forming cells. *J. Immunol. 104:* 148-165.

Hege, J. S. and Cole, L. J. (1966). A mathematical model relating circulating antibody and antibody forming cells. *J. Immunol. 97:* 34-40.

Heidelberger, M. (1939). Chemical aspects of the precipitin and agglutin reactions. *Chem. Rev. 24:* 323-343.

Heidelberger, M. and Kendall, F. E. (1935). The precipitin reaction between type III pneumococcus polysaccharide and homologous antibody. III. A quantitative study and a theory of the reaction mechanism. *J. Exp. Med. 61:* 563-591.

Honjo, T., Packman, S., Swan, D., and Leder, P. (1976) Quantitation of constant and variable region genes for mouse immunoglobulin λ chains. *Biochem. 15:* 2780-2785.

Hood, L., Campbell, J. H., and Elgin, S. C. R. (1975). The organization, expression, and evolution of antibodies and other multigene families. *Ann. Rev. Genet. 9:* 305-353.

Hood, L. and Talmage, D. W. (1970). Mechanism of antibody diversity: germ line basis for variability. *Science 168:* 325-334.

Hozumi, N. and Tonegawa, S. (1976). Evidence for somatic rearrangement of immunoglobulin genes coding for variable and constant regions. *Proc. Nat. Acad. Sci. (USA) 73:* 3628-3632.

Hsu, I-D. and Kazarinoff, N. D. (1977). Existence and stability of periodic solutions of a third order nonlinear autonomous system simulating immune response in animals. *J. Roy. Soc. Edinburgh* (in press).

Humphrey, J. H. and Dourmashkin, R. R. (1969). The lesions in cell membranes caused by complement. *Adv. Immunol. 11:* 75-115.

Jacobson, H. and Stockmayer, W. H. (1950). Intramolecular reaction in polycondensation. I. The theory of linear systems. *J. Chem. Phys. 18:* 1600-1606.

Jerne, N. K. (1955). The natural-selection theory of antibody formation. *Proc. Nat. Acad. Sci. (USA) 41:* 849-856.

Jerne, N. K. (1971). The somatic generation of immune recognition. *Eur. J. Immunol. 1:* 1-9.

Jerne, N. K. (1973). The immune system. *Sci. Am. 229/1:* 52-60.

Jerne, N. K. (1974). Towards a network theory of the immune system. *Ann. Immunol. Inst. Pasteur 125C:* 373-389.

Jerne, N. K. (1976). The immune system -- a web of V domains. *Harvey Lectures, 70:* 93-110. Academic, New York.

Jerne, N. K. and Nordin, A. A. (1963). Plaque formation in agar by single antibody-producing cells. *Science 140:* 405.

Jerne, N. K., Nordin, A. A., and Henry, C. (1963). The agar plaque technique for recognizing antibody-producing cells. In *Cell Bound Antibodies* (B. Amos, and H. Koprowski, eds.). Wistar Institute Press, Philadelphia, pp. 109-125.

Jerne, N. K., Henry, C., Nordin, A. A., Fuji, H., Koros, A. M. C., and Lefkovits, I. (1974). Plaque forming cells: methodology and theory. *Transplant. Rev. 18:* 130-191.

Jilek, M. (1971a). The number of immunologically activated cells after repeated immunizations. (A mathematical model). *Folia Microbiol. 16:* 12-23.

Jilek, M. (1971b). On contacts of immunocompetent cells with antigen. (Note to a probability model.) *Folia Microbiol. 16:* 83-87.

Jilek, M. (1973). Immune response and its stochastic theory. In *Identification and System Parameter Estimation,* Proc. Third IFAC Symp., Hague, Netherlands, pp. 209-212.

Jilek, M. and Sterzl, J. (1970). A model of differentiation of immunologically competent cells. In *Developmental Aspects of Antibody Formation and Structure.* Academia, Prague, pp. 963-981.

Jilek, M. and Sterzl, J. (1971). Modelling of the immune processes. In *Morphological and Functional Aspects of Immunity, Adv. Exp. Med. Biol.,* vol. 12. (K. Lindahl-Kaessling, G. Alm, and M. G. Hanna, Jr., eds.). Plenum, New York, pp. 333-349.

Jilek, M. and Ursínoyá, Z. (1970a). The probability of contact between the immunocompetent cell and antigen. *Folia Microbiol. 15:* 294-302.

Jilek, M. and Ursínoyá, Z. (1970b). On the distribution of the epoch of the first contact of immunocompetent cell with antigen. *Folia Microbiol. 15:* 492-499.

Jones, J. M., Amsbaugh, D. F., and Prescott, B. (1976). Kinetics of the antibody response to type III pneumococcal polysaccharide. II. Factors influencing the serum antibody levels after immunization with an optimally immunogenic dose of antigen. *J. Immunol. 116:* 52-64.

Karush, F. (1962). Immunologic specificity and molecular structure. *Adv. Immunol. 2:* 1-40.

Kendall, F. E. (1942). The quantitative relationship between antigen and antibody in the precipitin reaction. *Ann. New York Acad. Sci. 43:* 85-105.

Kim, Y. T., Weblin, T. P., and Siskind, G. W. (1974). Distribution of antibody affinities. II. Fractionation of antibody with respect to its hapten binding affinity. *Immunochem. 11:* 685-690.

Klinman, N. R. and Press, J. L. (1975). The B cell specificity repertoire: its relationship to definable subpopulations. *Transplant. Rev. 24:* 41-83.

Langer, W. L. (1976). Immunization against smallpox before Jenner. *Sci. Am. 234:* 112-117.

Lederberg, J. (1959). Genes and antibodies. *Science 129:* 1649-1653.

Leschly, W. (1914). *Studiev over Komplement,* Stiftsbortrykkeriet, Aarhus.

Marrack, J. R. (1934). *Chemistry of Antigens and Antibodies,* 2nd ed. His Majesty's Stationery Office, London.

Mayer, M. M. (1961). Development of the one-hit theory of immune hemolysis. In *Immunochemical Approaches to Problems in Microbiology* (M. Heidelberger and O. Plescia, eds.). Rutgers University Press, New Brunswick, New Jersey, pp. 268-279.

Mayer, M. M. (1972). Mechanism of cytolysis by complement. *Proc. Nat. Acad. Sci. (USA) 69:* 2954-2958.

Mayer, M. M. (1973). The complement system. *Sci. Am. 229:* 54-66.

Merrill, S. (1977). A geometric study of B cell stimulation and humoral immune response. In *Proc. Int. Conf. on Nonlinear Systems and Applications.* (V. Lakshmikantham, ed.). Academic, New York (in press).

Mitchison, N. A. (1964). Induction of immunological paralysis in two zones of dosage. *Proc. Roy. Soc. B 161:* 275-292.

Möller, G. (1975). One non-specific signal triggers B lymphocytes. *Transplant. Rev. 23:* 126-137.

Morales, M. F., Botts, J., and Hill, T. (1948). Equilibrium equations for a model of antibody-antigen combination. *J. Am. Chem. Soc. 70:* 2339-2341.

Morgan, B. J. T. (1971). On the solution of differential equations arising in some attachment models of virology. *J. Appl. Prob. 8:* 215-221.

Nisonoff, H., Hopper, J. E., and Spring, S. B. (1975). *The Antibody Molecule.* Academic, New York.

Nisonoff, A. and Pressman, D. (1958). Heterogeneity and average combining constants of antibodies from individual rabbits. *J. Immunol. 80:* 417-428.

Ohta, T. (1976). Simple model for treating evolution of multigene families. *Nature 263:* 74-76.

Ohta, T. (1977). Genetic variation in multigene families. *Nature 267:* 515-517.

Palmiter, M. T. and Aladjem, F. (1963). The antigen-antibody reaction. IV. A quantitative theory of antigen-antibody reactions. *J. Theor. Biol. 5:* 211-235.

Palmiter, M. T. and Aladjem, F. (1968). On the composition of insoluble antigen-antibody complexes. *J. Theor. Biol. 18:* 34-52.

Pauling, L. (1940). A theory of the structure and process of formation of antibodies. *J. Am. Chem. Soc. 62:* 2643-2657.

Pauling, L., Pressman, D., Campbell, D. H., and Ikeda, C. (1942). The serological properties of simple substances. II. The effects of changed conditions and of added haptens on precipitin reactions of polyhaptenic simple substances. *J. Am. Chem. Soc. 64:* 3003-3009.

Perelson, A. S. and Bell, G. I. (1977). Mathematical models for the evolution of multigene families by unequal crossing-over. *Nature 265:* 304-310.

Perelson, A. and DeLisi, C. (1975). A systematic and graphical method for generating the kinetic equations governing the growth of aggregates. *J. Chem. Phys. 62:* 4053-4061.

Perelson, A. and Goldstein, B. (1977). Antigen modulation of antibody forming cells: the relationship between direct plaque size, antibody secretion rate and antibody affinity. *J. Immunol. 118:* 1649-1654.

Perelson, A., Mirmirani, M. and Oster, G. (1976). Optimal strategies in immunology. I. B-cell differentiation and proliferation. *J. Math. Biol. 3:* 325-367.

Perelson, A., Mirmirani, M., and Oster, G. (1977). Optimal strategies in immunology. II. B memory cell production. *J. Math. Biol.* (in press).

Pimbley, G. H., Jr. (1974a). Periodic solutions of predator-prey equations simulating an immune response, I. *Math. Biosciences 20:* 27-51.

Pimbley, G. H., Jr. (1974b). Periodic solutions of predator-prey equations simulating an immune response, II. *Math. Biosciences 21:* 251-277.

Pimbley, G. H., Jr. (1974c). Periodic solutions of third order predator-prey equations simulating an immune response. *Arch. Rat. Mech. Anal. 55:* 43-123.

Poland, D. and Scheraga, H. A. (1970). *Theory of Helix-Coil Transitions in Biopolymers*, Academic, New York.

Porschke, D. and Eigen, M. (1971). Cooperative non-enzymic base recognition. III. Kinetics of the helix-coil transition of the oligoribouridylic-oligoriboadenylic acid system and of oligoriboadenylic acid alone at acidic pH. *J. Molec. Biol. 62:* 361-381.

Pruitt, K. M., Turner, M. E., and Boackle, R. J. (1974). A kinetic model for the quantitative analysis of complement. *J. Theor. Biol. 44:* 207-217.

Rapp, H. J. and Borsos, T. (1970). *Molecular Basis of Complement Action.* Appleton-Century-Crofts, New York.

Rescigno, A. and DeLisi, C. (1977). Immune surveillance and neoplasia. II. A two-stage mathematical model. *Bull. Math. Biol.* (in press). (in press).

Scatchard, G. (1949). The attractions of proteins for small molecules and ions. *Ann. New York Acad. Sci. 51:* 660-672.

Sercarz, E. and Coons, A. H. (1962). The exhaustion of specific antibody producing capacity during a secondary response. In *Mechanisms of Immunological Tolerance* (M. Hasek, A. Lengerová, and M. Vojtísková, eds.). Academic, New York, pp. 73-83.

Sips, R. (1948). On the structure of a catalyst surface. *J. Chem. Phys. 16:* 490-495.

Smith, G. P. (1973). Unequal crossover and the evolution of multi-gene families. *Cold Spring Harbor Symp. Quant. Biol. 38:* 507-513.

Smith, G. P. (1976). Evolution of repeated DNA sequences by unequal crossover. *Science 191:* 528-535.

Smithies, O. (1967). Antibody variability. *Science 157:* 267-273.

Stockmayer, W. H. (1943). Theory of molecular size distributions and gel formation in branched-chain polymers. *J. Chem. Phys. 11:* 45-55.

Szilard, L. (1960). The molecular basis of antibody formation. *Proc. Nat. Acad. Sci. (USA) 46:* 293-302.

Talmage, D. W. (1957). Allergy and immunology. *Ann. Rev. Med. 8:* 239-256.

Thom, R. (1975). *Structural Stability and Morphogenesis.* Benjamin, Reading, Massachusetts.

Tonegawa, S. (1976). Reiteration frequency of immunoglobulin light chain genes: further evidence for somatic generation of diversity. *Proc. Nat. Acad. Sci. (USA) 73:* 203-207.

von Krough, M. (1916). Colloidal chemistry and immunology. *J. Infect. Dis. 19:* 452-477.

Waltman, P. E. and Butz, E. (1977). A threshold model of antigen-antibody dynamics. *J. Theor. Biol. 65:* 499-512.

Watson, G. S. (1958). On Goldberg's theory of the precipitin reaction. *J. Immunol. 80:* 182-185.

Weblin, T. P. and Siskind, G. W. (1972). Distribution of antibody affinities: technique of measurement. *Immunochem. 9:* 987-1011.

Wells, H. G. (1925). *Chemical Aspects of Immunity.* The Chemical Catalog Co., Inc., New York.

Whittle, P. (1965). Statistical processes of aggregation and polymerization. *Proc. Comb. Phil. Soc. 61:* 475-495.

Wu, T. T. and Kabat, E. A. (1970). An analysis of the sequences of the variable regions of Bence Jones proteins and myeloma chains and their implications for antibody complementarity. *J. Exp. Med. 132:* 211-250.

Part II

THE PHILOSOPHY OF THEORETICAL IMMUNOLOGY

Chapter 2

"GESTALT IMMUNOLOGY": A LESS REDUCTIONIST APPROACH TO THE SUBJECT

A. J. Cunningham*

Department of Microbiology
John Curtin School of Medical Research
Australian National University
Canberra, Australia

The whole is more than the sum of the parts. Aristotle

*Present affiliation: Division of Biological Research, Ontario Cancer Institute, Toronto, Ontario, Canada

The major, unsolved problems of immunology concern the regulation of immune responses. Experimentally, these problems are difficult to attack without thinking about the immune system in terms of smaller units, usually cells and molecules. This reductionism, the breaking down of a complex whole into parts, has its advantages, but also exacts certain penalties: some properties of the whole lymphoid population are unavoidably lost. The immunological case is only one instance of the general difficulty, discussed by many authors, of studying complex organized entities.

Some examples are given of the apparently misleading application of reductionism to immunological problems. In considering alternative approaches, it is suggested that "laws" of lymphocyte population behavior might usefully be sought. Analogies drawn with other disciplines may be helpful: for example, there are similarities between the behavior of lymphocytes in the body and the evolution of a free-living species of protozoa. Finally, the application of general systems theory to immunology is advocated. A simple example of its influence is the prediction that, since stable equilibria are invariably maintained as a balance of opposing forces, immunological self-tolerance will be found to rely on suppression rather than cell deletion mechanisms.

I. INTRODUCTION

Many of the most important questions in immunology are about control: How can the immune system respond to almost any antigen, yet control its own operations so that there is no reaction against "self"? For practical purposes we need to be able to predict and to influence what response a given set of conditions will provoke. Many unsolved diseases are abnormalities of immune control, for example various autoimmune and allergic conditions. Tissue transplantation is still bedeviled by rejection problems. Effective immune control of many viral and metazoan parasites, and of cancer, has not yet been achieved. In these areas we have not advanced much since Pasteur, although our knowledge of immune *mechanisms* has increased enormously since his time.

The difficulty probably arises from great complexity of control processes in the immune system. It is the theme of this chapter that many immune functions, such as control, may be impossible to understand if we rely entirely on the "classical" scientific method of reducing the system to its simplest elements and attempting to predict the behavior of the whole from the properties of the parts. "Gestalt immunology" is proposed as a possible additional approach.

Gestalt is a German word meaning the way a thing is put together, its pattern or form. The school of gestalt psychology (Kohler, 1947) maintained that the way in which an object is perceived depends on the things with which it is associated; that an analysis of parts alone cannot provide a total understanding of a functional whole. By analogy, gestalt biology would be the doctrine that the functions of a living organism can only be meaningfully dealt with at a higher level than chemistry or physics. Gestalt immunology is a way of expressing the idea that we should avoid always trying to reduce the immune system to its elements, and look at larger functional aggregates, such as cell populations, as units in their own right. It suggests certain kinds of experiments which are different from those fashionable at present.

II. UNDERSTANDING COMPLEX SYSTEMS

A. Organized Complexity

Compare the following objects, each weighing about 20 g: a diamond, a piece of clay, and a mouse. The structure of the crystal is relatively simple and uniform throughout. That of the clay is complex, but it is a relatively *unorganized* complexity: many different samples of the material will have different detailed structures but essentially the same properties. The complexity of the mouse is different in kind: it is highly *organized*, and the details of its organization are essential to its nature.

Living things have been described as a "hierarchy of systems" (Koestler, 1967; Weiss, 1969; von Bertalanffy, 1969), with many "levels" of organization, for example, atoms, molecules, cells, tissues, organs. At the highest level, individuals may be organized into a society. There are rich interconnections between the units of any one level: for example, a single kind of protein may take part in several different metabolic pathways within a cell. Connections obviously also exist between levels: what a part does may influence the whole (e.g., overproduction of thyroid hormone), and vice versa. It is the exacting task of biology to understand this complexity.

B. The Reductionist Philosophy

The classical method of Western science, introduced by Descartes, Newton, Galileo, and others, is to reduce things to their simplest units in an attempt to understand the whole. This is sometimes called "reductionism." It works well for some simple systems. Most of us have been educated to believe that this is an essential procedure in any scientific investigation, for example, "vary the factors one at a time."

However, many of the problems which now confront mankind concern highly organized, complex entities, not only living things, but also communication networks, automated factories, large companies, many facets of human society (e.g., economic patterns), and so on. There is a strong tendency for the relentless application of reductionism to all such entities. Yet reductionism does not work well for analysis of many complex things. Waddington (1975), writing about biology, describes the "present epidemic intellectual disease" as the belief that "the reality of anything is proportional to the precision with which it can be defined in molecular or atomic terms." A tune is far more than the sum of its notes, or a painting than the chemistry of its pigments. The essence of a living creature is its organization, the way its parts are put together. One biochemistry can lead to many different biologies, as indeed, common biochemical mechanisms underlie the operations of numerous species. Some authors (Jacob, 1970; Elsasser, 1975), would go so far as to say that we still do not understand most of the very principles upon which living organisms are constructed. We know something of the DNA and of molecular processes within cells, and quite a lot about organization at the morphological level, but very little in between.

The inadequacy of reductionism has been discussed by many authors. In a recent book, *The Logic of Living Systems*, Francois Jacob (1970) outlines very clearly the difficulties of understanding biological organization. He likens an organism to a nest of Russian dolls: each doll, when taken apart, reveals another inside it, down through several layers. At each level of organization of a living creature "novelties appear in both properties and logic." By logic he means that each level has a series of laws of operation which have little meaning at lower levels. For example, the concept of natural selection refers to individuals within a population; one does not think of this process as operating directly on atoms, or molecules. (It will *affect* molecules, of course, but only by acting at a much higher level, on individuals.) Similarly "to reproduce," says Jacob, "is not within the power of any single molecule by itself. This faculty appears only with the simplest integron deserving to be called a living organism, that is, the cell." Cells generally show a range of properties characteristic of their particular level of organization: adhesion of like to like, phagocytosis, mitosis, active movement. All these things naturally have molecular and atomic explanations, but could hardly be predicted from simple biochemical analysis of the constituents of a cell. At a higher level, studying isolated cells alone will rarely predict the properties of an organ: only an optimist would expect to understand consciousness simply by culturing isolated neurons.

The phenomena of irreducible complexity appear also in apparently simple physical and mathematical systems. The gravitational effects of three physical bodies acting on one another are said to still be without a detailed solution. The outcome is not predictable by studying interactions between two bodies only. Apter (1966) cites work on simple mathematical models which rapidly generated complex patterns. In most cases it was impossible to discover the simple generating rules after the pattern had been completed except by trying all possible rules. This seems analogous to the biological case: we understand much of the molecular workings, but just why a tissue or individual is organized in the particular way it is would require a knowledge of evolutionary history and environmental agents acting on the individual, a host of factors over and above simple composition at one point in time.

Some scientists and philosophers believe that a complex whole may have properties which *in principle* are unpredictable from the parts. To me, it is unclear whether if one knew everything about every atomic particle in the universe, it would be possible to predict all events in the future. But for practical purposes, it is abundantly clear that the parts do not fully explain the whole. I think the difficulty may be that no entity exists in isolation: a living thing is ultimately inseparable from its environment, and the environment has shaped its nature over evolutionary time.

III. THE COMPLEXITY OF IMMUNE PHENOMENA

It used to be thought that immune induction was a simple affair: antigen became attached to a receptor-bearing cell and stimulated its clonal proliferation. Then came the idea (Claman et al., 1966; Mitchell and Miller, 1968; Bretscher and Cohn, 1970; Mitchison, 1971) that cell interactions were essential for induction. More recently still, it has been realized (e.g., Gershon, 1974a) that interactions between cells are necessary to suppress as well as to induce immune responses. Immune regulation daily looks more complex. Yet the predominant methodology of the subject, as in most current biology, is reductionism. This has worked well for simple questions dealing with structure and effector functions of lymphocytes and their products — What kinds of cell make antibody? What is the nature of the T-cell receptor? — but it will probably not be sufficient by itself to elucidate more complex phenomena. Fractionation procedures may destroy the subtle balance between cell populations.

To translate this argument into concrete terms we can consider several examples of the misleading effects of reductionism in immunology. The first is very simple. T-helper cell function often appears much more cross-reactive than antibody (e.g., Hoffmann and Kappler, 1973). It is often said that this implies "less specific" receptors on T than on B cells. This preoccupation with one element of the system, the reaction between an antigenic determinant and a single antibody combining site, neglects the rather obvious difference between the thermodynamics of antigen interacting with a free-floating divalent antibody, or with a cluster of receptors on the surface of a T cell. The same antibody molecules could react with quite different overall avidities in the two situations. Other factors may also be important. Similarly, in attempting to predict what antibody an antigen will induce, there is a tendence to concentrate on the fine structure of the antigen, and to ignore such higher-order but often crucial factors as the relation of the antigen to self components, antigenic history of the animal, role of chance in immune induction, and so on. This particular question has been discussed in detail elsewhere (Cunningham, 1974a). The way in which recognition of an antigenic determinant is critically influenced by the rest of the antigen is strikingly reminiscent of the way in which visual perception of an object is said, by gestalt psychologists, to be influenced by associated objects.

The second example concerns the high proportion of cells which takes part in reactions between allogeneic populations of lymphocytes. The conventional, and essentially reductionist explanation for this phenomenon is that there exist many more immunocompetent cells with receptors for alloantigens than for xenoantigens (antigens of other species), a hypothesis which in turn led to the theory of immune surveillance. Consideration of the main experimental facts about allogeneic reactions at a higher level than antigen-antibody combination suggests another view: mixed lymphocyte reactions could be simply abnormal forms of immune induction. A stimulator cell probably has two properties over and above mere possession of antigen. The antigen may be attractively displayed as a matrix on the cell surface, so that multipoint binding converts weak individual antigen-receptor reactions into a strong overall binding; and the stimulator cell, which needs to be metabolically active and lymphoid in type, can give "signal 2" to the responder. These two characteristics might well raise the efficiency of induction by several orders of magnitude. Other aspects of this hypothesis are discussed elsewhere (Lafferty and Cunningham, 1975; Cunningham, 1975a). For the present, it doesn't matter whether the idea is correct, only that it illustrates how other possible explanations for puzzling phenomena may emerge from considering them at several levels.

A third example at a different level of organization: invertebrates manage to protect themselves against many harmful environmental antigens, therefore, some say, they must have at least a rudimentary immune system of the vertebrate type. But consider that individual invertebrates usually do not show *adaptive* immunity. In other words, such individuals don't learn immunologically from their experiences. Faced with a new pathogen, most members of a species die (or fail to reproduce), while resistant variants survive the conventional evolutionary strategy. By contrast, vertebrate individuals do learn. They exploit the evolutionary potential of an internal population of lymphocytes among which variants appear and are positively selected by antigen. Thinking about the differences between vertebrates and invertebrates at the level of natural selection suggests that a fruitful comparison can be drawn between the individual invertebrate and the individual lymphocyte (Cunningham, 1976).

Many more examples could be given where examining events at a very detailed level obscures possible explanations which become obvious when higher levels of organization are considered. What of cell interactions and control of immune responses? It would be a pity to restrict our hypotheses to simple additive effects between, say, helper and suppressor cells. Higher-order factors like absolute cell numbers per unit volume, circulation of cells, length of time which antigen, helper cells, and suppressor cells have spent together, may be decisive, as many immunologists realize. The process of fractionating cells must destroy the organization of the whole population. The standard experiment for detecting suppressor cells is to culture dissociated cells from a tolerant animal together with another population from a normal donor. This often gives useful information, but is a crude procedure. A negative result (no suppression of the normal population's response) need not mean that suppressor cells were absent within the tolerant donor. It is important that we try to find more sophisticated experimental approaches to questions like this.

IV. ALTERNATIVES TO REDUCTIONISM

Having insisted on the limitations of reductionism, one is bound to try and find alternatives. As a first step, a plea for "holism" should be entered; considering the whole often has advantages, as shown by the examples in the previous section. It is obviously very difficult to suggest *specific* techniques for understanding complex systems, partly because of the nature of the problem, and partly because science has just begun to concern itself with organized complexity. Below, three possible kinds of approach are outlined. They overlap one another considerably.

A. Searching for Laws at Different Levels

As pointed out by Jacob (1970), we can expect characteristic laws to emerge from the study of different levels of organization in a complex whole. Some examples at the single-cell level have already been given. The generalization that one cell makes one antibody is another case, one which has been very useful in immunology.

It seems to me that at the present stage of development of the subject, we should look for laws of behavior of *populations* of lymphocytes, without always worrying about what individual cells are doing. Gershon (1974b) has put forward a "law" of this kind: "for every T cell dependent augmentation, there is an equal and opposite T cell suppression." Such a statement would be regarded by many as incomplete. They would want to know why this occurs at the cellular and perhaps the molecular (although probably not the atomic!) levels. More detailed analysis might be worthwhile. But if Gershon's law is generally true, then I suggest that as it stands it represents a useful systematization of knowledge. It could have clinical repercussions, for example.

Another example of population behavior, nonimmunological this time: the rate of glycolytic metabolism of certain yeasts depends on cell density. At certain densities, rapid oscillation is observed (Aldridge and Pye, 1976). This interesting phenomenon would have little meaning at the single-cell level, that is, it is a property of the whole population. It would not appear in single-cell cultures, nor would it be predictable from studying isolated cells. Similar examples of cellular synchronization occur in slime molds. We should expect to discover analogous phenomena among lymphocytes.

B. Modeling

It is often useful to try to abstract certain important features of a complex system, and make simple mathematical predictions about their interactions which can then be tested experimentally. A well-known case, cited by Haken (1973), is the Lotka-Volterra analysis of predator-prey relations in animals. A species of small fish have an unlimited food supply, but are liable themselves to be eaten by larger predator fish. Simple equations can be written to predict how the numbers of the two kinds of fish vary. These equations have an oscillatory solution, that is, numbers of each species fluctuate regularly. The oscillations are out of phase. As big fish increase, little fish disappear, which in turn causes the numbers of big fish to drop, and so on. We might expect to find something similar in competing populations of helper and suppressor lymphocytes.

The science of genetics, from Mendel's time until recently, operated very successfully using a series of simple abstract concepts whose real mechanistic basis was unknown. "Characters" were inherited according to certain laws. Useful and accurate predictions could be made. Knowing the structure of DNA has in fact made little difference to the study of, for example, animal breeding.

An interesting model currently being discussed in immunology is the idiotype "network" of Jerne (1974) and Lindenmann (1974). Antibodies, being themselves antigenic, provoke anti-antibodies, and so on in a expanding net. Some insights into the possible operation of such a system might be gained by experimenting with electronic model circuits, or by applying the mathematical theory of nets. Other kinds of immune network can be imagined, involving reaction against exogenous antigens rather than idiotypes.

Comparisons between widely different disciplines may often be useful, for example between lymphocyte populations and electronic circuitry or predator-prey cycles. There is a generalization in the ecology of forests that trees bigger than their neighbors will have an advantage and tend to grow still bigger relative to the average. This suggests certain similarities with dominant lymphocyte clones. Perhaps in this case the resemblance is too superficial to be helpful, but many useful analogies which might illuminate lymphocyte behavior may be found in other fields concerned with different kinds of human and animal populations. The accumulated wisdom on natural selection must be relevant to lymphocytes.

Modeling could be seen as having some reductionist elements, but in fact it puts relatively little emphasis on mechanisms. The aim seems to be to predict the behavior of a whole from manipulation of parts at only "one level down" in detail. It is a process of building up, as opposed to the reductionist's tearing down.

C. Applying General Systems Theory

Statistics is a series of techniques for treating unorganized complexity (see Section II). Its methods are applicable to a wide range of problems, regardless of the actual nature of the material studied. Less well-known is the growing body of knowledge dealing, in an abstract way, with organized complexity. This is called general systems theory. The insight that complex organized entities, whether animate or inaminate, should obey the same laws, is attributed to von Bertalanffy (reviewed by von Bertalanffy, 1972). Systems theory is said to include, among other things, cybernetics, information theory, set, graph, and network theory, regional mathematics, game and decision theory, and computer simulation. Its theoretical formulations have already been applied in many fields, among them psychology, physiology, metabolism, economics, aesthetics, management science, sociology, and the distribution of medical care. The process of modeling, and the comparison of the behavior of widely different systems discussed in the last section, could be thought of as examples of systems theory methodology.

This "science of organization" should have great relevance to immunology. Cybernetics is that branch of systems theory dealing with *control* in both machines and living things (this subject has had a developmental history rather independent of general systems theory, and was pioneered by Norbert Wiener, 1954). I would like to consider briefly two related examples of general laws in cybernetics which seem directly translatable into immunological terms.

1. *Dynamic Equilibria*

It is said that any dynamic equilibrium must be maintained as a balance between opposing forces. Immunological self-tolerance is a stable equilibrium. Yet the ruling theory is that it is achieved, not really as a balance but as a deletion of self-reactive cells. Cybernetic considerations should make us suspicious of this conclusion, however difficult active suppressor mechanisms may be to demonstrate experimentally. Simple deletion would probably not ensure stability. For example, once any localized concentration of cells had begun to react with self antigens there would seem to be no way of preventing a rapid, generalized autoimmunity. The converse problem with a deletion mechanism is that it might eventually destroy all the lymphocytes of the immune system. There are thousands of self antigens and, because of the degeneracy of cell-antigen combinations, discussed earlier, all lymphocytes, whatever their receptors, will probably bind to some of these antigens with at least low avidity (probability). Flypaper has a very low probability of catching a particular fly in a short time, yet this kind of deletion mechanism is, or used to be, an efficient way of ridding a room of flies!

As a concrete example of the impact of cybernetic considerations on what is actually done in the laboratory, it may be of interest to describe briefly some recent experiments on self-tolerance from our own laboratory. We became convinced, by the arguments cited above and others, that self-tolerance must be maintained by active suppression. We then looked for, and found, cells making antibody to internal antigens within isologous erythrocytes in normal mice (Cunningham, 1974b). These antibody plaque-forming cells were quite numerous, about 5000 per spleen. A "cybernetic" hypothesis was advanced, that this relatively constant level of antibody-forming cells must be a product of two opposing forces: constant autoantigenic stimulation on the one hand, and some suppressor mechanism on the other. Two main lines of evidence were found to support this view. (a) When a large amount of the exposed internal autoantigen was injected into a mouse, the number of specific antibody forming cells was not usually raised. This argues against the competing hypothesis, that the level of antibody forming cells actually seen simply reflects constant low-level stimulation by limiting amounts of antigen without any suppression. (b) When antilymphocyte serum, an agent which kills recirculating lymphocytes, was administered to normal mice, the number of cells making antibody to the internal autoantigen rose 20-fold (Cunningham, 1975b). This increased activity caused by killing some lymphocytes seems most simply explained as a removal of suppressor cells.

2. *Oscillations*

If an immune response were normally terminated by simple removal of antigen, one ought to see an exponential decline in amounts of antibody or antibody forming cells. On the other hand, if every response provokes an "anti-response," cybernetic considerations predict a damped, oscillating curve, as is seen in many other systems. Examples have in fact been described in immunology (reviewed by Weigle, 1975). Figure 1 shows another. Oscillations imply opposing forces. We should find them in many immune events, but it will need careful measurements at short time intervals. Cyclic variations are of course familiar in many other fields, for example, electronics and economics.

Goodwin (1969) has provided an interesting discussion of oscillations in cells. After describing oscillations in variables concerned with metabolite synthesis, he suggests that cells have actively exploited these regular fluctuations to organize themselves. Complex but stable coupling can occur between two or more oscillators, and can be used for temporal ordering of dynamic processes. For Goodwin, the cell is not passive, but a vibrant entity, a kind of resonating system which cycles continuously through a set of metabolic states.

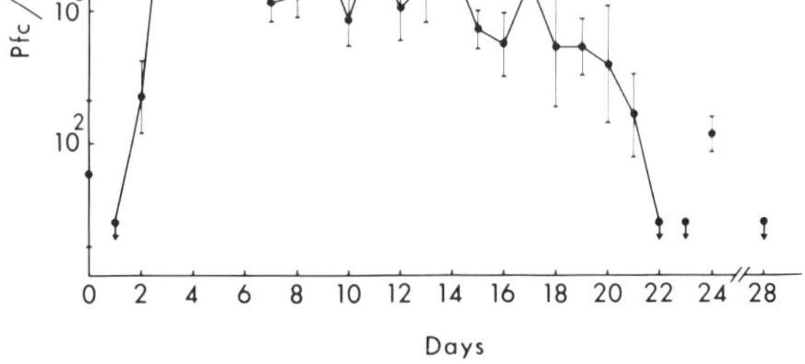

FIG. 1. The response of CBA mice to an intravenous injection of 0.2 ml of 10% rat RBC. All members of the group were injected at the same time, and four individuals were assayed on each day. Direct plaques only are shown. (Indirect plaques were seen only occasionally.) Geometric means ± 2 S.E.

V. CONCLUSIONS

I have tried to make the argument that (a) many of the properties of complex organized entitites are lost by reductionist analysis, (b) that the immune system is probably highly organized and very complex; and (c) that we therefore need new approaches, in addition to reductionism, to help solve the outstanding problems of immunology. There is of course no reason to abandon reductionism (not that there is much danger that the majority of workers will do so!). Ultimately we would like to understand the immune system at every level. But it is always worthwhile to think about the most efficient strategy to apply to unsolved questions. More holistic or gestalt experiments could be valuable additions to the current range of experimental approaches.

In practical terms, the suggestion has been made that some time should be spent thinking about the lymphocyte population as a unit, rather than always about single cells or molecules. We should respect the probable subtlety of immune control, and plan experiments which disturb balances as little as possible. For example, instead of looking for suppression by mixing cells and transferring to a third-party host, one might consider challenging tolerant animals with coupled antigens. If a mouse has suppressor tolerance to X, then a response to Y coupled to X will be suppressed, while the response to Y in a simple mixture of the two antigens should be unaffected. Suppressor control of self-tolerance is predictable. We have found an example of this (Cunningham, 1975b) after being stimulated to look for it by the cybernetic literature. Time spent reading about problems analogous to immune control, but in totally different fields, need not be wasted. Finally, the application of general systems theory to immunology is indicated. The examples given in this paper are very simple ones, almost intuitively obvious, but deeper insights might come from collaboration with experts in systems methodology.

ACKNOWLEDGMENTS

I am grateful to Drs. E. Steele, K. Lafferty, P. Bretscher, A. Bellett, G. Ada, and to Mr. A. Mullbacher, for reading the manuscript. Dr. Steele expressed a reluctance to criticize the parts for fear of destroying the whole!

REFERENCES

Aldridge, J. and Pye, E. K. (1976). Cell density dependence of oscillatory metabolism. *Nature 259:* 670.

Apter, M. J. (1966). *Cybernetics and Development*, Pergamon Press, Oxford.

Bretscher, P. A. and Cohn, M. (1970). A theory of self-nonself discrimination. *Science 169:* 1042.

Claman, H. N., Chaperon, E. A., and Triplett, R. F. (1966). Thymus-marrow cell combinations. Synergism in antibody production. *Proc. Soc. Exp. Biol. Med. 122:* 1167.

Cunningham, A. J. (1974a). Predicting what antibodies an antigen will induce: the inadequacy of the determinant model. *Curr. Topics Microbiol. Immunol. 67:* 97.

Cunningham, A. J. (1974b). Large numbers of cells in normal mice produce antibody to components of isologous erythrocytes. *Nature 252:* 749.

Cunningham, A. J. (1975a). Why do so many cells take part in mixed lymphocyte reactions? *Cell. Immunol. 19:* 368.

Cunningham, A. J. (1975b). Active suppressor mechanism maintaining tolerance to some self components. *Nature 254:* 143.

Cunningham, A. J. (1976). Evolution in microcosm: the rapid somatic diversification of lymphocytes. *Ann. Immunol. Inst. Pasteur 127C:* 531.

Elsasser, W. M. (1975). *The Chief Abstractions of Biology*. Elsevier, New York.

Gershon, R. K. (1974a). T cell control of antibody production. *Contemp. Topics Immunobiol. 3:* 1.

Gershon, R. K. (1974b). T cell regulation: the "second law of thymodynamics." In *The Immune System: Genes, Receptors, Signals* (E. E. Sercarz, A. R. Williamson, and C. F. Fox, eds.). Academic Press, New York and London, p. 471.

Goodwin, B. C. (1969). A statistical mechanics of temporal organisation in cells. In *Towards a Theoretical Biology*, Vol. 2. Edinburgh University Press, p. 140.

Haken, H. (1973). Introduction to Synergetics. In *Synergetics* (H.H. Haken, ed.). B. G. Teubner, Stuttgart, p. 9.

Hoffmann, M. and Kappler, J. W. (1973). Regulation of the immune response. II. Qualitative and quantitative differences between thymus- and bone-marrow-derived lymphocytes in the recognition of antigen. *J. Exp. Med. 137:* 721.

Jacob, F. (1970). *The Logic of Living Systems* (translated by B. E. Spillman, 1974). Allen Lane, London.

Jerne, N. K. (1974). Toward a network theory of the immune system. *Ann. Immunol. Inst. Pasteur 125C:* 373.

Koestler, A. (1967) *The Ghost in the Machine*, Hutchinson, London, and Macmillan, New York.

Kohler, W. (1947). *Gestalt Psychology*, Liveright Publ. Co., New York.

Lafferty, K. J. and Cunningham, A. J. (1975). A new analysis of allogeneic interactions. *Aust. J. Exp. Biol. Med. Sci. 53:* 27.

Lindenmann, J. (1974). Speculations on idiotypes and homobodies. *Ann. Immunol. Inst. Pasteur 124C:* 171.

Mitchell, G. F. and Miller, J. F. A. P. (1968). Immunological activity of thymus and thoracic-duct lymphocytes. *Proc. Nat. Acad. Sci. (USA) 59:* 296.

Mitchison, N. A. (1971). The carrier effect in the secondary response to hapten-protein conjugates. *Eur. J. Immunol. 1:* 18.

von Bertalanffy, L. (1969). Chance or Law. In *Beyond Reductionism*, (A. Koestler and J. R. Smythies, eds.). Hutchinson, London, p. 56.

von Bertalanffy, L. (1972). The history and status of general systems theory. In *Trends in General Systems Theory* (J. Klir, ed.). Wiley-Interscience, New York, p. 21.

Waddington, C. H. (1975). Fifty years on. *Nature 258:* 20.

Weiss, P. (1969). The living system. In *Beyond Reductionism* (A. Koestler and J. R. Smythies, eds.). Hutchinson, London, p. 1.

Weigle, W. O. (1975). Cyclical production of antibody as a regulatory mechanism in the immune response. *Adv. Immunol. 21:* 87.

Wiener, N. (1954). *The Human Use of Human Beings*, Houghton Mifflin Co., Boston.

Chapter 3

CLONAL SELECTION AND AFTER

F. M. Burnet

Department of Microbiology
University of Melbourne
Parkville, Victoria, Australia

This is an historically oriented approach to the requirements for immunological theory from the angle of a biologist with a strongly darwinian attitude toward all biological phenomena. The clonal selection theory as elaborated and modified since 1957 is accepted as the core of modern immunological theory. Current difficulties in reaching accepted interpretations of the generation of antibody diversity, the number and characteristics of lymphocyte subpopulations, and the homeostatic and self-monitoring qualities of the immune system are discussed. It is concluded that the special quality of immune specificity has allowed a deeper investigation of the immune system than has yet been possible for any other area of mammalian biology. The complexity of the cellular and molecular components, and of the overall control of the system generated by their interactions, may indicate a block to new meaningful and clinically relevant developments in the relatively near future, and perhaps presage something equivalent in other biological fields.

I. EARLY IMMUNOLOGICAL THEORIES

In this paper I am concerned with the broad concepts which from the beginnings of immunology have been put forward as an aid to understanding the observed phenomena. An interpretation necessarily had to be in terms of the current level of understanding of other aspects of biology, and particularly of biochemistry. This automatically limits our interest to the present century, beginning with Paul Ehrlich's address to the Royal Society in London in 1900 (Ehrlich, 1900). The "side chain" theory of antitoxic immunity that he advanced on that occasion was the first general immunological theory to have a serious vogue. In recent years it has sometimes been claimed as the first "selection" theory of antibody production, but in fact it was concerned essentially with antitoxic immunity. As expressed by Bulloch (1938) in his history of bacteriology:

> When the sidechains of particular cells have been brought under the influence of a toxin through the intermediation of the haptophoric complex [equivalent to antigenic determinant] of the latter, the cell was thereby rendered physiologically defective. In order to compensate the physiological defect Ehrlich believed that the living protoplasm replied with regeneration of like side-chains...[which] being ultimately cast into the bloodstream constituted what had been called antitoxin.

The cells that produce the antitoxic side chains are the same cells that are sensitive to damage by toxin. Clearly, Ehrlich's approach in 1900 could have no more than contemporary usefulness, and even at its own level was soon largely displaced by the concepts of Jules Bordet and Elie Metschnikov.

Biochemistry developed rapidly, and interest in the side chain theory of Ehrlich faded away when Landsteiner in the 1920's showed that an unlimited number of organic substances could serve as haptens when combined with a protein such as serum or egg albumin (Landsteiner, 1946). Preexistent side chains with normal physiological functions could not be of an infinite number of types.

The next step was the appearance of what came to be known as the direct template hypothesis, put forward around 1932 by several workers and given its definitive form by Pauling in 1940 (Pauling, 1940). By this time it was well understood that proteins were made up of linear sequences of amino acids in peptide linkage, and that the primary polypeptide chain underwent secondary configurational changes to take on the character of a soluble "spherical" protein such as antibody. Pauling's theory was that all antibodies were of the same amino acid constitution and differed one from the other only in their secondary folding. This, by hypothesis, took place against the antigen which served as a physical template inside the globulin producing cell. Pauling pictured one end of the polypeptide being folded against the significant molecular configuration of the template and fixed, possibly by H bonds, in that position. It was then released, inverted, and the same process carried on at the other end of the polypeptide. The bivalent antibody, on release, was thus able to recognize and unite with the same antigen if it were subsequently met in the body. In addition to the very awkward requirement that both ends of the polypeptide had to be folded and released, presumably from the same template molecule, there were already a number of biological difficulties, which I discussed in a monograph written in 1941 (Burnet, 1941). In terms of modern knowledge, the idea that a single protein could be twisted into the whole repertoire of antibodies is ridiculous, but it seemed reasonable in 1940. It is only too evident that even such intellectual giants as Ehrlich and Pauling cannot hope to escape the limitations of contemporary scientific ideas.

II. THE CLONAL SELECTION THEORY

The rise of molecular biology can be dated from 1943, when Avery showed that DNA acted as a transforming principle for pneumococci; after that the modern approach to protein synthesis kept in pace with the chemical interpretation of the gene. The first selection theory of antibody formation was due to Jerne (1955), and although it had at least two totally unsatisfactory features, the concept was intrinsically attractive and was a major stimulus for me to produce what proved to be a more durable clonal selection theory 2 years later. This was published in extenso in 1959 (Burnet, 1959). The main new features postulated were:

1. Generation of new random genetic changes, subsequently expressed as diverse antibody patterns by a form of accelerated somatic mutation in "mesenchymal stem cells" (including precursors of lymphocytes and plasma cells)
2. Phenotypic restriction of one pattern to one differentiated cell and retention of that pattern by clonal descendants
3. Elimination of newly differentiated immunocytes reactive with antigenic patterns carried by self components
4. Proliferation, plasma cell change, and antibody production, on contact of mature immunocyte with antigen in the body
5. The concept of forbidden clones resistant to early elimination by self antigens as the basis of autoimmune disease.

A. Subsequent Modification and Elaboration

After nearly 20 years, every one of the main contentions has been modified or elaborated, but I believe that it is justifiable to claim that the clonal selection theory played a major role in the transformation of immunology that took place in the 1960's. Since the Cold Spring Harbor Symposium on Antibodies in 1967, it has been accepted essentially as the basic theoretical background for further development.

A few notes about the more important modifications of those five points is probably all that is called for on the present occasion.

1. No one doubts that diversity of immune pattern, with its physical basis in changes in the variable regions of light and heavy chains, is produced by a genetic mechanism, but opinion still differs widely on almost every detail, and in particular as to the relative parts played at the germline level and as a result of somatic change. One can accept completely the summary of Hood et al (1975): "Germ line diversity, somatic variability, combinatorial association, and multispecificity probably all contribute to the diversity of immune responses, [functional antibodies] although the relative contribution of each is entirely unknown." I believe that most immunologists favor a predominantly somatic generation of diversity, but the necessary mechanism is still obscure. My own attachment to the process, suggested by Baltimore (1974), will be mentioned at a later stage.

2. Some qualifications of phenotypic restriction have had to be accepted.

a. There is no doubt that a single cell can undergo change in the quality of the constant segments of heavy chain without change in the V segments or idiotype. The indications are that change from IgM to IgG is normal but not mandatory, and this probably holds also for the IgG to IgA switch. The significance of IgD, which is frequently present with IgM in the same cell, is uncertain. The genetic and other controlling factors governing these switches are obscure.

b. When due notice is taken of differing affinities of antigenic determinant for antibody or receptor combining site, it becomes apparent that phenotypic restriction is in regard to the chemical structure of the two V segments making up the combining site; this does not necessarily mean that its reactivity is limited to a single antigenic determinant. Kreth and Williamson (1973), using isoelectric focusing to differentiate and identify monoclonal antibodies against NIP-hapten as a determinant in a pure-line mouse strain, calculated that this strain could make 8,000 ± distinguishable antibodies active against the hapten. The converse also holds. A considerable number of myeloma proteins react as antibody of moderate affinity against DNP as hapten. If some of these are tested against a range of related haptens, each antibody protein shows its own patterns of reactivity and not infrequently a hapten other than DNP will react with greater affinity than it does. The half-unconscious assumption of one antibody for each antigenic determinant and vice versa that was held in 1950 has been replaced by recognition of a much wider range of reactivity on both sides.

3. The elimination of newly differentiated B cells by contact with antigen has been experimentally demonstrated and given the name clonal abortion by Nossal and Pike (1975). They consider that this must still be regarded as a standard means of ensuring natural tolerance to self components. There are, however, many other ways by which an expected immune response may be inhibited, and suppressor T-cell action has been widely studied in this respect.

4. Even with mature immunocytes, the result of exposure to antigen will differ according to such factors as the concentration, affinity, and method of presentation of antigen, and the presence of nonspecific mitogens, including those arising from specific stimulation of T cells. The result may be positive with functional activation or negative with "tolerization," inhibition, or destruction. In general, T cells are tolerized by concentrations of antigen much lower than are needed for B cells. Under appropriate circumstances, B cells capable of reacting in principle with a self antigen may persist indefinitely owing to the absence through tolerization of any appropriate helper T cells.

5. The etiology of autoimmune disease is known to be much more complex than it seemed in 1957. A direct genetic component is important, and the relative accessibility of the autoantigen can plan an important role. This, as well as other aspects of general immunology that were not known of or were considered irrelevant, are further considered in the next section, which will deal with what seem to be the essential contemporary features of immunology.

III. LIMITATIONS OF IMMUNOLOGICAL THEORY

I ended the first full-length discussion of clonal selection (Burnet, 1959) with the following words: "The approach that I have used has led to a rather simple picture in terms which are not those of chemistry and physics, but of biology. And it is an article of my scientific faith that there is intrinsic virtue in simplicity, if it aids understanding without doing violence to the facts of observation and experiment."

Implicit in those last words is a scepticism about ever reaching truth in biology. Now more than ever I am convinced that the whole truth in the sense of full molecular specification will never be possible for biological units more complex than one of the larger bacterial viruses. Crick once talked of an *Escherichia coli* project to interpret that workhorse of molecular biology in full at the molecular level, but the project seems to have been shelved. The molecular interpretation of any mammalian function is, and is likely to remain, extremely limited. There is of course literally no limit to the amount of acceptable biochemical work that can be done in any area, but largely as a result of experience in immunology, it is now evident that the delicacy and fine structure of control processes are as yet totally beyond handling at a molecular level. We must be content to settle for something that lies between the practicing surgeon's common sense understanding of macroscopic anatomy and physiology on the one hand and a complete molecular interpretation on the other. The categories within which aspects of immune phenomena will need to be interpreted will be governed by expediency and will change from one decade to the next as knowledge advances and conceptual approaches changes.

The pragmatic view would be that what is to be aimed at is to present the situation in any area of scholarly effort in such terms as will facilitate the effective handling of real (i.e., socially significant) problems in that area. The classical demand is that, in the long term, new knowledge should be relevant to the prevention and cure of human disease and disability, to the improvement and extension of the industrial fermentation industries, and so forth. It is of the essence of the problem that in practice the men and women who must carry out the actual handling of human disease, of cattle breeding, or of cheese manufacture will necessarily be people of reasonable but not exceptional intelligence and motivation. They must be educated, and if they are to become competent practitioners in whatever specialty they espouse, their teachers and their textbooks must provide what is needed in a form that the student can use. It is a joy to a good teacher to have a good story to tell, and a good story in his sense must be basically a simple story.

To me the outstanding finding of current immunological research is that there is no set of simple and useful generalizations emerging or showing any promise of doing so. The chemical nature and mode of synthesis of antibody and immunoglobulins has been developed satisfyingly and is the greatest achievement of immunology. But it is significant that the origin of the diversity of antibody pattern has remained elusive.

A. B and T Cells

At the functional level, the most important and almost the only "simple" generalization since 1958 has been the definition of B and T lymphocytes. The differentiation was a gradual one. In 1958 three distinct types of immune response were well recognized. They were (a) classical antibody production and antibody-mediated tissue responses such as the Arthus reaction, (b) hay fever type skin reactions and serum reagin, and (c) tuberculin-type responses transferable only by cells; it was recognized that skin sensitization to simple chemicals and homograft immunity were probably also of this type. These three types of response correspond very closely to what we now recognize as the respective activities of (a) B lymphocytes and plasma cells, (b) B cells producing IgE, and mast cells/basophils carrying it as a passive receptor, and (c) T cells.

The first experimental indication that distinct categories of cells were concerned in antibody production (a) and homograft reactions (c) was by Warner and Szenberg (Warner et al., 1962) working in my laboratory. They showed that "hormonal bursectomy" during embryonic life destroyed the subsequent capacity of chickens to produce antibody, but left intact their power to reject skin homografts and to produce chorioallantoic membrane pocks in a graft-vs.-host reaction. The special association of the bursa with antibody production, and the work of Miller (1961) soon afterwards showing that neonatal thymectomy in the mouse removed capacity to reject homografts, gave rise to the B (for bursa) and T (for thymus) nomenclature. Then, first Claman et al. (1966) and a little later but from a different angle Mitchell and Miller (1968) showed that cooperation between B cells and helper T cells was necessary for antibody production. Nearly 10 years' work since then has produced an unprecedented number of competent papers on theoretical immunology, but as yet no comprehensive new interpretation in reasonably simple terms.

B. The Character of Current Theoretical Work

In an attempt to sort out the reasons why immunology seems to have lost much of its intellectual excitement in the last decade, I have tried to look critically at the character of what is currently being done in the laboratories. Admittedly, such comments on the general nature of good, theoretically oriented primary papers, as they appear in 1975, are probably unfair, since they are made by one who has been away from significant experimental work since 1965, but they may be relevant to the current impasse in immunology. To each comment I have added an illustrative quotation selected from the discussion or summary of experimental papers appearing in a single number of a journal published in August 1975.

1. Most experiments are done with mice that for good experimental reasons have been made biologically abnormal in such ways as be being (a) genetically pure-line or F1 hybrids, (b) neonatally thymectomized, or (c) lethally irradiated and rescued by cells from a syngeneic or allogeneic donor. All these are manipulations of the whole animal and must or may involve functions other than those intended.

> Cells from the semiallogeneic radiation chimeras respond normally to third party determinants, give a definite though reduced MLR with host-type determinants, but this is *not* associated with differentiation into cytotoxic lymphocytes as it is with third party cells.

2. The fact that an experimental paper has been accepted for publication in a journal of repute almost automatically signifies that with a new experimental procedure an unexpected result has been obtained. In other words, a new degree of complexity and a more rigid requirement for reproducible results has been introduced.

> the 2-locus (K and D) model is an over-simplication...discovery of the related but distinct Ia antigens...a third strong locus has been discovered in the I region...loci coding for weak transplantation antigens may be dispersed through the whole H2 complex....

3. Attempts to work with pure subpopulations of cells rarely allow more than 95% uniformity, and for this or other reasons very few experiments give better than 90% of the expected and accepted results.

> Adoptively transferred carrier immune T cells interact with nonimmune T cells or recipients in a fashion which generates immunosuppression, although both immune and normal cells function quite well as helper cells when not admixed.

4. Evidence is frequently found that a certain subpopulation of cells will, with minor experimental changes, show a wide spectrum of activity.

> the spectrum of T cell regulation from facilitation (i.e., help) at one end to suppression at the other, which has been well documented in T-B cell interactions, is also followed in T cell regulation of other T lymphocytes.

As a result of such a survey, one can sense an increasing recognition of the complexity of the cellular interactions that are taking place and of the "soft-edged" quality of most of the experimental observation. The experimental studies chosen to provide representative quotations were all obviously competent pieces of experimental work in which every effort had been made to standardize the conditions and eliminate irrelevant variables. Whatever information can be gained about the interaction of defined subpopulations of cells under such circumstances represents the sort of information that will contribute to any broader understanding of control mechanisms in the immune system. The deeper question, however, is whether the dynamic, unstructured quality of the system is such as to allow large numbers of such experimental studies to provide even in principle an understanding of the actual functioning of the system. It is even more difficult to see how they could lead to clinical manipulations of a malfunctioning system with a view to its correction.

Rightly or wrongly, I believe that such difficulties indicate that we are approaching the limit of practical understanding, and that it is rather highly unlikely that immunologically-based, as contrasted with empirical, procedures will ever be effectively used in the treatment of such conditions as autoimmune and lymphoproliferative diseases. This may be simply an indication that we have come farther in immunology than in any other "real" biological field: if so, it could presage a similar block at equivalent points in other biological sciences.

IV. AN ATTEMPT AT A COMPREHENSIVE APPROACH

Since my retirement from active association with experimental work in 1965, I have tried to keep reasonably in touch with current experimental and clinical work in immunology, primarily because of a deep and continuing interest in the way immunological theory was developing. It seemed conceivable that someone not directly associated with an active experimental group might be in a better position to contribute theoretical ideas than an experimentalist who must always find himself to some degree tied to the experimental system he is familair with. The remainder of this chapter represents an attempt, essentially unsuccessful, to use this sort of approach to extract the essence of immunological research in the last decade and convey it to students. In the background, and becoming of increasing importance with each successive year, was the need to find why this seems to be on the road to becoming impossible.

A. Genetic Aspects

The most active new area of research in immunology is at the genetic level. There are two distinct sets of phenomena that call for genetic elucidation. The first is the generation of the diversity which allows a virtually infinite number of distinct immune patterns to be coded for by the V genes. The second derives from the finding, initially in mice, that certain functional differences between mouse strains in their capacity to respond to marginal antigens were correlated with major histocompatibility antigens. These seem to be controlled on quite different chromosomes and can be considered separately.

The process by which antibody diversity is generated remains a matter of controversy, and to an outsider there seems to be a curious failure to discuss what may well be the most productive approach, Baltimore's (1974) suggestion that a stripped-down DNA polymerase, his terminal nucleotidyl transferase, is concerned in the concentration of amino acid diversity on the hypervariable segments of the V regions. As a result of a deep interest in error-proneness of DNA polymerases, I have tried to spell out the position in more detail than Baltimore would probably consider justifiable, but I must stress that whole approach is his. In human myeloma proteins the hypervariable segments are well defined: three in $V\kappa$ or $V\lambda$, four in V_H; and what evidence is available points strongly to their providing the points of contact for antigenic determinants in the joint V_L-V_H combining site. Particularly in V_L regions, each hypervariable site is dominated by the exceptionally high variability of one specific position in V_L segments (Wu and Kabat, 1970; Capra and Kehoe, 1974a,b). Having regard to processes of DNA repair and the action of restriction endonucleases, the presence of one exceptionally variable position suggests very strongly that it serves as a recognition point for the initiation of a limited excision of nucleotides, followed by repair that has little or no fidelity in replacing the correct nucleotides in the strand involved. This application of an extremely error prone DNA polymerase to a physiological need has a proper biological feel, and if the number of V genes transmitted through the germ line is of the order 20 to 100, the application of this hypervariation process over a few cell generations would produce the required diversity. Since the terminal transferase has been found in thymus and in cells of acute lymphoblastic leukemia, there is an a priori case for this being the error prone DNA polymerase, but for the present the concept is no more than a speculative hypothesis. It is, however, a hypothesis that should be susceptible to experimental test by available techniques for molecular genetics.

The influence of loci in the H2-I region on whether mice are responders or nonresponders to certain antigens is well established (McDevitt and Benacerraf, 1969), and much detailed work on the location of the genes concerned has been reported. It is not nearly so easy to find a rational interpretation of what often seem rather trivial degrees of modulation of marginal immune responses.

B. Controls Needed in a Functioning Immune System

One may also approach the problem from a consideration of what might be required in the way of genetic control to allow the effective functioning of a mammalian immune system. Such a system is in essence a mobile system of cells adapted to make contacts with one another and with a variety of soluble agents, mostly macromolecular. When certain contacts take place, signals are generated in one or both cells, modifying their subsequent function. These functional changes result in control of the whole mechanism, so that it retains its character as a homeostatic and self-monitoring system. In a real sense this is an information-processing control system which, instead of utilizing a neural or pseudoneural circuitry, makes use of the unstructured system of random contact that is consummated in signal production when steric recognition between patterned macromolecules takes place. Elaboration of such a system follows.

The primary cellular units are T and B lymphocytes, each represented by genetically and/or adaptively different subpopulations with other, largely fixed populations of monocyte-macrophages. The significant macromolecules in solution are antibody, and antibody fragments such as monomeric IgM and free light chains, foreign antigens and potential self-antigens, lymphokines of various types, and other hormones of which cortisol and insulin appear to be significant.

The structure of the lymphoid system is such as to ensure a constant entry of recruits to the various subpopulations of B and T lymphocytes from sources in bone marrow and in early life in the thymus, as well as from germinal centers and other sites of proliferation in the peripheral lymphoid system. It also provides opportunity for great potentialities of contact between cells in spleen, lymph nodes, etc. The turnover of cells in an activated lymph node suggests that every lymphocyte has a substantial likelihood of meeting during its lifetime a cell of the subpopulation with which circumstances call for it to interact. Equally, monocyte-macrophage cells presenting antigen on their surfaces are also present in strategic localities where large numbers of lymphocytes can make tentative contacts.

Most antigens require cooperation of T cells if they are to stimulate a B cell to antibody production. It is accepted that some production of IgM antibody by a B cell may take place on stimulation by antigen in the absence of a helper T cell of appropriate specificity. T-cell cooperation, however, is required to obtain a standard antibody response with B-cell proliferation and plasma cell production and the capacity to switch to IgG antibody. As a result, B cells potentially capable of reaction with self antigens remain inert in the absence of effective T cells, which under these circumstances are tolerized by much smaller effective contact with self antigen than B cells.

It is becoming increasingly probable that any definable subpopulation of lymphocytes, T or B, can be recognized by units in the immune system, and, if necessary, the subpopulation can be stimulated to proliferate or its activity suppressed. Without attempting to validate that statement in detail, one may cite work on suppressor T cells, feedback inhibition by antibody of the immune response, blocking antibody, antiidiotypic antibody, and antiallotypes, and also refer to a variety of studies of immunopathological states. This capacity implies that each immunologically significant cell type must be identifiable by one or more surface antigens, which could include those that mediate immune reactivity (idiotype) and functional cytotoxicity, as well as the antigens characteristic of autoimmune or malignant lymphoid cell clones. It would be in line with most current work to ascribe the *recognizing* cells to suppressor T-cell populations, but it might be wise not to exclude soluble antibody or B-cell activities. A recognition of the importance of this self-monitoring function of the immune system brings much more order into one's understanding of "suppressor T cells" and gives a simple explanation of why, when malignant disease appears with abnormal frequency and at an unusually early age in persons under immunosuppressive drugs or suffering from subacute immunodeficiency disease, the tumors are of predominantly lymphomatous type. This is precisely what would be expected if lymphoid cells were both relatively prone to malignant transformation and readily recognized and eliminated by the self-monitoring function, presumably exercised by T-cell subpopulations.

It is a useful, though probably not wholly correct, generalization to say that B cells and their descendent plasma cells are specialized antibody producers whose activity as such is controlled by T cells and factors liberated from them. T cells, on the other hand, are concerned mainly with the *control* of the immune system, chiefly by localized or general liberation of lymphokines but partly by direct cellular contact. The range of genetically and/or functionally differentiable T cells has not been defined nor is the nature of their specific immune receptors fully understood. This is important enough for a separate paragraph.

A consideration of the available data leads me to suggest that no simple interpretation of T-cell receptors may be possible. In the most primitive forms, cyclostomes, antibody is produced and homografts rejected, although there is only a very rudimentary thymus. In goldfish (Warr et al., 1976) and larval frogs (Du Pasquier, 1973), immunoglobulin can be shown to be present and easily demonstrable by immunofluorescence on the surface of thymocytes. In mammals and birds, T cells show no "obvious" immunoglobulin, but with refined methods they have of the order of one-hundredth of the amount carried by a B-cell surface. There is evidence both in rats and mice that some (or all?) of this is passively received from B cells. Phylogenetically it seems probable that the primitive vertebrate immunocyte subserved both B and T functions, and perhaps at more than one point in evolution "split" into the two distinct categories of B and T cells. In the B lines, function was concentrated on the diversification of V pattern eventually by Baltimore-type hypervariation, and the synthesis and secretion of the various classes of immunoglobulin. On the other hand, T cells, we may assume, allowed those functions to degenerate or at least did not develop the specialized mechanisms for diversification and synthesis characteristic of B cells. Receptors would still be necessary. One interpretation of the T-cell receptors that is compatible with the facts but might be almost impossible to confirm or refute experimentally is to assume that the T cell continues to produce V gene coded immunoglobulin receptors, probably of IgM1 quality but vestigial in function and number. Some additional form of receptor would be required, and most of the highly specific quality of T cells to react with foreign antigens would on this view depend on activated T cells taking up IgM1 passively from B cells in the initial stages of antibody production. There is a good deal of circumstantial but no decisive experimental evidence in favor of this passive "arming" of T cells.

The allogeneic reactivity of T cells appears to demand a clonal system of a different quality from the Ig-receptor antibody system of B cells. Subject to possible differences between major histocompatibility antigens as detected by serological (SD) or mixed lymphocyte reactions (LD), these can be interpreted as directed against the whole range of major histocompatibility antigens (MHCA) characteristic of the species. From the data of Nisbet et al (1969), Hunt and Williams (1974), Ford et al. (1975), and others, one can postulate perhaps 100 receptor patterns carried in the germ line and distributed (derepressed) at random, with phenotypic restriction of one pattern per cell. Maintaining a strict analogy with what is known of B cells, it is assumed that stimulation by the corresponding MHCA induces clonal proliferation, and there is effective tolerance to all MHCA carried by the individual. The nature of the receptor is unknown. It would make an elegant story if the germ-line V genes, postulated above gave rise directly to these receptors, but there is no evidence one way or the other. One would be hopeful that study of T-cell lymphomas of mice might help to decide the possibility. Some are known to synthesize an immunoglobulin, and, conceivably, a transplantable or readily cultured tumor might produce enough monoclonal immunoglobulin for chemical and sequencing stuides. It should be emphasized, however, that the allogeneic receptors may be totally unrelated to immunoglobulin.

A matter of great interest is the implication, direct from the facts of mixed lymphocyte reactions and graft-vs.-host reactions, that large numbers of allogeneic receptors are produced genetically against MHCA of whose structure the genome responsible should possess no information. A satisfactory, if rather complex, explanation can be obtained by assuming two systems of multigenes with appropriately different mechanisms of derepression and distribution (cf Hood et al., 1975).

C. Immunopathology and the Self-monitoring Function

Any theory of immunity, if it is to be worth proposing, must be applicable to immunopathological as well as to normal situations. One of the most important developments in the last 5 years for clinical medicine has been the recognition that, in Caucasians, two HLA antigens, HLA-B8 and HLA-B27, are present in highly significant excess in patients diagnosed as suffering from one or another of a number of autoimmune diseases or some immunopathological condition involving a foreign antigen (McDevitt and Bodmer, 1974). Less striking associations have also been recorded, notably HLA-B7 and the corresponding LD7a antigen in multiple sclerosis, and W15 with systemic lupus erythematosus. No such findings have been established for any clinical condition unrelated to immunopathology. This group of phenomena, then, provides direct evidence that genetic factors are needed to allow the appearance of a clinically manifested malfunction of the immune system and must therefore also be directly concerned in maintaining the normal system in a state of healthy function.

Another direct pointer in the same direction is that the only autoimmune diseases that it is practicable to examine for monoclonality of the immunocytes responsible are the autoimmune hemolytic anemias. Most or all of those tested in warm, cold, or Donath-Landsteiner varieties were found to be monoclonal. In other words, genetic change in a single B cell (or its precursor) was responsible for the appearance of the "forbidden" B-cell clone. The evidence, both of HLA group associations with the autoimmune disease in man, and of the inheritance of the autoimmune manifestations in NZB mice, suggests that for a somatic mutation to be effective in initiating an autoimmune clone a preexisting (germ-line) genetic anomaly must be present in the cell line concerned.

Such findings are to be expected if the picture of the homeostatic and self-monitoring system described above is approximately correct. The steric configuration of every receptor and effector concerned (except those of foreign antigens) is genetically determined, either directly by structural germ-line genes or indirectly with the intervention of a somatic process of diversification. They include not only the products coded for by the V genes and functioning as immunoglobulin receptors, antibody combining sites, and idiotypic antigens, but, as well, the major histocompatibility antigens, normal antigens of the lymphocyte surface, including complement- and Fc-receptors, and any modified surface antigens that are associated with malignancy or with the autoimmune state.

No doubt there are many other points still unknown where correct genetically coded configurations are equally necessary for effective function. Enough has been said to indicate both the scope for genetic error and the likelihood that there are second-line, fail-safe mechanisms to handle effectively at least some of the temporary lapses from proper function. If, as seems inescapable, we accept the main impact of aging as the essentially random accumulation of genetic error in all types of somatic cells, it is easy to see how this would lead to the typical inefficiency of many immune functions in the aged.

More to the point is the well-established increase in signs of low-grade autoimmune manifestations in the old, which include the presence, usually without symptoms, of one or more of the autoantibodies routinely tested for in clinical immunology, hyperglobulinemia, and minor degrees of amyloidosis. This is precisely what would be expected if the main factors in development of autoimmune conditions are genetic predisposition expressed through T-cell lines, and accumulating genetic error in some of the cell lines concerned with the self-monitoring function of the immune system.

D. Concluding Remarks

Possibly the most intriguing aspect of the point of view I have been supporting is the possibility that it may offer an explanation of the disappointing character of current research on theoretical immunology. I am fully aware that to those actively immersed in experimental work with a system which in their hands is "working well," the excitement of good experiments that answer the question asked and open up new avenues for exploration is as great as ever it was, but, to a teacher or general biologist who must have a working understanding of immunology as a whole, current primary papers and technical reviews are unhelpful. As I have tried to indicate on other occasions, there are two approaches to a scientific understanding of immunological phenomena. On the one hand, T and B lymphocytes, with their myriad subpopulations, can be regarded almost as autonomous organisms, arising, interacting, and dying in a darwinian evolutionary system at the cellular level. As in the orthodox evolutionary situation, we can identify genetic variation, proliferation, and death (including something analogous to predation) among the lymphocytes. Intellectually, this provides an important road to understanding but little practical enlightenment. On the other side, we have the standard biochemical and cytological approaches of the laboratory, with which this volume is almost wholly concerned. Here, also, there has been a prolific harvest of facts and ideas, and most of what I have to say in these concluding remarks must be at these more conventional levels.

In immunology, more than in any other branch of biology, nature has provided inbuilt markers in the form of immune patterns, and this has allowed us to get closer to seeing how a biological system works than ever before. The essence of what we have found is a highly complex system of interlocking controls to maintain *both* routine homeostasis *and* a system of emergency and fail-safe mechanisms to deal with major episodes such as serious bacterial or viral infections, and the results of internal genetic errors such as malignancy or incipient autoimmune disease. It is probably not a coincidence that what we now find in immunology is curiously similar to what the car manufacturers are aiming for in the next generation of automobiles to run in a world that is becoming more crowded and more oil-hungry with each decade. Progressively greater degrees of automation to replace inexpert human control of the engine and slovenly or dangerous driving will be introduced. Complexity will be greatly increased, and the minicomputer that will be in control may eventually monitor even the driver's physiological fitness to be at the wheel. From the beginning, every living organism has been an automated system "on its own." Evolution has had more than three billion years to develop not only the gross form and function of organisms, but also to recognize and develop the fine controls equivalent to the minicomputers of the automobile of the next decade without which effective function in an ever changing environment would be impossible. In two areas of biology at least, we may have reached the point where the nature of the "fine controls" of biological material must be faced and interpreted and the task is one for which we are not yet equipped. One of those fields is immunology, the other is the most fundamental of all: the enzymological control of DNA replication, repair, and correction of informational errors.

The essence of the immune system is its cellular heterogeneity and the virtually unrestricted mobility of its units, two qualities that militate strongly against the effective application of the standard methods of experimental science. We accept the dogma that the functioning immunocytes are of clonal nature, but there is no way in which a clone can be isolated from a normally responding animal under immunization. It was only the accident that semimalignant change, as in myeloma (and some rare occurrences in experimentally immunized rabbits), gave rise to a demonstrably monoclonal product that confirmed the credibility of a clonal appraoch which made the hypothesis acceptable. Initially, it was as untestable as is the present concept of "a homeostatic and self-monitoring information-processing system, of freely mobile functional units which interact by random exploratory contact followed by recognition through complementary steric interaction between effector and receptor macromolecules." Add to that the concept of almost infinite refinement of control by the introduction of new feedback links in what is by its nature a very open-ended system, and we have an intellectual concept that may be very difficult to express in any form of mathematical or mechanical model, and which, as far as I can see, is extremely unlikely to be capable of experimental refutation. I hope I am wrong, but unless I am, this may mean the end of the road for the contribution that immunology has made, and is making, to general biology.

REFERENCES

Baltimore, D. (1974). Is terminal deoxynucleotidyl transferase a somatic mutagen in lymphocytes? *Nature 248:* 409-411.

Bulloch, W. (1938). *The History of Bacteriology,* Oxford University Press, London.

Burnet, F. M. (1941). *The Production of Antibodies,* Walter and Eliza Hall Institute Monograph No. 1, Macmillan, Melbourne.

Burnet, F. M. (1959). *The Clonal Selection Theory of Acquired Immunity,* Vanderbilt University Press, Nashville, and Cambridge University Press, Cambridge, England.

Capra, J. D. and Kehoe, J. M. (1974a). Variable region sequences of five human immunoglobulin heavy chains of the V_H III subgroup: Definitive identification of four heavy chain hypervariable regions. *Proc. Nat. Acad. Sci. (USA) 71:* 845-848.

Capra, J. D. and Kehoe, J. M. (1974b). Structure of antibodies with shared idiotypy: The complete sequence of the heavy chain variable regions of two immunoglobulin M anti-gamma globulins. *Proc. Nat. Acad. Sci. (USA) 71:* 4032-4036.

Claman, H. N., Chaperon, E. A. and Triplett, R. F. (1966). Immunocompetence of transferred thymus-marrow cell combinations. *J. Immunol. 97:* 828-832.

Du Pasquier, L. and Weiss, N. (1973). The thymus during the ontogeny of the toad *Xeropus laevis:* growth, membrane-bound immunoglobulins and mixed lymphocyte reaction. *Eur. J. Immunol. 3:* 773-777.

Ehrlich, P. (1900). On immunity with special reference to cell life. *Proc. Roy. Soc. Lond. 66:* 424-448.

Ford, W. L., Simmonds, S. J. and Atkins, R. C. (1975). Early cellular events in a systemic graft-vs-host reaction. II. Autoradiographic estimates of the frequency of donor lymphocytes which respond to each Ag-B-determined antigenic complex. *J. Exp. Med. 141:* 681-696.

Hood, L., Campbell, J. H. and Elgin, S. C. R. (1975). The organization, expression, and evolution of antibody genes and other multigene families. *Ann. Rev. Genet. 9:* 305-353.

Hunt, S. V. and Williams, A. F. (1974). The origin of cell surface immunoglobulin of marrow-derived and thymus-derived lymphocytes of the rat. *J. Exp. Med. 139:* 479-496.

Jerne, N. K. (1955). The natural-selection theory of antibody formation. *Proc. Nat. Acad. Sci. (USA) 41:* 849-857.

Kreth, H. W. and Williamson, A. R. (1973). The extent of diversity of anti-hapten antibodies in inbred mice: anti-NP (4-hydroxy-5-iodo-3-nitro-phenacetyl) antibodies in CBA/H mice. *Eur. J. Immunol. 3:* 141-147.

Landsteiner, K. (1946). *The Specificity of Serological Reactions*, revised ed. Harvard University Press, Cambridge, Massachusetts.

McDevitt, H. O. and Benacerraf, B. (1969). Genetic control of specific immune responses. *Adv. Immunol. 11:* 31-74.

McDevitt, H. O. and Bodmer, W. F. (1974). HL-A, immune-response genes, and disease. *Lancet i:* 1269-1275.

Miller, J. F. A. P. (1961). Immunological function of the thymus. *Lancet ii:* 748-749.

Mitchell, G. F. and Miller, J. F. A. P. (1968). Immunological activity of thymus and thoracic-duct lymphocytes. *Proc. Nat. Acad. Sci. (USA) 59:* 296-303.

Nisbet, N. W., Simonsen, M. and Zaleski, M. (1969). The frequency of antigen-sensitive cells in tissue transplantation. A commentary on clonal selection. *J. Exp. Med. 129:* 459-467.

Nossal, G. J. V. and Pike, B. L. (1975). Evidence for the clonal abortion theory of B-lymphocyte tolerance. *J. Exp. Med. 141:* 904-917.

Pauling, L. (1940). A theory of the structure and process of formation of antibodies. *J. Am. Chem. Soc. 62:* 2643-2657.

Warner, N. L., Szenberg, A. and Burnet, F. M. (1962). The immunological role of different lymphoid organs in the chicken. I. Dissociation of immunological responsiveness. *Aust. J. Exp. Biol. Med. Sci. 40:* 373-387.

Warr, G. W., DeLuca, D. and Marchalonis, J. J. (1976). Phylogenetic origins of immune recognition: lymphocyte surface immunoglobulins in the goldfish, *Carassius auratus*. *Proc. Nat. Acad. Sci. (USA) 73:* 2476-2480.

Wu, T. T. and Kabat, E. A. (1970). An analysis of the sequences of the variable regions of Bence Jones proteins and myeloma light chains and their implications for antibody complementarity. *J. Exp. Med. 132:* 211-250.

Part III

ANALYSIS OF EXPERIMENTAL TECHNIQUES (ASSAYS)

Chapter 4

LIMITATIONS OF THE JERNE HEMOLYTIC PLAQUE TECHNIQUE

Byron Goldstein

Theoretical Division
University of California
Los Alamos Scientific Laboratory
Los Alamos, New Mexico

After reviewing the mathematical theory of hemolytic plaque formation, I use the theory to clarify a number of misconceptions concerning plaque experiments. Special emphasis is given to fallacies associated with the interpretation of plaque inhibition experiments. I also employ the theory to investigate how sensitive the plaque growth rate is to changes in the antibody secretion rate of a plaque forming cell during the course of a plaque experiment.

I. INTRODUCTION

The hemolytic plaque assay originally was used solely to detect cells which secreted antibodies against red blood cell (RBC) antigens (Jerne and Nordin, 1963; Jerne et al., 1963; Ingraham and Bussard, 1964). The antibody forming cells (AFC) detected by this technique were overwhelmingly IgM producers.[*]

In a typical experiment, a thin agar layer is prepared which contains sheep RBC and spleen cells from a mouse immunized with sheep RBC. The layer is incubated at 37°C for 1 hr and then complement is added. RBC with sufficient bound antibody are lysed by the complement, causing the formation in the layer of clear areas, direct plaques, which have at their center AFC.[**]

This assay has undergone considerable modification since its introduction. Now it is routinely used to detect AFC which secrete either IgM or IgG against a wide variety of antigens (see the review article by Jerne et al., 1974).

---

[*] This is because IgM fixes complement much more efficiently than IgG. In the presence of complement it takes only one IgG, but approximately 800 IgG molecules, bound to a sheep RBC to cause lysis (Humphrey, 1967).

[**] Indirect plaques are obtained by adding heterologous anti-Ig serum to the layer prior to the addition of complement. This increases the sensitivity of the plaque assay for AFC that produce low efficiency hemolytic IgG antibodies.

The plaque assay has also been modified to measure quantities other than numbers of AFC. At present, the only assay used to determine affinity at the level of a single cell is the plaque inhibition technique (Andersson, 1970). Plaque experiments have been carried out which test AFC against a mixture of two different types of RBC. Results of such experiments have been cited as evidence that antibody diversity is generated after B cells have been stimulated to proliferate (Cunningham and Fordham, 1974; Cunningham and Pilarski, 1974a,b; Pilarski and Cunningham, 1974,1975), and that two antibody molecules of different specificities can be secreted by a single AFC (Couderc, Bleux, Birrien, and Liacopoulos, 1975; Couderc, Bleux and Liacopoulos, 1975). Schrader and Nossal (1974) and Schrader (1975) compared the size, the time development, and the number of plaques produced by AFC that have, or have not, been incubated with multivalent forms of antigen which the AFC produce antibodies against. Their results suggest a new mechanism for B-cell tolerance, called effector cell blockade, where the binding of antigen to the AFC specifically reduces its rate of antibody secretion.

These later modifications of the plaque technique require a detailed understanding of the physical process of plaque growth in order to ensure that the results of experiments employing the techniques are correctly interpreted. Simple intuitive arguments can be misleading. For example, the following statements appear in the literature on plaque experiments, but are either sometimes, or always, *incorrect*:

1. Cells that secrete high affinity antibodies produce smaller plaques than cells that produce low affinity antibodies.
2. The area of a plaque is directly proportional to the rate at which antibodies are secreted by the AFC.
3. The plaque inhibition curve is a measure of the AFC affinity distribution.
4. Plaques produced by high affinity antibodies will be inhibited by less free hapten than plaques produced by low affinity antibodies.

5. $2/H_{50}$, where H_{50} is the hapten concentration needed to inhibit 50% of the plaques, is a measure of the average affinity.

The claim that statements 1-5 are either sometimes, or always, incorrect, is based primarily on the results of the mathematical theory of plaque development, although recent experiments concerning statements 3 (Goidl et al., 1975) and 5 (North and Askonas, 1974) also lend support.

Two mathematical descriptions of plaque growth have been presented by DeLisi and Bell (1974) and Jerne (Jerne et al., 1974). DeLisi and Bell's mathematical formulation, based on diffusion-reaction equations, has been extended to a wide variety of plaque experiments including plaque inhibition experiments (DeLisi and Goldstein, 1974, 1975; DeLisi, 1975a,b, 1976); modified plaque experiments which use two types of RBC (Goldstein, 1975; DeLisi and Bell, 1976); and experiments where plaques develop in the presence of an electric field (Goldstein and Perelson, 1976).

II. THE TIME DEVELOPMENT OF PLAQUES

Experiments have been performed that followed the time development of single direct plaques. The plaques were produced in thin layers which contained both RBC and complement so that plaque growth could be observed continuously. After an initial lag period, the plaque radius R was found to obey the following equation (Ingraham and Bussard, 1964; Nossal et al., 1970; Nossal and Lewis, 1971; Schrader and Nossal, 1974; Esrig et al., 1977):

$$R^2 = k(T - T_0) \tag{1}$$

where k is a constant for a given plaque. Equation (1) holds for $T \geqslant T_0$, where T = 0 is the time at which the AFC is placed in the layer, and T_0 is the lag time. For $T \leqslant T_0$, no plaque is seen. In most experiments, Eq. (1) correctly described plaque growth up to $T \simeq 1$ hr, after which the plaque either grew more slowly or stopped growing. However, plaques have been observed which obeyed Eq. (1) for times as long as 4 hr (Nossal et al., 1970).

How plaques develop in time depends to a large extent on the type of binding that antibodies undergo at the RBC surface; whether it is predominantly monovalent or multivalent. Theory predicts that if single-site attachment is the dominant type of binding, and the AFC secretes antibodies at a constant rate, the plaque radius will grow as described by Eq. (1). Thus, the time studies of direct plaques imply that the dominant type of binding between IgM and sheep RBC determinants is single-site attachment (Ingraham and Bussard, 1964; Nossal et al., 1970; Nossal and Lewis, 1971; Esrig et al., 1977).

Let us look more carefully at the theory. Consider an AFC placed at time T = 0 in a thin layer of thickness h. The layer contains RBC and complement. ρ_{RBC} is the concentration of RBC and ρ_0 is the concentration of binding sites in the layer. $\rho_0 = e\rho_{RBC}$, where e is the number of sites per RBC (epitope density). Assume the AFC secretes IgM antibodies at a rate S(t), beginning at time T_0. The antibodies diffuse in the layer with a constant diffusion coefficient D. They can also undergo reversible binding to various sites on the RBC surface. K is the affinity for this reaction and it equals the ratio of the overall forward rate constant k_1, to the overall reverse rate constant k_2. If IgM forms only single-site attachments, $K = 10K_s$, where K_s is the affinity for the binding of a single IgM site to a site on the RBC surface.

The theory enables one to predict how plaque radii will grow for a given form of the AFC secretion rate and a given scheme for the kinetics of antibody-epitope binding. By comparing with experiment one can gain insight into the time behavior of the antibody secretion rate and the type of binding that the antibody undergoes at the RBC surface. The mathematical details of the theory are presented in the Appendix.

Except where otherwise stated, four assumptions were made in deriving the results presented in this paper. The first concerns the definition of the plaque radius, the second and third are related to the antibody-epitope binding kinetics, and the last has to do with the thickness of the layer. The assumptions are as follows:

1. At the plaque radius there are a fixed number N of antibodies bound per RBC [Jerne has estimated N to be between 1 and 10 for IgM (Jerne et al., 1974)].

If $c_b(r, T)$ is the concentration of bound antibodies a distance r from the AFC, T seconds after it was placed in the layer, then at the plaque radius, R,

$$N\rho_{RBC} = c_b(R, T) \tag{2}$$

To obtain an equation for the plaque radius, the concentration of bound antibodies must be calculated as a function of position and time. To do this, the detailed kinetics of binding must be considered.

2. The free and bound antibody concentrations are in local equilibrium.

This assumption will hold when the binding is monovalent. For such binding any bond that forms will rapidly dissociate since $k_2^{-1} \lesssim 10$ sec for single-site binding of IgM. [Measurements made on IgG indicate that for a single binding site $k_1 \sim 10^5$-10^7 M^{-1} sec^{-1} (Froese, 1968; Hornick and Karush, 1972; Barisas et al., 1975)]. For monovalent binding of IgM, typically $K \sim 10^5$ M^{-1}, but values from 10^2-10^7 M^{-1} have been reported (Voss and Eisen, 1968; Hornick and Karush, 1972; Kim and Karush, 1973; Mukkur et al., 1974; Oriol and Rousset, 1974a,b). For $K = k_1 k_2^{-1} = 10^5$ M^{-1}, $k_2^{-1} \sim 1.0$-10^{-2} sec.] Antibodies will go on and off the RBC surface many times before there is an appreciable change in the free antibody concentration. Under such conditions, local equilibrium will exist between the free and bound antibody concentrations.

3. The fraction of sites bound on any single RBC is small.

Because the free antibody concentration in the layer is produced by the emission of antibodies by a single AFC, it is never high enough to cause a large fraction of sites to be bound through single-site attachment (Perelson and Goldstein, 1977).

4. The layer is thin enough so that the diffusion can be treated as planar.*

With assumptions 1-4 the time development of a plaque can be predicted for any behavior of the AFC secretion rate. One of the simplest types of behavior is when the AFC secretes antibodies at a constant rate. That case is treated below, while some more complicated types of antibody secretion are treated in Section V.

If an AFC secretes no antibodies until time T_0, and then secretes at a constant rate S_0, theory predicts that the plaque radius will obey the following equation:

$$\frac{4\pi DhN}{KeS_0} = E_1\left(\frac{R^2}{4D^*t}\right) \tag{3}$$

where $t = T - T_0$ is the total time the AFC has secreted antibodies. $D^* = D/(1 + K\rho_0)$ is the hindered diffusion coefficient. D^* appears because the effect of binding is to slow the diffusion of free antibodies outward and make them appear to diffuse with a diffusion coefficient that is reduced by a factor of $1 + K\rho_0$. $E_1(\cdot)$ is the exponential integral of order one. $E_1(x)$ decreases monotonically as x increases. It is a tabulated function whose value can be determined for any value of its argument (see for example Gautschi and Cahill, 1964).

It is useful to define the following parameters, since they constantly appear in the theory.

$$\Theta = \frac{4\pi DhN}{KeS_0} \tag{4}$$

$$\beta = \frac{R^2}{4D^*(T - T_0)} \tag{5}$$

---

*The theory has been extended to a layer of finite thickness where both diffusion in the plane and perpendicular to is are included (Goldstein and Perelson, 1977). Assumption 4 will be valid for an average AFC and a thin layer with $h = 3 \times 10^{-3}$ cm for times greater than a few minutes.

The left side of Eq. (3), Θ, is a constant, and therefore the right side must be also. The only way this can be is if the argument of E_1 is a constant, that is,

$$\frac{R^2}{4D^*(T - T_0)} = \text{const} \tag{6}$$

This is the experimental result that has been found for direct plaques and RBC antigens.

If the layer contains two types of RBC, such as in the modified plaque experiments of Cunningham and his coworkers (Cunningham and Fordham, 1974), in general, there will be two plaque radii R_1 and R_2; to a distance R_1 type one RBC are lysed while to a distance R_2 type two RBC are lysed (see Fig. 1). If assumptions 2 and 3 hold for both types of RBC, then two equations identical in form to Eq. (6) hold for R_1 and R_2.* By taking the ratio of these equations one finds that

$$\frac{A_1}{A_2} = \text{const}$$

where $A_1 = \pi R_1^2$ and $A_2 = \pi R_2^2$.

This ratio has been used to define plaque morphology (Cunningham and Fordham, 1974) and therefore, the theory predicts that if an AFC secretes at a constant rate, and assumptions 1-4 hold, a single plaque's morphology will not change with time. The constancy of plaque morphology for direct plaques has been observed by Cunningham and Pilarski (1974b), and Esrig et al. (1977).

---

*In these equations the hindered diffusion coefficient will be given by the expression: $D^* = D/(1 + K_1\rho_{10} + K_2\rho_{20})$, where K_1 and K_2, and ρ_{10} and ρ_{20}, are the antibody-RBC affinities and the density of binding sites for the two types of RBC.

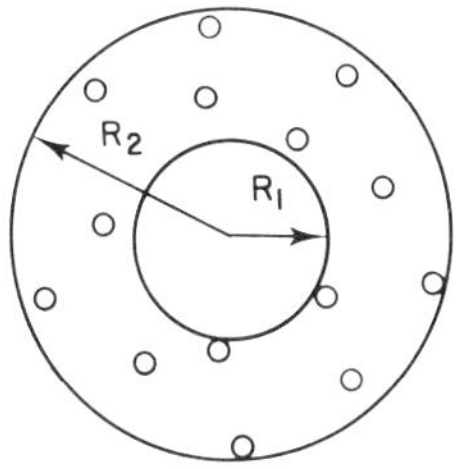

FIG. 1. Diagram of a plaque when two types of RBC are used. To a distance R_1 both types of RBC are lysed, between R_1 and R_2 only type 2 RBC are lysed, beyond R_2 neither type of RBC is lysed. The small open circles represent type 1 RBC. The RBC beyond R_2 are not shown.

III. PLAQUE SIZE AND PHYSICAL PARAMETERS

From the theoretical results of the previous section one can determine how the plaque radius depends on various parameters. As was pointed out, these results hold for direct plaques and RBC antigen, as well as for any other antibody-antigen combination where single-site attachment is the dominant type of binding; for example, for sparsely haptenated RBC where the average spacing between haptens on the RBC is large compared to the dimensions of an antibody.

In terms of the parameters β and Θ, Eq. (3) becomes

$$\Theta = E_1(\beta)$$

Since $E_1(\beta)$ decreases with increasing β, smaller values of Θ correspond to larger values of β. When $K\rho_0 << 1$, so that $D^* \simeq D$,

$$R^2 = 4D\beta(T - T_0)$$

and the smaller Θ is, the larger the plaque radius will be. For fixed D and h, increasing K, e, or S_0 will decrease the value of Θ. Thus, two AFC that secrete at the same rate and for the same length of time, but produce antibodies with different affinities for the same antigen, will produce plaques of different size. *If* $K\rho_0 << 1$, *the largest plaque will correspond to the AFC secreting antibodies with the largest affinity.* For monovalent binding of IgM,

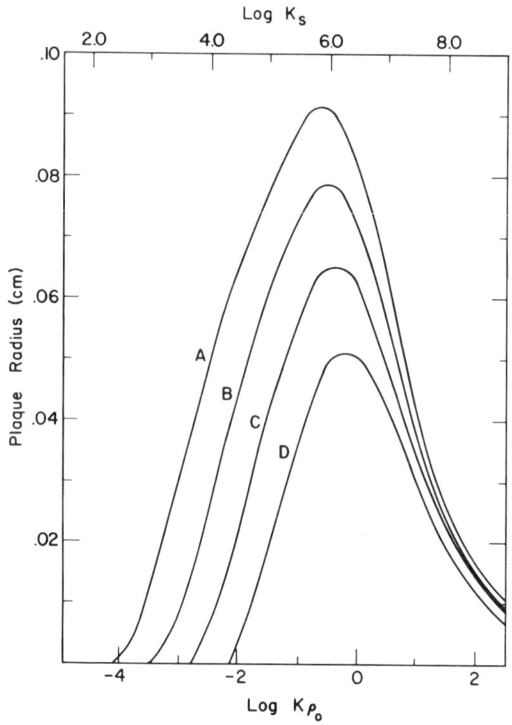

FIG. 2. Variation of plaque radius with antibody affinity for constant RBC density. Θ/K has the following values for the four curves: (A) 2.05×10^4 M^{-1}; (B) 8.20×10^4 M^{-1}; (C) 3.28×10^5 M^{-1}; (D) 1.31×10^6 M^{-1}. These values can be obtained with the following set of parameters: $D = 1.7 \times 10^{-7}$ cm^2/sec, $h = 5 \times 10^{-3}$ cm, $N = 2$, $e = 5 \times 10^4$ sites/RBC, and S_0 equaling 1.25×10^4, 3.13×10^3, 7.81×10^2, and 1.95×10^2 Ab/sec in curves A through D, respectively. The scale above the curves, where K_S is the affinity for a single IgM binding site, gives values of log K_S for ρ_0 constant and equal to 2×10^{13} sites/cm^3. This ρ_0 value corresponds to an RBC density of 4×10^8 RBC/cm^3 and $e = 5 \times 10^4$ sites/RBC. I have taken $K = 10\ K_S$.

$K \sim 10^5$ M^{-1} $= 1.7 \times 10^{-16}$ cm^3/molecule (Hornick and Karush, 1972). Typically, for RBC, $e \lesssim 10^6$ sites/RBC and $\rho_{RBC} = 2 \times 10^8$ RBC/cm^3 (Jerne et al., 1974). For $K = 10^5$ M^{-1}, $\rho_{RBC} = 2 \times 10^8$ RBC/cm^3, and $e = 10^5$ sites/RBC, $K\rho_0 = 3.3 \times 10^{-3}$, and $D^* = 0.997\ D$; for the same values of ρ_{RBC} and K, and $e = 10^6$ sites/RBC, $K\rho_0 = 3.3 \times 10^{-2}$ and $D^* = 0.968\ D$.

Figure 2 shows how the plaque radius varies with affinity. Different curves correspond to different values of the antibody secretion rate. For the physical range of parameters which characterize plaques, R increases with increasing Ke when $K\rho_0 \lesssim 0.2$ and R decreases with increasing Ke when $K\rho_0 \gtrsim 0.6$ (Perelson and Goldstein, 1977). Under typical experimental conditions where RBC antigens are used, or hapten densities are such that $e \lesssim 10^5$, $K\rho_0$ is usually less than 0.2, and I expect the size of direct plaques to increase with increases in either antibody affinity or epitope density. However, this argument only holds for single-site attachment. If e is increased to the point where multisite attachment occurs, Eq. (3) is not valid and the argument breaks down.

The antibody secretion rate enters Eq. (3) only through the parameter Θ. Increasing the secretion rate while keeping all other parameters fixed always increases the plaque radius. The relation between plaque area and secretion rate is given by Eq. (3). It is not a simple proportionality. *The area of a plaque is not directly proportional to the rate at which antibodies are secreted by the AFC* (see Fig. 3).

The diffusion coefficient of the antibody can be changed by changing the medium in which the plaque experiment is performed. Changing the diffusion coefficient will not affect all plaques in the same way. Increasing D will always decrease the antibody concentration near the AFC and increase the concentration far from the AFC. For a good emitter this increases the distance out to which the antibody concentrations are high enough to lyse RBC in the presence of complement. For a poor emitter this spreading-out of the antibodies has the opposite effect. If $\Theta \geqslant 0.655$, an increase in D will cause a decrease in the plaque radius, while if $\Theta \leqslant 0.655$ a decrease in D will cause a decrease in the plaque radius (to see how this result is obtained see the appendix). $\Theta \leqslant 0.655$ corresponds to AFC that are strong antibody secreters. From the published plaque radii studies of Merchant and Peterson (1968), Θ was estimated to range from 0.20 to 2.8, with a mean of 1.08. Switching from a gel

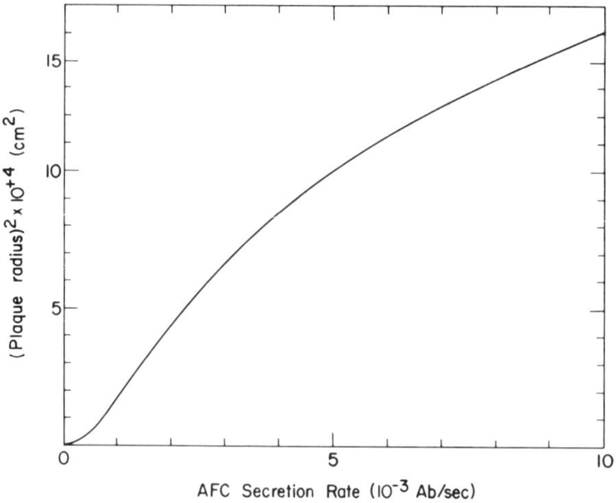

FIG. 3. Variation of the square of the plaque radius with AFC secretion rate, when $K\rho_0 \ll 1$. $\Theta/S = 1.5 \times 10^{-3}$ sec^{-1}. This value can be obtained with the following set of parameters: $D = 1.7 \times 10^{-7}$ cm^2/sec, $h = 6 \times 10^{-3}$ cm, $N = 2$, $e = 10^5$ sites/RBC, and $K = 10^5$ M^{-1}.

to a liquid medium of the same thickness would increase D and tend to increase the size of very small plaques and reduce the size of very large plaques. This assumes the secretion characteristics of the AFC population are the same in the two media.

IV. INTERPRETATION OF PLAQUE INHIBITION EXPERIMENTS

Plaque inhibition experiments are used primarily to study the affinity distribution of antibodies produced by a given cell population, but there is no a priori reason to assume that a plaque inhibition curve will reflect only this distribution. Indeed, I shall show that in many cases the inhibition curve is relatively insensitive to the affinity distribution and is determined primarily by the distributions in AFC secretion rates and lag times.

In a typical plaque inhibition experiment, haptenated RBC, spleen cells, and free hapten (hapten not coupled to RBC surfaces) are present in the same layer. From a single spleen a number of plates are prepared, each having a different concentration of free hapten. The free hapten competes for antibody binding sites with the hapten that is coupled to the RBC surfaces. At large hapten concentrations most of the antibody sites are bound by free hapten; there is insufficient binding of antibodies to the RBC to cause lysis, and plaques do not appear. Results of such experiments are usually presented in the form of plaque inhibition curves which are plots of the number of plaques, or the percent inhibition, vs. the free hapten concentration. If Np(H) is the number of plaques observed when the free hapten concentration in the layer is H, then the percent inhibition is simply

$$I = 1 - \frac{Np(H)}{Np(0)}$$

A. Monovalent Hapten and Single-site Binding at the RBC Surface

When there is free monovalent hapten in the layer, the equation for the plaque radius is again given by Eq. (3), but with K replaced by an effective affinity K_{eff}

$$K_{eff} = \frac{K}{1 + K_s H}$$

where K_s is the affinity for the binding of a free hapten to a single antibody binding site. If the binding of an antibody site to both the free and coupled hapten can be described by the same affinity, then for IgM, $K = 10K_s$ and for IgG, $K = 2K_s$.

When K is replaced by K_{eff} in Eq. (3) the following equation is obtained

$$\frac{1 + K_s H}{KS} \frac{4\pi DhN}{e} = E_1\left(\frac{R^2}{4D^*t}\right) \tag{7}$$

where $D^* = D/(1 + K_{eff}\rho_0)$.

In terms of Eq. (7), a plaque will be inhibited when its radius falls below some minimum value R_{min}. *Note that if two AFC start secreting antibodies at the same time and secrete them at the same rate, and if* $K\rho_0 \ll 1$ *so that* $D^* \simeq D$, *the AFC secreting the higher* *affinity antibodies will require a higher hapten concentration to be inhibited than the AFC secreting the lower affinity antibodies.** This is just the opposite of what is usually stated in the literature.

1. The Effect of Free Hapten on Plaque Size

Increasing H has two effects: it decreases K_{eff} and it increases D*. In the presence of free hapten only a fraction $[1/(1 + K_sH)]$ of the antibody sites are free to bind to sites on the RBC, and therefore the antibodies ability to bind to RBC, its effective affinity, is reduced. Because of this, on the average, an antibody spends less time bound on RBC surfaces and appears to diffuse more rapidly in the layer. In the limit that H approaches infinity, all antibody sites are filled with free hapten, there is no binding to RBC, and D* equals the true diffusion coefficient D.

For any AFC, no matter how rapidly it secretes antibodies and no matter how high the affinity of these antibodies, there exists a hapten concentration above which it cannot form a plaque. However, because D* increases as H increases, it is possible that at low hapten concentrations the radii of AFC that are strong antibody secreters will increase with increasing H. I show in the Appendix that for any AFC with $\Theta > 0.655$, its plaque radius will always decrease with increasing H. The behavior of plaques with $\Theta < 0.655$ depends on the value of $K\rho_0$, since it is $K\rho_0$ which determines by how much D and D* differ. For $K\rho_0 << 1$, all plaques within the range of physically realizable parameters will decrease in size with increase in H. For any value of $K\rho_0$ there will be a critical value of Θ such that if an AFC has $\Theta < \Theta_c$, its plaque will first increase with H to a maximum size and then decrease as H is increased further. For $K\rho_0 = 1$, $\Theta_c = 0.135$, while for $K\rho_0 = 2$, $\Theta_c = 0.289$. Although I expect that for typical direct plaque experiments $K\rho_0 \ll 1$, values of $K\rho_0 \geqslant 1$ are realizable. For $\rho_{RBC} = 2 \times 10^8$ RBC/cm^3, $e = 5 \times 10^5$

*This follows from Eq. (7). Since $(1 + K_sH)/K_s$ is a monotonically decreasing function of K_s, if K_s is increased, E_1 will decrease and the argument of E_1 will increase, i.e., $R^2/4Dt$ will increase.

sites/RBC, and $K = 6 \times 10^6\ M^{-1}$, $K\rho_0 = 1$. For $h = 10^{-2}$ cm, $D = 1.5 \times 10^{-7}\ cm^2/sec$, $N = 2$, any AFC which has $K \geqslant 6 \times 10^6\ M^{-1}$ and $S_0 \geqslant 56$ Ab/sec will have $\Theta \leqslant \Theta_c$.

2. Sensitivity of Inhibition Curves to Secretion Rate and Affinity Distributions

An interesting feature of Eq. (7) is that when $K_sH \gg 1$, the equation becomes independent of K_s, providing also that $K_{eff}\rho_0 \ll 1$. When these conditions are satisfied, the plaque inhibition curve reflects the secretion rate and possibly the lag time distribution, but not the affinity distribution.

From Eq. (7), plaque inhibition curves can be calculated for AFC populations whose distributions in S_0, K, and T_0 are known. In this way, the sensitivity of the plaque inhibition curves to various distributions can be tested. Shown in Fig. 4a is the inhibition curve that would be obtained if there were no spread in the values of T_0 or S_0 and a uniform distribution in K ranging from $3 \times 10^4\ M^{-1}$ to $3 \times 10^6\ M^{-1}$. Each AFC was assumed to secrete 10^3 Ab/sec for 50 min. For this curve, $2/H_{50} = 4.6 \times 10^3 M^{-1}$, which does not equal the average affinity, nor in this case even lie within the range of K values (the average affinity $\langle K \rangle = 1.5 \times 10^6\ M^{-1}$). In general, $2/H_{50}$ does not equal the average affinity.

In Fig. 4b, I have generated the inhibition curve that would be obtained if there was a monoclonal population of AFC, all with $K = 10^5\ M^{-1}$, no distribution in T_0, and a uniform distribution in S_0 ranging from 3×10^2 to 3×10^4 Ab/sec. In Fig. 4a a broad distribution in K values gave a very narrow inhibition curve, however in Fig. 4b a broad distribution in S_0 values yielded a broad inhibition curve. The region of the curve which represented the onset of inhibition is sensitive to both S_0 and K, but as H increases the curve rapidly becomes sensitive only to S_0.

Shown in Fig. 4c is the plaque inhibition curve that would be obtained if there was no spread in the values of T_0 and uniform distributions in both S_0 and K. Notice that the curves in Figs. 4b and 4c are almost identical. For this example, changing the affinity

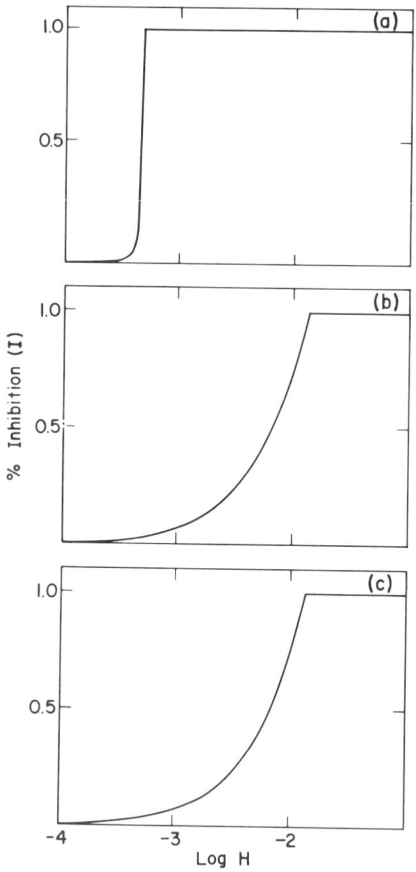

FIG. 4. Plaque inhibition curves generated from Eq. (7) for three different theoretical AFC populations which have no distribution in their lag times. Each AFC secretes antibodies at a constant rate for 50 min. For all cases the binding between antibody and free hapten, and antibody and RBC binding sites, is monovalent. (a) All AFC secrete 10^3 Ab/sec. The AFC population has a uniform distribution in affinity with K ranging from $3 \times 10^4\ M^{-1}$ to $3 \times 10^6\ M^{-1}$. (b) All AFC have $K = 10^5\ M^{-1}$, i.e., the population is monoclonal. The population has a uniform distribution in secretion rates with S_0 ranging from 3×10^2 to 3×10^4 Ab/sec. (c) The AFC population has a uniform distribution in both affinity ($3 \times 10^4\ M^{-1} \leqslant K \leqslant 3 \times 10^6\ M^{-1}$) and secretion rate ($3 \times 10^2$ Ab/sec $\leqslant S_0 \leqslant 3 \times 10^4$ Ab/sec). If this distribution is plotted in K and S_0 space, it will be a rectangle. Any point in the rectangle represents an AFC with K and S_0 values that are the point's coordinates.

distribution from a monoclonal to a broad uniform affinity distribution has almost no effect on the inhibition curve.

At any hapten concentration, Eq. (7) can be used to see if a particular AFC, which is characterized by the three parameters S_0, K, and T_0, will produce a plaque. This is done by substituting K and S_0 into the left side of Eq. (7) and solving for E_1. With E_1 known, β can be found (e.g., from tables) and R calculated from β by substituting the value of t into the equation

$$R^2 = \frac{4Dt\beta}{1 + [K\rho_0/(1 + KH)]}$$

If $R \leqslant R_{min}$, the plaque is inhibited.

When $K_{eff}\rho_0 \ll 1$, and there is no distribution in T_0, a simple condition is obtained for plaque inhibition. From Eq. (7) it follows that any AFC will be inhibited if its K and S_0 values satisfy the inequality below. (If the right side of the inequality is negative, the plaque is too small to be observed even when there is no free hapten in the layer.)

$$\frac{H}{10} \geqslant \frac{S_0}{\Omega} - \frac{1}{K} \tag{8}$$

where

$$\Omega = \frac{4\pi DhN}{eE_1(\beta_{min})} \tag{9}$$

and $\beta_{min} = R_{min}^2/4Dt$. For the following parameter values, $\beta_{min} = 3.7 \times 10^{-3}$ and $E_1(\beta_{min}) = 5.06$: $R_{min} = 0.002$ cm, $D = 1.5 \times 10^{-7}$ cm^2/sec, and t = 50 min. This value of D is appropriate for IgM in a liquid medium.

When $S_0/\Omega \gg 1/K$, Eq. (8) predicts that it is only the value of S_0 that determines whether or not a plaque will be inhibited at a particular hapten concentration. For $h = 10^{-2}$ cm, N = 2 and $e = 10^5$ sites/RBC, $\Omega = 7.45 \times 10^{-14}$ cm^3/sec. For this Ω value and $S_0 = 10^3$ Ab/sec, $S_0/\Omega \gg 1/K$ is satisfied for $K \gtrsim 10^5$ M^{-1}. In Fig. 4, the condition $S_0/\Omega \gg 1/K$ is met over a major portion of each of the inhibition curves. It is for this reason that $2/H_{50}$ is insensitive to the affinity distribution, and the curves of Figs. 4b and 4c are so similar.

The results that have been derived in this section only hold when both the binding of free hapten to antibody, and the binding of free antibody to sites on RBC surfaces, are equilibrium controlled. For such conditions, if there is no distribution in lag times, a plot of the slope of the inhibition curve vs. H will reflect primarily the secretion rate distribution. DeLisi and Goldstein (1975) showed that under these conditions, if $K_s H >> 1$, the secretion rate distribution is related to the slope $dI/d[\log(H)]$, in the following way:

$$g(S_0) = \frac{1}{\Omega}\frac{dI}{dH} = \frac{1}{\Omega H \ln 10} \times \text{slope}$$

where, for plaques produced by IgM, $S_0 = \Omega\ H/10$, and $g(S_0)$ is the normalized secretion rate distribution, that is, $g(S_0)dS_0$ equals the number of AFC that have secretion rates between S_0 and $S_0 + dS_0$. To obtain $g(S_0)$ from experiment requires knowing Ω, and this necessitates determining physical parameters (e, N_1, D_1, R_{min}) which are normally not determined in plaque experiments.

B. Monovalent Hapten and Multisite Binding at the RBC Surface

When can information about the affinity distribution be extracted from plaque inhibition experiments? DeLisi and Goldstein (1975) predict that if the binding of antibodies to sites on RBC surfaces is by multivalent attachment, while the binding to free hapten is by single-site attachment, the plaque inhibition curve will be quite sensitive to the affinity distribution, but influenced by the distributions in S_0 and T_0 as well.

This prediction rests on the assumption that once an antibody binds multivalently, it is bound for the remainder of the experiment, that is, multivalent binding of antibodies can be treated irreversibly for times less than, or on the order of, 1 hr. It is difficult to assess the validity of treating multisite attachment in this way, when time development studies of plaques produced by multivalent binding of antibodies to RBC have yet to be performed. The hypothesis can be tested by comparing the predicted time development [for multi-site binding the theory predicts a different result than those of Eq. (1)] with the experimentally determined one.

If it is correct to treat the binding of antibodies to RBC as irreversible, then the forward rate constant, and not the affinity constant, governs the binding reaction. Studies indicate that there is little variation in hapten-antibody forward rate constants (Froese, 1968; Barisas et al., 1975); the distribution in affinities seems to be due almost entirely to the wide spread in reverse rate constants. If, in addition to the forward rate constant distribution, the secretion rate and lag time distributions are also narrow, then in the absence of free hapten all the plaque radii will be approximately the same size. When this is so, the inhibition curve will reflect only the properties of the affinity distribution. Unlike the single-site attachment case (Fig. 4a), the range of hapten concentrations over which inhibition occurs will reflect the width of the affinity distribution, and a broad affinity distribution will yield a broad inhibition curve.

Unfortunately it does not appear that in plaque inhibition experiments, plaque radii are uniform in the absence of free hapten. North and Askonas (1974) attempted to use plaque inhibition of indirect plaques to measure the affinity of anti-DNP (2,4-dinitrophenyl) and anti-NIP (4-hydroxy-5-iodo-3-nitrophenacetyl) IgG antibodies produced in monoclonal responses. They found poor agreement between the affinity measured by plaque inhibition ($K = 2/H_{50}$) and, in the serum, by the Farr assay. Further, in some cases inhibition occurred over a narrow range of hapten concentrations, but in others the range was quite broad. With no free hapten present cells in some clones produced plaques which varied considerably in size. For example, in one clone, the plaque diameters ranged from 0.15 to 1.0 mm. If the response was truly monoclonal, the distribution in sizes could not be due to affinity differences between the AFC. One could thus conclude that the dispersion in plaque sizes was due to differences in emission rates and lag times. Yamada, Yamada, and

Hollander (1970) found that cells from the mouse myeloma MOPC-315, which secretes IgA that binds to DNP, also produced plaques of varying size (0.1-0.8 mm in diameter). These results cast doubt on the validity of plaque inhibition as a reliable assay for antibody affinity at the cellular level.

This is not to say that information about the affinity distribution cannot be obtained from plaque inhibition experiments. For example, when a monovalent inhibitor is used, and the antibodies bind multivalently at the RBC surfaces, the inhibition curve is sensitive to the affinity distribution. If the affinity distribution undergoes a systematic change over a period of time, while the other distributions do not, this change will be reflected in the inhibition curves. DeLisi (1976) has examined this in great detail for a variety of haptenation conditions.

To interpret an inhibition curve requires knowing what type of binding occurs between antibody and free hapten, and antibody and sites on the RBC. It would be most helpful if time studies of single plaques were carried out in conjunction with any inhibition study of direct plaques. Measurements of the plaque radius as a function of time should be made in layers, both with and without free hapten present. If both with and without the inhibitor Eq. (1) is obeyed, that is, R^2/t = constant, then Eq. (7) is correct, and the binding of antibody to both free hapten and sites on the RBC is equilibrium controlled. As was shown, for this case the inhibition curve will be relatively insensitive to the affinity distribution. If with H = 0 Eq. (1) is obeyed, but with free hapten in the layer it is not, the binding of antibody to RBC sites is equilibrium controlled, but the binding to inhibitor sites is not. This would be possible if a multivalent inhibitor is used.*

---

*The theory for inhibition of plaques with multivalent inhibitor has been published for thick gels (DeLisi, 1975a,b) but these results are not directly applicable for many inhibition studies. If a plaque obeys Eq. (1), the thin gel result must be used. The thin gel results can be obtained by using the equations of DeLisi and the solution given by Goldstein and Perelson (1977).

Weyer et al. (1972) performed time studies on direct plaques produced by AFC populations from mice immunized with sheep RBC. They observed a spread in times at which the AFC began secreting in the layer. In light of these results, inhibition experiments should be done as a function of time. If they truly assay for affinity, the inhitition curves should be independent of time, but if they do not, the effect of the distribution in lag times can be assessed.

V. SENSITIVITY OF PLAQUE GROWTH TO CHANGES IN AFC SECRETION RATES

I now turn from considerations of properties of cell populations to consider single AFC. In particular I investigate the following questions: How sensitive is plaque growth to changes in the AFC secretion rate? For example, if a metabolic inhibitor is added to a layer containing an AFC, that is producing a plaque, can the effects of the inhibitor be inferred from studying the growth of this plaque with time?

To gain some insight into this question, consider what happens to the plaque radius of an AFC that suddenly changes its secretion rate from S_0 to S_1 at $T = T_1$, that is,

$$S(t) = \begin{cases} 0 & T < T_0 \\ S_0 & T_0 \leqslant T < T_1 \\ S_1 & T_1 \leqslant T \end{cases}$$

From the Appendix, Eq. (A5), one can show that the plaque radius obeys the following equations:

$$\Theta = E_1(\beta) \qquad T_0 < T < T_1$$

$$\Theta = E_1(\beta) - \frac{1 - S_1}{S_0} E_1[\beta(\alpha + 1)] \qquad T_1 < T \tag{10}$$

where $\alpha = (1 - \Delta T/T)^{-1} - 1$, and $\Delta T = T_1 - T_0$. For $T < T_0$, $R = 0$ since $S(t) = 0$.

If $S_1 = 0$ (the AFC secretes antibodies for a time ΔT and then abruptly stops secreting at time T_1), R will grow to a maximum value and then recede. This is because R is defined as the distance from the AFC at which there is a fixed number, N, of antibodies bound per RBC. Shortly after the AFC stops secreting, the free antibody concentration will start to drop everywhere within the plaque radius. One must move closer to the AFC to find a concentration high enough to bind N antibodies. With complement present during the entire experiment, R will grow to a maximum value and stop. If complement is added at the end of the experiment, the size of the plaque will depend on how soon after the AFC stopped secreting antibodies the complement was added. This is illustrated in Fig. 5.

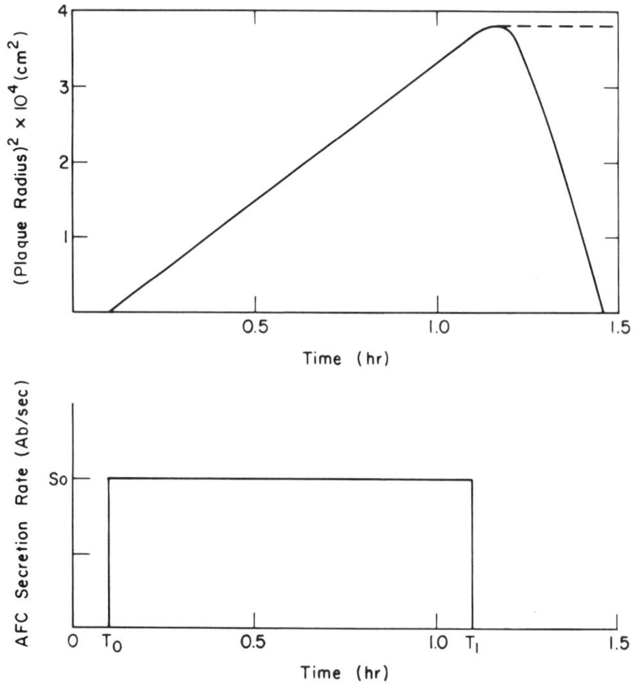

FIG. 5. An AFC secretes antibodies at a constant rate S_0 from T_0 = 0.1 hr to T_1 = 1.1 hr. Θ = 1.36, D = 1.5 $\times$ 10^{-7} cm^2/sec, and $K\rho_0 \ll 1$. For $T \leqslant T_1$ the solid and dashed curves are identical. The solid curve is for the case when complement is added at the end of the experiment; the dashed curve is for the case when complement is always present.

Notice in Fig. 5 that very soon after the AFC shuts off, the plaque radius stops increasing. The smaller Θ (small Θ values correspond to high secretion rates), the longer the delay between the time the AFC stops secreting and the time the plaque stops growing. The delay time depends only on Θ and ΔT. It can be seen from Fig. 6 that considerable delays can occur for high secreters of antibody.

If the AFC, instead of stopping antibody secretion entirely at $T = T_1$, changes to a new nonzero secretion rate S_1, some interesting types of plaque growth can occur. From Eq. (10), R as a function of T can be obtained for given values of Θ, D*, T_0, T_1 and S_1/S_0. In Fig. 7, R^2 vs. T is plotted for an AFC that secretes at a constant rate S_0 for the first half hour, after which it secretes at a constant rate S_1. If there is a 20% decrease in the secretion rate

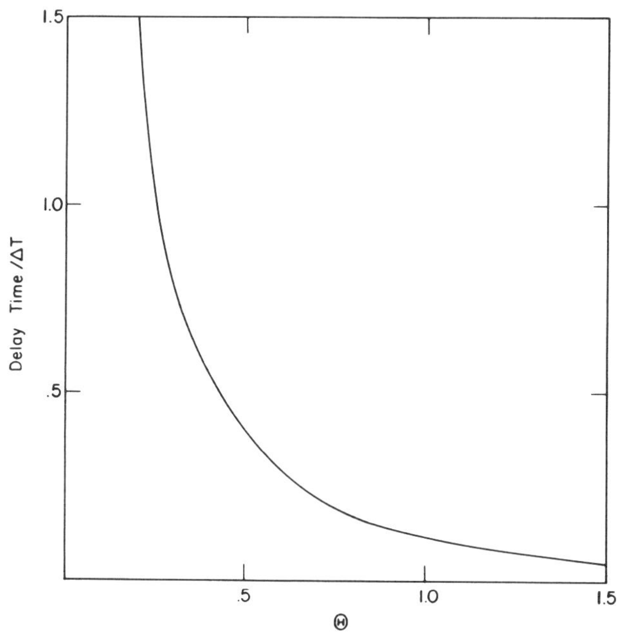

FIG. 6. $\Delta T = T_1 - T_0$ is the total time the AFC secretes antibodies. The delay time equals the difference between the time the AFC stops secreting and the time the plaque stops growing. $\Theta = 4\pi DhN/KeS_0$.

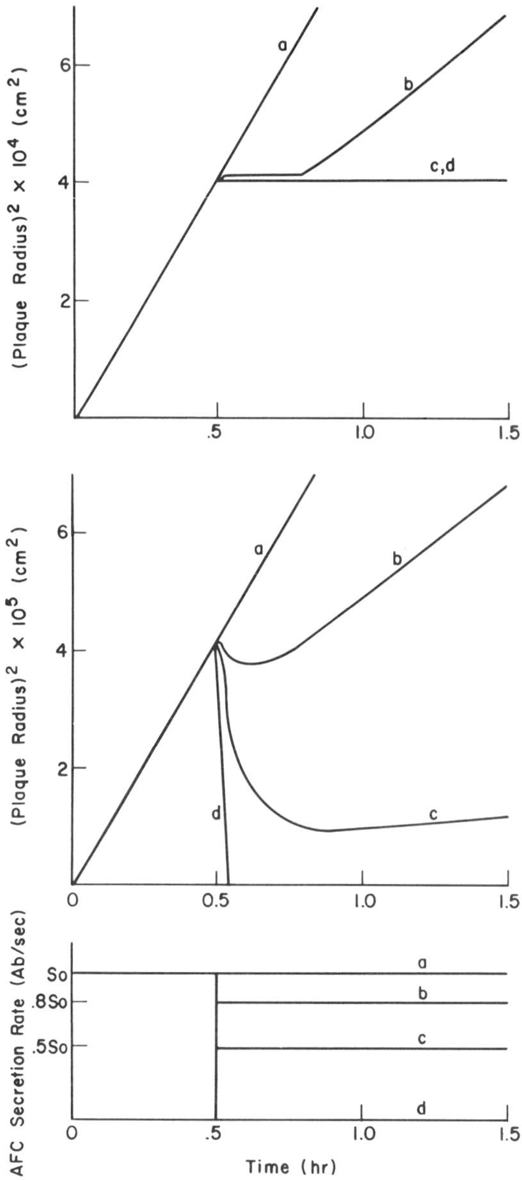

FIG. 7. Curves for four AFC that start at time $T_0 = T$ to secrete antibodies at a rate S_0. $\Theta = 2.72$, $D = 1.5 \times 10^{-7}$ cm^2/sec, and $K\rho_0 \ll 1$. At $T_1 = 0.5$ hr the secretion rate of the AFC: (a) undergoes no change, (b) drops to 0.8 S_0, (c) drops to 0.5 S_0, or (d) drops to zero. The top figure is for the case when complement is always present. The middle figure is for the case when complement is added at the end of the experiment.

(S_1/S_0 = 0.8), and if complement is present, the plaque will grow for the first 0.52 hr and then stop. At 0.79 hr it will begin to grow again at a slower rate. If S_1/S_2 = 0.5, the plaque will stop growing almost exactly at 0.5 hr and not begin growing again until 80 hr have elapsed. *The fact that a plaque stops growing does not necessarily mean that the AFC has stopped secreting antibodies, but only that its secretion rate has decreased since the start of the experiment.*

With complement present one can determine how the plaque radius changes with time. However, as can be seen from Fig. 7, from such a plot the time course of the AFC emission rate cannot be uniquely determined (curves c and d are identical although their S(t) functions are different).

A sudden change in the secretion rate will not always lead to a period when the plaque does not grow. For certain values of the parameters the plaque will continue to increase in size, but the rates of growth before and after the change will be different. This behavior was observed in a study done by Nossal and Lewis (1971). Figure 8 shows the results from one of their plaque studies; for Θ = 1.66 and S_1/S_0 = 0.86, a 14% decrease in the secretion rate, a good fit is obtained. If the value of the hindered diffusion coefficient is known, Θ and S_1/S_0 can be unambiguously determined from the experimental curve. As yet D* has not been measured. I have simply taken D* = 1.5×10^{-7} cm^2/sec, a value somewhat smaller than the diffusion coefficient of IgM in water, $D_{20,W}$ = 1.7×10^{-7} cm^2/sec (Kabat and Petersen, 1938; Suzuki and Deutsch, 1967). Although a different choice of D* will change the values of Θ and S_0/S_1, the conclusion will be the same: that the AFC has undergone a sudden change in secretion rate during the course of the experiment.

The plaque experiment tells us nothing about the cause of this sudden change. There was no sudden outside perturbation of the system during the experiment. If the AFC reduced its output of IgM and began secreting IgG, a curve similar to Fig. 8 would be obtained; however, more mundane explanations can also be found. If known perturbations are introduced, then the theory should be of considerable aid in understanding their effects on antibody secretion.

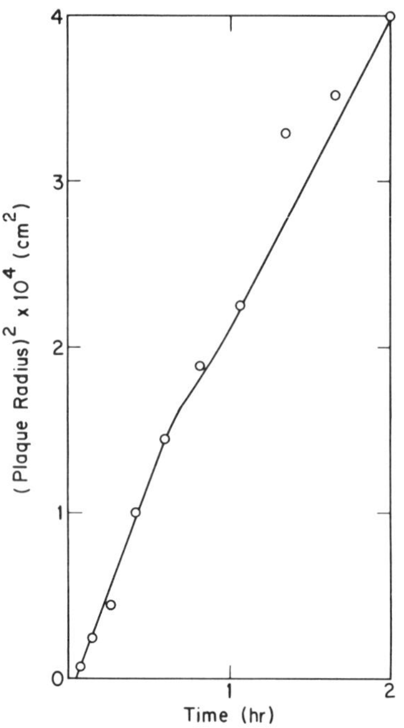

FIG. 8. The solid line is the theoretical curve for an AFC with $\Theta = 1.66$. The AFC starts at time $T_0 = 2.4$ min to secrete antibodies at a rate S_0. At $T_1 = 36.0$ min its secretion rate suddenly decreases to $S_1 = 0.86\ S_0$. D was taken equal to 1.5×10^{-7} Ab/sec. The open points are data points from Fig. 1 of a study by Nossal and Lewis (1971) of single AFC.

APPENDIX

A. General Equations

For a thin layer (planar diffusion), the free antibody concentration c obeys the equation:

$$\frac{\partial c}{\partial t} = D\nabla^2 c - \frac{\partial c_b}{\partial t} + \frac{S(t)}{h}\,\delta(r) \qquad \text{(A-1)}$$

where c_b is the bound antibody concentration and $\delta(r)$ is the two-dimensional Dirac delta function $[\delta(r) = \delta(x)\ \delta(y)]$. The surface integral of $\delta(r)$ equals one when it is over any area which includes the origin.

Equation (A-1) states that the free antibody concentration changes with time due to diffusion, due to the loss (or gain) of antibodies through binding to (or loss from) RBC sites, and at the origin by the production of antibodies at a rate S(t).

To solve Eq. (A-1) an additional equation is needed which describes how the bound antibody concentration changes with time. For the case of single-site attachment, I assume that the free and bound antibody concentrations are in local equilibrium, in which case

$$\rho(r, t) = \frac{\rho_0 Kc(r, t)}{1 + Kc(r, t)} \qquad \text{(A-2)}$$

ρ is the bound site concentration and ρ_0 is the initial free site concentration.

If the fraction of sites bound on any RBC is small, that is, $\rho/\rho_0 << 1$, then

$$\rho(r, t) = \rho_0 Kc(r, t) \qquad \text{(A-3)}$$

For single-site attachment, the number of bound antibodies equals the number of bound sites, $\rho = c_b$, so Eq. (A-3) can be differentiated and substituted directly into Eq. (A-1). When this is done

$$-\frac{S(t)}{Dh}\,\delta(r) = \frac{1}{D^*}\,\frac{\partial c}{\partial t} + \nabla^2 c \qquad \text{(A-4)}$$

where $D^* = D/(1 + K\rho_0)$.

This is just the diffusion equation which has the following solution:

$$c(r, t) = \frac{1}{4\pi Dh}\int_0^1 S(t - tu)\,\frac{\exp(-r^2/\,D^*Tu)}{u}\,du \qquad \text{(A-5)}$$

At the plaque radius R there are N antibodies bound per RBC. An equation for the plaque radius is obtained by evaluating Eq. (A-5) for a particular form of S(t), and substituting the result into Eq. (A-3). Since $\rho_0 = e\rho_{RBC}$ at the plaque radius, Eq. (A-3) becomes

$$N = eKc(R, t) \qquad \text{(A-6)}$$

From Eq. (A-5) it follows that for a constant secretion rate S_0

$$c(r, t) = \frac{S_0}{4\pi Dh} \int_0^1 \frac{\exp(-r^2/4D^*tu)}{u} du \tag{A-7}$$

If the change of variables u = 1/x is made, Eq. (A-7) becomes

$$c(r, t) = \frac{S_0}{4\pi Dh} \int_1^\infty \frac{\exp(-\beta x)}{x} dx \tag{A-8}$$

where the integral equals $E_1(\beta)$ (Gautschi and Cahill, 1964). If Eq. (A-8) is substituted into Eq. (A-6), Eq. (3) is obtained.

B. Hapten and the Plaque Radius

Equation (7) describes how the plaque radius grows as a function of time in the presence of hapten. By differentiating Eq. (7) the following result is obtained:

$$2 \frac{d \ln R}{dH} = \frac{K_S}{1 + K_S H} \left[\frac{K\rho_0}{1 + K_S H + K\rho_0} - \exp(\beta) E_1(\beta) \right] \tag{A-9}$$

When the quantity in brackets is positive

$$\frac{K\rho_0}{1 + K_S H + K\rho_0} > \exp(\beta) E_1(\beta) \tag{A-10}$$

R increases with H.

The left side of Eq. (A-10) is always less than 1. When $\beta = 0.43$, the quantity $\exp(\beta)E_1(\beta) = 1$. For this value of β it follows from Eq. (7) that $\Theta(1 + K_S H) = 0.65$. For any plaque with $\Theta \geqslant 0.65$, R will always decrease with H since the inequality cannot be satisfied.

C. The Diffusion Coefficient and the Plaque Radius

If Eq. (3) is differentiated with respect to D, and dR/dD set equal to zero, one finds that $1 = \exp(\beta)E_1(\beta)$, that is, $\beta = 0.43$ and $\Theta = 0.65$. If $\Theta < 0.65$, then $dR/dD > 0$, while if $\Theta > 0.65$, then $dR/dD < 0$.

REFERENCES

Andersson, B. (1970). Studies on the regulation of avidity at the level of the single antibody-forming cell. *J. Exp. Med. 132:* 77-88.

Barisas, B. G., Singer, S. J., and Sturtevant, J. M. (1975). Kinetics of binding of 2,4-dinitrophenyl and 2,4,6-trinitrophenyl haptens to homologous and heterologous rabbit antibodies. *Immunochem. 12:* 411-421.

Couderc, J., Bleux, C., Birrien, J. L., and Liacopoulos, P. (1975). The potentiality of antibody-producing cells. I. Bispecific cell occurence in double stimulated cultures of syngeneic or allogeneic spleen cells of the mouse. *Immunology 29:* 653-664.

Couderc, J., Bleux, C., and Liacopoulos, P. (1975). The potentiality of antibody-producing cells. II. Evidence for two antibody molecules of different specificities secreted by micromanipulated bispecific mouse spleen cells. *Immunology 29:* 665-674.

Cunningham, A. J. and Fordham, S. A. (1974). Antibody cell daughters can produce antibody of different specificities. *Nature 250:* 669-671.

Cunningham, A. J. and Pilarski, L. M. (1974a). Generation of antibody diversity. I. Kinetics of production of different antibody specificities during the course of an immune response. *Eur. J. Immunol. 4:* 319.326.

Cunningham, A. J. and Pilarski, L. M. (1974b). The generation of antibody diversity. II. Plaque morphology as a simple marker for antibody specificity at the single-cell level. *Eur. J. Immunol. 4:* 757-761.

DeLisi, C. (1975a). The kinetics of hemolytic plaque formation. III. Inhibition of plaques by antigen. *J. Theor. Biol. 51:* 337-345.

DeLisi, C. (1975b). The kinetics of hemolytic plaque formation. IV. IgM plaque inhibition. *J. Theor. Biol. 52:* 419-440.

DeLisi, C. (1976). Hemolytic plaque inhibition: the physical chemical limits on its use as an affinity assay. *J. Immunol. 117:* 2249-2257.

DeLisi, C. and Bell, G. I. (1974). The kinetics of hemolytic plaque formation. *Proc. Nat. Acad. Sci. (USA) 71:* 16-20.

DeLisi, C. and Bell, G. I. (1976). Plaque morphology as an antibody specificity marker: an analysis of the physical chemical foundation of the method. *Immunochem. 13:* 21-28.

DeLisi, C. and Goldstein, B. (1974). The mechanism of hemolytic plaque inhibition. *Immunochem. 11:* 661-665.

DeLisi, C. and Goldstein, B. (1975). The kinetics of hemolytic plaque formation. II. Inhibition of plaques by hapten. *J. Theor. Biol. 51:* 313-335.

Esrig, S. M., Racis, S. P., Lichtblau, H., Kruger, R., and Goldstein, B. (1977). A computer method for determining plaque size and plaque morphology. *J. Immunol. Methods* (in press).

Froese, A. (1968). Kinetic and equilibrium studies on 2,4-dinitrophenyl hapten-antibody systems. *Immunochem. 5:* 253-264.

Goidl, E. A., Birnbaum, G., and Siskind, G. W. (1975). Determination of antibody avidity at the cellular level by the plaque inhibition technique: effect of valence of inhibitor. *J. Immunol. Methods. 8:* 47-52.

Goldstein, B. (1975). Effect of antibody emission rates on plaque morphology. *Nature 253:* 637-639.

Goldstein, B. and Perelson, A. S. (1976). The electrophoretic hemolytic plaque assay - theory. *Biophysical Chem. 4:* 349-362.

Goldstein, B. and Perelson, A. S. (1977). The hemolytic plaque assay: theory for finite layers. *Biophysical Chem.* (in press).

Gautschi, W. and Cahill, W. F. (1964). Exponential integral and related functions. In *Handbook of Mathematical Functions* (M. Abramowitz and I. A. Stegun, eds.). National Bureau of Standards, Washington, p. 228.

Hornick, C. L. and Karush, F. (1972). Antibody affinity. III. The role of multivalence. *Immunochem. 9:* 325-340.

Humphrey, J. H. (1967). Haemolytic efficiency of rabbit IgG anti-forssman antibody and its augmentation by anti-rabbit IgG. *Nature 216:* 1295-1296.

Ingraham, J. S. and Bussard, A. (1964). Application of a localized haemolysin reaction for specific detection of individual antibody-forming cells. *J. Exp. Med. 119:* 667-684.

Jerne, N. K., Henry, C., Nordin, A. A., Fuji, H., Koros, A. M. C., and Lefkovits, I. (1974). Plaque forming cells: methodology and theory. *Transplant. Rev. 18:* 130-191.

Jerne, N. K. and Nordin, A. A. (1963). Plaque formation in agar by single antibody-producing cells. *Science 140:* 405.

Jerne, N. K., Nordin, A. A., and Henry, C. (1963). The agar plaque technique for recognizing antibody-producing cells. In *Cell-Bound Antibodies* (B. Amos and H. Korpowski, eds.). Wistar Institute Press, Philadelphia, pp. 109-125.

Kabat, E. A. and Petersen, K. O. (1938). The molecular weights of antibodies. *Science 87:* 372.

Kim, Y. D. and Karush, F. (1973). Equine anti-hapten antibody. VII. Anti-lactoside antibody induced by a bacterial vaccine. *Immunochem. 10:* 365-371.

Merchant, B. and Peterson, B. (1968). Comparative sensitivities of the hemolytic plaque in agar and microchamber assays for detection of rabbit immune cells. *J. Immunol. 110:* 860-867.

Mukkur, T. K. S., Szewczuk, M. R., and Schmidt, D. E. (1974). Determination of total affinity constant for heterogeneous hapten-antibody interactions. *Immunochem. 11:* 9-13.

North, J. R. and Askonas, B. A. (1974). Analysis of affinity of monoclonal antibody responses by inhibition of plaque-forming cells. *Eur. J. Immunol. 4:* 361-366.

Nossal, G. J. V., Bussard, A. E., Lewis, H., and Mazie, J. C. (1970). In vitro stimulation of antibody formation by peritoneal cells. I. Plaque technique of high sensitivity enabling access to the cells. *J. Exp. Med. 131:* 894-916.

Nossal, G. J. V. and Lewis, H. (1971). Functional symmetry amongst daughter cells arising in vitro from single antibody-forming cells. *Immunol. 20:* 739-753.

Oriol, R. and Rousset, M. (1974a). The IgM antibody site. I. Increase of binding affinity of rat 19S and 7S anti-dinitrophenyl antibodies. *J. Immunol. 112:* 2227-2234.

Oriol, R. and Rousset, M. (1974b). The IgM antibody site. II. Comparison of the two populations of IgM antibody sites and analysis of the behavior of the low affinity population of equilibrium with a dinitrophenylated hapten. *J. Immunol. 112:* 2235-2240.

Perelson, A. S. and Goldstein, B. (1977). The relationship between direct plaque size and antibody affinity. *J. Immunol. 118:* 1649-54.

Pilarski, L. M. and Cunningham, A. J. (1974). The generation of antibody diversity. III. Variation in the specificity of antibody produced within single clones of antibody-forming cells in vitro. *Eur. J. Immunol. 4:* 762-767.

Pilarski, L. M. and Cunningham, A. J. (1975). Generation of antibody diversity. IV. Variation within single clones of antibody-forming cells developing in vivo. *Eur. J. Immunol. 5:* 10-16.

Schrader, J. W. (1975). Effector-cell blockade. II. A demonstration of the reversible masking of an immune response by blockade of antibody forming cells. *Eur. J. Immunol. 5:* 808-812.

Schrader, J. W. and Nossal, G. J. V. (1974). Effector cell blockage; a new mechanism of immune hyporeactivity induced by multivalent antigens. *J. Exp. Med. 139:* 1582-1598.

Suziki, T. and Deutsch, H. F. (1967). Dissociation, reaggregation and subunit studies on some human γqM-globulins. *J. Biol. Chem. 242:* 2725-2738.

Voss, E. W., Jr. and Eisen, H. N. (1968). Valence and affinity of IgM antibodies to the 2,4-dinitrophenyl (DNP) group. *Fed. Proc. 27:* 684.

Weyer, J., Bourgaitt, J. J., and Bussard, A. E. (1972). Kinetics of antibody production by single cells. I. Automatic recording of plaque production in the local haemolysis system. *Immunol. 22:* 347-359.

Yamada, H., Yamada, A., and Hollander, V. P. (1970). 2,4-dinitrophenyl-hapten specific hemolytic plaque-in-gel formation by mouse myeloma (MOPC-315) cells. *J. Immunol. 104:* 215-255.

Chapter 5

FACTORS AFFECTING THE RELIABILITY OF CAPILLARY MIGRATION INHIBITION FACTOR ASSAYS

Ralph Nossal

Physical Sciences Laboratory
Division of Computer Research and Technology
National Institutes of Health
Bethesda, Maryland

A simple mathematical model is used to investigate the relative importance of noise sources which influence in vitro capillary migration assays of cellular immune sensitivity. Analytic expressions for the migration inhibition index I_∞ are derived from a model of planar locomotion which incorporates concentration-dependent mobility coefficients. Several sources of experimental variability are considered, including (a) uncertainties in loading of cells into the capillaries, (b) variable culture conditions, and (c) migration inhibition factor (MIF) absorption by extraneous erythrocytes.

I. INTRODUCTION

When a biological parameter is probed by an in vitro assay, the value obtained generally reflects factors introduced by the measurement process itself. Ancillary "noise," deriving either from irregularities in technique or changes in uncontrolled parameters, limits the resolution with which underlying phenomena can be measured. The following work is directed toward understanding how such extrinsic experimental variability affects capillary migration assays of cellular immune sensitivity.

Hopefully, insight gained from the analysis will serve in improving the reliability of such assays when they are used for clinical diagnosis. Thus, specific attention is given here to the direct migration inhibition factor (MIF) assay utilizing human white blood cells. In this instance, peripheral blood leukocytes are packed into capillaries and then allowed to migrate onto the surfaces of tissue culture dishes covered with media containing antigens to which a patient might have become sensitized. Some of the lymphocytes contained in the cell population produce soluble migration inhibition factors, which cause a decrease in the area subtended by the migrating leukocytes, as compared with migration of cells into media which lack the putative antigen. Recent applications of this in vitro technique include detection of human colonic adenocarcinomas (Bull et al., 1973), diagnosis of parasitic infection (Lelchuk et al., 1974), and determinations of autoimmune involvement in thyroid disease (Mahieu and Winand, 1972; Munro et al., 1973).

The assay has been described in considerable detail elsewhere (see, e.g., Bloom and Glade, 1971; David, 1973; Morley, 1974; Remold and David, 1974). Many of its parameters are difficult to control or are easily influenced by technical error. Among these are the conditions of the culture medium, proportions of the various leukocytes appearing in the extracted cell population, and the total number of cells contained in each capillary. Since mobility coefficients can be functionals of cell concentration (Patten et al., 1973; Zigmond and Hirsch, 1973), the latter is of particular concern. Not only may the density of the cell suspension vary among different leukocyte preparations, but techniques used in preparing the capillaries can cause uncertainty in cell titer even among the supposedly identical capillaries used for a specific test series [e.g., the capillaries are filled, centrifuged in order to pack the cells into a dense mass, and then rather imprecisely cut at the "cell-medium" interface (Bloom and Glade, 1971)]. In addition to direct effects on mobility, variation in cell titer also might lead to modification of assay results via associated changes in culture conditions.

Consequently, in clinical application, assay plates typically are prepared in triplicate. Nonetheless, a rather wide spectrum of responses frequently is discerned, not only for sensitized patients but also when the assay is applied to normal controls. Responses of some individuals of the control group usually overlap some of those of the sensitized group, even though the mean response of the patient group clearly demonstrates MIF-related inhibition (see Fig. 1). Such dispersion tends to limit the usefulness of the assay for diagnostic purposes so that, for example, an average migration inhibition exceeding 20% usually is required for a test to be scored as positive.

A simplified theory recently has been proposed for analyzing dose-response relations occurring in capillary migration assays (Nossal, 1977). That exposition is based on a mathematical description of cell migration analogous to a linear diffusion equation. The theory now shall be modified to account for concentration-dependent mobilities, and used for determining the relative importance of several sources of experimental variability.

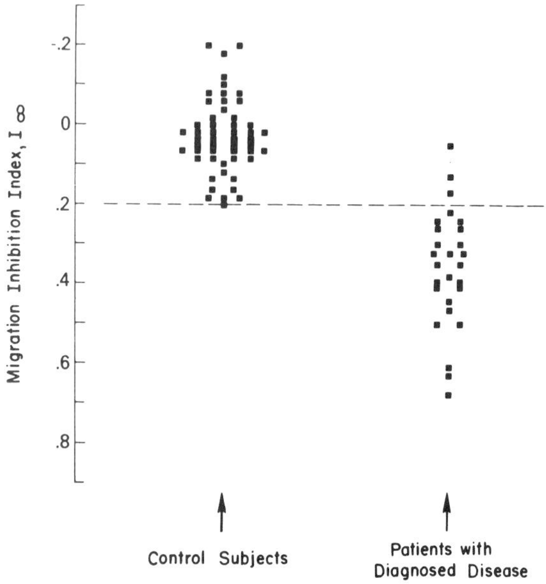

FIG. 1. Typical MIF assay results. These data, originally presented by Bull et al. (1973), were obtained for patients with diagnosed adenocarcinomas of the colon. Although they indicate that in vitro cellular sensitivity to adenocarcenoma tissue antigens on the average is correlated closely with the patients' disease, variability within subject groups is considerable.

II. CELL KINETICS

A. Migration Inhibition Index

Results of capillary migration assays usually are expressed in terms of some variant of the inhibition index I, defined as

$$I = 1 - \frac{A_M}{A_0} \qquad (1)$$

In this expression, A_M represents the area of migration of cells migrating from capillaries which are incubated in media containing the test antigen, and A_0 is the area discerned for cells moving in media lacking the antigen. As indicated elsewhere (Nossal, 1977), the migration area is approximately proportional the mean square radius $\langle r_t^2 \rangle$ of the cell concentration. Thus, I(t) can be represented as

$$I \simeq 1 - \frac{\langle r_t^2 \rangle_M}{\langle r_t^2 \rangle_0} \tag{1a}$$

where $\langle r_t^2 \rangle$ is defined as

$$\langle r_t^2 \rangle = \frac{2\pi \int_0^\infty dr\, r[r^2 C(r, t)]}{2\pi \int_0^\infty dr\, rC(r, t)} \tag{2}$$

C(r, t) being the density of cells within a differential annulus of width dr located at distance r from the origin. The latter is taken to be identical with the location of the mouth of the capillary (i.e., where cells are inserted onto the surface along which they subsequently migrate), and an essentially radial symmetry has been assumed.

B. Expression for $\langle r_t^2 \rangle$

As before (Nossal, 1977), we describe the migration of cells by a planar diffusion equation, viz.,

$$\frac{\partial C(r, t)}{\partial t} = \frac{1}{r} \frac{\partial}{\partial r} \left[r\mu(r, t) \frac{\partial C(r, t)}{\partial r} \right] + S(r, t) \tag{3}$$

subject to the condition $\lim_{r\to\infty} C(r, t) = 0$. Here, S(r, t) is a source term which, for migration from the mouths of narrow bore capillaries, can be approximated by a delta function

$$S(r, t) \simeq \frac{S(t)\ \delta(r)}{2\pi r} \tag{4}$$

Correspondingly, as an initial condition we take C(r, 0) = 0, r > 0. The mobility coefficient μ(r, t) is an empirical macroscopic constant which, if cells interact through collisions and adhesions, can have a strong dependence upon cell concentration. When such is the case, Eq. (3) becomes a nonlinear partial differential equation for which solutions generally are elusive. However, a useful expression for $\langle r_t^2 \rangle$ nonetheless can be obtained, based essentially on an approximate iterative solution to Eqs. (3) and (4).

For this purpose we write the mobility coefficient as

$$\mu(r, t) = \bar{\mu}(t)\{1 - f[C(r, t)]\} \tag{5}$$

where $\bar{\mu}(t)$ is the mobility coefficient which would occur if the cell concentration were to remain at a high constant value (e.g., at the density at which the cells are packed into a capillary), and f(C) expresses deviations from this value. Even in the absence of effects related to cell density, one expects that the mobility varies with time due to MIF production and other changes occurring in the culture medium. These are accounted for by expressing $\bar{\mu}(t)$ as (Nossal, 1977)

$$\bar{\mu}(t) = \mu_\infty h(t)\{1 - k[M(t)]^\alpha\} \tag{6}$$

where μ_∞ is the intrinsic high concentration mobility coefficient, M(t) is the MIF concentration in the culture medium, k and α are positive constants, and h(t) is a dimensionless quantity which accounts for changes in mobility deriving from changes in the conditions of the culture medium other than lymphokine production [the latter being the products of sensitized lymphocytes when activated by appropriate antigen (David et al., 1964; Dumonde et al., 1969)]. The derivation of Eq. (6), which is part is based on data presented by Dumonde et al. (1972), is further discussed elsewhere (Nossal, 1977). Using Eq. (5) one can rewrite Eq. (3) as

$$\frac{\partial C}{\partial t} = \frac{\bar{\mu}(t)}{r}\frac{\partial}{\partial r}\left(r\,\frac{\partial C}{\partial r}\right) + S_{eff}(r, t) \tag{7}$$

where $S_{eff}(r, t)$ has the formal definition

$$S_{eff}(r, t) = S(r, t) - \frac{\bar{\mu}(t)}{r}\frac{\partial}{\partial r}\left[rf(C)\,\frac{\partial C}{\partial r}\right] \tag{8}$$

If we multiply both sides of Eq. (7) by r^2 and integrate, Eq. (2) yields (cf Nossal, 1977)

$$\langle r_t^2 \rangle = \frac{\int_0^t d\tau \int_0^\infty dr\, r\left[4\bar{\mu}(\tau)\int_0^\tau S(r, y)\, dy + r^2 S_{eff}(r, \tau)\right]}{\int_0^t d\tau \int_0^\infty dr\, rS(r, \tau)} \tag{9}$$

Thus, upon invoking Eq. (4) and performing some simple partial integrations, we find

$$\langle r_t^2 \rangle = \frac{4}{W(t)}\int_0^t d\tau\bar{\mu}(\tau)\left\{W(\tau) - 2\pi\int_0^\infty dr\, rF[C(r, \tau)]\right\} \tag{10}$$

where W(t) and F[C] are defined as

$$W(t) = \int_0^t S(\tau)\, d\tau \tag{11}$$

and

$$F[C] = \int_0^C f(c)\, dc \tag{12}$$

The exact solution for C(r, t) in principle could be obtained by using the iteration scheme implied by Eqs. (7) and (8) (Crank, 1956). In the following we evaluate the (first-order) correction in Eq. (10) with the zero'th order expression for the concentration (Crank, 1956)

$$C_0(r, t) = \int_0^t dyS(t - y)\, \frac{\exp[-r^2/\theta(y)]}{\pi\theta(y)} \tag{13}$$

where θ(y) is

$$\theta(t) \equiv 4\int_0^t \bar{\mu}(\tau)\, d\tau \tag{14}$$

Usually, S(t) is taken to be a delta function in time, that is,

$$S(t) = S_0 \, \delta(t) \tag{15}$$

since a more faithful specification of S(t) does not seem to be important (Nossal, 1977). In this case θ(t) is the mean square radius which would follow from Eqs. (3) to (7) if $f \equiv 0$.

C. Kinetics of MIF Production

The MIF concentration M(t) is herein specified by assuming, first, that MIF, having a molecular weight of 23,000 (Rocklin, Remold and David, 1972), diffuses so rapidly compared with the motion of the cells that its spatial variation can be neglected. Second, we presume that a simple mass action equation suffices for representing essential aspects of the phenomenology, in which case we have (Nossal, 1977)

$$M(t) = M_{st}[1 - \exp(-\xi t)] \tag{16}$$

where M_{st} and ξ are given as

$$M_{st} = \frac{bC_E}{\lambda_I C_I + \lambda_A C_A} \tag{17}$$

and

$$\xi = \lambda_I C_I + \lambda_A C_A \tag{18}$$

Here, C_E represents the number of MIF producing lymphocytes, C_I is the number of migrating cells which respond to MIF, and C_A represents other cells which might degrade MIF. λ_I, λ_A, and b are constants, the latter assumed to be proportional to the antigen concentration.

III. CONCENTRATION-DEPENDENT MOBILITY

A. Mobility Coefficients

In principle, to fully characterize the migration of cells, one would need to measure the cell density C(r, t) as a function of position. Routinely, however, in performing the MIF assay, one merely estimates the position of the "outermost boundary" of the cell mass, from which the "area of cell migration" is computed. Fortunately, these boundaries usually appear rather sharp, thus minimizing the subjectivity with which boundary determinations might otherwise be encumbered. However, the apparent sharpness of the boundary of the migrating cell population strongly suggests that the cells interact with one another, that is, that the mobility coefficient μ is a function of the cell density.

Direct evidence for the concentration dependence of mobility appears in a study of Patten et al. (1973), concerning the manner in which cell concentration influences both the passive migration of leukocytes in capillaries and their chemotactic response as measured by filter assays. In both cases locomotion was greater at higher cell densities. Migration was found to be relatively insensitive to concentration for cell densities greater than a threshold concentration C^*, but decreased more or less linearly to a value of half maximum when the cell density approached zero concentration.

Such concentration dependence can be modeled by Eq. (5) with f(C) given as

$$f(C) = \begin{cases} \frac{\Delta}{C^*}(C^* - C) & \text{for } 0 \leqslant C \leqslant C^* \\ 0 & \text{for } C > C^* \end{cases} \qquad (19)$$

Δ being a constant which is related to the ratio of the high and low values of the mobility coefficient according to $\Delta = [1 - \mu(0)]/\mu_\infty$. Although Δ is approximately equal to 0.5 for the data presented by Patten et al. (1973), we are not here concerned so much with the precise specification of f(C) as with choosing a representative function to illustrate the effects of nonlinear terms when they appear in Eq. (7).

B. Cell Migration

Using Eq. (12) we find from Eq. (19)

$$F(C) = \begin{cases} \dfrac{\Delta}{C^*}\left(C^*C - \dfrac{C^2}{2}\right) & \text{if} \quad C \leqslant C^* \\ \dfrac{\Delta}{2}\, C^* & \text{if} \quad C > C^* \end{cases} \tag{20}$$

so that the second integral appearing on the right side of Eq. (10) is

$$U(\tau) = 2\pi \int_{r^*(\tau)}^{\infty} rF[C(r, \tau)]\, dr + \pi[r^*(\tau)]^2\, F(C^*) \tag{21}$$

where $r^*(\tau)$ is that value of the radius beyond which $C(r) \leqslant C^*$. Using the approximate form for $C(r, \tau)$ obtained from Eqs. (13) and (15), namely,

$$C_0(r, \tau) = \frac{S_0}{\pi\theta(\tau)} \exp \frac{-r^2}{\theta(\tau)}$$

we immediately determine that $r^*(\tau)$ can be expressed as

$$r^*(\tau) = \begin{cases} \left[\theta(\tau)\ \ln \dfrac{S_0}{\pi\theta(\tau)C^*}\right]^{1/2} & \text{if} \quad \dfrac{S_0}{\pi\theta(\tau)} \geqslant C^* \\ 0 & \text{if} \quad \dfrac{S_0}{\pi\theta(\tau)} < C^* \end{cases} \tag{22}$$

and, from Eq. (20) and (21),

$$U(\tau) = \begin{cases} \dfrac{1}{2}\, S_0\Delta R\theta(\tau)\left[\dfrac{3}{2} - \ln(R\theta(\tau))\right] & \text{if} \quad \theta(\tau) \leqslant R^{-1} \\ S_0\Delta\left\{1 - [4R\theta(\tau)]^{-1}\right\} & \text{if} \quad \theta(\tau) > R^{-1} \end{cases} \tag{23}$$

where R is defined as

$$R = \frac{\pi C^*}{S_0} \tag{24}$$

Finally, from Eqs. (10), (11), (14) and (23) we see that $\langle r_t^2 \rangle$ can be expressed as

$$\langle r_t^2 \rangle = \theta(t) - S_0^{-1} \int_0^t U[\theta(\tau)]\, d\theta(\tau) \tag{25}$$

so that, for the function given in Eq. (23),

$$\langle r_t^2 \rangle = \begin{cases} \theta(t)\left\{1 - \frac{R\Delta\theta(t)}{4} [2 - \ln(R\theta(t))]\right\} & \text{if} \quad \theta(t) \leqslant R^{-1} \\ (1 - \Delta)\theta(t) + \frac{\Delta}{4R}[2 + \ln(R\theta(t))] & \text{if} \quad \theta(t) > R^{-1} \end{cases} \tag{26}$$

If instead of the expression given by Eq. (19) we were to use a step function

$$f(C) = \begin{cases} \Delta & \text{for} \quad 0 \leqslant C \leqslant C^* \\ 0 & \text{for} \quad C > C^* \end{cases} \tag{27}$$

we would find by the same arguments

$$\langle r_t^2 \rangle = \begin{cases} \theta(t)\left\{1 - \frac{R\Delta\theta(t)}{2} \left[\frac{3}{2} - \ln(R\theta(t))\right]\right\} & \text{for} \quad \theta(t) \leqslant R^{-1} \\ (1 - \Delta)\theta(t) + \frac{\Delta}{4R} & \text{for} \quad \theta(t) > R^{-1} \end{cases} \tag{28}$$

The expressions given by Eqs. (26) and (28) are analytically quite similar, differing in essence only by the slowly increasing logarithmic term present in Eq. (26) for large values of t.

To illustrate these results, we have plotted in Fig. 2 the time dependence of $\langle r_t^2 \rangle$ as given by Eq. (26), for various values of R and Δ. Note that the abscissa is $\theta(t)$, so that $\langle r_t^2 \rangle$ here also reflects changes which might be occurring in the culture milieu. If, however, culture conditions were constant, we would have $\theta(t) = 4\mu_\infty t$, in which case $\theta = 0.02\ \text{cm}^2$ would correspond to $t \simeq 9$ hr if $\mu_\infty = 15\ \mu\text{m}^2/\text{sec}$.* The value $\langle r_t^2 \rangle = 0.02\ \text{cm}^2$ (which corresponds

---

*Using preparative techniques commonly employed for MIF assays, Nossal and Chang (1976) have measured $\mu(0) = 7.5\ \mu\text{m}^2/\text{sec}$ for the mobility of noninteracting human polymorphonuclear leukocytes [see also discussion following Eq. (19)].

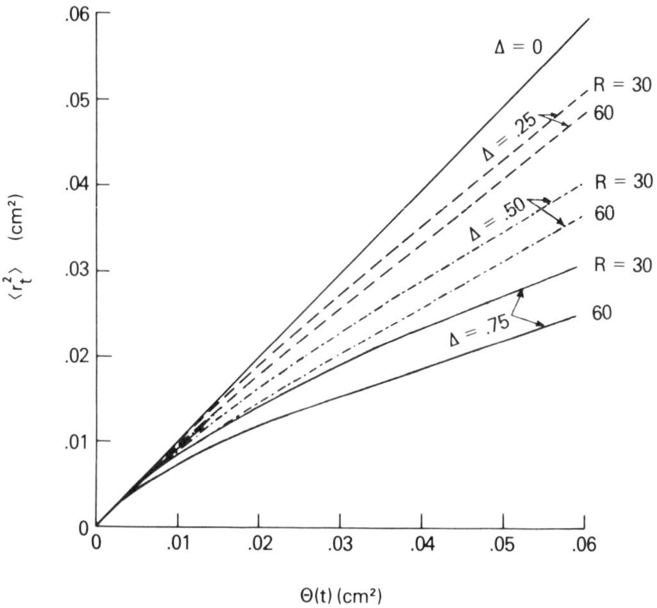

FIG. 2. Deviations from simple diffusion due to concentration-dependent mobility: $\langle r_t^2 \rangle$ vs. the reduced variable $\theta(t)$ according to the expressions given in Eq. (26). The curves depend upon the parameters Δ and $R = \pi C^*/S_0$, where Δ is the ratio of the mobilities occurring at high and low concentration, S_0 is the cell titer, and C^* is the critical concentration below which the concentration dependence of the mobility becomes apparent [see Eq. (19)]. When Δ is small, a change in initial cell titer S_0 results in small variation in migration area; on the other hand, when Δ is large, a change in S_0 leads to marked change in the migration area.

to a migration radius of approximately 5 mm; see Nossal, 1977) would be achieved at that time if only simple linear diffusion were occurring.

When Δ is small, deviations from linear diffusion due to concentration dependence of the mobility coefficient are relatively insignificant, whatever the value of S_0. However, when Δ is large, migration area strongly depends upon the initial cell titer through the latter's effect on the parameter $R = \pi C^*/S_0$. As an example, we note that $R = 30\ \text{cm}^{-2}$ could correspond to a capillary load S_0 of 10^6 cells and a concentration threshold C^* of 10 cells/100 μm^2 (i.e., a layer approximately five cells thick).

IV. MIGRATION INHIBITION

A. Analytical Considerations

In order to calculate the migration inhibition index, we next need to determine the expression for $\langle r_t^2 \rangle_M$ and $\langle r_t^2 \rangle_0$ to be used in Eq. (1a). First, we ascertain $\theta(t)$ by assuming that h(t) is given in Eq. (6) as a simple exponential, viz.,

$$h(t) = \exp(-\chi t) \tag{29}$$

since cell migration tends to diminish with time even in the absence of MIF production. In this case, by expanding $[M(t)]^\alpha$ in a power series as [cf Eq. (16)]

$$[M(t)]^\alpha = [M_{st}]^\alpha \left\{ 1 - \alpha \sum_{j=1}^{\infty} a_j \exp(-j\xi t) \right\} \tag{30}$$

we find from Eqs. (6) and (14) that $\theta(t)$ is given as

$$\theta_M(t) = 4\mu_\infty \left\{ (1 - k[M_{st}]^\alpha) \left[\frac{1 - \exp(-\chi t)}{\chi} \right] + \alpha k [M_{st}]^\alpha \times \sum_{j=1}^{\infty} a_j \frac{[1 - \exp -(\chi + j\xi)t]}{\chi + j\xi} \right\} \tag{31}$$

where the $\{a_j\}$ are defined as

$$a_1 = 1 \quad a_n = \frac{(n - 1 - \alpha)(n - 2 - \alpha)\cdots\cdots(1 - \alpha)}{n!} \quad n \geqslant 2 \tag{32}$$

The subscript M in Eq. (31) refers to the case where MIF is being produced; for control capillaries incubated in medium lacking antigen we set $k = 0$ in that expression and obtain, simply,

$$\theta_0(t) = 4\mu_\infty \frac{1 - \exp(-\chi t)}{\chi} \tag{33}$$

It is sometimes convenient to define a reduced variable $\tau = 4\mu_\infty t$, in which case the expression given by Eq. (29) becomes $h = \exp(-\tau/Q)$, where Q is given as $Q = 4\mu_\infty/\chi$. For illustration, we note that the 1/e decay of h(t) would occur at approximately 13.5 hr when $Q = .03\ \mathrm{cm}^2$, assuming that the mobility had the value $\mu_\infty = 15\ \mu\mathrm{m}^2/\mathrm{sec}$.

I(t) now can be obtained from Eq. (1a) by straightforward computation, employing the expressions for θ_M and θ_0 given in Eqs. (31) and (33) and appropriate expressions for $\langle r_t^2 \rangle$. Due to its simpler analytic form, we here use Eq. (28) for the latter and find

$$I(t) = \begin{cases} 1 - \dfrac{\theta_M(t)\left\{2 - R\Delta\theta_M(t)\left[\frac{3}{2} - \ln(R\theta_M(t))\right]\right\}}{\theta_0(t)\left\{2 - R\Delta\theta_0(t)\left[\frac{3}{2} - \ln(R\theta_0(t))\right]\right\}} & \text{if } 0 \leq \theta_0(t) \leq R^{-1} \quad (34a) \\ 1 - \dfrac{\theta_M(t)\left\{4 - R\Delta\theta_M(t)\left[3 - 2\ln(R\theta_M(t))\right]\right\}}{4(1 - \Delta)\theta_0(t) + R^{-1}\Delta} & \text{if } \theta_M(t) \leq R^{-1} \leq \theta_0(t) \quad (34b) \\ 1 - \dfrac{4(1 - \Delta)\theta_M(t) + R^{-1}\Delta}{4(1 - \Delta)\theta_0(t) + R^{-1}\Delta} & \text{if } R^{-1} < \theta_M(t) \quad (34c) \end{cases}$$

This expression increases rapidly with time and for plausible parameter values, approaching an approximately constant plateau after only 6 to 8 hr (Nossal, 1976). Since assay plates typically are read after an 18 to 24 hr period, the parametric dependence of the MIF assay can be investigated by concentrating on the asymptotic value of I obtained when $t \to \infty$. For example, if $\theta_M(\infty) > R^{-1}$, we find from Eq. (34c) that I_∞ (the asymptotic value) is given as

$$I_\infty = \frac{T_0 - T_1}{T_0 + 0.25\Delta R^{-1}(1 - \Delta)^{-1}} \qquad (35)$$

where T_0 and T_1 are defined as [cf Eqs. (31) and (33)].

$$T_0 \equiv \theta_0(\infty) = 4\mu_\infty \chi^{-1} \qquad (36)$$

$$T_1 \equiv \theta_M(\infty) = T_0 - k[M_{st}]^\alpha T_0 \left(1 - \alpha \sum_{j=1}^{\infty} \frac{a_j}{1 + j\chi^{-1}\xi}\right) \qquad (37)$$

and R and Δ are defined in Eqs. (24) and (27).

Asymptotic expressions for Eqs. (34a) and (34b) can be given in like manner. However, since we also wish to examine the consequences of variation in initial capillary titer S_0, we present here more general expressions of which Eq. (35) and its analogs are but special cases. Suppose that the number of cells loaded into a test capillary (S_0^{MIF}) differs from that used for the control (S_0^0), such that $S_0^{MIF} = (1 + \delta)S_0^0$. We find by a trivial extension of the arguments which lead to Eq. (35) that the apparent inhibition would be given by the following: (a) if $\delta > 0$

$$I_\infty = \begin{cases} 1 - \dfrac{T_1\left\{2 - R_M T_1 \Delta\left[\frac{3}{2} - \ell n(R_M T_1)\right]\right\}}{T_0\left\{2 - R_0 T_0 \Delta\left[\frac{3}{2} - \ell n(R_0 T_0)\right]\right\}} & \text{if } T_1 < R_M^{-1},\ T_0 < R_0^{-1} \quad (38a) \\ 1 - \dfrac{T_1\{4 - R_M T_1 \Delta[3 - 2\ell n(R_M T_1)]\}}{4(1 - \Delta)T_0 + R_0^{-1}\Delta} & \text{if } T_1 < R_M^{-1},\ R_0^{-1} < T_0 \quad (38b) \\ 1 - \dfrac{4T_1(1 - \Delta) + R_M^{-1}\Delta}{4T_0(1 - \Delta) + R_M^{-1}\Delta} & \text{if } R_M^{-1} < T_1,\ R_0^{-1} < T_0 \quad (38c) \end{cases}$$

where R_M and R_0 pertain to the test and control capillaries, respectively, (b) If $\delta < 0$, the expressions given by Eqs. (38a) and (38c) still apply but, instead of Eq. (38b), we have

$$I_\infty = 1 - \frac{4(1 - \Delta)T_1 + R_M^{-1}\Delta}{T_0\{4 - R_M T_0 \Delta[3 - \ell n(R_0 T_0)]\}} \qquad \text{if } R_M^{-1} < T_1,\ T_0 < R_0^{-1} \quad (39)$$

When antigen is absent we have $T_1 = T_0$, and the conditions given in Eqs. (38b) and (39) need to be replaced by $R_0^{-1} < T_0 < R_M^{-1}$ and $R_M^{-1} < T_0 < R_0^{-1}$, respectively. Slight variations of Eqs. (38) and (39) pertain, also, when the cell load is constant (i.e., $R_0 = R_M$) but culture conditions differ, in which case T_1 is computed with a value of χ which differs from that used to compute T_0.

B. Effects of Variations in Cell Titer

The cell titer S_0 is one of the parameters which is most difficult to control in the capillary assay. In this respect two types of variability need to be considered. First, all capillaries might be filled with precisely the same number of cells, but the number could differ from that used on some other occasion. Second, S_0 might vary among the capillaries of a specific test series due to technical inaccuracies introduced during their preparation.

In Fig. 3 we show computed values of I_∞ when S_0 is changed equally for control and test capillaries. These computations, based on Eq. (35) and its equivalents, indicate that a uniform variation in the cell load is likely to change assay results in a significant manner only when very large changes in cell titer are affected. Thus, little advantage is gained by trying to adjust the cell titer in order to optimize assay results. In order to conserve assay material, one should use as few cells as possible for loading the capillaries, that is, the minimum number necessary for accurate determinations of the migration areas.

Variation of cell concentrations among capillaries within a given assay set are somewhat more significant. In Fig. 4 we see the errors which might arise in this instance. The abscissa is the relative change in S_0 as compared with the control titer, and the ordinate shows the apparent migration inhibition. We note, however, that irregularities in S_0 are attenuated by the assay. For example, a 20% error in loading leads to a deviation in I_∞ of only 0.04 (see curve 4c).

C. Variations in Rate Constants

The results portrayed in Figs. 3 and 4 are direct manifestations of changes in cell concentration, deriving from the concentration dependence of the mobility coefficients. However, variations in cell concentration also may affect I_∞ *indirectly* since a larger number of cells will deplete metabolites more rapidly and produce higher levels of toxins. When this happens, rate constants pertaining to the culture medium are affected, with consequent change in the determined rate of migration inhibition index.

In Fig. 5 we show that marked error in I_∞ can result if the rate constant for a test capillary differs from that for a control. The apparent variations in this case are easily large enough to explain the 15% variability about zero migration inhibition often discerned among the results for "normal" controls in MIF assay

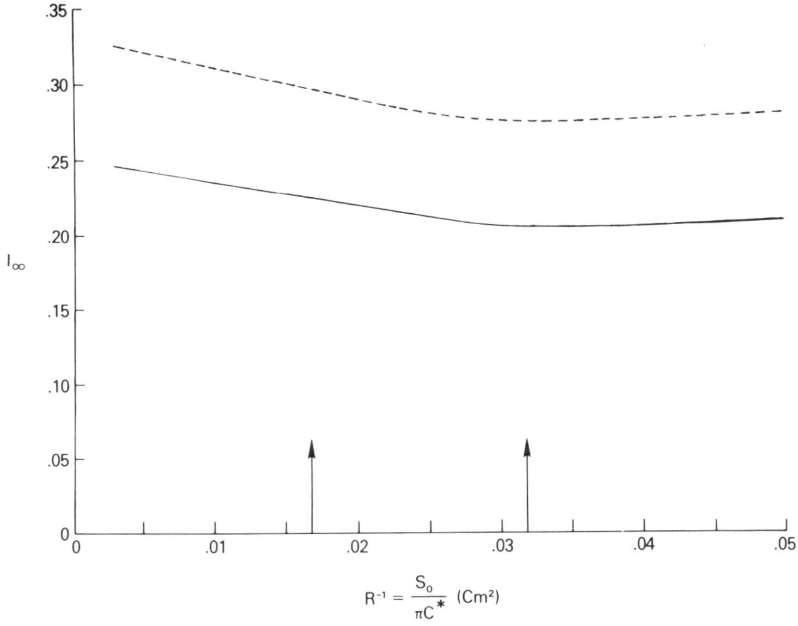

FIG. 3. Effects of cell concentration on migration index: I_∞ vs. $R^{-1} = S_0/\pi C^*$, calculated from Eqs. (35) to (39) for standard parameter values ($\alpha = 0.25$, $\Delta = 0.5$, $4\mu_\infty\chi^{-1} = 0.03\ \text{cm}^2$, $\xi\chi^{-1} = 1.5$). The dotted curve pertains to an intrinsic biological response $I_0 \equiv k[M_{st}]^\alpha = 0.4$, whereas the solid curve pertains to $I_0 = 0.3$. The two arrows correspond to $R = 30\ \text{cm}^{-2}$ and $R = 60\ \text{cm}^{-2}$, values which are likely to be representative of actual assay conditions (see Fig. 2).

studies (see Fig. 1). On the other hand, the inset to Fig. 5 suggests that I_∞ is insensitive to *uniform* changes in culture conditions. Although migration kinetics depend upon χ (Nossal, 1977), test and control capillaries are essentially equally affected by changes in that parameter, and the differential index I_∞ remains unchanged.

Thus, variation in the protocol for preparing the capillaries can be tolerated if all capillaries within a given test set are treated equally. (For example, it does not matter very much if the preincubation period, i.e., between the harvesting of the cells and their being placed in the capillaries, varies in duration.) However, nonuniformity in handling the cells used for a particular series of

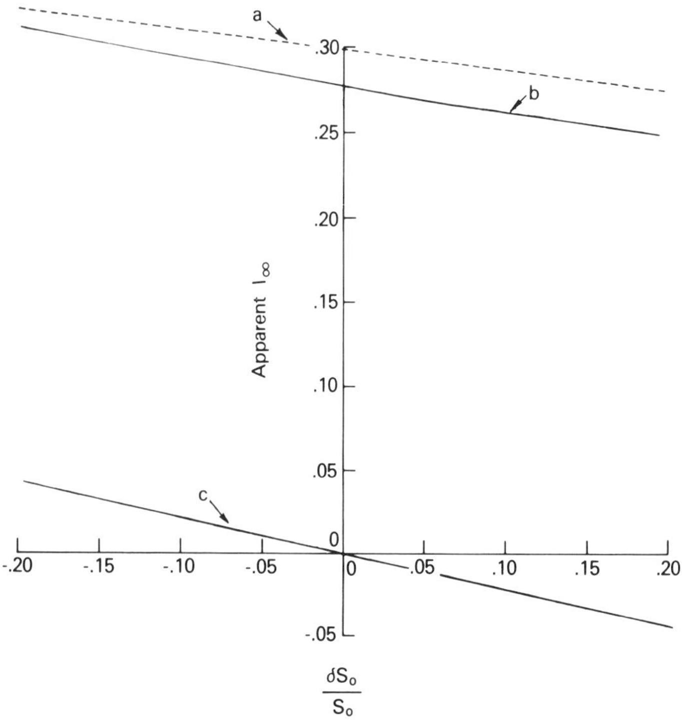

FIG. 4. Influence of variability in cell loading among the capillaries comprising the same assay set: I_∞ vs. $\delta S_0/S_0$, where S_0 is the nominal cell titer, and $\delta S_0/S_0$ is the fractional variation in S_0. (Conditions as in Fig. 3, except: (a) $I_0 = 0.4$, $R = 60\ cm^{-2}$; (b) $I_0 = 0.4$, $R = 30\ cm^2$; and (c) $I_0 = 0$ (no MIF), $R = 30\ cm^{-2}$.)

capillaries can lead to serious difficulties regarding the reproducibility and reliability of the assay. Care should be taken to place the capillaries in the incubation medium immediately after they are centrifuged and cut, and inconstancies in capillary loading due, for example, to the clumping of cells or cutting error, should be minimized.

D. Contaminant Cells

We have seen how various attributes of the MIF assay tend to attenuate the "true" biological response in the sense that they lead to a value of I_∞ which is lower than that which would be measured were simple

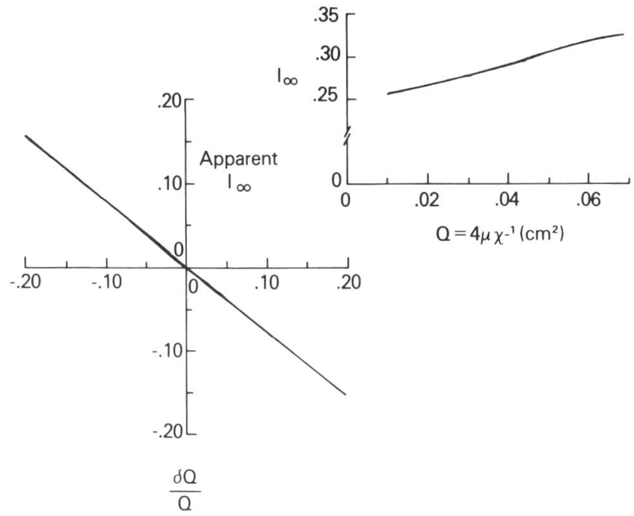

FIG. 5. Apparent migration inhibition index I_∞ vs. fractional variation in the kinetic parameter $Q = 4\mu_\infty\chi^{-1}$. Parameter values are the same as those used for Fig. 4(c). (That is, in this example $I_0 = 0$, so there would be no indication of migration inhibition were the capillaries to be loaded and incubated under identical conditions.) The inset, computed for $I_0 = 0.4$, shows the change in I_∞ when culture conditions vary uniformly for all capillaries including the controls.

linear diffusion to occur. Since the reliability of the assay thus can be improved by strengthening the detected signal, we have examined the pertinence of eliminating extraneous cells which might be present, that is, cells which neither produce MIF nor act as indicators for its presence.

Such contaminant cells, as well as miscellaneous debris, appear in the final cell suspension in uncertain amounts. Leukocytes are harvested by sedimentation from whole blood, followed by alternate centrifugation and resuspension in buffer. Thus, once they have appeared in the initial step, erythrocytes, for example, would be carried along in the various stages of the harvesting procedure. They would be present among the cells which are loaded into the capillaries unless previously subjected to lysis by hypotonic shock, and even then a few would remain.

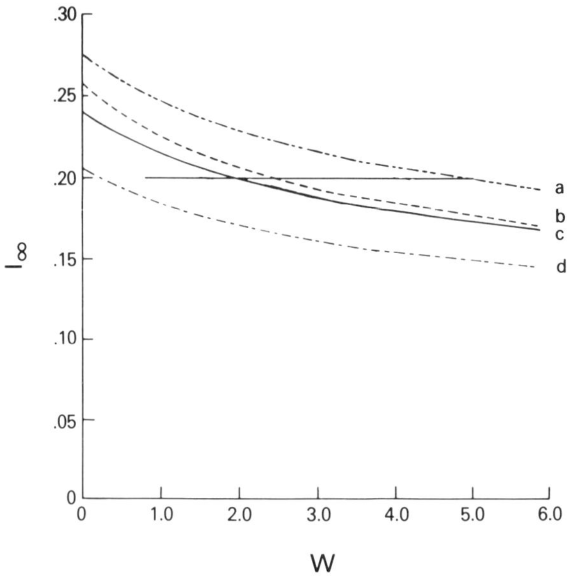

FIG. 6. Effects of extraneous MIF absorption. I_∞ vs. $W = \lambda_A[C_A - C_{A(0)}]/[\lambda_I C_I + \lambda_A C_{A(0)}]$, where $\lambda_A[C_A - C_{A(0)}]$ represents the rate of MIF absorption due to contaminants and $[\lambda_I C_I + \lambda_A C_{A(0)}]$ represents the intrinsic absorption [see Eq. (18)]. Parameter values used here are $R = 30\ cm^{-2}$, $4\mu_\infty\chi^{-1} = 0.03\ cm^2$, $\alpha = 0.25$, $\Delta = 0.5$; and (a) $I_0 = 0.4$, $\xi\chi^{-1} = 1.5$; (b) $I_0 = 0.35$, $\xi\chi^{-1} = 3.0$; (c) $I_0 = 0.35$, $\xi\chi^{-1} = 1.5$; and (d) $I_0 = 0.3$, $\xi\chi^{-1} = 1.5$. The solid line represents a criterion that 20% inhibition be surpassed for a test to be scored as positive (see also discussion related to Fig. 1).

In a related investigation (Nossal, 1977), it was found that MIF absorption by contaminants will significantly alter the outcome of the assay. Those calculations have been repeated now that we include here concentration dependence of mobility which previously was ignored. Results are shown in Fig. 6. The abscissa W is a relative measure of excess absorption, being defined as $W = \lambda_A[C_A - C_{A(0)}]/[\lambda_I C_I + \lambda_A C_{A(0)}]$ [see Eq. (18)]. Here, $C_{A(0)}$ is a reference number of absorbant cells, appropriate to that value of $I_0 \equiv k[M_{st}]^\alpha = k\{bC_E/[\lambda_I C_I + \lambda_A C_{A(0)}]\}^\alpha$ which would pertain if the contaminant cells were eliminated. [In more general terms, the quantity $\lambda_A[C_A - C_{A(0)}]$ represents any contaminant abosrption rate.]

The various curves in Fig. 6 relate to different values of I_0 and also different values of rate constant for MIF absorption (see Fig. 6, legend). It is apparent that absorption due to contaminants in certain instances might cause an intrinsically positive test to be incorrectly scored as negative.

REFERENCES

Bloom, B. R. and Glade, P. R. (1971). *In Vitro Methods in Cell Mediated Immunity.* Academic, New York.

Bull, D. M., Leibach, J. R., Williams, M. A. and Helms, R. A. (1973). Immunity to colon cancer assessed by antigen-induced inhibition of mixed mononuclear cell migration. *Science 181:* 957-959.

Crank, J. (1956). *The Mathematics of Diffusion.* Clarendon, Oxford.

David, J. R. (1973). Lymphocyte mediators and cellular hypersensitivity. *N. Engl. J. Med. 288:* 143-149.

David, J. R., Lawrence, H. S. and Thomas, L. (1964). Delayed hypersensitivity in vitro. II. Effect of sensitive cells on normal cells in the presence of antigen. *J. Immunol. 93:* 274-278.

Dumonde, D. C., Page, D. A., Matthew, M., and Wolstencroft, R. A. (1972). Role of lymphocyte activation products (LAP) in cell mediated immunity: I. Preparation and partial purification of guinea-pig LAP. *Clin. Exp. Immunol. 10:* 25-47.

Dumonde, D. C., Wolstencroft, R. A., Panayi, G. S., Matthew, M., Morley, J., and Howson, W. T. (1969). 'Lymphokines.' Non-antibody mediators of cellular immunity generated by lymphocyte activation. *Nature 224:* 38-42.

Lelchuk, R., Patrucco, A. and Manni, J. A. (1974). Studies of cellular immunity in Chagas disease: Effect of glutaraldehyde-treated specific antigen on inhibition of leukocyte migration. *J. Immunol. 112:* 1578-1581.

Mahieu, P. and Winand, R. (1972). Demonstration of delayed hypersensitivity to retrobulbar and thyroid tissues in human exophthalmos. *J. Clin. Endocrinol. Metab. 34:* 1090-1092.

Morley, J. (1974). Cell migration inhibition: an appraisal. *Acta Allergol. 29:* 185-208.

Munro, R. E., Lamki, L., Row, V. V. and Volpé, R. (1973). Cell-mediated immunity in the exophthalmos of Graves' disease as demonstrated by the migration inhibition factor (MIF) test. *J. Clin. Endocrinol. Metab. 37:* 286-292.

Nossal, R. (1977). Mathematical analysis of a capillary migration assay for cellular immune sensitivity. *J. Theor. Biol. 64:* 703-722

Nossal, R. and Chang, Y. T. (1976). A procedure for determining mobility parameters for cells moving along surfaces. *J. Mechanochem. Cell Mot. 3:* 247-251.

Patten, E., Gallin, J. I., Clark, R. A. and Kimball, H. R. (1973). Effects of cell concentration and various anticoagulants on neutrophil migration. *Blood 41:* 711-719.

Remold, H. G. and David, J. R. (1974). Migration inhibition factor and other mediators in cell-mediated immunity. In *Mechanisms of Cell-Mediated Immunity* (R. T. McCluskey and S. Cohen, eds.) John Wiley and Sons, New York, pp. 25-42.

Rocklin, R. E., Remold, H. G. and David, J. R. (1972). Characterization of human migration inhibition factor (MIF) from antigen-stimulated lymphocytes. *Cell. Immunol. 5:* 436-445.

Zigmond, S. and Hirsch, J. G. (1973). Leukocyte locomotion and chemotaxis. New methods for evaluation and demonstration of a cell-derived chemotactic factor. *J. Exp. Med. 137:* 387-410.

Part IV

INTERACTIONS OF ANTIGEN WITH ANTIBODIES AND CELLS

Chapter 6

LYMPHOCYTE SURFACE IMMUNOGLOBULIN: ITS DISPOSITION ON THE MEMBRANE AND ITS ROLE IN B-LYMPHOCYTE PHYSIOLOGY

Kenneth A. Ault and Emil R. Unanue

Department of Pathology
Harvard Medical School
Boston, Massachusetts

The importance of the surface immunoglobulin of B lymphocytes is discussed with emphasis on its functional role. Some aspects of patching, capping, synthesis of surface immunoglobulin, and its importance in cell motility are presented. The need for more quantitative approaches and for testable models is discussed. Finally, the current state of knowledge about the distribution of surface immunoglobulin on the cell surface is presented, in detail, with speculations about the significance of the distribution and improved experimental approaches expected to be available in the near future.

I. INTRODUCTION

The discovery of a population of lymphocytes that have immunoglobulin (Ig) on their surface opened up a new era in immunology. It also has had widespread implications for cell biology that are only beginning to be explored. This discovery fulfilled a theoretical prediction based on the exquisite specificity exhibited by the immune system. The cells that were ultimately responsible for synthesis of antibody had to be able to recognize the presence of corresponding antigen. The specificity of the cells for the antigen had to be at least as great as that of the antibody they were to produce. The most economical way to accomplish this was for the precursors of antibody secreting cells to have on their surfaces molecules of the same specificity as their antibody secreting progeny. That the molecule is antibody itself has been concluded from a large and ever-increasing body of experimental results. It is our purpose here to recount a small part of this information, which bears on the role of surface immunoglobulin (sIg) in B-lymphocyte physiology. For the immunologist, the central question is how the interaction of antigen with Ig receptors stimulates the lymphocyte to begin proliferation and differentiation leading to antibody production. For the cell biologist, there is the opportunity to study the trigger mechanism for a well-defined series of cellular metabolic changes that may offer insights into the control of cell proliferation and the general mechanisms of differentiation. Biochemists have become interested in the opportunity to study the interaction of a chemically well-defined molecule with the cell membrane and the cytoplasmic control of membrane functions. The biophysicist might make use of the ability to identify a specific molecule in the membrane to study the physical properties of the membrane. In fact, the lymphocyte has become one of the best models for the study of the biology of eukaryotic cells. We will try to discuss some topics which illustrate this, with emphasis on

---

Abbreviations used in this chapter: Fab, antigen combining region of antibody molecules; Ig, immunoglobulin; sIg, surface immunoglobulin.

areas in which the study of lymphocyte sIg lends itself to quantitation, or in which a theoretical approach is needed. It is gratifying to realize that immunology has progressed so rapidly in what is still its relative youth to permit some degree of quantitation and the application of more basic physical sciences which has been rare in biology in general.

Ig was first discovered on the cell surface by noting the effects on lymphocytes of anti-Ig antibody. In tissue culture, lymphocytes from rabbit blood were induced to proliferate by exposure to antiallotypic antibody (Sell and Gell, 1965). This tantalizing observation, which suggested that interaction with the putative antigen receptor was the direct trigger of proliferation, proved not to be a general phenomenon. Indeed, lymphocytes from other sources, such as mouse spleen or human blood, cannot be stimulated to proliferate significantly by anti-Ig alone. The exact reason for the phenomenon in rabbits has not been explained, but it nonetheless showed that there was Ig on the surface and, that at least under some circumstances the sIg could influence interior events.

It is now common to demonstrate sIg more directly by immunofluorescence. When living lymphocytes are reacted with fluorescent anti-Ig antibody, their surface is brightly labeled (Taylor et al., 1971). This method permits easy counting of the Ig-bearing lymphocytes, and gives a general idea of the distribution of the Ig on the cell surface (Fig. 1). The resolution of the fluorescence microscope is limited and this method does not lend itself to quantitation, although some investigators have used instruments to measure the intensity of fluorescence. Nevertheless, the simplicity of the technique, and the graphic demonstration that results, have made it the major method which has been used. The fluorescent method is subject to several errors, including the potential for nonspecific uptake of fluorescent antibody by clumps of cells, dead cells, and phagocytic cells. In addition, the presence of Fc receptors on macrophages, monocytes, and on lymphocytes of both B and T type raises the possibility of binding of the antibody to cells in a nonspecific fashion, especially if it is partially aggregated. It is,

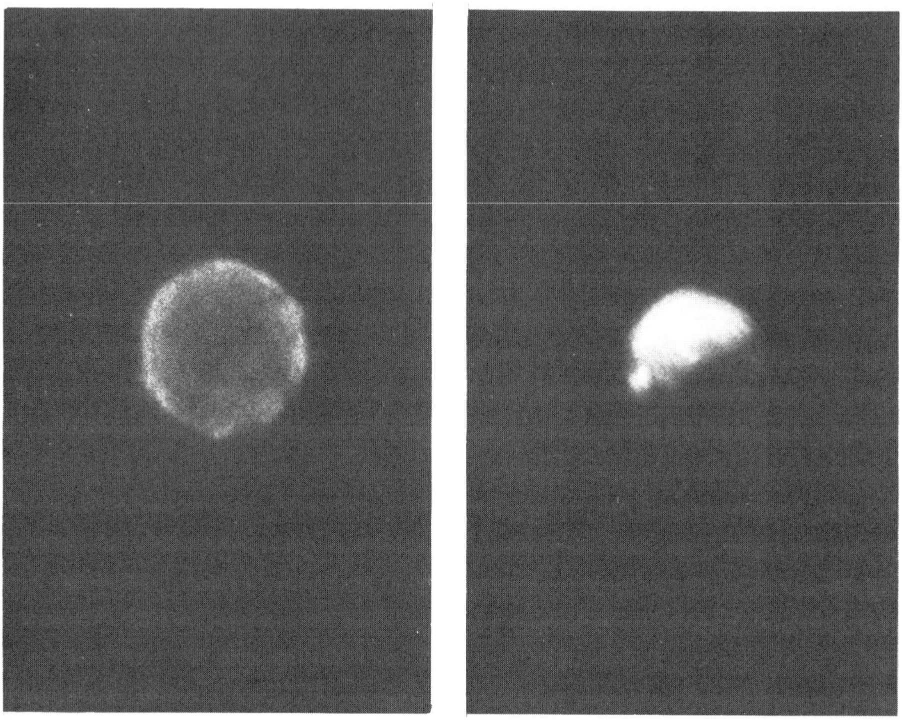

FIG. 1. The lymphocyte on the left has been labeled by fluorescein-coupled anti-Ig antibody and fixed in the cold. The label is diffuse with only the beginning of some patch formation along one edge. The cell on the right has been labeled and then warmed to 37°C. It shows a typical cap. (Reproduced with permission of Academic Press Inc.)

therefore, necessary to demonstrate the specificity of the antibody, not only immunochemically, but also in the actual labeling reaction which is being used. It is also necessary to demonstrate that sufficient amounts of antibody have been used to detect all the sIg present.

The use of anti-Ig antibody coupled to markers that can be detected in the electron microscope makes it possible to extend considerably the resolution with which one can study sIg. The two major types of markers that have been used are the electron-dense marker ferritin which can be seen in the transmission electron

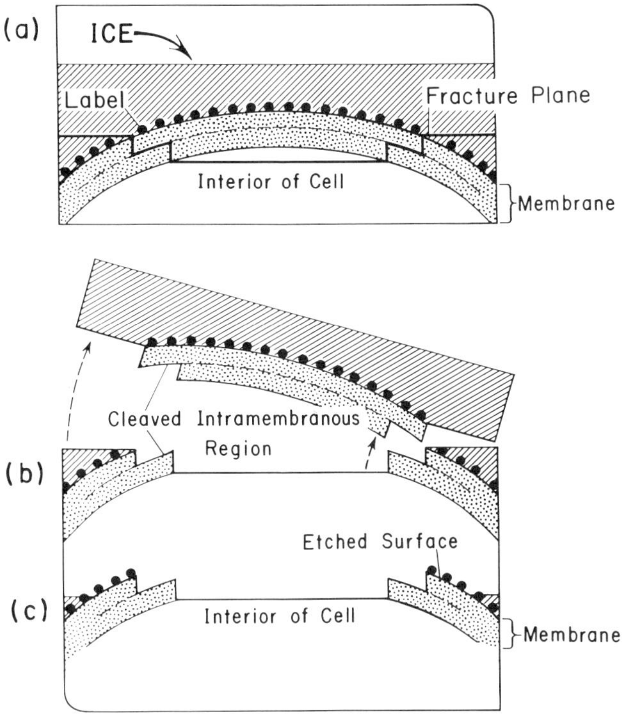

FIG. 2. The method of freeze-etching consists of imbedding the cell in ice (a) and then fracturing the cell, revealing part of the interior of the membrane and the interior of the cell (b). After subliming away part of the ice (c), the exterior surface of the cell can be identified and a carbon-platinum replica made for examination in the electron microscope. (Reproduced with permission of Academic Press Inc.)

microscope and allows a one-dimensional visualization of the membrane in thin sections (DePetris and Raff, 1973), or markers which have a distinctive shape, such as ferritin, hemocyanin, or viruses, to allow visualization by making replicas of the cell surface. These can be examined in the transmission electron microscope and allow two-dimensional mapping of the surface. Figure 2 demonstrates the freeze-etch method of making surface replicas that has been used to make maps of surface Ig. As yet the scanning electron microscope has not been used extensively to study sIg because of the lack of adequate resolution. However, technical improvements will soon make this an important method. Since most lymphocyte populations available consist of mixtures of different types of lymphocytes (B and T cells plus subclasses of T and perhaps B cells and a variable number of non lymphocytes), the electron microscope methods, in general, suffer from a sampling problem. It is important to demonstrate that the relatively few cells examined in the electron microscope are representative of the population under discussion. In the case of the freeze-etch techniques, only a small part of the cell surface is available for examination, and this, too, may not be representative, since we are aware of marked inhomogeneities in the distribution of sIg under some circumstances.

Several elegant biochemical methods have been devised to study sIg. These include selective radiolabeling of surface proteins, followed by dissolution of the membrane and isolation of the sIg by immunoprecipitation and electrophoresis (Vitetta and Uhr, 1973). Similar isolation and analysis techniques can be applied to cellular Ig that has been labeled by incorporation of radiolabeled amino acids or sugars (Melchers and Andersson, 1973). These studies have led to information on the molecular form of sIg (predominantly monomeric IgM and perhaps IgD) and to its rate of synthesis, rate of loss from the membrane, variations in turnover during activation of the lymphocytes, etc. These techniques are limited by the difficulty of obtaining a high degree of specificity in immunoprecipitation reactions and by the necessity of using homogeneous populations of cells which are very difficult to obtain. Nevertheless, it seems certain that biochemical approaches will lead to better understanding of the molecular mechanisms that control the synthesis of sIg and the mechanisms of activation. Questions that might be answered in this way are: What molecules support or anchor the sIg molecules in the membrane, and by what molecular mechanisms does sIg communicate with the cell interior? We now have strong evidence that sIg is connected to other cellular elements under some conditions, but as yet no biochemical information about these connections has been obtained.

A composite picture revealed by these techniques is that the resting B lymphocyte has about 10^5 molecules of Ig diffusely distributed over its surface. This Ig is turning over with a half-time of 20 to 80 hr, with a significant amount being shed off into the environment. On any particular B lymphocyte, the sIg is all of the same light chain class, it all has the same combining sites for antigen, and it represents the major antigen-specific trigger system of the cell. It is a sample of the antibody that the progeny of the B cell will produce as plasma cells. One intriguing recent discovery is that in the human, most B lymphocytes display both IgM and IgD on their surface. In the mouse, a second heavy chain, distinct from that of IgM, has also been described on the B-cell surface. The proportion of lymphocytes bearing IgD in the human is much greater than the relative amount of IgD found in serum. Thus, it seems that IgD may play a special role as a membrane molecule of as yet unknown function. It has been demonstrated that on cells having both IgM and IgD. these Igs have the same antibody specificity (Stern and McConnell, 1976) and the same idiotype (Fu et al., 1975). Current speculation centers on the possibility that these two molecules may both serve as antigen receptor but represent different stages of B-lymphocyte differentiation (Vitetta and Uhr, 1975), or that they may communicate different messages to the cell. There is as yet not enough evidence to decide. We would now like to describe the events that take place when these antigen receptor sIg molecules are bound by anti-Ig antibody or by antigen.

II. PATCHING

If great effort is made to minimize the disturbing effects of the methods used to study sIg, it can be shown that sIg is present diffusely over the cell surface (see below). However, if antibody is bound which can interconnect the sIg, or if multivalent antigens are bound, there is a very prompt change in the distribution of the sIg. This can be seen in both the fluorescent and the electron microscope as the formation of many small micropatches (Fig. 1).

This "patching" phenomenon has been fairly well studied and has proven to be very difficult to prevent. It is absolutely dependent on the ability of the ligand to cross-link sIg molecules. It takes place more slowly at low temperatures but can be seen even when the cells are held on ice. It is not possible to prevent patching by depriving the cell of metabolic energy (Loor et al., 1972; Unanue and Karnovsky, 1973). The most likely explanation for patching is that it is the thermodynamic result of forming bonds between sIg molecules that are able to diffuse in the plane of the membrane. It can be considered the two-dimensional analogy of precipitation from a liquid. Because patching may be a relatively simple physical phenomenon, it lends itself to further study. For example, the temperature dependence of the rate of patching should yield information on the diffusivity of sIg in the membrane and the energy required to cross-link sIg molecules. A study of the steady-state outcome of prolonged patching could yield information on the restrictions to free diffusion which may be imposed by the membrane and he rates of competing processes. Unfortunately, these studies remain largely undone, primarily because of the difficulty of quantitating patching as a function of time and because, under most experimental conditions, patching is but a prelude to much more dramatic and forceful changes in the cell membrane. Some observations that have been made include the demonstration of patching in ethylene glycol solutions at 4°C but not at -7°C (Raff and DePetris, 1973) and inhibition of patching by very high concentrations (0.5 M) of D-mannose and D-galactose (Loor et al., 1972). The conclusion of these latter investigators was that such inhibition was due to increased viscosity of the membrane, but this has not been shown directly.

There have been many estimates made of the apparent viscosity of both natural cell membrane and artificial lipid bilayers using electron spin magnetic resonance methods and fluorescence (Edidin, 1974). These estimates are complicated by the difficulty in determining the relative contribution of the viscosity of the extracellular medium and the submembrane cytoplasm. Similar methods have been used to estimate diffusion constants for proteins in membranes (Edidin et al., 1976).

It seems that the patching phenomenon of lymphocytes would be an ideal situation for studying the diffusion of sIg if it could be better quantitated. The structure of sIg is known, and good estimates of the degree to which it protrudes from the membrane into the extracellular fluid could be made. The energy of interaction of anti-Ig antibody and the span over which it cross-links is known, and the possibility of detailed mapping of single sIg sites on the membrane exists. Thus it would be entirely within the realm of possibility to study the rate of aggregation of sIg as a function of temperature under the influence of a known amount of cross-linking antibody. Comparison of the observed sIg distribution with statistical models of the patching phenomenon could be very helpful. The major difficulty would be the possibility that sIg is associated with another as yet unknown molecule in the membrane. The evidence for this is that sIg behaves like an intrinsic membrane protein during attempts to isolate it by detergent dissolution of the membrane (Melchers et al., 1975), but it has been demonstrated that only a very small part of the sIg molecule is buried in the membrane (Fu and Kunkel, 1974). The only way for a molecule to be almost fully exposed on the surface and yet behave as if it had a large hydrophobic component in the membrane, would be for it to be attached to another largely lipid-soluble molecule, but this has not yet been shown to be the case.

III. CAPPING

If sIg is bound by antibody or antigen and the cell is observed at physiological temperatures, the early patching of sIg is rapidly replaced by a coordinated mass movement of all the sIg to one pole of the cell (see Fig. 1). The result is a crescent-shaped distribution which has been called a "cap" (Taylor et al., 1971). Capping is a dramatic process that can be distinguished from patching in several ways. It also requires a cross-linking or multivalent ligand. It is not seen when the cells are held near ice temperatures but proceeds at room temperature and takes only a few minutes at 37°C. Capping is much more strongly inhibited by low temperature than is patching. This suggests that interference with energy production by lowered temperature is more important than changes in membrane viscosity.

Although capping is more easily quantitated than patching (e.g., by estimating the fraction of the circumference of the cell that is occupied by the cap), there have been very few attempts to correlate the rate of capping with temperature or other parameters (Lewis et al., 1974). There is some evidence that capping proceeds at different rates in different species and even in different mouse strains (Fram et al., 1976).

The best current estimates of the diffusion constant for movement of protein in the membrane are about 10^{-9} to 10^{-10} cm^2/sec (Edidin et al., 1976). We have estimated that if capping were to be explained on the basis of diffusion and cross-linking of sIg (i.e., if it were a special case of patching), the diffusion constant would have to be on the order of 10^{-7} to 10^{-8} cm^2/sec.

Capping requires energy and thus is prevented by metabolic inhibitors. It requires a certain threshold amount of sIg cross-linking. For example, at very low doses of anti-Ig antibody, it is possible to observe patching but not capping. Some polymeric antigens produce much more dramatic capping than others (Ault and Unanue, 1974). Finally, capping seems to be a specialized cell function, for although it has been described in many cell types with many different cell surface markers, it takes place with much greater ease for some than for others. Recent evidence indicates that capping is under cytoplasmic control (Schreiner and Unanue, 1976).

Capping has been described with other membrane elements such as protein antigens, carbohydrate lectin binding sites, and even lipids. However, it is important to make clear the conceptual difference between one possible outcome of patching, namely, the formation of a single large aggregate at one point on the cell surface, and the organized and progressive movement which is typical of sIg capping. The speed and uniformity of sIg capping make it virtually unique. It seems quite likely that, although one or more caps can be produced on a cell by extensive cross-linking of almost any membrane element, the capping seen with sIg is controlled and facilitated by cellular mechanisms for an as yet unidentified reason. Evidence to support this includes the fact that the sIg cap always forms over the region of the cell occupied by the Golgi apparatus, whereas other types of caps do not seem to be so specific in their location (Stackpole et al., 1974). The formation of the sIg cap occurs independently of any locomotion of the cell (Unanue et al., 1974), whereas some other types of caps seem to form only after the cell has begun to move and thus may be secondary to the cell motion (Unanue and Karnovsky, 1974). Finally, there is accumulating evidence that the formation of the cap is under cytoplasmic control, in that it can be modified by altering the distribution of calcium ions in the cell, and by drugs which affect the state of contractile elements such as microfilaments (Schreiner and Unanue, 1976). Most dramatic is the observation that the fully formed cap can be disrupted by a drug (ionophore) which admits calcium to the cell, and by membrane-active agents that act as local anesthetics. The disruption by Ca^{2+} influx requires energy, and thus seems to demonstrate that there are active contractile elements in the cell which dictate the formation, the location, and perhaps the subsequent fate of the cap. Disruption of the cap by local anesthetics seems to take place even in the presence of metabolic inhibitors (Schreiner and Unanue, 1976). If this is the case, it may be possible to conclude that energy deprivation stops capping by interfering with the active movement of sIg, rather than by producing a secondary change in the membrane such as increased viscosity which prevents sIg movement. It seems likely that a better understanding of physical properties of the cell membrane will result from careful study of the kinetics of capping and the role of various membrane-active agents.

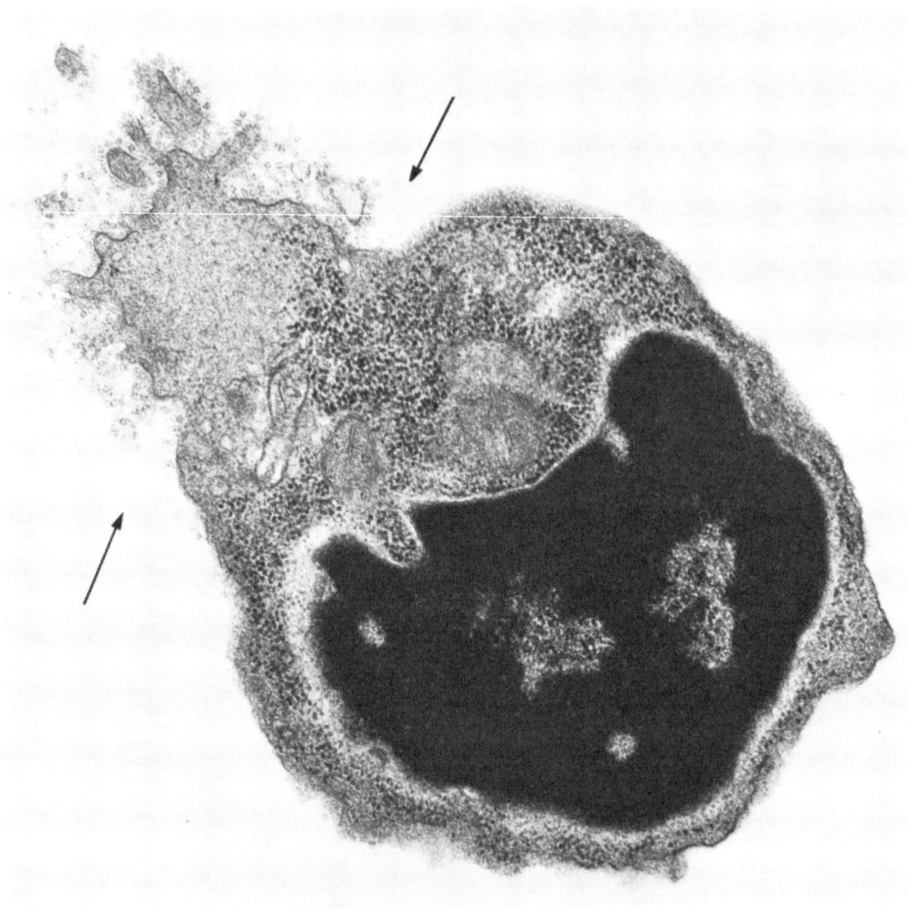

FIG. 3. A lymphocyte that has been labeled with anti-Ig coupled to hemocyanin, a large square molecule, is shown in the motile form. On the uropod there are many folds of membrane and the hemocyanin molecules attached to the surface show the location of the cap. Note the apparent zone of constriction at the base of the uropod (arrows). (Reproduced with permission of Academic Press Inc.)

Extensive interactions between capping molecules and drugs that affect microtubules and microfilaments have been described (Edelman et al., 1973). For example, the lectin concanavalin A binds to the cell and in some conditions prevents subsequent capping of sIg by anti-Ig antibody. This inhibition can be reversed by colchicine and the effects of colchicine can be prevented by cytochalasin B (Unanue and Karnovsky, 1974). Colchicine is known to cause depolymerization of microtubules, and cytochalasin B is thought to interfere with microfilaments and, therefore, presumably contractile mechanisms in the cell. Unfortunately, this type of reasoning is all indirect and depends upon unproven assumptions about the intracellular effects of the drugs. Possible secondary effects on the cell, such as on metabolism or cell motility, are difficult to take into account.

Examination of the surface in the region of the forming cap with the electron microscope seems to show streaming of labeled Ig sites into the cap. It is possible that a detailed analysis of the time course of formation of these apparent lines of flow could reveal something of the underlying mechanism. It is now known that the static distribution of Ig sites is not random (Abbas et al., 1975). Virtually nothing is known of the dynamic changes in distribution that occur after ligand binding, except on the relatively large scale that we have just described.

Electron microscopy of the cap region shows that the membrane is thrown up in exaggerated folds (Fig. 3). This may be related to the capping itself, or it may be more closely related to the phenomenon of cell locomotion described below. In any case it certainly suggests the intimate involvement of sub-membrane contractile elements.

IV. LOSS AND REPLACEMENT OF SURFACE IMMUNOGLOBULIN

Subsequent to patching and concomitant with capping, the lymphocyte is endocytosing large amounts of cap material (complexes of sIg and ligand). Much of this endocytosed material is degraded, some appears in the environment as large complexes (Engers and Unanue, 1973). After a period on the order of an hour, if the amount of ligand was sufficient to involve all of the sIg, the cell surface is virtually free of both sIg and ligand. At this stage, the cell is unable to bind antigen until new sIg is synthesized and placed into the membrane

(Ault and Unanue, 1974). This process begins to be detectable at about 6 hr and is usually complete by 24 hr. This period is not well understood but may be crucial for immunity and tolerance. There is no evidence that the number, the type, or the specificity of the new receptors has changed. Direct observation of antigen-binding cells does not show an obvious increase in the amount of antigen bound, and the amount of sIg does not change detectably . We know, however, that the cell has been at least temporarily changed by its cycle of receptor clearance. It seems to have decreased in density as judged by equilibrium centrifugation, and perhaps to have increased its rate of protein synthesis (Ault, unpublished observations). The cell also shows a prolonged (at least 48 hr) unresponsiveness to mitogen stimulation which persists well beyond the time required to replace its sIg (Sidman and Unanue, 1976). However, it has not been triggered to proliferate or differentiate. The binding of anti-Ig antibody or of most antigens (the exceptions being the T-independent antigens that seem to possess the intrinsic ability to activate the B cell directly) is not sufficient to trigger the B cell. Nevertheless, some crucial signal has been given which is necessary but not sufficient for the immune response. There is a large body of evidence that indicates that some aspects of the receptor-ligand interaction may affect the subsequent immune response. For example, there are several systems in which the degree of polymerization of the antigen profoundly changes its effect on the B cell (Diener and Feldmann, 1972; Miranda et al., 1972). These systems seem to be largely T-cell independent. Thus, although the low molecular weight forms of the antigen are fully capable of interacting with sIg, they may produce less cross-linking, perhaps less patching, or less complete capping, and thus change the outcome of the interaction. As yet, no simple interpretation seems possible because the effects of molecular size and antigen dose are different for different antigens, but it seems likely that a more quantitative understanding of the effects of different degrees of sIg cross-linking on membrane behavior will allow a unified interpretation.

V. STIMULATED MOVEMENT

In addition to the obvious importance of sIg in the initiation of the immune response, an additional role for it in B-lymphocyte physiology has recently been explored. As implied above, sIg is intimately involved in the control of lymphocyte movement. The fact that lymphocytes appear in large numbers at sites of inflammation, and the apparent necessity for multicellular interaction with antigens, implies that lymphocytes must be motile cells under some conditions. The appropriate B lymphocyte must be present with its antigen and whatever other cells (T cells and macrophages) are necessary for the immune response to begin. This multicellular interaction probably requires the cells to be in close proximity, perhaps in actual contact.

It has long been known that moving lymphocytes display a distinctive shape known as uropod formation (Fig. 3). It has now been shown that the majority of splenic lymphocytes which spontaneously display this shape are T cells and that B cells are stimulated to change their shape by the interaction of ligand with sIg (Unanue et al., 1974). This change of shape has been correlated with random translational movement that is triggered by the interaction with sIg, that continues for a period of several minutes, and then ceases before the complete cycle of receptor clearance has finished. It is known that the triggering of movement involves the activation of a serine esterase, that it requires intact contractile mechanisms in the cell, that it is inhibited by cytochalasins, and that it is modulated by the level of Ca^{2+} in the cell and by cyclic nucleotides (Schreiner and Unanue, 1976). It thus has much in common with other cell functions that are under the control of surface interactions. It is quite possible that the stimulation of movement is an integral part of the beginning of the immune response. In any case, it is a clearly definable consequence of the interaction with sIg and may prove to be a part of an entire sequence of discrete events that together constitute the triggering of the B cell.

It has not yet been possible to clearly demonstrate directed chemotaxis in response to a gradient of antigen or anti-Ig antibody. Nevertheless, the circumstantial evidence is strong that such chemotaxis must exist. If chemotaxis can be demonstrated, there will be a tremendous opportunity to study the way in which well-defined interactions at the surface with a known receptor molecule guide cell motion.

VI. MAPPING OF SURFACE IMMUNOGLOBULIN

Having mentioned several times that it is possible to make detailed maps of the position of sIg molecules on the membrane, we would like to discuss in some detail how this is done and what information is available from such maps. As shown in Fig. 2, the freeze-etching technique makes it possible to produce replicas of part of the surface of cells. If these surfaces are labeled with a marker of sufficient size and of distinctive shape, the marker can be seen and a map made. The major difficulties are those of applying the marker without disturbing the position of the molecules to be marked and of overcoming the sampling problem that arises because only a small part of the surface of relatively few cells can be examined.

We, in association with Abbas and Karnovsky, have reported a technique that at least begins to solve these problems satisfactorily (Abbas et al., 1975). It makes use of a two-layer or "sandwich" labeling method. The sIg is first labeled by a monovalent (Fab fragment) anti-Ig antibody that has been conjugated with fluorescein. This has the advantage of being non-cross-linking. Fab fragments can be shown not to produce patching of sIg, and thus it can be assumed that the original distribution is not disturbed by this label. In addition, this label is fluorescent, which allows confirmation of the fraction of cells which are labeled in a population for comparison with the fraction of labeled cells seen in subsequent electron microscope examination. It is also possible to obtain molecules of fluoresceinated Fab anti-Ig that have, on the average, only one fluorescein molecule per Fab molecule. This is done on an ion exchange column, taking advantage of the alteration of the charge of the Fab molecule by the binding of fluorescein to ε-amino groups of lysine.

The second part of the labeling involves the use of a ferritin-conjugated Fab fragment of an antifluorescein antibody. This marker binds to the fluorescein as a hapten. It has the advantage that the ferritin is visible both in thin section as an electron-dense marker and in the freeze-etch replica method because of its size (120 Å). It, too, is not cross-linking and can be prepared with an average molecular ratio of ferritin to Fab of about one or less. Thus, the second layer of the sandwich reveals the position of the sIg on the membrane in the electron microscope. Thin sections can be examined for the fraction of cells labeled and the saturation of sIg sites can be confirmed by grain counts. Freeze-etch replicas can be photographed and enlarged and then copied to make maps of sIg prepared under various conditions. Figure 4 shows a photograph of such a freeze-etch replica and Fig. 5, a map drawn from an enlargement of such a photograph.

The major difficulty with this mapping technique is the possibility of having several anti-Ig Fab molecules binding to one sIg site. Although the one-to-one ratio of ferritin to antifluorescein and of fluorescein to anti-Ig help to insure that this error will not be amplified, there is nevertheless the possibility that a small cluster of ferritin molecules will represent one sIg molecule. Steric considerations make it unlikely that this will take place to a very great extent.

The fact that this technique does not significantly alter the distribution of sIg has been demonstrated by labeling the cells in the cold (0°C), fixing them, and then showing that the resulting distribution is indistinguishable from that obtained at 20°C, where the sIg is much more likely to redistribute if it were being significantly cross-linked.

The existence of such maps of sIg, and the ease with which the method can be generalized to other surface molecules (it is much easier to make fluorescein conjugates of antibodies than to make

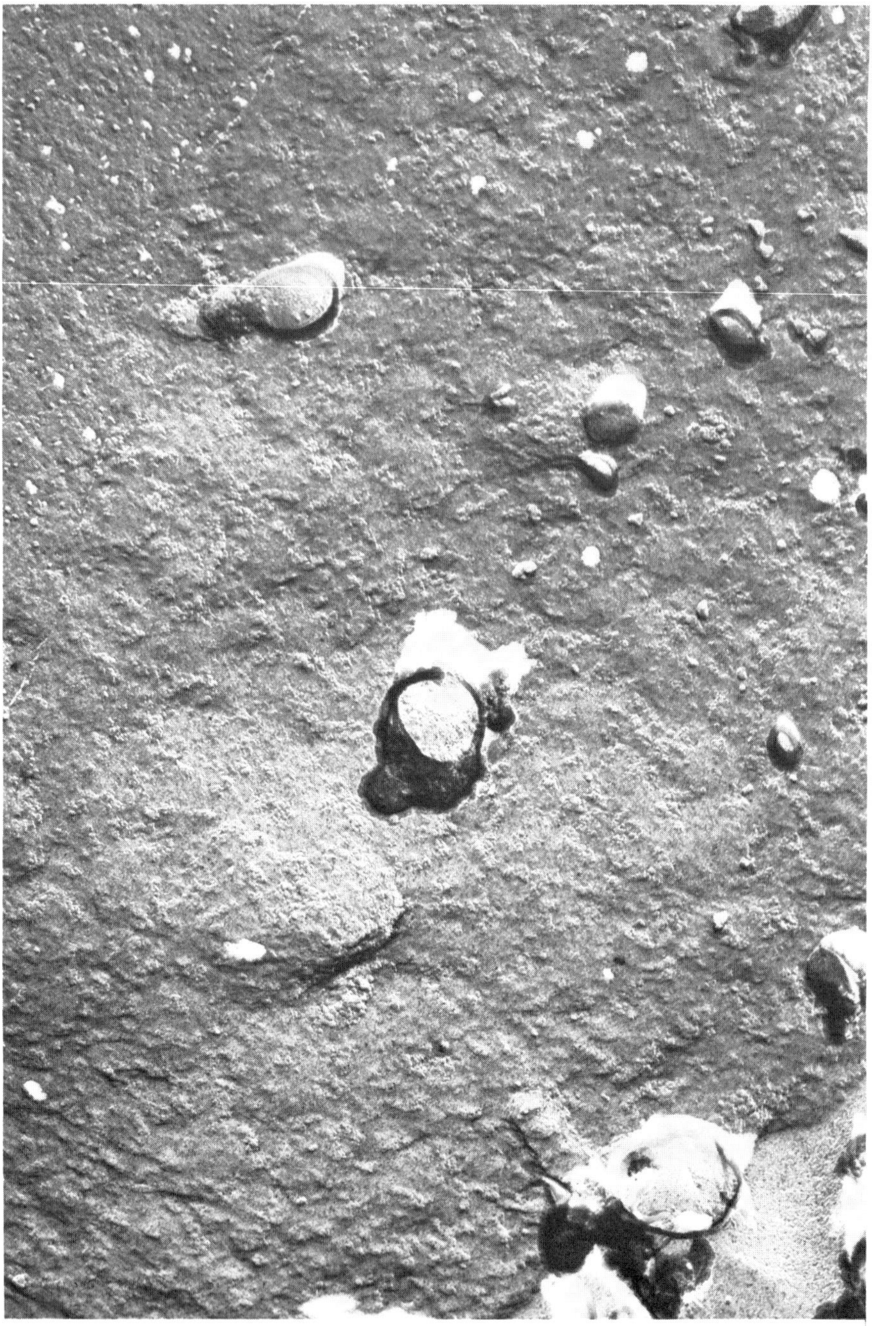

FIG. 4. A freeze-etch replica showing ferritin-labeled anti-Ig on the surface of a lymphocyte. The ferritin molecules are small nodules in clusters and chains. The defects in the surface are due to ice crystal artifacts. (Reproduced with permission of Academic Press Inc. and Williams and Wilkins Co.)

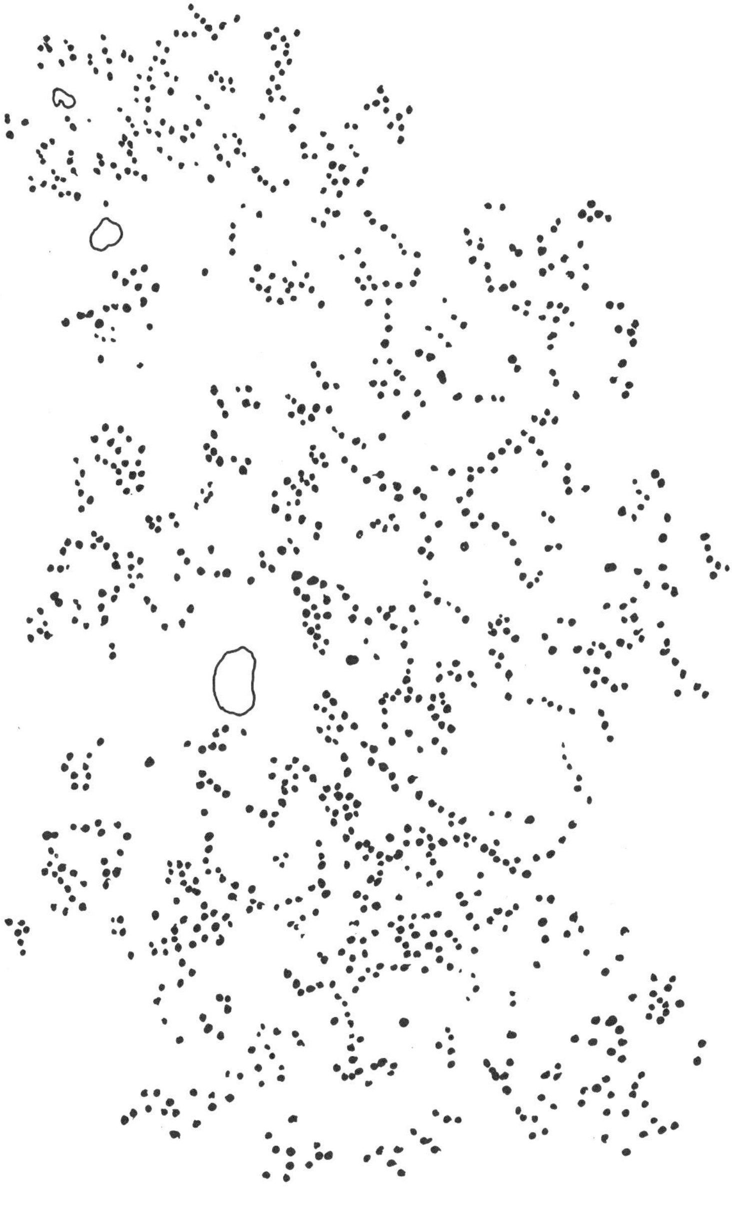

FIG. 5. A map made by tracing an enlargement of a replica such as the one in Fig. 4. (Reproduced with permission of Academic Press Inc. and Williams and Wilkins Co.)

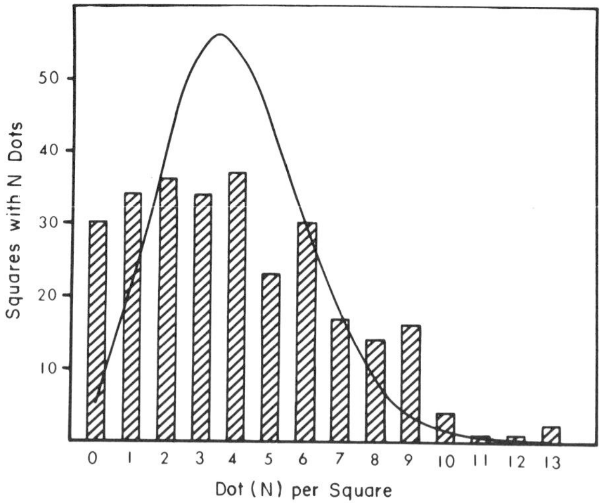

FIG. 6. The vertical bars represent the results of an analysis of a surface map obtained by counting dots in each box of a rectangular grid placed over the map. The smooth line is the Poisson distribution of a random array of dots of the same average density. The differences are statistically significant using a chi-square test. (Reproduced with permission of Williams and Wilkins co.)

ferritin conjugates directly), should present a new opportunity for statistical analysis of the disposition of molecules on the cell surface. We have succeeded in demonstrating that sIg is not randomly distributed in the undisturbed state and that its distribution deviates in the direction of a tendency to clump into small regions of increased density with intervening areas of "bare" membrane. This was done by comparing the observed distributions with the expected (Poisson) distribution for the random placement of sites on a surface (Fig. 6). In 19 out of 20 maps made from 19 different cells, the observed distribution was significantly nonrandom by the chi-square test, and in every case the variance was greater than the mean, indicating a tendency toward clumping. In collaboration with Perelson of the Los Alamos Scientific Laboratory more sophisticated tests are being applied to these maps (Perelson, Chap. 7).

The greatest use will be made of these techniques when it is possible to test hypotheses about membrane organization by comparing theoretical to observed distributions. For example, one might have predicted on theoretical grounds that antigen receptor sites should be grouped in order to facilitate interaction with multivalent antigens. The avidity of cells for antigen is much greater than the affinity of soluble antibody for the same antigen (Bystryn et al., 1973). This is due to the multipoint cooperative interaction of antigen with receptors on the cell surface (Davie and Paul, 1972; DeLisi, Chap. 8; Perelson, Chap. 7). The majority of naturally occurring antigens are polymeric (consider, for example, virus and bacterial surfaces). Thus, it seems reasonable to predict that cells responsible for recognizing small amounts of antigen would have developed a method of grouping individual receptors for maximum binding efficiency to the antigen. We do not yet know how this is accomplished, but it is possible to construct hypotheses that would predict some type of sIg distribution and then compare it to the observed distribution. All such comparisons will have to be statistical because there certainly are stochastic processes superimposed on whatever structure exists in the membrane. For example, we know that sIg probably interacts with linear structures such as microfilaments or microtubules. It is possible that sIg is actually located at random intervals along linear structures which are themselves arranged in some as yet unknown way beneath the membrane. Such speculations could be used to construct models for comparison with surface maps.

Another area of application for mapping techniques is in examining dynamic changes in sIg, for example after patching or during the early stages of capping. Such maps may reveal a great deal of the structure of the membrane and permit more complex theories to be tested. Similarly, the effects of drugs on distributions at the molecular level could be very helpful in understanding membrane organization.

If we were to speculate about the ideal technique for studying the cell surface, it might be one which would take into account the curving and folding of the surface, as freeze-etch replicas do not.

It might also be one which would visualize the membrane in three dimensions rather than two. Such a technique does not seem to be too far from reality. The scanning electron microscope certainly allows us to see the folding of the surface and the scanning beam could be used to probe beneath the surface to submembrane components. Slightly better resolution is required to permit use of molecular markers which do not obscure the surface map and the development of internal markers to reveal structures inside the cell. The use of backscatter techniques have already permitted visualization of tubules, vesicles, and nuclei in cells with the scanning electron microscope (Becker and DeBruyn, 1976). If there were heavy metal markers specific for microfilaments or microtubules, and if backscatter methods were combined with surface mapping in the scanning electron microscope, we might be able to visualize directly the relation of sIg to submembrane structures.

Such a marriage of techniques seems quite possible. What will be needed is a theoretical framework that will allow predictions to be made and tested. As biology probes deeper into the structure of life, it will no longer be possible to rely on simple observation. To be able to *see* complex structures does not always allow one to understand them. It will be necessary to construct theories, make models, and compare them with what we see in order to fully understand how patterns are produced and how dynamic changes take place.

ACKNOWLEDGMENTS

We are grateful to all of our colleagues who have shared in the work and the ideas discussed herein, especially to Professor M. J. Karnovsky for his excellent electron microscopy and for many of the figures reproduced here. Some of this work was supported by National Institute of Health Grant number AI10091 and by National Cancer Institute Grant number 14723.

REFERENCES

Abbas, A. K., Ault, K. A., Karnovksy M. J., and Unanue, E. R. (1975). Nonrandom distribution of surface immunoglobulin on murine B lymphocytes. *J. Immunol. 114:* 1197-1204.

Ault, K. A. and Unanue, E. R. (1974). Events after the binding of antigen to lymphocytes: removal and regeneration of the antigen receptor. *J. Exp. Med. 139:* 1110-1124.

Becker, R. P. and DeBruyn, P. P. H. (1976). Backscattered electron imaging of endogenous and exogenous peroxidase activity in rat bone marrow. In *Scanning Electron Microscopy* (O. Johari and R. P. Becker, eds.). Illinois Institute of Technology Research Institute, pp. 171-178.

Brystryn, J. C., Siskind, G. W., and Uhr, J. W. (1973). Binding of antigen by immunocytes I. Effect of ligand valences on binding affinity of MOPC315 cells for DNP conjugates. *J. Exp. Med. 137:* 301-316.

Davie, J. M. and Paul, W. E. (1972). Reception on immunocompetent cells. IV. Direct measurement of cell receptors and cooperative binding of multivalent ligands. *J. Exp. Med. 135:* 643-659.

de Petris, S. and Raff, M. C. (1973). Normal distribution, patching and capping of lymphocyte surface immunoglobulin studied by electron microscopy. *Nature New Biology 241:* 257-259.

Diener, E. and Feldmann, M. (1972). Relationship between antigen and antibodyinduced suppression of immunity. *Transplant. Rev. 8:* 76-103.

Edelman, G. M., Yahara, I., and Wang, J. L. (1973). Receptor mobility and receptor cytoplasmic interactions in lymphocytes. *Proc. Nat. Acad. Sci. (USA) 70:* 1442-1446.

Edidin, M. (1974). Rotational and translational diffusion in membranes. *Ann. Rev. Biophys. Bioeng. 3:* 179-201.

Edidin, M., Zagyansky, Y., and Lardner, T. J. (1976). Measurement of membrane protein lateral diffusion in single cells. *Science 191:* 466-468.

Engers, H. D. and Unanue, E. R. (1973). The fate of anti-immunoglobulin surface immunoglobulin complexes on B lymphocytes. *J. Immunol. 110:* 465-475.

Fram, R., Sidman, C. L., and Unanue, E. R. (1976). Genetic Control of ligand induced events in B lymphocytes. *J. Immunol. 117:* 1456-1463.

Fu, S. M. and Kunkel, H. G. (1974). Membrane immunoglobulins: Inability to detect certain characteristic IgM and IgD antigens. *J. Exp. Med. 140:* 895-903.

Fu, S. M., Winchester, R. J. and Kunkel, H. G. (1975). Similar idiotypic specificity for membrane IgD and IgM of human B lymphocytes. *J. Immunol. 114:* 250-252.

Lewis, G. K., Cruse, J. M., and Crawford, L. V. (1974). Kinetic analysis of antigen induced cell receptor movement (abstract). *Fed. Proc. 33:* 765.

Loor, F., Forni, L., and Pernis, B. (1972). The dynamic state of the lymphocyte membrane. Factors affecting the distribution and turnover of surface immunoglobulins. *Eur. J. Immunol. 2:* 203-212.

Melchers, U., Eidels, L., and Uhr, J. W. (1975). Are immunoglobulins integral membrane proteins? *Nature 258:* 434-435.

Melchers, F. and Andersson, J. (1973). Synthesis, surfaces, deposition and secretion of IgM in bone marrow derived lymphocytes before and after mitogenic stimulation. *Transplant. Rev. 14:* 76-130.

Miranda, J. J., Zola, H., and Howard, J. G. (1972). Studies on immunological paralysis. X. Cellular characteristics of the induction and loss of tolerance to Levan (Polyfructose). *Immunology 23:* 843-855.

Raff, M. C. and de Petris, S. (1973). Movement of lymphocyte surface antigens and receptors; the fluid nature of the lymphocyte plasma membrane and its immunological significances. *Fed. Proc. 32:* 48-54.

Schreiner, G. F. and Unanue, E. R. (1976). Membrane and cytoplasmic changes in B lymphocytes induced by ligand-surface immunoglobulin interaction. *Adv. in Immunol.* (in press).

Sell, S. and Gell, P. G. H. (1965). Studies on rabbit lymphocytes in vitro. I. Stimulation of blast transformation with an anti-allotype serum. *J. Exp. Med. 122:* 423-439.

Sidman, C. L. and Unanue, E. R. (1976). Control of B lymphocyte function. I. Inactivation of mitogenesis by interactions with surface immunoglobulin and Fc receptor molecules. *J. Exp. Med.* (in press).

Stackpole, C. W., Jacobson, J. S. and Lardis, M. P. (1974). Two distinct types of capping of surface receptors on mouse lymphoid cells. *Nature 248:* 232-234.

Stern, C. and McConnell, I. (1976). Immunoglobulins M and D as antigen binding receptors on the same cell, with shared specificity. *Eur. J. Immunol. 6:* 225-227.

Taylor, R. B., Duffus, W. P. H., Raff, M. C., and de Petris, S. (1971). Redistribution and pinocytosis of lymphocyte surface immunoglobulin molecules induced by anti-Ig Ab. *Nature New Biology 233:* 225-229.

Unanue, E. R., Ault, K. A., and Karnovsky, M. J. (1974). Ligand induced movement of lymphocyte surface macromolecules. IV. Stimulation of cell motility by anti-Ig and lack of relationship to capping. *J. Exp. Med. 139:* 295-312.

Unanue, E. R. and Karnovsky, M. J. (1973). Redistribution and fate of immunoglobulin complexes on surface of B lymphocytes: functional implication and mechanisms. *Transplant. Rev. 14:* 184-210.

Unanue, E. R. and Karnovsky, M. J. (1974). Ligand induced movement of lymphocyte membrane macromolecules. V. Capping, cell movement, and microtubular function in normal and lectin-treated lymphocytes. *J. Exp. Med. 140:* 1207-1220.

Vitetta, E. S. and Uhr, J. W. (1973). Synthesis, transport, dynamics and fate of cell surface immunoglobulin and alloantigens in murine lymphocytes. *Transplant. Rev. 14:* 50-75.

Vitetta, E. S. and Uhr, J. W. (1975). Immunoglobulin receptors revisited. *Science 189:* 964-969.

Chapter 7

MODELS OF THE EVENTS RESPONSIBLE FOR ANTIBODY PRODUCTION BY B LYMPHOCYTES

Alan S. Perelson

Theoretical Division
University of California
Los Alamos Scientific Laboratory
Los Alamos, New Mexico

A variety of mathematical techniques and models are used to study the distribution of immunoglobulin molecules on the surface of B lymphocytes and some aspects of B-cell triggering, proliferation, and differentiation.

I. INTRODUCTION

Tremendous progress in immunology has been brought about by the adoption of the paradigm of clonal selection and the elucidation of the molecular structure of the immunoglobulins, but detailed understanding of the basic cellular and biochemical events that regulate the behavior of the cells of the immune system is still lacking. According to the clonal selection hypothesis, antigen selects a subpopulation of cells and stimulates them to divide and differentiate into antibody-secreting cells. Although this function almost certainly requires the interaction of antigen with cellular receptors, the nature of the interaction and the conditions under which the cells then proliferate and differentiate are unclear. In an effort to explain the underlying cellular control mechanisms, I shall develop mathematical models of three aspects of the events preceeding antibody production by mature plasma cells. First, I shall describe the spatial distribution of immunoglobulin on the surface of B lymphocytes. In the absence of cross-linking agents, the distribution is nonrandom, and its statistical properties can be delineated by studies of the radial distribution function, power spectrum, and various indices of clumping. Next, I study the interaction of antigen and various ligands with these immunoglobulin receptors. By employing a model developed by Bell, I shall show that the binding of multivalent ligand to cells depends primarily upon receptor density and not receptor affinity. Using a modification of this model, the rate of patching is studied and its dependence on antigen concentration, antigen valence, and receptor-antigen affinity computed. Further, the biological implications of assuming that ligand-induced redistribution of surface receptors is a necessary first step for lymphocyte triggering are explored.

Last, using optimal control theory, I determine the sequence of proliferation and differentiation events that lead to the elimination of antigen in minimal time. Hypothesizing that the mammalian immune system has been optimized over evolutionary time by natural selection, this study suggests possible mechanisms for controlling the proliferation and differentiation of large lymphocytes and the formation of plasma cells.

II. SURFACE IMMUNOGLOBULIN

B lymphocytes have on their surface immunoglobulin molecules which function as receptors for antigen (Warner, 1974). Presumably this immunoglobulin has the same specificity for antigen as the antibodies secreted by the B cell when it differentiates into a plasma cell. The amount of surface immunoglobulin (sIg) can be quantitated immunochemically. In the mouse one finds a mean content of approximately 10^5 molecules per cell (Rabellino et al., 1971), which have been estimated to occupy less than 10% of the total membrane surface (Unanue, 1974). The precise spatial distribution of sIg has been difficult to measure because of technical difficulties in cell labeling and ultrastructural examination (Abbas et al., 1975). Studies of the distribution of surface immunoglobulin on B cells labeled with a monovalent ligand and then examined by immunofluorescence, which is a low resolution technique, or by electron microscopy of thin section, which only reveals the pattern in the plane of the section, have disclosed patterns described as random (Taylor et al., 1971; de Petris and Raff, 1973). Studies by the freeze-etch method, which permits the examination of large areas of the cell surface, have shown that immunoglobulin molecules are distributed nonrandomly in microclusters of varying size (Karnovsky et al., 1972; Ault et al., 1973; Abbas, et al., 1975). The microaggregates are composed of at most five to ten molecules and are separated from each other by areas of bare membrane (Unanue, 1974). Similar observations have recently been made about the distribution of Ia antigens on murine B lymphocytes (Abbas et al., 1976).

Investigations of cell surface immunoglobulin by scanning immunoelectronmicroscopy (Libscomb et al., 1975) and immunofluorescence microscopy (Loor and Hägg, 1975) have revealed the presence of microvilli with Ig molecules on their surface. In the studies of Libscomb et al. (1975) using tobacco mosaic virus (TMV) as a morphological marker, the sIg was described as randomly distributed on the surface, appearing both on the microvilli and the smooth surface of the cell. Due to the large size of TMV, the resolution in these studies was probably not sufficient to reveal small microclusters.

III. MATHEMATICAL ANALYSIS OF SURFACE IMMUNOGLOBULIN DISTRIBUTION

In the experiments by Abbas et al. (1975), electron micrographs obtained by the freeze-etch procedure were analyzed by statistical tests in order to ascertain whether immunoglobulin molecules are distributed nonrandomly on B-lymphocyte surfaces. A two-antibody indirect labeling procedure was utilized in these studies; murine B lymphocytes were labeled first with fluorescein conjugates of monovalent (Fab) antiimmunoglobulin, then treated with monovalent antifluorescein antibody coupled to ferritin. The method avoids the use of bivalent molecules which could cross-link and aggregate surface Ig, but creates the risk that several ferritin grains may label each Ig molecule. By comparing the pictures that result from using different fluorochrome protein ratios, the possibility of having more than one ferritin molecule per Fab anti-Ig molecule was excluded. In the analysis performed by Abbas et al. (1975), tracings were made of the ferritin grains on each electron micrograph, then overlain with a transparent grid which divided the picture into several hundred squares. The number of ferritin grains in each square was counted. If the grains were distributed randomly one would expect the probability of finding n grains in a single square, P_n, to be given by the Poisson distribution:

$$P_n = \frac{\lambda^n \exp(-\lambda)}{n!} \tag{1}$$

where λ is the mean number of grains per square. A characteristic property of the Poisson distribution is that the variance of the distribution, σ^2, is equal to the mean. If the variance is greater than the mean, the distribution deviates toward clustering. Distributions with the variance less than the mean tend toward regularity (Zar, 1974). A total of 20 photographs were studied by Abbas et al. (1975). In all cases the variance was greater than the mean, implying clustering.

Various quantitative measures of the degree of aggregation have been proposed. These measures have not yet been used to analyze receptor distributions, but could be very useful for comparing different receptor patterns, especially in experiments designed to assay changes in receptor distribution with time or ligand concentration. David and Moore (1954) have defined an index of clumping

$$I = \frac{\sigma^2}{\lambda} - 1 \qquad (2)$$

For the data presented by Abbas et al. (1975), I varies between 1.04 and 4.65. The degree of receptor aggregation on two cells, labeled 1 and 2, may be compared by choosing a sample area containing N ferritin grains from freeze-etch micrographs of each cell and then computing

$$w = \frac{1}{2} \ln \left(\frac{\sigma_1^2/\lambda_1}{\sigma_2^2/\lambda_2} \right) \qquad (3)$$

If the absolute value of w is greater than $2.5/\sqrt{N - 1}$, then the indices of clumping for the two cells differ significantly at the 5% confidence level (David and Moore, 1954). The index of clumping has the property that it decreases if the total number of receptors on a cell decreases by a random process such as shedding (Pielou, 1969). Lloyd (1967) has proposed two other measures of aggregation which do not change if receptors are gained or lost at random; an *index of crowding* m* and an *index of mean patchiness* p*. If one defines X_i as the number of grains that share a square with ferritin grain i, then

$$m^* = \frac{\sum_{i=1}^{N} X_i}{N} \tag{4}$$

and

$$p^* = \frac{m^*}{\lambda} \tag{5}$$

where N is the total number of grains. A detailed discussion of the relative merits of these indices can be found in Pielou (1969).

A. Radial Distribution Function

Further information about the clustering and the "forces" among surface Ig molecules responsible for their nonrandom distribution, may be obtained by computing the *radial distribution function* g(r) for the ferritin grain patterns. This function, which is commonly used in the study of the structure of matter (Egelstaff, 1967; Hill, 1956), has also been employed to analyze the spatial organization of connective tissue (Farrell and Hart, 1969), and the distribution of pores on nuclear membranes (Markovics et al., 1974). Given a distribution of ferritin grains on an electron micrograph, the radial distribution function is defined as the ratio of the average local number density at a distance r from an arbitrary grain to the average overall density of grains (Reed and Gubbins, 1973). For an area A containing N grains (density $\rho = N/A$), the local distribution function, $g_i(r)$, for the i'th grain is

$$g_i(r) = \frac{n_i(r)}{\rho A_i(r)} \tag{6}$$

where $n_i(r)$ is the number of grains lying in an annulus of width Δr, $\Delta r \ll r$, with area $A_i(r)$, totally contained within the area A, and whose boundaries are at distances $(r - \Delta r/2)$ and $(r + \Delta r/2)$ from the i'th grain. The radial distribution function is a weighted average of the $g_i(r)$

$$g(r) = \frac{\sum_{i=1}^{N} A_i(r) g_i(r)}{\sum_{i=1}^{N} A_i(r)} \tag{7}$$

For a random distribution of a large number of particles the local density is the same as the overall density, and $g(r) = 1$. Any order in the distribution is reflected in deviations from unity. For example, for molecules distributed on a two-dimensional square lattice (e.g., two-dimensional crystal) with spacing a, g(r) would be zero everywhere except at $r = a, \sqrt{2}a, 2a, \sqrt{5}a, 2\sqrt{2}a, 3a, \ldots$.* For more liquid structures in which the molecules undergo random thermal motion, the discrete distribution characteristic of a crystal is transformed into a continuous distribution. Short-range order between molecules is preserved, but at large distances the net effect of thermal motion is to destroy any long-range correlations in the relative positions of the molecule; hence $g(r) \to 1$ as $r \to \infty$.

From the 20 photographs studied by Abbas et al. (1975), I arbitrarily chose five and computed the radial distribution function for each from Eqs. (6) and (7). All the pictures yielded qualitatively similar radial distribution functions. One of them and the corresponding ferritin grain pattern, are illustrated in Fig. 1 and Fig. 2a. In these figures the radial distribution function is plotted as a function of the dimensionless distance $x = r/r_0$, where $r_0 = \rho^{-1/2}$ is the mean separation distance between grains. Notice that the peak in the distribution occurs at x well below 1 and approaches unity for x greater than 1. This type of radial distribution function is characteristic of a clustered pattern. The distance along the axis between the peak and x = 1, and the sharpness of the peak, determine the amount of cluster character in the

---

*If the computational scheme outlined by Eqs. (6) and (7) were used to compute g(r), the radial distribution function would also be nonzero for distances within $\Delta r/2$ of these values.

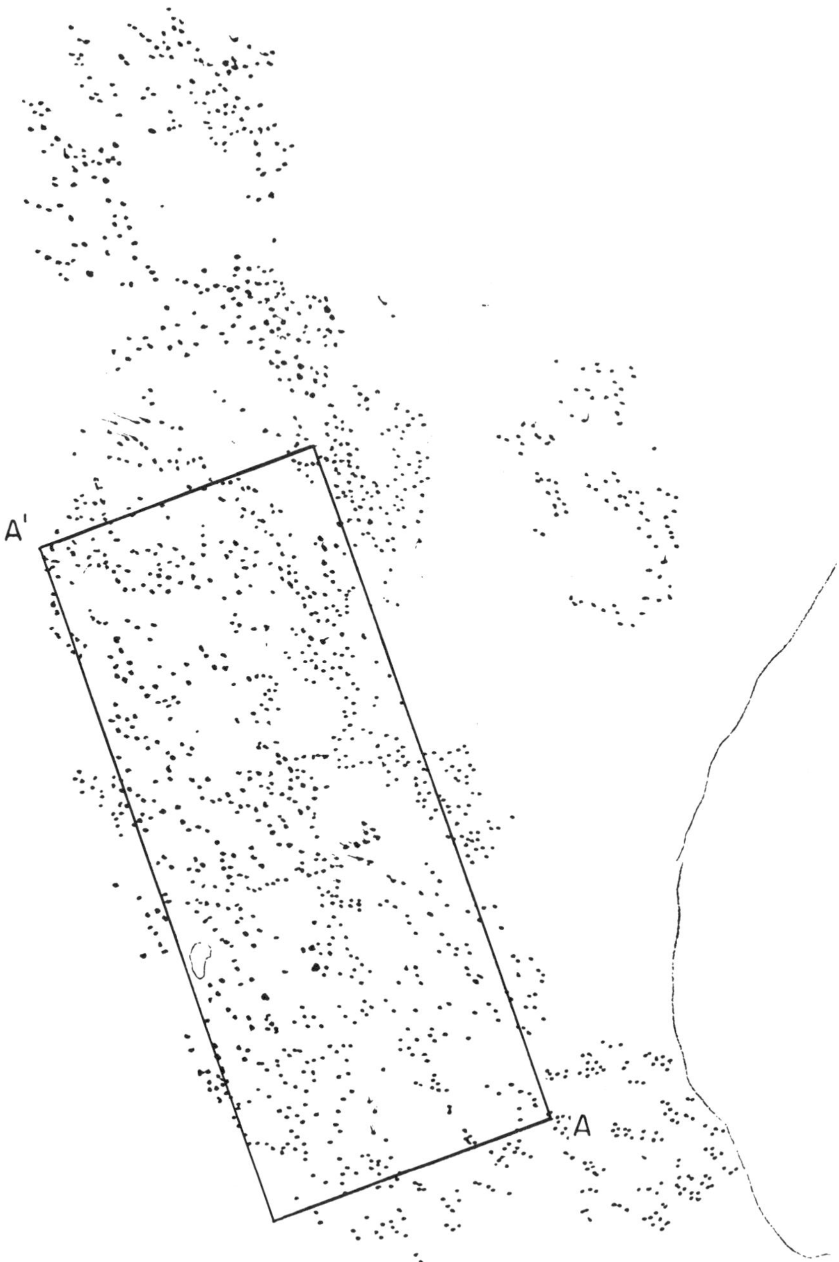

FIG. 1. The ferritin grain pattern traced from a freeze-etched replica (magnified X 109,000) of a B lymphocyte. Only the area enclosed by the rectangle was analyzed.

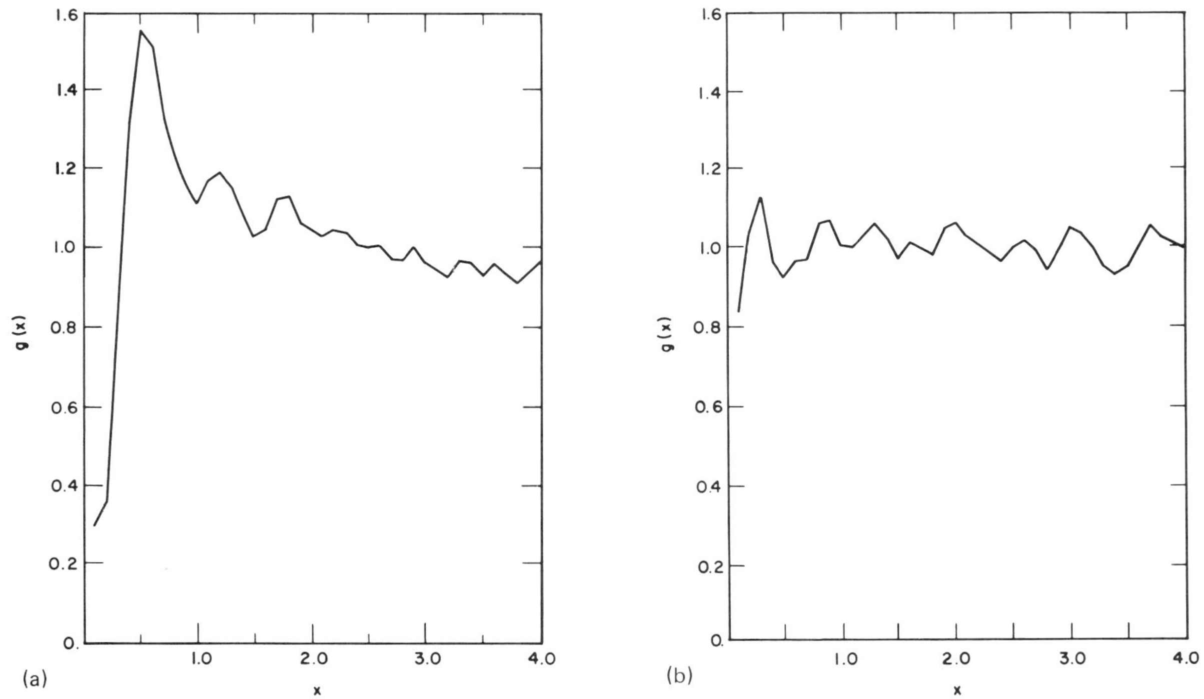

FIG. 2. (a) The radial distribution function of the portion of the ferritin grain pattern enclosed by the rectangle in Fig. 1, plotted as a function of the dimensionless distance $x = r/r_0$, where $r_0 = \rho^{-1/2}$ is the mean separation distance between grains, N = 653. (b) The radial distribution function for N = 653 points placed at random on a rectangle of identical size to that studied in (a)

distribution (Markovics et al., 1974). At small values of x, g(x) is much smaller than 1, presumably because molecules cannot get arbitrarily close. However, because the ferritin grains are much larger than the surface Ig molecules and two overlapping grains may not easily be resolved, one cannot obtain reliable information at small distances. Moreover, because the number of grains that appear close together is small, the computation of the average radial distribution function is not very accurate and is subject to random fluctuations for values of x near zero.

It is possible that the clustering reflects the manner in which the Ig is inserted into the membrane. However, since receptors are believed to diffuse within the plane of the membrane, any memory of the dynamic scheme by which the pattern was initially formed should quickly be lost. If the movement of the Ig is subject to some intermolecular interaction, then a degree of short-range order is not inconsistent with the fluid mosaic model of membrane structure (Singer and Nicholson, 1972). Assuming that the interaction between surface immunoglobulins is occurring at local equilibrium and that it can be described by an intermolecular potential energy, u(r), the techniques developed to study the structure of liquids can be applied.

For a dilute gas

$$g(r) = \exp \frac{-u(r)}{kT}$$

while for a denser system a correction term $\tau(r)$ is needed

$$g(r) = \exp \frac{-u(r)}{kT} \tau(r)$$

where k is Boltzman's constant and T is the absolute temperature (Egelstaff, 1967). The maximum in g(r), therefore, occurs at a minimum of the potential u(r). The typical form for g(r) of a dense liquid and a dilute gas are shown in Fig. 3. At small r, g(r) is zero, due to the high energies required to force the electron shells of atoms to overlap [i.e., u(r) is repulsive for small r]. At a distance near the atomic diameter, u(r) has a minimum, and there is a peak in g(r) due to the sphere of nearest neighbors.

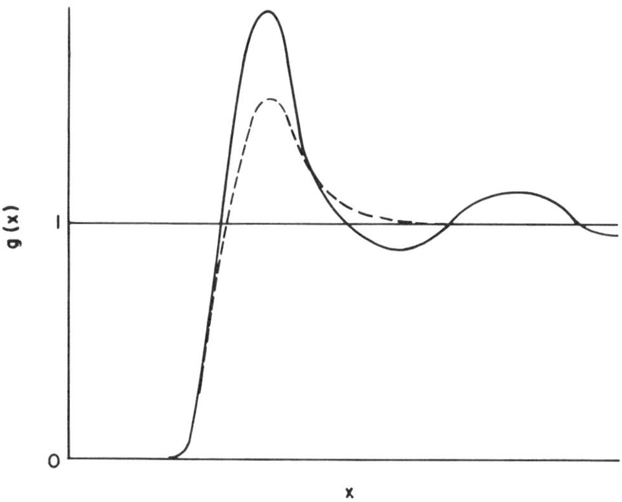

FIG. 3. The radial distribution function for a simple monatomic fluid: (——) dense liquid showing some short-range order, (- - - -) dilute gas showing a single peak. Adapted from Reed and Grubbins (1973).

In liquids, more distant neighbors are represented by subsequent peaks which give g(r) an oscillating character. These oscillations decrease as r increases and eventually g(r) approaches 1.

Although the radial distribution for sIg in Fig. 2a appears to exhibit maxima after the nearest neighbor peak, these may not be statistically significant. The radial distribution function for the same number of points placed at random on an identical-sized rectangle is shown in Fig. 2b. From the figure one can see that fluctuations in g(r) of $\pm$ 0.1 are not uncommon,* and hence one cannot assign any significance to these distant peaks. Increasing the number of receptors used to calculate g(r) would decrease the statistical fluctuations and would allow a more accurate evaluation

---

*Using a statistical analysis developed by Markovics et al. (1974) I estimated S.E., the standard error of g(r). One expects 95% of the values to lie within $\pm$ 2 S.E. of the mean. For Fig. 2a, 2 S.E. varies from 0.14, near the first peak to 0.08 for $x \geqslant 2.2$.

of the radial distribution function. The absence of noticeable maxima after the first peak would indicate that $g(r)$ resembles the radial distribution function of a gas more than that of a liquid, and hence that long-range forces between immunoglobulins are negligible.

The number of ferritin grains used to calculate $g(r)$ is limited by the presence of ice crystals and other structures, possibly microvilli, that prevent the selection from the freeze-etch micrographs of large areas of smooth membrane for study. Other preparations may allow more detailed calculations of $g(r)$ and a better study of inter-Ig forces.

B. Nearest Neighbor Analysis

Further information about the organization of sIg on B lymphocytes can be obtained by determining the average number of first nearest neighbors surrounding each ferritin grain. If we let $n(r)\Delta r$ be the average number of ferritin grains at distances between $r + \Delta r/2$ and $r - \Delta r/2$ from a given grain then one can show that $n(r)$ is approximately given by

$$n(r)\Delta r = 2\pi\rho r \, \Delta r \, g(r) \tag{8}$$

The function $n(r)$ is 0 at $r = 0$, increases as r increases, usually through a maximum, and then continues to increase with possible subsequent maxima. The peaks in $n(r)$ are caused by the higher than average density of particles in the nearest neighbor shells. In a liquid the nearest neighbor shells overlap making it difficult to identify the positions of all but the first nearest neighbor shell. By summing $n(r)\Delta r$ from $r = 0$ to a position R at the end of the first nearest neighbor peak one obtains z, the average number of first nearest neighbors surrounding a ferritin grain, that is,

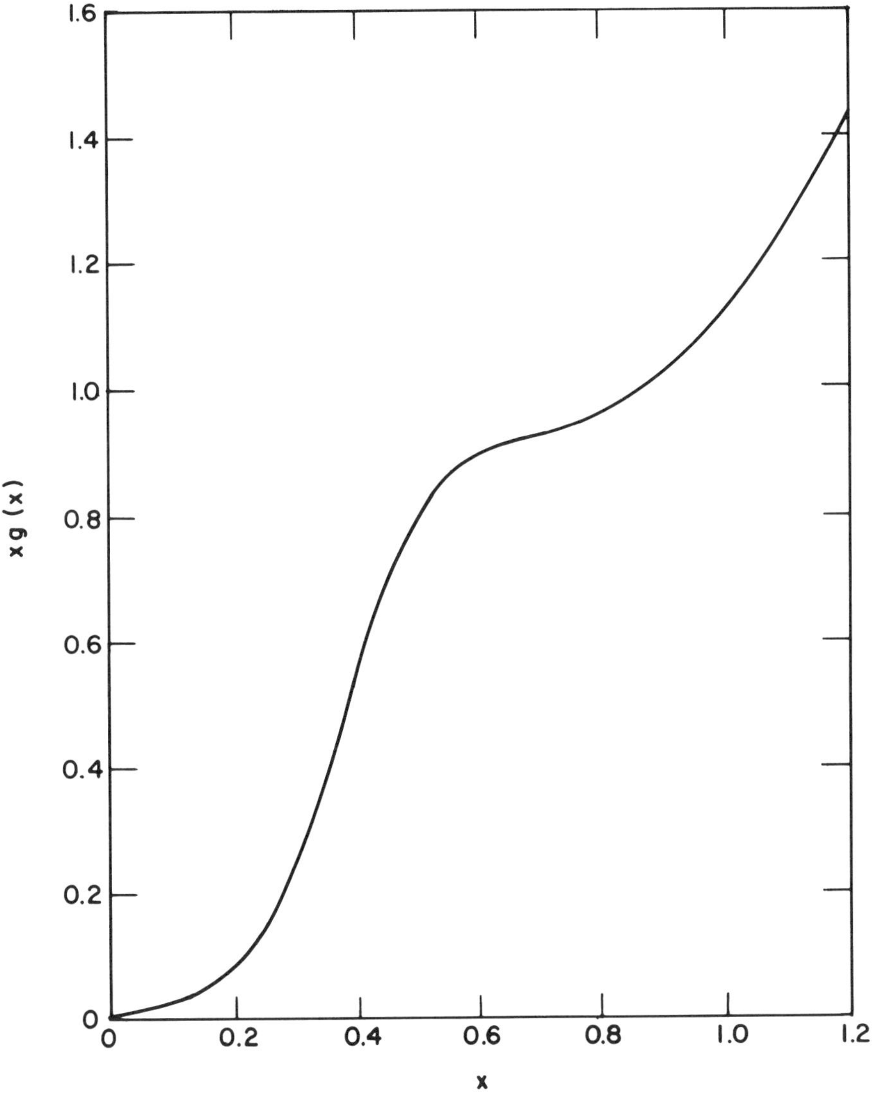

FIG. 4. The average number of ferritin grains at a distance x from a given grain is proportional to xg(x). The first nearest neighbor peak was assumed to terminate at x = 0.7.

$$z = \sum_{r_i=0}^{R} n(r_i)\Delta r = 2\pi\rho\ \Delta r \sum_{r_i=0}^{R} r_i g(r_i) \tag{9}$$

where r_i and R are chosen as multiples of Δr so as to avoid multiple counting of ferritin grains.

In Fig. 4, xg(x), which is proportional to n(r), is plotted for the ferritin grain pattern shown in Fig. 1. Although there is no true maxima in the curve, I chose the position x = 0.7 as the end of the first nearest neighbor shell. Using Eq. (9) one then finds z = 2.2. Doing the same calculation for all 5 ferritin grain patterns, one finds that z varies from 1.5 to 3.0, with mean 2.2. According to Mikolaj and Ping (1968) this method of computing z may give an overestimate since some particles in the second nearest neighbor shell may lie at positions $r < R$.

For a pattern in which ferritin grains were organized along well separated lines or curves, each ferritin grain would have two nearest neighbors. The grains in Fig. 1 have the appearance of being associated with lines connecting the A and A' corners of the marked rectangle. Further analysis is required to verify the hypothesis of linearity in the pattern.

IV. PATCHING AND CAPPING

Reactions between surface immunoglobulin and ligand can be studied using either antigen or antiimmunoglobulin antibody. The events that take place in vitro following ligand-receptor interaction are quite striking.*

1. Ligand-receptor complexes are formed over the entire cell surface. In studies utilizing fluorescent-tagged anti-Ig, the fluorescence which is first seen uniformly distributed over the cell, quickly coalesces into aggregates called "patches" or "spots" (Taylor et al., 1971).

---

*Loor and Hägg (1975) have suggested that this sequence of events may not represent the in vivo situation.

2. The receptor-ligand complexes or patches rapidly move to one pole of the cell forming a "cap" (Taylor et al., 1971).

3. Simultaneous with the formation of a cap the cell starts translatory movement and adopts an ameboid shape (Unanue et al., 1974).

4. The receptor-ligand complexes forming the cap are rapidly endocytosed and shed (Engers and Unanue, 1973). Within a few minutes the lymphocyte returns to its native round shape, but now with a surface membrane lacking antigen receptors.

5. New receptors are reexpressed within 6 to 12 hr (Ault and Unanue, 1974).

These events have been extensively reviewed (see Ault and Unanue, Chap. 6; Unanue, 1974; Unanue and Karnovsky, 1973).

Ligand-induced redistribution of membrane receptors is by itself not sufficient to induce B cells to proliferate and differentiate (Katz and Unanue, 1972). However, the cross-linking of receptors by multivalent antigen may be the initial step in the activation process. For example, Kishimoto and Ishizaka (1975) found that triggering occurred if the cell-free supernatant from a culture of primed rabbit lymph node cells was added to a culture of rabbit mesenteric lymphocytes *after* their receptors had been cross-linked by anti-Ig. Since the supernatant was most effective when added 24 hr after the anti-Ig, and no response was observed if the supernatant was added together with the anti-Ig, Kishimoto et al. (1975) suggested that cross-linking of surface-Ig receptors and their removal by the capping, shedding, interiorization process, induces either the formation or exposure of surface receptors for a soluble factor contained in the supernatant.

Other experiments indicate that the clearing of patches and caps may be important in triggering. Dinitrophenylated (DNP)-D-GL, a synthetic copolymer made exclusively of the d-amino acids d-glutamic acid and d-lysine, has been found to be a highly potent tolerogen (Katz

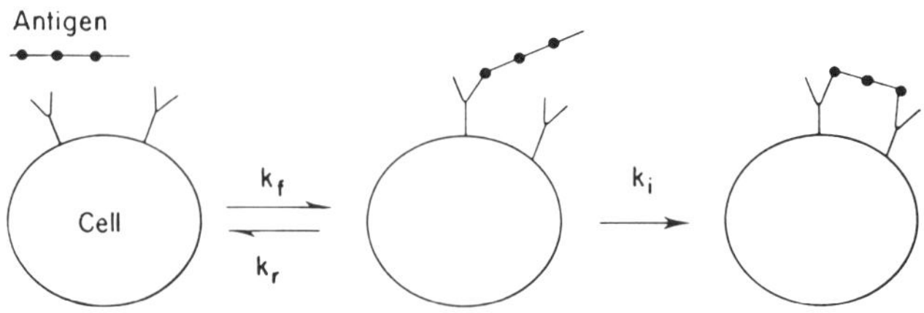

FIG. 5. The binding of multivalent ligand to cellular receptors. First, the ligand binds to a single receptor site with rate constant k_f. The ligand then either dissociates with rate constant k_r or irreversibly cross-links receptors with rate constant k_i. Reproduced from DeLisi and Perelson (1976).

et al., 1971). Once this polymer binds to a cell a majority of it remains on the cell surface and is not interiorized (Ault and Unanue, 1974). New anti-DNP receptors are never reexpressed on these B cells (Unanue and Ault, 1974). These results suggest that interfering with the ability of a B cell to clear its surface of receptor-antigen complexes prevents effective stimulation of the cell (Unanue, 1974).

The ligand-induced redistribution of receptors may also have an important role in facilitating the binding of multivalent ligands to a cell. By aggregating receptors, the lymphocyte can concentrate binding sites and hence form more bonds with a given antigen, binding it more stably. Using a model for the binding of multivalent antigens to cells developed by Bell (1974), I shall show below that for highly multivalent ligands, such as T-independent antigens, it is the receptor density and not the receptor-antigen affinity that determines the number of antigens bound per cell.

V. BINDING OF MULTIVALENT LIGANDS TO CELLULAR RECEPTORS

In Bell's model (Fig. 5), ligand is assumed to bind first to a single receptor site with rate constant k_f. This singly bound antigen is then assumed either to dissociate with rate constant k_r or to irreversibly bind other receptor molecules, with rate constant k_i, thereby becoming multivalently bound and causing the cross-linking of two or more receptors. With ρ and ρ_0, the concentrations of free and total receptor sites, respectively, and C, m, and M the concentrations of unbound, singly bound, and multiply bound antigen molecules, respectively, the equations of the model are

$$\rho(t) = \rho_0 - m(t) - nM(t) \tag{10}$$

$$\frac{dm}{dt} = k_f C\rho - k_r m - k_i m\rho \tag{11}$$

$$\frac{dM}{dt} = k_i m\rho \tag{12}$$

where n is the average number of bonds holding the multiply bound antigen to the cell. If the rate of dissociation of singly bound antigen is sufficiently rapid compared to the rate of cross-linking ($k_r >> k_i\rho_0$), local equilibrium will be established between free and singly bound antigen when $t >> 1/(k_f C + k_r)$. For typical parameter values ($k_r = 10\ \text{sec}^{-1}$, $k_f = 2 \times 10^8\ M^{-1}$, $C = 10^{-9}$ M), this takes less than a few seconds. In this local equilibrium limit $dm/dt = 0$ and from Eq. (11)

$$m = KC\rho \tag{13}$$

where $K \equiv k_f/k_r$ is the receptor-ligand equilibrium constant (affinity). If antigen is first introduced at t = 0, and C is thereafter constant, one can show (Bell, 1974)

$$M = \frac{\rho_0}{n} \frac{\alpha\rho_0 t}{1 + \alpha\rho_0 t} \tag{14}$$

where

$$\alpha = \frac{nk_i KC}{(1 + KC)^2} \tag{15}$$

I shall now show that after a reasonable length of time the concentration of multiply bound antigen is independent of affinity and depends predominantly on the receptor density ρ_0. One cannot use the model for large t since the assumptions that the cross-linking of receptors is irreversible will eventually break down. Notice that if $\alpha\rho_0 t >> 1$, then from Eq. (14) $M \sim \rho_0/n$ and the concentration of multiply bound ligand would not depend on the receptor affinity K. From Eq. (15),

$$\alpha\rho_0 t = nk_i\rho_0 t \frac{KC}{(1 + KC)^2} \tag{16}$$

Bell (1974, 1975) estimates, using 5×10^{-11} cm^2 sec^{-1} as a typical receptor diffusion coefficient, that with approximately 10^5 receptors per B cell $k_i\rho_0 \gtrsim 0.03$ sec^{-1}. More recent evidence suggests that protein diffusion coefficients are approximately 2.6×10^{-10} cm^2 sec^{-1} (Edidin et al., 1976), and hence I shall assume $k_i\rho_0 \gtrsim 0.1$ sec^{-1}. I also suppose $n \geqslant 10$, and that the multivalent binding of a ligand to a cell and the crosslinking of receptors is substantially completed when $t \geqslant 30$ min (1800 sec). Using these parameter values

$$\alpha\rho_0 t = 1800 \frac{KC}{(1 + KC)^2} \tag{17}$$

For $DNP_{2.7}$-polymerized flagellin (POL), Feldmann (1972) has found that antigen (not hapten) concentrations of 10^{-9} M to 10^{-10} M were the most effective in stimulating antibody production in vitro. In vivo experiments using the T-independent antigen $DNP_{1.4}$-lysine (lys)-levan (LE) also show that antigen concentrations of approximately 10^{-9} M are maximally stimulating.* Presuming that optimal stimulation by these T-independent antigens occurs only after substantial ligand binding, I shall suppose $C = 10^{-9}$ M. $DNP_{2.7}$-POL with molecular weight 10^7 contains 2.7 DNP groups per MON (molecular weight 40,000) or 675 DNP groups per molecule. Affinities are usually defined as the equilibrium constant between a receptor and

---

*Klaus and Humphrey (1974) found that the optimal does in a mouse was approximately 50 μg. Assuming an immune system volume of 1.25 ml and a molecular weight of 10^7 for DNP-lys-LE, this does correspond to a concentration of 4×10^{-9} M.

a single DNP group. Therefore, K = 675 K', where K' is the affinity of a receptor for a single DNP group.* Substituting these values for C and K into Eq. (17), one finds $\alpha\rho_0 t$ is greater than one for K' between 10^3 M^{-1} and 10^9 M^{-1}, and substantially greater than one for 10^4 $M^{-1} \leqslant K' \leqslant 10^8$ M^{-1}. Thus, over most of the range of biologically reasonable values for K', binding of multivalent antigen to cell surfaces is independent of affinity. From Eq. (17) it is clear that the range of K' values depends upon C. Thus for $C = 10^{-10}$ M, $\alpha\rho_0 t \gg 1$ when 10^5 $M^{-1} \leqslant K' \leqslant 10^9$ M^{-1}, while for $C = 10^{-8}$ M, $\alpha\rho_0 t \gg 1$ when 10^3 $M^{-1} \leqslant K' \leqslant 10^7$ M^{-1}. Increasing either the time allowed for interaction t or the average number of bonds per antigen n by an order of magnitude will increase the range of K' by two orders of magnitude. For example, with t = 5 hr, n = 10, $C = 10^{-10}$ M, $\alpha\rho_0 t \gg 1$ when 10^4 $M^{-1} \leqslant K' \leqslant 10^{10}$ M^{-1}.

The rate of dissociation of singly bound antigen will not be rapid compared to the cross-linking rate in all circumstances. However, if one assumes $k_i\rho_0 \gg k_r$, then Bell (1974) has shown that

$$\frac{dM}{dt} = k_f C\rho \tag{18}$$

In this limit, singly bound antigens will rapidly form additional attachments. Consequently, I assume m is negligible compared with nM, and thus Eq. (10) becomes

$$\rho = \rho_0 - nM(t) \tag{19}$$

Substituting Eq. (19) into Eq. (18) and integrating with the initial condition M(t = 0) = 0, one finds

---

*This relation may be derived as follows. From Eq. (13) $K = m/C\rho$. By definition, K', the affinity of a receptor for a single DNP group is $K' = m'/675C\rho$, where 675C is the concentration of free DNP groups and m' is the concentration of bound DNP groups. Since we have assumed that in the equilibrium step the ligand binds by only a single site, m' = m, and thus K = 675K'.

$$M(t) = \frac{\rho_0}{n} [1 - \exp(-nk_f Ct)]$$

Thus once again M is independent of the receptor affinity and is proportional to ρ_0/n.* A process such as patching, which can increase the local density of receptors, will effectively increase ρ_0 and hence M.

VI. MODEL FOR PATCH FORMATION

Patch formation can be considered as a two-dimensional polymerization reaction. In three-dimensional systems, the polymerization theory of Flory (1941) and Stockmayer (1943) has been used by Goldberg (1952) to compute the equilibrium probability distribution of aggregate sizes when homogeneous populations of antigens and bivalent antibodies interact. The crucial parameter in such theories is the extent of reaction, p, which may be defined as the probability that an antibody combining site picked at random is bound. For systems which contain a fixed number of bivalent antibodies and f-valent antigen molecules, p determines the probability that an antigen site picked at random is bound. (This follows from the fact that the number of bound antibody sites must equal the number of bound antigen sites.) The extent of reaction will also determine the likelihood of finding any given antigen-antibody complex, providing all sites of a given type (antigen or antibody) are equally reactive, and intramolecular bonding or cycle formation can be neglected. This result is shown in Fig. 6. The effects of including intramolecular reaction can be estimated using percolation theory (Bell, 1971).

A slight modification of the Flory-Stockmayer condensation polymerization theory allows one to calculate the probability of finding antigen-receptor complexes of any size on the surface of a

---

*The case in which $k_i\rho_0 \approx k_r$ is more complex and has not been analyzed.

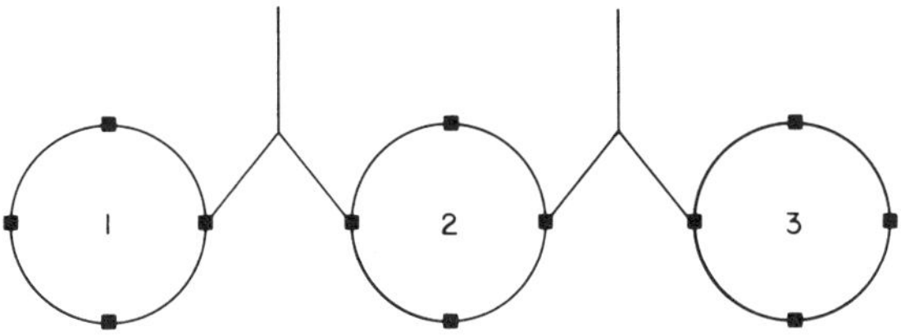

FIG. 6. An antigen-antibody aggregate composed of three tetravalent antigens and two bivalent antibodies. If p is the probability that an antibody site is bound and p_ℓ is the probability that an antigen site is bound, then the concentration of this antigen-antibody aggregate is proportional to $[(1 - p_\ell)^3 p_\ell]p[(1 - p_\ell)^2 p_\ell]p(1 - p_\ell)^3$. The factor $(1 - p_\ell)^3 p_\ell$ is the probability of finding antigen 1 with three free sites and one bound site. The next factor, p, represents the probability that the antibody bound to antigen 1 has its other site bound (to antigen 2). The factor $(1 - p_\ell)^2 p_\ell$ is probability of antigen 2 having two of its other sites free and one bound. The remaining factors are determined in a similar way.

lymphocyte (DeLisi and Perelson, 1976). In a phenomenon such as patching the extent of reaction p changes with time, and consequently so does the aggregate size distribution. If p increases beyond some critical value, p_c, then there is a finite probability of finding an infinite size aggregate (in a system containing an infinite number of antigens and receptors). One can approximate the time it takes a cell to patch by the time, t_c, at which p reaches p_c. The effects of factors such as the antigen valence, antigenic concentration, and receptor affinity, on the rate of patching can then be ascertained by studying the physical parameters that influence how p changes with time.

The extent of reaction p(t) can be calculated by generalizing Bell's model of antigen binding to cells. Again, assume that free antigen is in the bulk medium surrounding the lymphocytes at a concentration, C, which remains approximately constant during the course of the experiment. Suppose that the interaction between the antigen and the lymphocyte occurs in two steps (Fig. 5), and that the first is equilibrium controlled. (The equilibrium constant $K = k_f/k_r$, is the *affinity* of the whole antigen for a single receptor site.)

No assumptions are made about the average number of bonds per multivalent antigen.

The antigen-receptor interaction can be described by the following system of three differential equations

$$\frac{dS}{dt} = -k_f CS + k_r m - k_i LS$$

$$\frac{dm}{dt} = k_f CS - k_r m - (f - 1)k_i mS \tag{20}$$

$$\frac{dL}{dt} = (f - 1)(k_f CS - k_r m) - k_i LS$$

where S and L are the concentrations of free antibody and free antigen sites on the membrane, respectively, m is the concentration of antigen with precisely one site bound to the membrane, and f is an effective antigen valence.* When equilibrium is established between free and bound antigen

$$k_f CS = k_r m \tag{21}$$

and the three differential equations reduce to

$$m = KCS \tag{22}$$

$$\frac{dS}{dt} = -k_i LS \tag{23}$$

$$\frac{dL}{dt} = -k_i LS \tag{24}$$

From Eqs. (23) and (24) one can conclude S - L = constant = S(t = 0) - L(t = 0),** and thus

---

*In these equations the cross-linking rate k_i is measured on a per site basis and hence differs from Bell's k_i.

**From the assumption of equilibrium between free and bound antigen, it follows that $L(t = 0) \equiv L_0 = fKCS_0/(1 + KC)$ (DeLisi and Perelson, 1976).

$$\frac{dS}{dt} = -k_i S(S - \text{const}) \tag{25}$$

The extent of reaction p is given by the fraction of receptor sites which are bound, that is,

$$p(t) = \frac{S_0 - S(t)}{S} \tag{26}$$

where S_0 is the total concentration of receptor sites (free plus bound). Solving Eq. (25) with the initial condition $S(t = 0) = S_0$ and substituting the result into Eq. (26) determines p(t).

In Fig. 7 the dependence of a dimensionless critical patching time, $k_i S_0 t_c$, on KC is plotted for various values of the antigen valence. The curves show two asymptotes given by $KC = f - 1$ and $KC = 1/(f - 1)^2$. For values of KC greater than $1/(f - 1)^2$, or less than $f - 1$, large aggregates do not ever form, for intermediate values the patching time varies, reaching a minimum near $KC \approx 1$. When $f = 2$, infinite linear aggregates can form only when $KC = 1$.

Although most patching experiments use anti-Ig as a ligand, f should not be set equal to 2. Anti-Ig can combine with many sites on the receptor molecule and permit branched structures to form.

The valence f should not be regarded as the total number of antigenic determinants on an antigen because steric hindrance and the rigidity of the antigen molecule interfere with the availability of antigenic determinants for lattice formation. As a rough estimate, $f - 1$ equals the number of antigenic determinants on a membrane-bound antigen able to simultaneously interact with receptors. Thus the valence of DNP_{16}-human gamma globulin might be represented by a number considerably less than $f = 16$.

The rate $k_i S_0$ to establish a bond between one receptor and another will depend on the rate of diffusion of receptors in the membrane. Estimating this quantity by $k_i S_0 \gtrsim 0.1\ \text{sec}^{-1}$, Fig. 7 predicts minimum patching times on the order of 2 to 24 sec.

The hypothesis that patching is a necessary first step in lymphocyte activation may lead to a number of important conclusions. First, if patching must occur within a certain time period in order

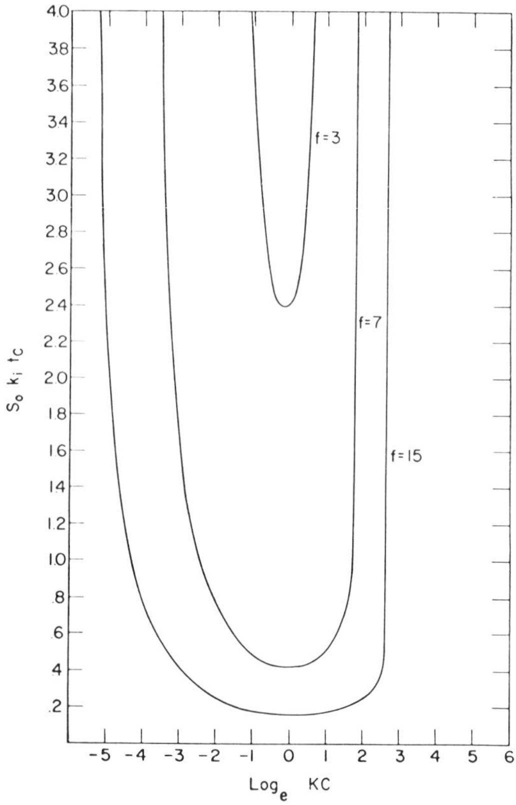

FIG. 7. The dependence of the rate of patching on antigen valence f, antigen concentration C, and receptor affinity K. The patching rate is plotted in a dimensionless form as $k_i S_0 t_c$. Notice that patching only occurs for a limited concentration range and that the size of the range increases with antigen valence. For any valence the minimum patching time occurs near ln KC = 0 or KC = 0. Reproduced from DeLisi and Perelson (1976).

to be an effective first stimulus, then Fig. 7 shows that there may be a limiting valence, f_c, below which triggering could not occur. This may mean that for an antigen with valence below f_c to trigger a B cell, an accessory cell would be needed in order to increase its effective valence. Second, from Fig. 7 one can see that for fixed f, patching occurs most rapidly when $KC \approx 1$ ($\ln KC \approx 0$), or $K \approx 1/C$. Assuming that the events subsequent to patching in the triggering process occur with little variation in rate, then one can associate differences in patching rates with differences in triggering rates. Thus, as C decreases during an immune response, the optimal value of K for rapid triggering of cells increases. The more rapid triggering of high affinity cells and the consequent proliferation of these cells would lead, over time, to an increase in the average serum antibody affinity. Such increases have been observed (Siskind and Benacerraf, 1969). This particular mechanism for the maturation of the immune response differs from those usually proposed (Siskind and Benacerraf, 1969), because it predicts the possibility of maturation even when antigen is in excess (DeLisi and Perelson, 1976). Third, since patching can occur only within a specified affinity-concentration range, one would also expect that triggering occurs only over a limited concentration range that is determined by the affinity of the B-cell receptor. Fourth, from the curves in Fig. 7 one would expect that there is an optimal antigen valence.

A variety of experimenters have obtained results consistent with some or all of these predictions. For example, Kishimoto and Ishizaka (1975) compared the responses to anti-Ig and DNP-ragweed fraction D (Rag) or DNP-Asc (Asc, *Ascaris suum* extract). For both classes of ligands they found an optimal concentration range for stimulation, which was narrower for anti-Ig than for DNP-carrier. This is in agreement with the predictions of Fig. 7, since anti-Ig has a lower effective valence than the DNP-carrier used. Recognizing that valence might be important, Kishimoto and Ishizaka (1975) then compared the responses to anti-Ig and polymerized anti-Ig. They found that the polymerized form stimulated lymphocytes over a larger concentration range than the monomer, and that for both monomer and polymer, 50 μg/ml was the most effective dose tested. Both of these observations are in agreement with Fig. 7, a higher valence gives a broader dose-response curve, and the optimal concentration is insensitive to valence always being near KC = 1. Not all data support the predictions of Fig. 7. For example, Feldmann (1972) has found that with a high substitution rate DNP-POL in vitro is tolerogenic rather than immunogenic.

Experiments on histamine release give additional support for the qualitative conclusions of this patching model. The reactions of either antigen or anti-IgE with cell-bound IgE on basophils and mast cells activates enzyme sequences for the release of histamine from these cells (Ishizaka and Ishizaka, 1969). Since bivalent $(Fab')_2$ fragments, but not monovalent (Fab') fragments, of pepsin-digested anti-IgE lead to histamine release, it has been suggested that cross-linking of cell bound IgE is necessary for histamine release (Ishizaka, 1963). When basophils of ragweed-sensitive individuals were incubated with either ragweed antigen E or anti-IgE the following observations were made: (a) the optimal concentration of anti-IgE for maximal histamine release was 10- to 1000-fold more than the corresponding concentration of antigen E, and (b) the optimal range of anti-IgE concentrations was much narrower than the range of antigen E concentrations needed for histamine release (Lichtenstein and Osler, 1964; Ishizaka et al., 1969). If the DeLisi-Perelson patching model applies, then the 10- to 1000-fold difference in optimal concentrations could be explained by corresponding differences in the affinity of surface-bound IgE for antigen E and anti-IgE. Similarly, the patching model would predict that since anti-IgE probably has a lower effective valence than antigen E, it would have a narrower optimal concentration range. It has been observed that membrane-bound IgE molecules can be redistributed into patches and caps by anti-IgE and antigen E, but not by monovalent anti-IgE (Sullivan et al., 1971; Becker et al., 1973). However, gross patching and capping were seen at high concentration of anti-IgE, while maximum histamine release occurred at lower concentrations with little redistribution (Becker et al., 1973). This suggests that if receptor redistribution is important in triggering histamine release, only small clusters may be required (Raff, 1975).

VII. B-CELL PROLIFERATION AND DIFFERENTIATION

After stimulation by either a specific antigen or a nonspecific mitogen, a small B lymphocyte, usually in a resting or G_0 phase of its cell cycle, undergoes blast transformation and becomes a large lymphocyte. A large B lymphocyte divides rapidly with generation times estimated to be between 6 and 48 hr (Eisen, 1973), and secretes modest amounts of antibody.* Such cells can further differentiate into terminal, nondividing, antibody secreting cells known as plasma cells. Plasma cells, which morphologically resemble secretory gland cells, can secrete antibody at rates estimated to be as high as 20,000 molecules per second (Conrad and Ingraham, 1974). However, plasma cells have relatively short mean lifetimes, estimated to range between 2 and 4 days (Ehrich, 1965), and die after a few or no cell divisions (Eisen, 1973, p. 470; Kuhlmann et al., 1975).

The mechanisms that determine whether a B cell proliferates or differentiates have not been fully elucidated. Recent experiments by Dutton (1974, 1975), Dutton and Hunter (1974), Hunter and Kettman (1974), Paul et al., (1974) and Hünig et al. (1974) have suggested that antigen alone is sufficient to cause B-cell proliferation, but that T cells are necessary to initiate differentiation and the start of immunoglobulin synthesis. The T-cell help appears to be mediated by a diffusible nondialysable factor, but the mechanisms regulating the secretion of this T-cell factor are unknown. No similar regulatory molecules have been isolated for responses due to T-independent antigens.

VIII. AN OPTIMAL CONTROL MODEL OF B-CELL PROLIFERATION AND DIFFERENTIATION

One method of determining possible regulatory mechanisms for B-cell proliferation and differentiation is to ascertain the optimal sequence of differentiation and proliferation steps available to the immune system when it responds to an antigenic challenge. However, such studies must be interpreted with care for there is

---

*The faster generation time seems more likely since stimulated lymphocytes in vitro have doubling times estimated to be between 4 and 8 hr (Dutton and Mishell, 1967); in vivo, Perkins et al. (1969) have found 6-hr doubling times.

certainly no a priori reason why the immune system, or any other biological system, should operate in an optimal fashion. Indeed, one may question whether the notion of an optimum can be given an operational meaning for many biological systems. Typically, an organism is forced to cope with a number of competing influences, so that improvement in one direction may involve a sacrifice in another. For example, while antibodies and the complement proteins help fight pathogenic organisms, they may also damage self components. Thus, in biology, optimum may have to be interpreted in some broad sense as a best compromise solution (for example, see Rocklin and Oster, 1976).

In the case of B cells, one may ask whether evolution has optimized them so that they proliferate and differentiate in a manner which leads to the quickest removal of antigen. Questions of this type can be answered by first constructing a mathematical model of the system, formulating an optimization criterion, and then using optimal control theory to compute the best strategy. If the calculated strategy is in accordance with observed behavior, then some insight has been gained about the evolution of the system and its current operating principles. If there is no agreement between reality and the model, then something else has been learned, either the system is not behaving optimally or the postulated objective criterion was incorrect. The biology may then be reassessed to determine if the model or the optimization criterion needs to be modified, or if natural selection, which generally makes improvements only on existing mechanisms, has become trapped in a "local maximum," where to reach a state of higher overall fitness would require a temporary, but possibly fatal, decrease in fitness.

A sequence of models, increasing in their realism and consequently their complexity, has been formulated of the immune response to a single injection of a nonreplicating T-independent antigen such as DNP-lys-LE (Perelson et al., 1976). To illustrate the techniques involved in computing the optimal behavior only the simplest model will be discussed; the strategy computed from the simple model is preserved in the full variety of structurally related models that have been studied.

A. The Model

Let S, L, and P denote the numbers of small B lymphocytes, large B lymphocytes, and plasma cells, respectively. Suppose small lymphocytes secrete no antibody, large lymphocytes secrete k antibodies/sec and plasma cells secrete γk antibodies/sec, where $\gamma \geqslant 1$. Then if A is the number of antibodies in the experimental animal, the rate of antibody secretion is given by

$$\frac{dA}{dt} = k(L + \gamma P) \tag{27}$$

Assume the injection of antigen has caused a fraction of the virgin B lymphocytes to undergo blast transformation resulting in a responding population at $t = 0$ of L_0 large lymphocytes. This population of large lymphocytes can proliferate with constant birth rate b, or they can differentiate into mature plasma cells at constant rate d. Lymphocytes and plasma cells "die" (i.e., are removed from the antibody-secreting state) at rates μ_L and μ_P, respectively. Plasma cells are assumed to be nondividing. Memory cells have not been included since the antigen is T independent. Thus for the large lymphocytes and plasma cells:

$$\frac{dL}{dt} = bu(t)L - d[1 - u(t)]L - \mu_L L \tag{28}$$

$$\frac{dP}{dt} = d[1 - u(t)]L - \mu_P P \tag{29}$$

where u(t) is the fraction of cells that remain large lymphocytes, and $1 - u(t)$ is the fraction that differentiates into plasma cells (see Fig. 8). As initial conditions, we assume $A(0) = P(0) = 0$ and $L(0) = L_0$.

In order to formulate an optimization criterion, suppose that an amount of antibody A^* is sufficient to neutralize the antigenic assault. Since the presence of the antigen can be assumed to be harmful to the organism, the optimal strategy (Perelson et al., 1976) examined is to choose u(t) so as to minimize the total time T required to secrete the amount of antibody A^*. Stated formally the optimization criterion is

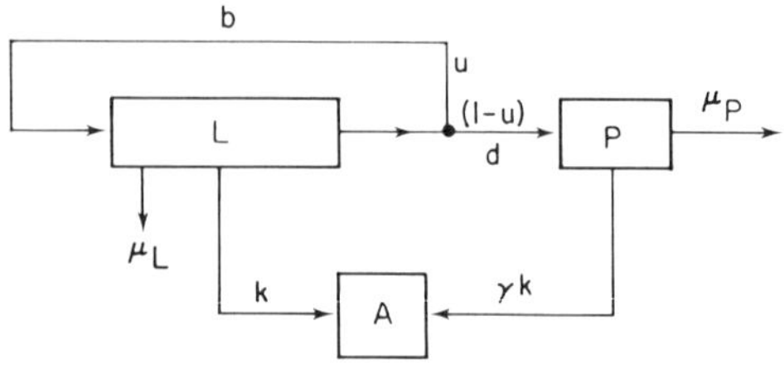

FIG. 8. Model of lymphocyte proliferation, differentiation, and antibody secretion. Large lymphocytes (L) divide at rate b, differentiate into plasma cells (P) at rate d, die at rate μ_L, and secrete antibody at rate k. The fraction of daughter cells that remain large lymphocytes is u, and 1 - u is the fraction that differentiates into plasma cells. Plasma cells do not divide, die at rate μ_P, and secrete antibody at rate γk. Reproduced from Perelson et al. (1976).

$$\min_u \int_0^T dt \tag{30}$$

where T is given by

$$A(T) = A^* \tag{31}$$

B. Optimal Strategy

Equations (27) to (31) constitute a bilinear optimal control problem which is amenable to solution by Pontryagin's maximum principle (cf Leitmann, 1966). In general, the maximum principle gives only necessary conditions for an optimal control. However, in this case the control satisfies a sufficiency condition as well (Perelson et al., 1976). Using reasonable assumptions about the parameter values, one can show that the strategies which produce the critical amount of antibody A* in shortest time are as follows.

1. If $(\gamma - 1)d \leqslant b$, then produce only large lymphocytes, that is, choose $u(t) = 1$, $0 \leqslant t \leqslant T$. This case, which has parameter values for which plasma cells hold no advantage over large lymphocytes, is not very realistic biologically. Either γ is near 1, so plasma cells secrete antibodies at nearly the same rate as lymphocytes, or d is small compared to b, so that it takes substantially

longer to differentiate into a plasma cell than to proliferate, or both. Clearly, when comparing the relative efficacies of lymphocytes and plasma cells over a given period of time, one must take into consideration that the lymphocytes are dividing and hence increasing their accumulated ability to secrete antibody, while the plasma cells are nondividing and dying and hence, as a population, producing ever-decreasing amounts of antibody. In the other case, which shall now be considered, plasma cells do have some advantage over lymphocytes but not necessarily for long periods of time.

2. If $(\gamma - 1)d > b$ then convert lymphocytes into plasma cells. The time at which this differentiation occurs depends on the antigen concentration, that is, the choice of A^*. If A^* is sufficiently small (roughly, small enough that one generation of plasma cells can produce A^*), choose $u(t) = 0$, $0 \leqslant t \leqslant T$, that is, immediately begin differentiating into plasma cells. The most realistic case occurs when A^* is large. Under these circumstances choose

$$u(t) = \begin{cases} 1 & 0 \leqslant t < t^* \\ 0 & t^* < t \leqslant T \end{cases} \tag{32}$$

In other words, the lymphocytes should first proliferate without differentiating. Then, at a critical time t^*, all proliferation should cease and the entire lymphocyte population should commence differentiating into plasma cells. The switching time t^* depends upon the values of the parameters $(b, d, \mu_L, \mu_P, k, \gamma)$, the antibody concentration A^*, and initial lymphocyte population size L_0. Intuitively, the switching time depends upon how long it takes to build up a substantial enough lymphocyte population so that the remaining antibody secretion can be performed by plasma cells. Let $\tau^* = T - t^*$. Thus τ^* is the time interval over which plasma cells are produced, while t^* is the interval over which large lymphocytes proliferate. Figure 9 shows that τ^* increases with γ and decreases with μ_P. Since $1/\mu_P$ is the mean plasma cell lifetime, τ^* increases somewhat with the plasma cell lifetime. In Fig. 10 we see that at high plasma cell secretion rates $(\gamma > 10)$, τ^* becomes nearly constant.

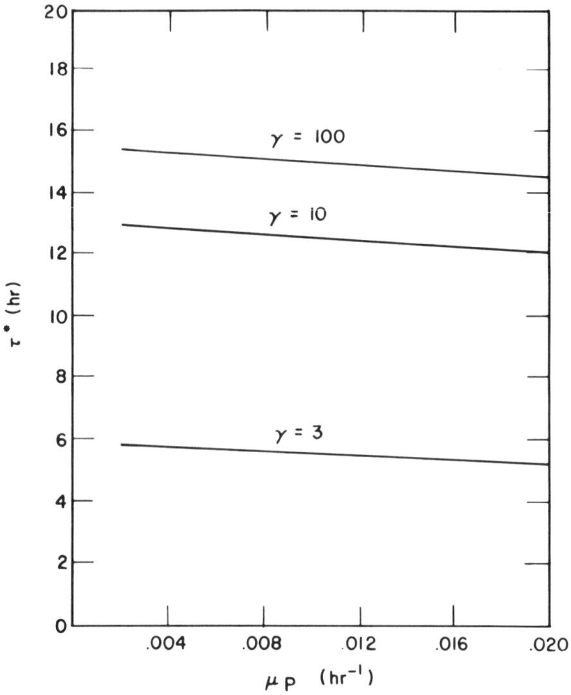

FIG. 9. The optimal length of time devoted to plasma cell production plotted as a function of the plasma cell death rate, for various values of μ_L and γ, the ratio of the plasma cell to the lymphocyte antibody secretion rate, with $b = 0.1\ hr^{-1}$. For each value of γ the curves for $\mu_L = 10^{-3}$, 10^{-4}, 10^{-5}, and $10^{-6}\ hr^{-1}$ are identical and are superimposed. Reproduced from Perelson et al. (1976).

Thus, regardless of how much faster plasma cells secrete antibodies than large lymphocytes, their finite lifetimes, when weighed against the benefits of being able to proliferate as a large lymphocyte, limit the length of time that should be devoted to plasma cell production. Figure 10 also shows that τ^* is not very dependent on the lymphocyte birth rate, but that increasing b decreases the total amount of time needed to secrete the critical amount of antibody. Since $t^* = T - \tau^*$, increasing b decreases t^*.

The type of solution in which the control takes just the two values 0 and 1 is known as *bang-bang control* in engineering or the *all-or-none principle* in biology. In engineering applications it

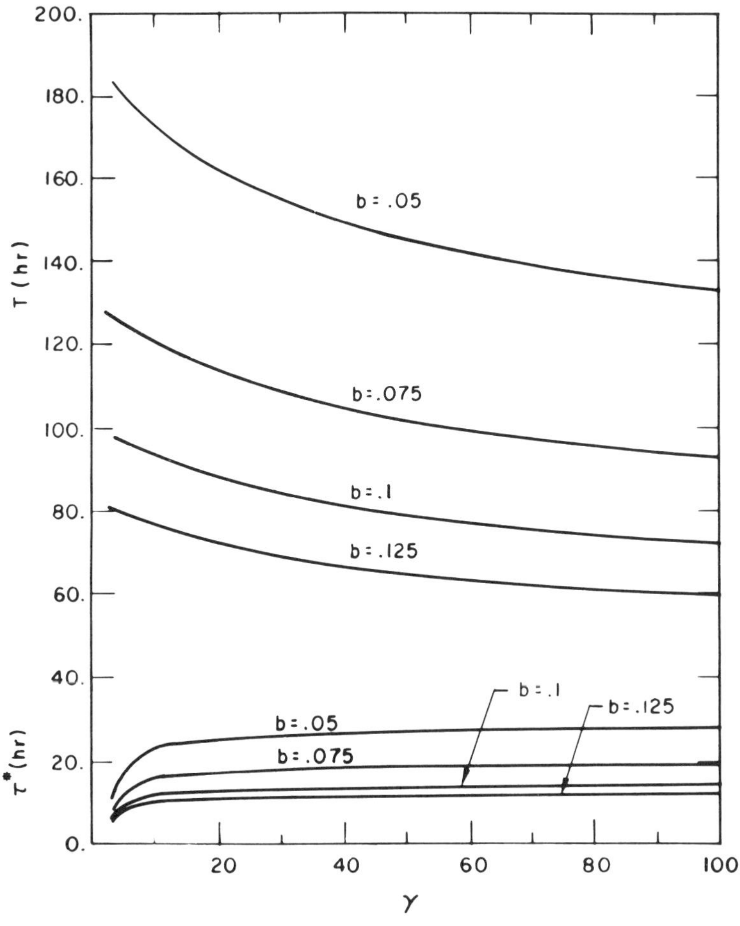

FIG. 10. The total time T it takes to secrete A* antibodies, and the length of time devoted to plasma cell production τ* when the optimal strategy is followed, plotted against γ for various values of the lymphocyte birth rate b measured in hr^{-1}, with $\mu_P = 0.02\ hr^{-1}$, $\mu_L = 10^{-5}\ hr^{-1}$, $L_0 = 4 \times 10^4$, $k = 10^3$ Ab $cell^{-1}\ sec^{-1}$, and $A^* = 5 \times 10^{-8}$ moles. Reproduced from Perelson et al. (1976).

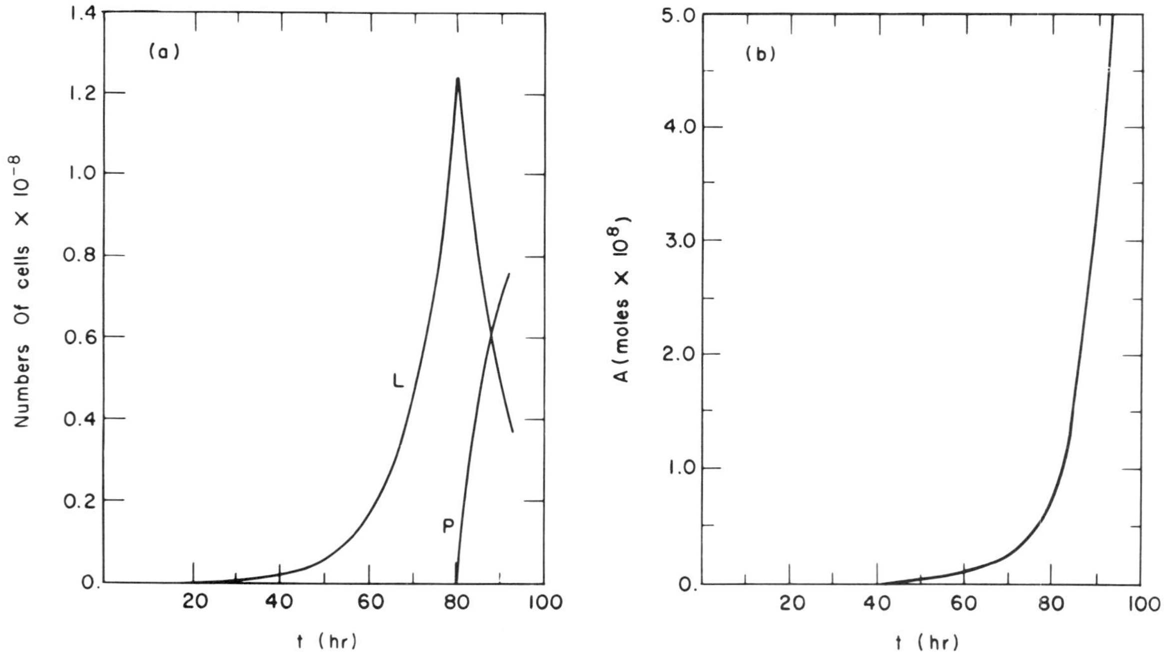

FIG. 11. The computed optimal dynamics of the immune response to a single injection of 50 μg DNP-lys-LE, a T-independent antigen. L, P, and A represent large lymphocytes, plasma cells, and antibody (IgM), with $\gamma = 10$, $d = b = 0.1\ hr^{-1}$, $\mu_P = 0.02\ hr^{-1}$, $\mu_L = 10^{-5}\ hr^{-1}$, $L_0 = 4 \times 10^4$, $k = 10^3$ Ab $cell^{-1}\ sec^{-1}$, and $A^* = 5 \times 10^{-8}$ moles. Reproduced from Perelson et al. (1976).

generally has been found to be less expensive to provide the capability of being in two extreme states than in all intermediate states. Similar consideration may play a role in optimizing by natural selection.

One word of caution is necessary. Although the control u(t) is bang-bang, all large lymphocytes do not immediately turn into plasma cells when u goes from 1 to 0 [see Eqs. (28) and (29), and Fig. 11].

The bang-bang strategy of lymphocyte proliferation and differentiation remains optimal under a variety of modifications of the basic model. Perelson et al. (1976) consider the following cases: (a) a time-varying rate of recruitment for large lymphocytes from the small lymphocyte pool is included; (b) antigen is explicitly considered and the goal is to reduce the antigen level to some tolerable level in minimal time; (c) the secretion rate k, or antibody affinity is allowed to increase with time; (d) time delays due to lymphocyte maturation are taken into account; and (e) the heterogeneity of the lymphocyte population is considered. In all cases except the last, the control is strictly bang-bang. However, differences between cells in birth and death rates or γ, the relative lymphocyte-plasma cell secretion rate, can cause individual cells to switch at different times. If such cell-to-cell variation is small, then the whole population will behave as if u(t) were a steep sigmoidal function going from 1 to 0 in a small time interval centered around $t = t^*$. This type of control would yield population behavior almost indistinguishable from the strict bang-bang case. Differences in the affinity of the antibody secreted by different cells, which could be large, do not produce any variation in the switching time in these models. Hence it was concluded that no graded response is as efficient as the all-or-none response for eliminating antigen in minimal time.

In order for lymphocytes to operate optimally there must exist a cellular switch which determines when proliferation and differentiation are to occur. Since the optimal control model deals only with cell populations, there is no need to specify detailed mechanisms at the cellular or molecular level to justify the model, so long as its conclusions do not contradict the accepted facts of cellular immunology. Although many models could be constructed, I shall briefly mention one model in order to demonstrate that such cellular switches are plausible. By best estimates, $(\gamma - 1)$ d is greater than b and hence one can rule out the case of no plasma cell development. For the remaining cases, the bang-bang control model predicts lymphocyte proliferation when the antigen concentration is high and differentiation into plasma cells when the antigen concentration is reduced to a level that could be eliminated by the plasma cells during their short lifetime. Assume an antigen is given in a high enough dose to cross-link receptors and trigger a cell, but not so high as to render the cell tolerant. By the mechanisms of patching and capping followed by the shedding and endocytosis of receptors, the receptor-antigen complexes are cleared from the cell surface. After about 8 hr new receptors are reexpressed on the membrane, and if the antigen concentration is in the appropriate range, capping and clearing can occur again (Unanue and Ault, 1974). Eventually the antigen concentration will fall and the cross-linking of new receptors will cease. This cessation of capping could then trigger differentiation. If the antigen dose is initially high enough to trigger the cells, but then falls below that needed to sustain capping, the cells would not proliferate before differentiating. This would correspond to the behavior predicted for low values of A*.

Direct experimental verification of the bang-bang control strategy may be difficult to obtain. The models we have developed all assume that antigen triggers an unspecified number, L_0, of large lymphocytes. If the antigen and its dose were such that the majority of clones capable of responding to the antigen were stimulated, then the predictions of the bang-bang control model would imply tolerance by immunological exhaustion (Howard, 1974), since in the model all stimulated lymphocytes become plasma cells. Hence after the response has subsided, one should find the animal depleted of cells capable of responding to a second challenge with the same antigen. Howard and Courtenay (1974) have obtained data which support this proposal. Following immunization with optimal doses of the T-independent antigens, levan or dextran B1355, they found that mice were unable to respond to a subsequent antigenic assault. Sterzl (1966) has also proposed immunological exhaustion as a mechanism for high zone tolerance.

At low antigen concentrations the optimal strategy again predicts that all responding cells differentiate into plasma cells. Except in this case, L_0 can not be expected to represent all possible responding clones. Since low antigen doses do preferentially stimulate high affinity cells, one would expect their elimination to leave only low affinity cells. Only a weak secondary response could ensue. Although most T-independent antigens do not show low zone tolerance, Waldmann and Pope (1975) have demonstrated this effect with lipopolysaccharide.

The hypothesis that the immune system responds to a T-independent antigen in a bang-bang fashion could most easily be disproved by kinetic studies. For example, if one could demonstrate substantial plasma cell production occurring simultaneously with lymphocyte proliferation, the predictions of the bang-bang strategy would be contradicted. One might expect some disagreement with kinetic experiments, since we have used an oversimplified model in which there are only three cell types; small lymphocytes, large lymphocytes, and plasma cells, and have neglected all intermediate states of differentiation. If necessary, more complicated models including other intermediate cell types, or even a continuum of differentiation states, can be devised and analyzed with optimal control theory.

ACKNOWLEDGMENTS

I would like to thank Leon Glass for suggesting that I examine the radial distribution function of surface immunoglobulin, and both Byron Goldstein and him for their helpful comments on the computation and interpretation of g(r). I also would like to thank Don Janney, Mike Cannon, and other members of the image analysis group at Los Alamos for their help and continuing interest.

This work was performed under the auspices of the U.S. Energy Research and Development Administration.

REFERENCES

Abbas, A. K., Ault, K. A., Karnovsky, M. J., and Unanue, E. R. (1975). Nonrandom distribution of surface immunoglobulin on murine B lymphocytes. *J. Immunol. 114:* 1197-1204.

Abbas, A. K., Dorf, M. E., Karnovsky, M. J., and Unanue, E. R. (1976). The distribution of Ia antigens on the surfaces of lymphocytes. *J. Immunol. 116:* 371-378.

Ault, K. A., Karnovsky, M. J., and Unanue, E. R. (1973). Studies on the distribution of surface immunoglobulin on human B lymphocytes. *J. Clin. Invest. 52:* 2507-2516.

Ault, K. A. and Unanue, E. R. (1974). Events after the binding of antigen to lymphocytes: removal and regeneration of antigen receptor. *J. Exp. Med. 139:* 1110-1124.

Becker, K. E., Ishizaka, T., Metzger, H., Ishizaka, K., and Grimely, P. M. (1973). Surface IgE on human basophils during histamine release. *J. Exp. Med. 138:* 394-409.

Bell, G. I. (1971). Mathematical model of clonal selection and antibody production. II. *J. Theor. Biol. 33:* 339-378.

Bell, G. I. (1974). Model for the binding of multivalent antigen to cells. *Nature 248:* 430-431.

Bell, G. I. (1975). B lymphocyte activation and lattice formation. *Transplant. Rev. 23:* 23-36.

Conrad, R. E. and Ingraham, J. S. (1974). Rate of hemolytic antibody production by single cells in vivo in rabbits. *J. Immunol. 112:* 17-25.

David, F. N. and Moore, P. G. (1954). Notes on contagious distributions in plant populations. *Ann. Bot. London N. S. 18:* 47-53.

DeLisi, C. and Perelson, A. S. (1976). The kinetics of aggregation phenomena. I. Minimal models for patch formation on lymphocyte membranes. *J. Theor. Biol. 62:* 159-210.

de Petris, A. and Raff, M. C. (1973). Normal distribution, patching and capping of lymphocyte surface immunoglobulin studies by electron microscopy. *Nature New Biology 241:* 257-259.

de Petris, S. (1975). Concanavalin A receptors, immunoglobulins, and θ antigens of the lymphocyte surface. *J. Cell Biol. 65:* 123-146.

Dutton, R. W. (1974) T-cell factor in the regulation of B-cell response. In *The Immune System: Genes, Receptors, Signals* (E. E. Sercarz, A. R. Williamson, and C. F. Fox, eds.), Academic, New York, pp. 485-496.

Dutton, R. W. (1975). Separate signals for the induction of proliferation and differentiation in the B-cell response to antigen. *Transplant. Rev. 23:* 66-77.

Dutton, R. W. and Hunter, P. (1974). The effects of mitogen stimulated T-cells on the response of B-cell to antigen and the mechanism of T-cell stimulation of the B-cell response. In *Cellular Selection and the Regulation of the Immune Response* (G. M. Edelman, ed.). Raven, New York, pp. 199-215.

Dutton, R. W. and Mishell, R. I. (1967). Cellular events in the immune response. The in vitro response of normal spleen cells to erythrocyte antigens. *Cold Spring Harbor Symp. Quant. Biol. 32:* 407-414.

Edelman, G. M., Yahara, I., and Wang, J. L. (1973). Receptor mobility and receptor-cytoplasmic interactions in lymphocytes. *Proc. Nat. Acad. Sci. (USA) 70:* 1442-1446.

Edidin, M., Zagyansky, Y., and Lardner, T. J. (1976). Measurement of membrane protein lateral diffusion in single cells. *Science 191:* 466-468.

Egelstaff, P. A. (1967). *An Introduction to the Liquid State.* Academic, New York.

Ehrich, W. E. (1965). Lymphoid tissues: their morphology and role in the immune response. In *Immunological Diseases* (M. Samter and H. L. Alexander, eds.). Little, Brown, & Co., Boston, pp. 251-277.

Eisen, H. N. (1973). Immunology. In *Microbiology* 2nd ed. (B. D. Davis, R. Dulbecco, H. N. Eisen, H. S. Ginsberg, and W. B. Wood, eds.). Harper and Row, New York, pp. 349-624.

Engers, H. D. and Unanue, E. R. (1973). The fate of anti-Ig-surface Ig complexes on B lymphocytes. *J. Immunol. 110:* 465-475.

Farrell, R. A. and Hart, R. W. (1969). On the theory of the spatial organization of macromolecules in connective tissue. *Bull. Math. Biophys. 31:* 727-760.

Feldmann, M. (1972). Induction of immunity and tolerance in vitro by hapten protein conjugates. I. The relationship between the degree of hapten conjugation and the immunogenecity of dinitrophenylated polymerized flagellin. *J. Exp. Med. 135:* 735-753.

Flory, P. J. (1941). Molecular size distributions in three dimensional polymers. *J. Am. Chem. Soc. 63:* 3083-3100.

Goldberg, R. J. (1952). A theory of antibody-antigen reactions. I. Theory for reactions of multivalent antigen with bivalent and univalent antibody. *J. Am. Chem. Soc. 74:* 5715-5725.

Hill, T. (1956). *Statistical Mechanics.* McGraw-Hill, New York.

Howard, J. G. (1974). Three categories of B-cell tolerance induced by polysaccharides: characteristics, interrelationship and general implication. In *Immunological Tolerance: Mechanisms and Potential Therapeutic Applications* (D. H. Katz and B. Benacerraf, eds.). Academic, New York, pp. 163-180.

Howard, J. G. and Courtenay, B. M. (1974). Induction of B cell tolerance to polysaccharides by exhaustive immunization and during immunosuppression with cyclophosphomide. *Eur. J. Immunol. 4:* 603-608.

Hünig, T., Schimpl, A., and Wecker, A. (1974). Autoradiographic studies on the proliferation of antibody-producing cells in vitro. *J. Exp. Med. 139:* 754-760.

Hunter, P. and Kettman, J. R. (1974). Model of action of a T-cell supernatant activity which nonspecifically stimulates the humoral immune response. *Proc. Nat. Acad. Sci. (USA) 71:* 512-516.

Ishizaka, K. (1963). Gamma globulin and molecular mechanisms by hypersensitivity reaction. *Prog. Allergy 7:* 32-106.

Ishizaka, K. and Ishizaka, T. (1969). Immune mechanisms of reversed type reaginic hypersensitivity. *J. Immunol. 103:* 588-595.

Ishizaka, T., Ishizaka, K., Johansson, S. G. O., and Bennich, H. (1969). Histamine release from human leukocytes by anti-γE antibodies. *J. Immunol. 102:* 884-892.

Karnovsky, M. J., Unanue, E. R., and Leventhal, M. (1972). Ligand-induced movement of lymphocyte membrane macromolecules. II. Mapping of surface moieties. *J. Exp. Med. 136:* 907-930.

Katz, D. H., Davie, J. M., Paul, W. E., and Benacerraf, B. (1971) Carrier function in anti-hapten antibody responses. IV. Experimental conditions for the induction of hapten-specific tolerance or for the stimulation of anti-hapten anamnestic responses by "nonimmunogenic" hapten-polypeptide conjugates. *J. Exp. Med. 134:* 201-223.

Katz, D. H. and Unanue, E. R. (1972). The immune capacity of lymphocytes after cross-linking of surface immunoglobulin receptors by antibody. *J. Immunol. 109:* 1022-1030.

Kishimoto, T. and Ishizaka, K. (1975). Regulation of antibody response in vitro. IX. Induction of secondary anti-hapten antibody release by antiimmunoglobulin and enhancing soluble factor. *J. Immunol. 114:* 585-591.

Kishimoto, T., Miyake, T., Nishizawa, Y., Watanabe, T., and Yamamura, Y. (1975). Triggering mechanism of B lymphocytes. I. Effects of anti-immunoglobulin and enhancing soluble factor on differentiation and proliferation of B cells. *J. Immunol. 115:* 1179-1184.

Klaus, G. G. B. and Humphrey, J. H. (1974). The immunological properties of haptens coupled to thymus independent carrier molecules. I. Characteristics of the immune response to DNP-lysine-substituted SIII and levan. *Eur. J. Immunol. 4:* 370-377.

Kuhlmann, W. D., Bouteille, M., and Avrameas, S. (1975). Correlation of cell division and specific protein production during the course of lymphoid cell differentiation. *Exp. Cell Res. 76:* 335-343.

Leitmann, G. (1966). *An Introduction to Optimal Control.* McGraw-Hill, New York.

Lichtenstein, L. M. and Osler, A. G. J. (1964). Studies on the mechanisms of hypersensitivity phenomena. IX. Histamine release from human leukocytes by ragweed pollen antigen. *J. Exp. Med. 120:* 507-530.

Lipscomb, M. F., Holmes, K. V., Vitetta, E. S., Hammerling, U., and Uhr, J. W. (1975). Cell surface immunoglobulin. XII. Localization of immunoglobulin on murine lymphocytes by scanning immunoelectron-microscopy. *Eur. J. Immunol. 5:* 255-259.

Lloyd, M. (1967). Mean crowding. *J. Anim. Ecol. 36:* 1-30.

Loor, F. and Hägg, L. B. (1975). The modulation of microprojections on the lymphocyte membrane and the redistribution of membrane-bound ligands, a correlation. *Eur. J. Immunol. 5:* 854-865.

Markovics, J., Glass, L., and Maul, G. G. (1974). Pore patterns on nuclear membranes. *Exp. Cell Res. 85:* 443-451.

Mikolaj, P. G. and Pings, C. J. (1968). The use of the coordination number in the interpretation of fluid structure. *Phys. Chem. Liquids 1:* 93-108.

Paul, W. E., Karpf, M., and Mosier, D. E. (1974). Activation and tolerance induction in DNP specific B-cells: Analysis with three distinct DNP-carrier conjugates. In *Immunological Tolerance: Mechanisms and Potential Therapeutic Applications* (D. H. Katz and B. Benacerraf, eds.), Academic, New York, pp. 140-158.

Perelson, A. S., Mirmirani, M., and Oster, G. F. (1976). Optimal strategies in immunology. I. B-cell differentiation and proliferation. *J. Math. Biol. 3:* 325-367.

Perkins, E. H., Sado, T., and Makinodan, T. (1969). Recruitment and proliferation of immunocompetent cells during the log phase of the primary antibody response. *J. Immunol. 103:* 668-678.

Pielou, E. C. (1969). *An Introduction to Mathematical Ecology.* Wiley-Interscience, New York.

Rabellino, E., Colon, S., Grey, H. M., and Unanue, E. R. (1971). Immunoglobulins on the surface of lymphocytes. I. Distribution and quantitation. *J. Exp. Med. 133:* 156-167.

Raff, M. C. (1975). Histamine release from mast cells: An unusually accessible model of ligand-induced cell response. In *Regulation of Growth and Differentiated Function in Eukaryote Cells* (G. P. Talwar, ed.). Raven, New York, pp. 177-184.

Reed, T. M. and Gubbins, K. E. (1973). *Applied Statistical Mechanics.* McGraw-Hill, New York.

Rocklin, S. and Oster, G. (1976). Competition between phenotypes. *J. Math. Biol. 3:* 225-261.

Singer, S. J. and Nicholson, G. L. (1972). The fluid mosaic model of the structure of cell membranes. *Science 175:* 720-731.

Siskind, G. W. and Benacerraf, B. (1969). Cell selection by antigen in the immune response. *Adv. Immunol. 10:* 1-50.

Sterzl, J. (1966). Immunological tolerance as the result of terminal differentiation of immunologically competent cells. *Nature 209:* 416-417.

Stockmayer, W. H. (1943). Theory of molecular size distributions and gel formation in branched-chain polymers. *J. Chem. Phys. 11:* 45-55.

Sullivan, A. L., Grimely, P. M., and Metzger, H. (1971). Electron microscopic localization of immunoglobulin E on the surface membrane of human basophils. *J. Exp. Med. 134:* 1403-1416.

Taylor, R. B., Duffus, W. P. H., Raff, M. C., and de Petris, S. (1971). Redistribution and pinocytosis of lymphocyte surface immunoglobulin molecules induced by anti-immunoglobulin antibody. *Nature New Biology 223:* 225-229.

Unanue, E. R. (1974). Cellular events following binding of antigen to lymphocytes. *Am. J. Pathol. 77:* 2-22.

Unanue, E. R. and Ault, K. A. (1974). Functional relationships in antigen-receptor interaction in B lymphocytes. In *Immunological Tolerance: Mechanisms and Potential Therapeutic Applications* (D. H. Katz and B. Benacerraf, eds.). Academic, New York, pp. 301-310.

Unanue, E. R., Ault, K. A., and Karnovsky, M. J. (1974). Ligand induced movement of lymphocyte surface macromolecules. IV. Stimulation of cell motility by anti-Ig and lack of relationship to capping. *J. Exp. Med. 139:* 295-312.

Unanue, E. R. and Karnovsky, M. J. (1973). Redistribution and fate of Ig complexes on surface of B lymphocyte: functional implications and mechanisms. *Transplant. Rev. 14:* 184-210.

Waldmann, H. and Pope, H. (1975). Low dose unresponsiveness with a thymus independent antigen. *Nature 258:* 730-731.

Warner, N. L. (1974). Membrane immunoglobulins and antigen receptors on B and T lymphocytes. *Adv. Immunol. 19:* 67-216.

Yahara, I. and Edelman, G. M. (1973). Modulation of lymphocyte receptor redistribution by concanavalin A, anti-mitotic agents and alterations of pH. *Nature 246:* 152-155.

Zar, J. H. (1974). *Biostatistical Analysis.* Prentice Hall, Englewood Cliffs, New Jersey, p. 301.

Chapter 8

SOME PHYSICAL-CHEMICAL ASPECTS OF CELLULAR SELECTION IN AN IMMUNE RESPONSE

Charles DeLisi

Laboratory of Theoretical Biology
National Cancer Institute
National Institutes of Health
Bethesda, Maryland

The requirement that antigens form relatively stable complexes with B cell bound receptors, perhaps by cross-linking them, leads to a number of predictions related to the mean thermodynamic properties and inhibitability of the cells selected to respond. In this paper I pursue the physical-chemical consequences of the assumption that B-cell activation requires the initial rate of cross-linking to exceed some minimum value. The model predicts that the heterogeneity and mean affinity of the population of responders, as well as the inhibitability of the response, may be strongly dependent upon receptor density, membrane fluidity, and receptor hinge flexibility (and therefore, perhaps also class), as well as on antigenic dose. Moreover, it is shown that the *qualitative* features of the dose dependence of response characteristics can change as a function of the quantitative relations among the model parameters. The theory suggests that strong selective pressures may be generated during the response as a consequence of a subtle interplay among a variety of parameters, and not just by a decrease in antigen concentration. A number of easily testable predictions are made which may help clarify the role of these parameters under various experimental conditions.

I. INTRODUCTION

Immunoglobulins (Igs) are proteins consisting of paired heavy and light polypeptide chains as illustrated in Fig. 1. Studies of amino acid composition reveal that for any given chain, the sequence of the first 110 residues varies significantly from one Ig to the next, and that within this region a few subsequences are *hypervariable*. Since both local and long-range primary structure (sequence) are expected to have an important influence on three-dimensional geometry, such hypervariability might be expected to confer distinctive and diverse structural features on a large number* of immunoglobulins,

---

*For a theory of how large this number actually needs to be, see Inman, Chap. 9.

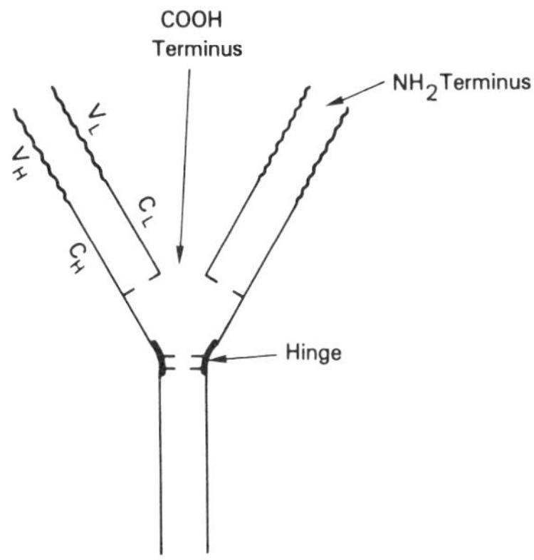

FIG. 1. Schematic of an immunoglobulin consisting of two heavy and two light polypeptide chains. The sequence in each can be divided into two regions: one in which the amino acid composition is peculiar to that particular molecule, (V_H and V_L) and another in which it is relatively invariant (C_H and C_L). The dashed lines represent the disulfide bonds which hold the chains together.

precisely the properties necessary if the immune system is to recognize the wide variety of antigenic determinants to which it may be exposed. Wu and Kabat (1970) were thus led to speculate that the spatial arrangement formed by the three-dimensional folding of these hypervariable regions with one another comprises the antigen binding site; a prediction which has since been verified by X-ray diffraction at a 2 Å level (Amzel et al., 1974; Edmundson et al., 1974), on several different immunoglobulins. All evidence indicates that there is one combining site for each heavy-light chain couple, and that all couples on a particular Ig are identical.

The remaining residues on each chain are relatively invariant and are therefore said to form the *constant* region. However, characteristic sequence and antigenic properties of heavy chain constant regions suggest that immunoglobulins can be grouped into five major *classes*, labeled, G, M, E, D, and A. In addition, a portion of this region, the *hinge*, exhibits conformational flexibility, thus allowing relative lateral combining site motion. It is evident that because the hinge is in the heavy chain constant region, the extent of its flexibility may be a class-dependent property.

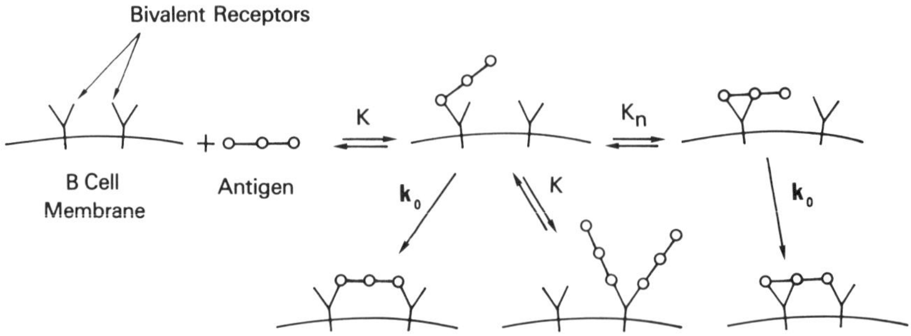

FIG. 2. A simple kinetic model for the binding of antigen to B cell bound receptor showing the possible states of antigen shortly after reaction has begun. K is the equilibrium constant for the antigen molecule receptor site interaction; K_n the intramolecular equilibrium constant, and k_0 the forward rate constant for receptor cross-linking.

Aside from their role as antibodies, immunoglobulins occur as receptors on the lymphocyte plasma membranes. According to current ideas, the precursors of antibody-secreting cells (B lymphocytes) are phenotypically committed, prior to antigenic contact, to the expression of a single light and single heavy chain variable region gene, the products of which serve as the amino terminal portion of B-cell receptors, as well as of antibodies ultimately secreted by B-cell progeny. The role of antigen is to select from the heterogeneous population of precursors, those possessing appropriately reactive membrane-bound receptors and to trigger these into clonal expansion and antibody production; the former process implying cellular proliferation and the latter differentiation.

It has, however, become apparent in recent years that rather than trigger activation, binding may lead to tolerance; i.e., to unresponsiveness to a subsequently administered normally immunogenic dose of antigen. Moreover, even when binding triggers activation, the relation between the extent of proliferation and differentiation may depend upon the details of the interaction as well as the concentrations of T cells (thymus-dependent lymphocytes), macrophages, and a variety of antigen-specific and nonspecific factors which they secrete. There is in fact considerable evidence indicating that for many antigens, an effective antibody response can occur only in the presence of T cells (see for example, Katz and Benacerraf, 1972; Feldmann and Nossal, 1972).

The effectiveness of a humoral (antibody-mediated) response will depend upon its intensity and its physical-chemical characteristics. The former refers to quantity of antibody produced in a given period of time; the latter to rate constant and affinity distributions, their time evolution, and dose dependence. Although T-cell factors affect response intensity, physical-chemical characteristics are expected to be strongly dependent upon the details of the interaction of B cells with antigen. In this paper, attention will be confined only to the physical-chemical aspects of the response, and only the interaction of B-cell receptors with antigen will be considered explicitly. However, as explained below, other factors may be included implicitly in the development.

When multivalent antigen interacts with bivalent receptor, there are several physically distinct binding possibilities. Antigen may be monovalently bound; multivalently bound by a single receptor (i.e., intramolecularly bound) or multivalently bound by two receptors, thus cross-linking them. These are the base states of the antigen; the fundamental complexes from which other surface aggregates can be composed (Fig. 2). The relative likelihood of each is expected to depend upon such things as: (a) antigen-receptor affinity, (b) antigenic structure and concentration, (c) receptor structure and concentration, and perhaps, (d) membrane fluidity; (a) through (d) will be referred to as the parameters of the model. As they change, the relative concentrations of the base states change, and this influrences the pattern of complexes on the surface of the membrane.

In order to relate these physical-chemical features to response characteristics, something must be said of the requirements for B-cell activation. A simple hypothesis which is consistent with current concepts and data is that the extent of cross-linking must exceed some critical value within some reasonable amount of time (see, e.g., Bell, 1975). This assumption does not imply that cross-linking is sufficient for activation nor does it imply that it provides a signal. What it says is that: (a) a certain amount of cross-linking is necessary for activation and (b) this certain amount must occur within a required time. As suggested by Coutinho and Möller (1974), cross-linking might be required merely to stabilize the antigen-cell complex. In any case, starting with the hypothesis embodied in (a) and (b), simple expressions can be developed relating the parameters of the model to the physical characteristics of the selected cells.

Before deriving explicit expressions, I would like to make a few remarks about the philosophical orientation of the paper. First, no attempt is made to present a quantitative theory. The purpose of the mathematical development is to allow a *qualitative* study of the logical consequences of the model while considering all parameters simultaneously. This provides some insight into possible relations among the parameters and leads to experimental predictions which might otherwise have gone unnoticed, and which in the present case turn out to be especially simple to test.

The attitude with regard to T-cell factors is that if they affect the physical-chemical characteristics of the response, they enter the theory parametrically through the rate constants. For example, specific T-cell factors might affect k_0 (Fig. 2) and therefore the rate of cross-linking. A theory of the dependence of rate constants on various ancillary factors is more fundamental and more difficult and will not be attempted here. Of course, T-cell factors may also have other effects; e.g., they might increase B-cell membrane permeability. However, effects of this sort which influence neither the binding of antigen to receptor nor the cross-linking rate, are expected to be involved in response intensity, rather than the physical aspects of selection.

II. THEORY

A. The Model

Figure 2 represents the simplest physical-chemical model of cross-linking in the presence of intramolecular bond formation. For heuristic reasons, the equilibrium constant K_n for this reaction will be written as the product of a geometrical factor A and a bimolecular equilibrium constant for the antigen receptor site interaction K (DeLisi and Crothers, 1971; Crothers and Metzger, 1972) so that

$$K_n = AK \tag{1}$$

The parameter A is expected to depend primarily on the structure of the hinge (and therefore antibody class), but its magnitude is not known a priori. Qualitatively, if the hinge is flexible, intramolecular bonding is expected to be relatively favorable and A relatively large. If the hinge is stiff, so that there are severe constraints placed upon the distance between combining sites, and this does not happen to coincide with the spacing between determinants, intramolecular bonding will be unlikely, and A will be small.

Antigen-receptor complexes are supposed to develop initially by pairwise interactions among the four species shown in Fig. 3a, except for the m_2, m_3 interaction, which is not possible. The resulting complexes may then interact among themselves forming larger aggregates, and so on. When monovalent hapten which can compete with antigen for receptors (but which cannot stimulate the cell) is also present, additional states must be allowed, as shown in Fig. 3b.

If it is supposed that reversible chemical reaction comes to equilibrium quickly on the time scale of cross-linkage formation

(a)

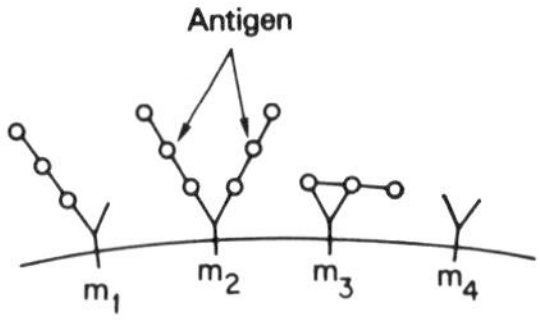

(b)

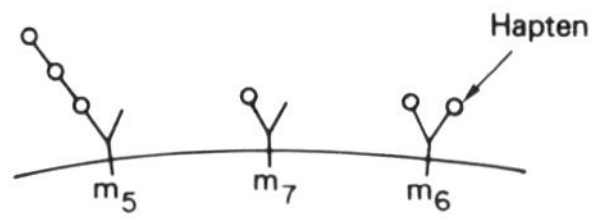

FIG. 3. The membrane complexes, allowed by the model, just prior to cross-linkage formation. The m_i are the concentrations of receptor molecules in state i; (a) possible states in the absence of inhibitory hapten, (b) additional states which must be allowed when hapten is present.

(Bell, 1974; DeLisi and Perelson, 1976), then R, the initial rate of cross-linking, is given by (Appendix A)

$$R = \frac{4k_0\rho_0^2 KcZ[Z + (f - 2)K_n/(f - 1)]}{(Z^2 + 2K_n Kc)^2} \tag{2}$$

where c is the concentration of antigen in solution, k_0 the forward rate constant for antigen receptor site interaction in the plane of the membrane, ρ_0 the total receptor density on a cell, f the effective antigen valence, and

$$Z \equiv 1 + Kh + Kc \equiv 1 + Kcy \tag{3}$$

h being the concentration of free (and in this case, also total) hapten in solution. Upon introducing the dimensionless cross-linking rate

$$\xi \equiv \frac{R}{4k_0\rho_0^2}$$

Eq. (2) becomes

$$\xi = \frac{KcZ[Z + (f - 2)K_n/(f - 1)]}{(Z^2 + 2K_nKc)^2} \tag{4}$$

When $K_n = 0$, Eq. (4) reduces to (Bell, 1975)

$$\xi = \frac{Kc}{Z^2} \tag{5}$$

If chemical reaction in the plane of the membrane is diffusion-controlled, then k_0 is expected to be a function of temperature and membrane fluidity, as well as the intrinsic reactivity of a receptor for the antigenic determinant under consideration.

B. The Parameters

The parameters under direct experimental control are c and h. Antigenic determinant concentrations used for in vitro stimulation commonly range from 10^{-5} to 10^{-11} M, and for any particular value, concentrations of monovalent hapten up to two orders of magnitude in excess may be introduced to produce varying degrees of response inhibition. Thus, reasonable constraints on c and y are

$$(10^{-11} \leqslant c \leqslant 10^{-5})\ \mathrm{M} \tag{6}$$

and

$$1 \leqslant y \leqslant 100 \tag{7}$$

For affinities I will assume that

$$(10^4 \leqslant K \leqslant 10^9)\ \mathrm{M}^{-1} \tag{8}$$

although certain parts of this range may be preferentially stimulated by a given antigenic dose.

The parameters A and ξ are more difficult to estimate. A will depend both on hinge structure and the density of antigenic determinants. For a freely jointed hinge and sufficiently high density (Crothers and Metzger, 1972), $A \approx 6 \times 10^{-4}$ M. An analysis of the binding of bivalent IgG to a dense array of determinants gives a result about half this large (DeLisi, 1976). However, receptors are often of the IgM or IgD class (Vitetta and Uhr, 1975). For the former, there is some evidence that the hinge region may be somewhat more restricted, so that A might be reduced by one or two orders of magnitude (DeLisi, 1975). For the latter class nothing is known. As a possible range I will take

$$(6 \times 10^{-4} \leqslant A \leqslant 6 \times 10^{-7})\ \mathrm{M} \tag{9}$$

Finally, variability in ξ_c, the threshold value of ξ below which activation is not possible, is expected to arise as a consequence of variations in ρ_0 and k_0. Bell (1974) has estimated that with 10^5 receptors per cell, $k_0\rho_0 \geqslant 0.03\ \mathrm{sec}^{-1}$. However, the possibility that ρ_0 may change with cell cycle and the state of differentiation should not be excluded. Similarly, membrane viscosity variations (and hence variations in diffusion coefficient) are possible. I will consider

$$(0.5 \leqslant k_0\rho_0 \leqslant 5 \times 10^{-3})\ \mathrm{sec}^{-1}$$

so that, for example, if activation requires 10% of the receptors cross-linked in 300 sec (typical patching times are a few minutes),

$$10^{-4} \leqslant \xi_c \leqslant 10^{-2} \tag{10}$$

More will be said, below, about the value of this parameter.

III. CELLULAR SELECTION

A. Mean Thermodynamic Properties

In order to obtain expressions for mean free energy and affinity, some assumption must be made about the distribution of precursor receptor free energies. From structural considerations one would expect the distribution in a virgin animal to be a monotonically decreasing function of free energy. The idea is that strong binding (i.e., high free energy and affinity) requires a rather precise fit between determinant and combining site, and one therefore expects relatively few receptors to possess the necessary structural features. As affi ity drops, the fit is not as precise, and consequently a larger number of receptors should be available. For simplicity I will suppose that the distribution drops exponentially as the free energy increases, so that n(G) dG, the fraction of cells having receptors with free energy between G and G + dG is

$$n(G)\ dG = B \exp \frac{-\alpha G}{RT}\ dG \qquad B > 0, \quad \alpha > 0 \tag{11}$$

where the thermal energy RT has been included for convenience. The distribution of receptor free energies should be clearly distinguished from the distribution of antibody affinity; the latter will reflect both the receptor distribution and the triggering mechanism and is expected to be peaked (DeLisi, 1976).

In terms of Eq. (11), the mean free energy $\langle G \rangle$ is given by

$$\langle G \rangle = \frac{\int_{G_1}^{G_2} G \exp(-\alpha G/RT)\ dG}{\int_{G_1}^{G_2} \exp(-\alpha G/RT)\ dG} \tag{12}$$

where G_1 and G_2 are the lowest and highest free energies associated with the response, that is, G_1 and G_2 delimit the range of cells selected. Carrying out the integration, one has that

$$\frac{\langle G \rangle}{RT} = \frac{1}{\alpha} + \frac{G_2}{RT} - \frac{(G_2 - G_1)w}{RT} \tag{13}$$

where

$$w \equiv \frac{1}{1 - \exp\ [-\alpha(G_2 - G_1)/RT]} \equiv \frac{1}{1 - (K_1/K_2)^{\alpha}} \tag{14}$$

with K_1 and K_2 representing the equilibrium constants associated with G_1 and G_2, respectively.

Defining a mean affinity $\langle K \rangle$ as

$$\langle K \rangle = \exp \frac{\langle G \rangle}{RT} \tag{15}$$

and substituting Eq. (13), one has that

$$\langle K \rangle = \exp \frac{1}{\alpha} K_2 \left(\frac{K_1}{K_2}\right)^w \tag{16}$$

It is at this point that specification of the model becomes important. For the particular one under consideration, an equation for the affinity cutoffs can be obtained by substituting $\xi = \xi_c$ into Eq. (4). The behavioral possibilities turn out to be rather varied and cannot all be considered in a short chapter. Therefore, rather than consider the entire range of every parameter, I will confine the analysis only to parameter domains for which particularly simple and interesting expressions can be obtained.

1. *Effectively Monovalent Receptors* (A = 0)

This case has its greatest range of validity when intramolecular reaction is relatively unfavorable, that is, when motion of the receptor hinge is highly restricted and/or antigenic determinant density is low. In Appendix B it is shown that

$$K_1 = \frac{g_1}{c} \tag{17}$$

and

$$K_2 = \frac{g_2}{c} \tag{18}$$

where g_1 and g_2 are functions of ξ_c and y as defined in Appendix B. Substituting Eqs. (17) and (18) into Eq. (16)

$$\langle K \rangle = \exp \frac{1}{\alpha} \quad g_2 \frac{(g_1/g_2)^w}{c} \tag{19}$$

For this case the model predicts a simple mass action type of expression

$$\langle K \rangle \; c = \text{const} \tag{20}$$

provided y is kept constant, with the constant having a form shown in Eq. (19) and being a function of receptor density, cross-linking rate constant, and perhaps, if diffusion limits the rate of chemical reaction, membrane viscosity (and therefore temperature; DeLisi and Metzger, 1976).

2. *Bivalent Receptors* ($A \neq 0$)

In this case (Appendix C)

$$K_1 = \frac{1}{2A'}\left[\left(\frac{1 + 4\xi_c A'}{c}\right)^{1/2} - 1\right] \tag{21}$$

and

$$K_2 = \frac{y(cy + A')}{\xi_c (cy^2 + 2A)^2} \tag{22}$$

so that

$$\langle K \rangle = \frac{\exp\ (1/\alpha(y(cy + A')}{\xi_c (cy^2 + 2A)^2}\left\{\frac{\xi_c [(1 + 4\xi_c A'/c)^{1/2} - 1](cy^2 + 2A)^2}{2A'y(cy + A')}\right\}^w \tag{23}$$

where w is given by Eq. (14) and is a function of the ratio K_1/K_2. Equation (23) may assume a number of different functional forms depending upon the quantitative relations among the parameters. For example

$$\langle K \rangle = \begin{cases} \exp \dfrac{1}{\alpha}\left(\dfrac{16\xi_c^3 A^4}{cy^2 A'^3}\right)^{w/2} \dfrac{yA'}{4\xi_c A^2} & c \ll \min\left\{\dfrac{2A}{y^2},\ 4\xi_c A'\right\} \quad \text{(24a)} \\[2ex] \exp \dfrac{1}{\alpha}\left[\dfrac{(\xi_c^3 c^3 y^6/A')^{1/2}}{cy + A'}\right]^w \dfrac{cy + A'}{\xi_c c^2 y^3} & \dfrac{1}{y^2} \ll \dfrac{c}{2A} \ll 4\xi_c \dfrac{f - 2}{f - 1} \quad \text{(24b)} \end{cases}$$

Equations 24 were obtained using

$$K_1 = \left(\frac{\xi_c}{A'c}\right)^{1/2} \qquad c \ll 4\xi_c A' \tag{25}$$

and

$$K_2 = \begin{cases} \dfrac{yA'}{4\xi_c A^2} & \dfrac{2A}{cy^2} \gg 1 \quad (26a) \\[2ex] \dfrac{cy + A'}{\xi_c c^2 y^3} & \dfrac{2A}{cy^2} \ll 1 \quad (26b) \end{cases}$$

which follow from Eqs. (21) and (22) under the indicated approximations. Since the restriction $1/y^2 \ll c/2A \ll 4\xi_c(f - 2)/(f - 1)$ requires $4\xi_c y^2 \gg (f - 1)/(f - 2)$, it is clear that Eq. (24b) can only hold for relatively large y. [For ξ_c in the range given by Eq. (10), y must exceed 2.5.]

B. Response Inhibition

In this section, the possible effects of systematically blocking antigen binding to B cells will be considered. The type of antigen I have in mind is a haptenated carrier such as dinitrophenylated keyhold limpet hemocyanin (DNP-KLH). The blocking agent is supposed to be identical to the hapten, and it therefore interacts specifically only with B cells having receptors for DNP. It does not affect the T cell-carrier interaction and T-cell factors are therefore assumed to be present at quantities necessary for activation.

In terms of the limiting free energies G_1 and G_2, the number of cells stimulated will be proportional to N(y) where

$$N(y) = \int_{G_1}^{G_2} \exp \frac{-\alpha G}{RT}\, dG \tag{27}$$

Integrating Eq. (27)

$$N(y) = \frac{RT}{\alpha}\left(K_1^{-\alpha} - K_2^{-\alpha}\right) \tag{28}$$

Under the conditions of Section III.A.1 (i.e., $A = 0$), Eq. (28) becomes (Appendix B)

$$N(y) \cong \frac{RT}{\alpha} c^{\alpha} \xi_c^{-\alpha} - \xi_c y^{2\alpha} \tag{29}$$

Introducing the *inhibition index*

$$I(y) \equiv \frac{N(y)}{N(1)} \tag{30}$$

which is the ratio of the number of stimulated cells in the presence of hapten to that in its absence (i.e., with $y = 1$) one has that, from Eq. (29)

$$I(y) = \frac{\xi_c^{-\alpha} - (\xi_c y^2)^{\alpha}}{\xi_c^{-\alpha} - \xi_c^{\alpha}} \tag{31}$$

Alternatively, when $A \neq 0$, Eqs. (21), (22), (28) and (30) give

$$I(y) = \frac{1 - \left(\left\{[(1 + 4\xi_c A'/c)^{1/2} - 1]\xi_c(cy^2 + 2A)^2\right\}/[2A'y(cy + A')]\right)^{\alpha}}{1 - \left(\left\{[(1 + 4\xi_c A'/c)^{1/2} - 1]\xi_c(c + 2A)^2\right\}/[2A'(c + A')]\right)^{\alpha}} \tag{32}$$

which has the limiting forms

$$I(y) = \begin{cases} \dfrac{1 - \left(16\xi_c^3 A^4/cy^2 A'^3\right)^{\alpha/2}}{1 - \left(16\xi_c^3 A^4/cA'^3\right)^{\alpha/2}} & c \ll \min\left\{\dfrac{2A}{y^2}, \; 4A'\xi_c\right\} \quad (33a) \\[2ex] \dfrac{1 - \left[\xi_c^3 c^3 y^6/A'(cy + A')^2\right]^{\alpha/2}}{1 - \left[\xi_c^3 c^3/A'(c + A')^2\right]^{\alpha/2}} & \dfrac{1}{y^2} \ll \dfrac{1}{2A} \ll 4\xi_c\left(\dfrac{f - 2}{f - 1}\right) \quad (33b) \end{cases}$$

IV. DISCUSSION: GENERAL REMARKS

The encounter between antigen and B cell bound receptors is widely believed to be a necessary first step in a series of steps leading to proliferation, differentiation, and antibody production. The model presented here assumes that receptor cross-linking is a subsequent *necessary* step in the process and leads to the prediction that the rate at which cross-linking occurs, and therefore (by hypothesis) the chance of cellular activation, is critically dependent upon the way the cell traps antigen, that is, on the details of the antigen-cell encounter. The possible types of interaction are enumerated and defined thermodynamically, and an expression for the initial cross-linking rate ξ, derived. The requirement that ξ exceed some threshold ξ_c in order that the amount of cross-linking necessary for triggering occur in a finite time (the time period may be set by a number of factors leading to cellular inactivation, including death), leads to specific predictions of response characteristics. The model thus distinguishes binding reactions from triggering reactions, since the magnitude of ξ will be a function of the relative frequencies of occurrence of the various types of interaction, and these in turn will depend upon such things as antigen-receptor affinity, antigen concentration, effective antigen valence and geometry, membrane fluidity, and receptor concentration. Since, depending upon the relations among parameters, certain types of interaction will be more likely than others, ξ_c may vary from close to zero through some maximum.

As a simple illustration of these ideas, consider the rate of cross-linkage formation as a function of antigen concentration when $A = 0$, that is, when the receptors are functionally monovalent. If the concentration of antigen in solution is relatively low (i.e., $c \ll 1/K$), the concentration of bound antigen will be low, and initially, almost entirely of the type m_1 (Fig. 3). Therefore, the rate of cross-linking will be slow since it depends on the collision frequency between m_1 and free receptors. Alternatively, when $c \gg 1/K$, there will be a rapid influx of antigen onto the cell, and many complexes of the type m_2 will form before cross-linking can begin. Cross-linking will again be slow, since there are now very few free receptors.

These ideas are reflected in Eq. (4). In its simplest form, with $K_n = h = 0$, $\xi = Kc/(1 + Kc)^2$. When $K \ll 1/c$, $\xi \cong Kc$, and since Kc is small, ξ will be small. When $K \gg 1/c$, $\xi \cong 1/Kc$, so that ξ decreases as Kc increases. In between, when $Kc \cong 1$, ξ goes through a maximum.

V. THE MEAN AFFINITY

A. Dependence on Concentration

In all cases considered, the mean affinity of stimulated cells was found to vary inversely as antigen concentration, so that as concentration decreases, mean affinity increases. Such behavior is in agreement with a wide range of data (Siskind and Benacerraf, 1969). However, the theory predicts that the precise functional relation between $\langle K \rangle$ and c will depend upon parameter values.

In the simplest case, with receptors considered functionally monovalent

$$\langle K \rangle c = \text{const} \tag{34}$$

Equation (34) looks familiar since it has the appearance of a mass-action expression, and it may therefore seem a not very surprising result. However, it should be remembered that $\langle K \rangle$ represents an average affinity, so the form of the expression is dependent upon the precursor distribution. The equation predicts, moreover, that a plot of mean free energy against ℓn c will be a straight line with slope 1.

It is not my intention to review here the rather extensive literature on the relation between antibody affinity and concentration of immunizing antigen. However, it should be pointed out that Eq. (34) is not in complete agreement with some of the most appropriate data available. Specifically, when Klinman's results (1972), obtained using DNP-hemocyanin, are plotted according to this theory, the curve is approximately, though not quite linear, over a fourfold range in concentration, and has an average slope of about 0.3.

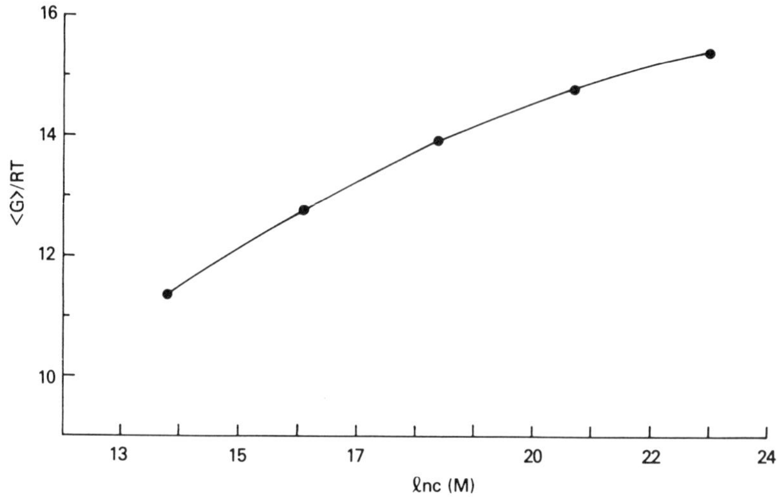

FIG. 4. Mean free energy as a function of immunogen concentration predicted by Eq. (23), $\xi_c = 10^{-3}$, $\alpha = 0.1$, $A' = A = 10^{-5}$ M, $y = 1$.

When $A \neq 0$, Eq. (23) is appropriate and the slope no longer equals 1, nor is it constant. As an illustration of the possibilities, for the parameters used to generate Fig. 4, the slope varies from 0.55 to 0.28 over a four-order of magnitude change in concentration. Thus the model predicts that for $y = 1$ and within some concentration range, there is a relation between mean affinity and concentration of the form

$$\langle K \rangle c^{\gamma} = \text{const} \quad \gamma \leqslant 1$$

where γ is often a slowly varying function so that a $\langle G \rangle$ vs. $\ln c$ plot has the appearance of a straight line over a wide intermediate concentration range.

Equation (23) will be invalid at extreme antigen concentrations and, in fact, Klinman's results show plateaus at high and low concentrations which cannot be accounted for by this equation. The deviations, however, are easily understood in terms of the restricted validity of the assumptions of the model.

For very high affinity receptors, the dissociation rate for antigen will be very slow and the equilibrium assumption becomes invalid. For this segment of the population, the mean time for dissociation is long compared to the time required to establish a cross-link, so that once the first bond is formed, irreversible binding occurs before the antigen can dissociate. Thus, the reverse rate constant plays no role. This means that above a certain free energy the rate of cross-linking becomes affinity-independent. Therefore, a continued decrease in concentration will not select for higher affinity cells, and a plateau in the mean free energy is expected.

At the low affinity end of the distribution, the assumption that cross-linking occurs irreversibly will break down. Thus, the affinity cutoffs cannot continue to decrease with concentration, and a plateau at high antigen concentrations is also expected.

B. Dependence on A and ξ_c

Equation (24a) predicts that $\langle K \rangle$ is a sensitive function of A, and decreases as A increases. The reason is that with increasing A, the high affinity cells can become more readily saturated with species of typc m_3 and this deters cross-linking. A, it will be recalled, is related to both hinge flexibility and antigenic determinant density, and although the former is not easily controlled experimentally, the latter is. Thus an easily testable prediciton is that $\langle K \rangle$ will decrease as epitope density increases. Such an experiment would also help clarify the role of cross-linking. If it assisted activation merely by stabilization, intramolecular reaction would also be expected to assist, albeit not as effectively, and a negative experimental result [$\langle K \rangle$ does not decrease with increasing epitope density] would tend to support this hypothesis. A positive result would be more difficult to interpret, since one could conclude that cross-linking leads to some sort of activation signal and/or that intramolecular binding supplies some sort of tolerogenic signal.

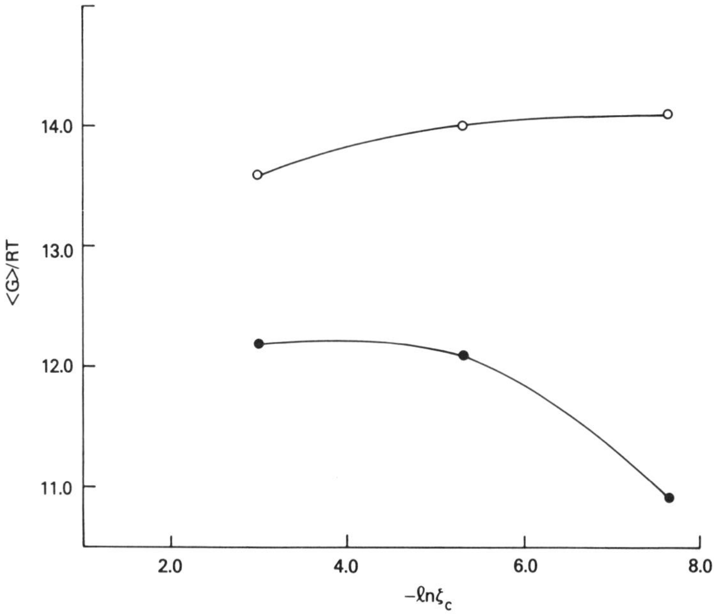

FIG. 5. Curves calculated according to Eq. (23) with $y = 1$, $A = A' = 10^{-5}$ M, $\alpha = 0.1$, $c = 5 \times 10^{-7}$ M (-●-), and 5×10^{-9} M (-0-).

The relation between $\langle G \rangle$ and ξ_c is more complicated. As illustrated in Fig. 5, $\langle G \rangle$ may increase or decrease with increasing ξ_c, depending upon antigen concentration and hinge flexibility. For example, when the antigen concentration is relatively high, decreasing ξ_c (increasing ρ_0 or k_0) will favor stimulation of low affinity cells and thus decrease the mean affinity.

C. The Ratio of Affinity Cutoffs

The ratio K_1/K_2 provides a measure of response heterogeneity. When Eq. (24a) is applicable,

$$\frac{K_1}{K_2} = \left(\frac{16\xi_c^3 A^4}{cy^2 A'^3}\right)^{1/2}$$

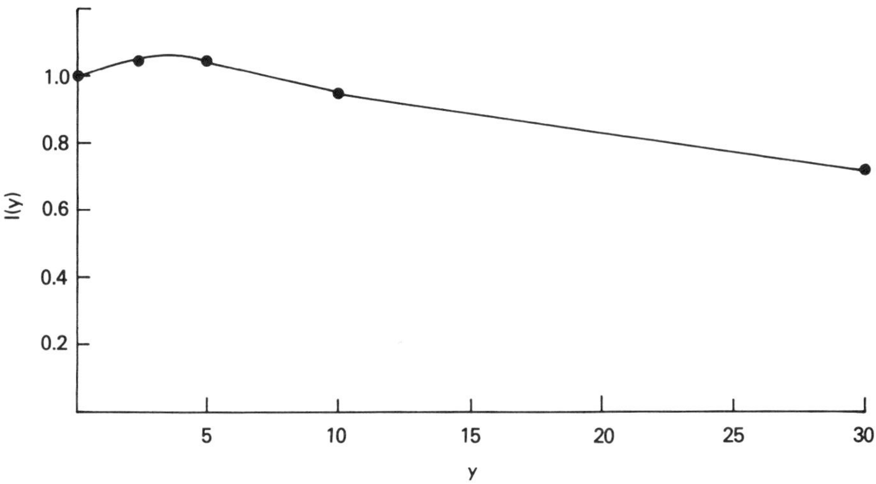

FIG. 6. Fraction of cells inhibited as a function of hapten-antigen ratio according to Eq. (35), $A = A' = 10^{-5}$ M, $c = 10^{-6}$ M, $\xi_c = 10^{-3}$, $\alpha = 0.1$.

so that as c increases, the distribution spreads, whereas as A or ξ_c increases, the distribution sharpens. The result indicates that the width will be especially sensitive to changes in ξ_c, and hence to receptor density. In fact, the ratio is proportional to ρ_0^{-3}, so that decreasing ρ_0 should dramatically sharpen the distribution. It is interesting that the response to large bacterial cell wall antigens is relatively homogeneous (Krause, 1970). Such restricted heterogeneity could be interpreted in terms of the results derived here if the receptors for these antigens were less dense than the usual immunoglobulin receptors. Undoubtedly there are also other factors involved, including antigen geometry, route of immunization, and prior sensitization. An experimental study attempting to disentangle these might prove rewarding.

D. Response Inhibition

Figure 6, which was generated using Eq. (32) illustrates the possibility of negative inhibition, that is, of increasing the magnitude of the response by adding free hapten. The phenomenon is favored by having 2A large compared to cy^2, so as y continues to increase, the enhancement must vanish and the response will eventually be completely inhibited as expected.

The reason for this unexpected enhancement can be traced to an increase in species of type m_6 and m_7 at the expense of m_3. This frees some receptor sites, but the slight advantage quickly disappears as hapten concentration increases and species of type m_6 predominates. The prediction is easily testable by inhibiting at reduced immunogen concentrations ($\sim 10^{-8}$ M), and the results should provide further insight into the role of intramolecular reaction.

Equation (32) also predicts that inhibition becomes more difficult as A increases or ξ_c decreases. Thus, increased difficulty in inhibition may reflect increased hinge flexibility, increased receptor density, or decreased viscosity. These predictions are in accord with intuitive expectations, since such changes favor more rapid formation of a stable receptor-antigen complex, while having no effect on the stability of a small hapten.

APPENDIX A: THE INITIAL RATE OF CROSS-LINKING

Multiply bound antigen can form by collision between free receptor sites and either singly or intramolecularly bound antigen. If ρ is the concentration of free receptor sites and m the concentration of singly bound antigen, then R, the initial rate of formation of multiply bound antigen, is

$$R = k_0 m\rho + k_0 \left(\frac{f - 2}{f - 1}\right) \rho m_3 \qquad \text{(A-1)}$$

f being the effective antigenic valence and k_0 the rate constant for interaction of singly bound antigen and free receptor site. In addition, prior to cross-linkage formation

$$\rho = m_1 + 2m_4 + m_7 \qquad \text{(A-2)}$$

and

$$m = m_1 + 2m_2 + m_5 \qquad \text{(A-3)}$$

With the assumption that reversible binding is equilibrium controlled on the time scale of cross-linkage formation, thermodynamic mass action requires that

$$m_1 = 2Kcm_4 \tag{A-4}$$

$$m_2 = (Kc)^2 m_4 \tag{A-5}$$

$$m_3 = 2K_n Kcm_4 \tag{A-6}$$

$$m_5 = 2KcKhm_4 \tag{A-7}$$

$$m_6 = (Kh)^2 m_4 \tag{A-8}$$

$$m_7 = 2Khm_4 \tag{A-9}$$

substituting Eqs. (A-4), (A-5), (A-7), and (A-9) into Eqs. (A-2) and (A-3), one finds that

$$\rho = 2Zm_4 \tag{A-10}$$

and

$$m = 2KcZm_4 \tag{A-11}$$

where

$$Z \equiv 1 + Kc + Kh \equiv 1 + Kcy$$

thus, from Eqs. (A-6), (A-10), and (A-11),

$$m = Kc\rho \tag{A-12}$$

$$m_4 = \frac{\rho}{2Z} \tag{A-13}$$

and

$$m_3 = \frac{K_n Kc\rho}{Z} \tag{A-14}$$

An expression for ρ in terms of physical chemical parameters can be obtained from the conservation condition for the total concentration of receptor molecules

$$\rho_0 = \sum_{i=1}^{7} m_i \tag{A-15}$$

Substituting Eqs. (A-4) and (A-9) into Eq. (A-15)

$$\rho_0 = m_4\left(Z^2 + 2K_n Kc\right) \tag{A-16}$$

or from Eq. (A-13)

$$\rho = \frac{2Z\rho_0}{Z^2 + 2K_n Kc} \tag{A-17}$$

Substituting Eqs. (A-12), (A-14), and (A-17) into Eq. (A-1), one finds that

$$R = \frac{4k_0\rho_0^2 KcZ}{(Z^2 + 2K_n Kc)^2}\left[Z + \left(\frac{f - 2}{f - 1}\right)K_n\right]$$

APPENDIX B: AFFINITY CUTOFFS IN THE ABSENCE OF INTRAMOLECULAR REACTION

With $A = 0$, Eq. (4) (Section II.A) becomes

$$\xi(1 + Kcy)^2 = Kc \tag{B-1}$$

The equations for the affinity cutoffs are found by substituting $\xi = \xi_c$ into Eq. (B-1), and solving the resulting quadratic equation for K_1 and K_2. The solutions are

$$K_1 = -\frac{1}{cy} + \frac{1}{2\xi_c cy^2}\left[1 - (1 - 4\xi_c y)^{1/2}\right] \equiv \frac{g_1}{c} \tag{B-2}$$

and

$$K_2 = -\frac{1}{cy} + \frac{1}{2\xi_c cy^2}\left[1 + (1 - 4\xi_c y)^{1/2}\right] \equiv \frac{g_2}{c} \tag{B-3}$$

When $(4\xi_c y)^2$ is much less than 1,

$$K_1 \cong \frac{\xi_c}{c} \tag{B-4}$$

and

$$K_2 \cong \frac{1}{c}\quad \frac{1}{\xi_c y^2} - \frac{2}{y} - \xi_c \quad \cong \frac{1}{\xi_c c y^2} \tag{B-5}$$

The last two equations were obtained by substituting

$$(1 - 4\xi_c y)^{1/2} \cong 1 - \frac{4\xi_c y}{2} - \frac{(4\xi_c y)^2}{8} - \cdots$$

into Eqs. (B-2) and (B-3) and neglecting powers of $\xi_c c$ greater than 1.

APPENDIX C: AFFINITY CUTOFFS WITH INTRAMOLECULAR BINDING

The equation of interest, obtained from Eq. (4) with $\xi = \xi_c$, is

$$f(K) \equiv \xi_c\left[(1 + Kcy)^2 + 2AK^2c\right]^2 - Kc(1 + Kcy)\left[1 + Kcy + \frac{(f - 2)AK}{(f - 1)}\right] = 0 \tag{C-1}$$

which can be written as

$$f(K) = \sum_{i=0}^{4} a_i K^i \tag{C-2}$$

where

$$a_0 \equiv \xi_c > 0$$

$$a_1 \equiv c(4y\xi_c - 1)$$

$$a_2 \equiv 2c^2y(3\xi_c y - 1) + Ac\left[4\xi_c - \frac{(f - 2)}{(f - 1)}\right]$$

$$a_3 \equiv c^3y^2(4\xi_c y - 1) + Ac^2y\left[8\xi_c - \frac{(f - 2)}{(f - 1)}\right]$$

$$a_4 \equiv \xi_c c^2(4A^2 + 4Acy^2 + c^2y^4) > 0$$

With $4\xi_c y \leqslant 1$ and for all allowed values of the other parameters, a_3 and a_2 are less than zero and $a_1 \leqslant 0$. Thus, under these circumstances, the sequence a_4, a_3, a_2, a_1, a_0 has two sign changes and the quartic has at most two real positive roots. It is evident from the allowed ranges of y and ξ_c that this covers most possibilities. Most of what remains falls under the condition $3\xi_c y \geqslant 1$. In this case, $a_1 > 0$ and there will be some ranges of the other parameters for which a_3 and a_2 are both greater than zero. In that case, the sequence of coefficients exhibits no sign changes; there are no real positive roots, and consequently there can be no stimulation. There are other possibilities, but they represent very special cases and will not be considered. I confine myself to the situation in which the quartic has at most two real roots; a case which covers most of the hypervolume in the space defined by ξ_c, c, A, and y.

It is straightforward but algebraically tedious and somewhat peripheral to the intention of this chapter to work out conditions under which there are exactly two real positive roots. Instead I will find approximate expressions for them sufficient to illustrate the ideas in the main text.

A. Upper Affinity Cutoff

It is reasonable to suppose that $K_2 c \gg 1$ (otherwise binding would always be weak) and numerical studies bear this out. Hence, for the purpose of finding a functional relation for K_2, Eq. (C-1) can be approximated by

$$\xi_c\left[(K_2 cy)^2 + 2AK_2^2 c\right]^2 = (K_2 c)^2 y\left[K_2 cy + \frac{(f - 2)}{(f - 1)} AK_2\right]$$

and, therefore

$$K_2 = \frac{\left[cy + \left(\frac{f - 2}{f - 1}\right)A\right]y}{\xi_c(cy^2 + 2A)^2} \tag{C-3}$$

B. Lower Affinity Cutoff

It is evident from Eq. (C-1) that $f(0) > 0$ and that with $4\xi_c y < 1$, $f(K)$ decreases as K increases from zero. Moreover, since $\xi_c \ll 1$, $f(K)$ will cut the abscissa when both K_1c and AK_1^2c are much less than one. In addition, K_1cy will also be much less than one for all but the largest values of y and ξ_c. This can be seen by noticing that in the absence of intramolecular reaction $K_1c \approx \xi_c$, and the effect of intramolecular bond will be to decrease K_1 (for a fixed c). Therefore, in the vicinity of K_1, Eq. (C-1) is approximately

$$\xi_c \cong K_1c + K_1^2cA'$$

from which

$$K_1 = -\frac{1}{2A'} + \frac{1}{2A'}\left(\frac{1 + 4\xi_cA'}{c}\right)^{1/2} \qquad \text{(C-4)}$$

where

$$A' \equiv A\,\frac{(f - 2)}{(f - 1)} \qquad \text{(C-5)}$$

REFERENCES

Amzel, L. M., Poljak, R. J., Saul, F., Varga, J. M., and Richards, F. F. (1974). The three dimensional structure of a combining region ligand complex of Ig NEW at 3.5 Å resolution. *Proc. Nat. Acad. Sci. (USA) 41:* 1427-1430.

Bell, G. I. (1974). Model for the binding of multivalent antigen to cells. *Nature 248:* 430-431.

Bell, G. I. (1975). B lymphocyte activation and lattice formation. *Transplant. Rev. 23:* 23-36.

Coutinho, A., and Möller, G. (1975). Immune activation of B cells: evidence for one nonspecific triggering signal not delivered by the Ig receptors. *Scand. J. Immun. 3:* 133-146.

Crothers, D. M. and Metzger, H. (1972). The influence of polyvalency on antibody binding properties. *Immunochem. 9:* 341-357.

DeLisi, C. (1975). A theory of precipitation and agglutination reactions in immunological systems. *J. Theor. Biol. 45:* 555-575.

DeLisi, C. (1976). *Antigen-Antibody Interactions.* Springer-Verlag, Berlin.

DeLisi, C. and Crothers, D. M. (1971). The influence of oligonucleotide chain conformation on nucleic acid stability. *Biopolymers 10:* 1809-1827.

DeLisi, C. and Metzger, H. (1976). Some physical chemical aspects of ligand receptor interactions. *Immunological Communications 5 (5):* 417-436.

DeLisi, C. and Perelson, A. (1976). The kinetics of aggregation phenomena. I. Minimal model of patch formation on lymphocyte membranes. *J. Theor. Biol. 62:* 159-210.

Edmundson, A. B., Ely, K. R., Abola, E. E., Schiffer, M., Westham, F. A., Fausch, M. D., and Deutch, H. F. (1974). Binding of 2,4-dinitrophenyl compounds and other small molecules to a crystalline λ-type Bence Jones Dimer. *Biochem. 13:* 3816-3827.

Feldmann, M. and Nossal, G. J. V. (1972). Tolerance, enhancement and the regulation of interactions between T-cells, B-cells and macrophages. *Transplant. Rev. 13:* 3-34.

Katz, D. H. and Benacerraf, B. (1972). Regulatory influence of activated T-cells. *Adv. Immunol. 15:* 1-94.

Klinman, N. (1972). The mechanism of antigenic stimulation of primary and secondary clonal precursor cells. *J. Exp. Med. 136:* 241-260.

Krause, R. M. (1970). The search for antibodies with molecular uniformity. *Adv. Immunol. 12:* 1-56.

Siskind, G. and Benacerraf, B. (1969). Cell selection by antigen in the immune response. *Adv. Immunol. 10:* 1-50.

Vitetta, E. and Uhr, J. W. (1975). Immunoglobulin receptors revisited. *Science 189:* 964-969.

Wu, T. T. and Kabat, E. (1970). *J. Exp. Med. 132:* 211.

Chapter 9

THE ANTIBODY COMBINING REGION: SPECULATIONS ON THE HYPOTHESIS OF GENERAL MULTISPECIFICITY

John K. Inman

Laboratory of Immunology
National Institute of Allergy and Infectious Diseases
National Institutes of Health
Bethesda, Maryland

A very general view of antibody-hapten binding is presented which is developed into a quantitative description of the hypothesis of general multispecificity. This hypothesis holds that any antibody combining region can bind a fraction of all possible haptens with an association constant greater than some defined minimum value. The group of molecules which bind consists of many families of haptens; within each family the haptens are quite similar in structure, yet between families their structures may be appreciably dissimilar. Haptens are best characterized as dissimilar if they are observed to bind in distinctly different ways to the antibody combining region. General multispecificity is treated in terms of the adequacy of antibody and serological specificity, and with regard to antigen-combining universality for a reasonably sized antibody repertoire. A theoretical, probability-based model is developed which describes the frequency of binding events that occur above any given association constant as a function of the latter when many immunoglobulins are tested against randomly selected haptens.

I. INTRODUCTION

Antisera raised against substances bearing known chemical structures (haptens) exhibit a high degree of specificity when tested with carriers to which haptens of similar structure are attached (Landsteiner, 1945; Kabat, 1976). Positive reactions, such as visible precipitation, are often obtained with very similar haptens and less often with less similar ones. Cross-reactions tend to be weaker than reactions with the eliciting hapten and are seldom stronger.

Taken together, these findings have led to the commonly held notion that antibodies react uniquely well with the eliciting hapten, and when cross-reactions occur, they do so *only* by virtue of structural similarity between eliciting and test haptens. The cross-reacting structures are visualized as fitting into a singular site on the antibody molecule which has a shape closely matching (but complementary to) that of the immunizing hapten. In this chapter I will refer to antibodies with the foregoing properties as being monospecific.

I will discuss in the following section a serious logical problem that arises from the assumption of monospecificity which, along with some evidence against it, has led a number of authors to propose or suggest an alternate hypothesis (Talmage, 1959; Eisen et al., 1967; Schubert et al., 1970; Glazer, 1970; Hood and Talmage, 1970; Rosenstein et al., 1972; Williamson, 1972; Hirschfeld, 1974; Inman, 1974). This hypothesis, which I will call general multispecificity, holds that most or all antibodies have the ability to combine well with occasional substances that bear little or no structural resemblance to the eliciting hapten. This circumstance will occur infrequently but regularly. The disparate structures that bind will do so in the same area (combining region) of the antibody as the homologous hapten but in different positions and/or orientations which involve separate selections of microscopic events for free energy minimization. In regard to this last point, demonstration of a difference in mode of binding provides a more operational and less subjective definition of multispecific binding than a mental-visual assessment of structural dissimilarity between haptens.

Below I will discuss the feasibility of multispecific binding by antibodies from the standpoint of events at the atomic and molecular levels, and I will develop a probability-based model that quantitatively describes the expected frequencies of occurrence of multispecific binding as a function of the association constant. The model is compatible with some data on screening of myeloma proteins and with thermodynamic and structural considerations. I will also present a model for expected frequencies of serological cross-reactions involving multispecific antibodies and give estimates of a minimum antibody repertoire needed for universal antigen combining capability.

I will not attempt to review all evidence bearing on general multispecificity. At present, it is not adequate. Several experimental programs, including one in my laboratory, are endeavoring to provide more data to test the generality of multispecificity. Meanwhile, much of the existing evidence has come from studies of myeloma proteins, some of which react with several disparate antigens; but cross-reactions between normally raised antibodies and dissimilar structures have also been reported. Examples of these several kinds of observations have been given by Schubert et al. (1970), Eisen et al. (1970), Underdown and Eisen (1971), Eisen (1971), Rosenstein et al. (1972), Riesen and Morell (1972), Varga et al. (1973), Varga et al. (1974), Richards et al. (1975), Tolleshaug and Hannestad (1975), and Cameron and Erlanger (1976).

II. THE ANTIBODY REPERTOIRE PARADOX

Specific antibodies have been raised in animals against hundreds of haptenic determinants of both natural and synthetic origin. When an animal has failed to respond, the result could usually be attributed to the selection of the immunogen carrier or the immunization procedure, or to a preexisting state of specific tolerance and not to an innate incapacity for forming a suitable antibody structure. Apparently, individual animals can produce specific antibodies reactive with almost any possible substance, since there is no reason to suppose that the haptens studied so far constitute a peculiar sample.

If antibodies are presumed to be monospecific, this means that any antibody with a recognized reactivity against an eliciting antigen will seldom or never react better with other antigens bearing only disparate structural features. Often an animal responds with many diverse antibodies reactive to the eliciting antigen, and accordingly would have a repertoire of antibodies approaching the number of all possible haptenic substances. It has long been feared that this number would be impossibly high even after allowance has been made for shared structural features. As a result, instructive theories of antibody formation (preantibody conforming to an antigen template) were proposed (Pauling, 1940). Cellular studies of antibody formation led to the distinctly different hypothesis of clonal selection (Burnet, 1959). In this view, a precursor lymphocyte becomes committed to a particular antibody Fab structure without instruction from an antigen. An antigen which can fortuitously combine with the selected antibody structure subsequently may serve as a specific stimulus for growth and differentiation to form a clone of antibody-secreting cells. One form or another of this hypothesis is now generally accepted. Simple instructive theories were clearly disproven by observations that antibodies could be completely unfolded and renatured in the absence of antigen with recovery of their specific combining properties (Haber, 1964; Whitney and Tanford, 1965; Jaton et al., 1968). Thus, information for specificity was shown to lie in the amino acid sequences of the component peptide chains. Because of this fact, and/or because of limitations set by the number of B-cell clones an animal can possess and generate within a limited time span, I wish to show that a nearly universal antibody specificity repertoire cannot be accounted for by assuming that antibodies are essentially monospecific.

First of all, it is interesting to see how large a lower limit can be set for the enumeration of all possible haptenic structures. An exact enumeration is clearly not feasible. To start with, one should estimate a lower limit to the number of organic compounds in the size range that normally complements the binding surfaces of antibodies. Studies have shown that antigens and corresponding antibodies interact with structural components spanning up to 20 or 30 Å which may involve, for example, five or six residues of amino acids or monosaccharides (Kabat, 1976, Chap. 6). Corresponding molecular weights will range from about 400 to 900. There are about 6×10^6 known and recorded compounds, so let us suppose that a third of these fall into the very common molecular weight range of 200 to 400, about half the required size. For any one of these compounds a chemist could easily write structures for a dozen or more variants which have never been synthesized or reported. That makes a minimum estimate of 3×10^7 half-sized structures. Conceivably, one can build haptens by joining any two of these compounds in, say, 10 different ways. The completion of this process leaves one with around $(3 \times 10^7)^2 \times 10 \approx 10^{16}$ as a lower limit for the number of all possible compounds with molecular weight 400 to 900.

The possible haptens should have a somewhat higher count for the following reason. The above compounds exist in solution in many conformations, some of which occur with low frequency; measurable binding to antibodies will seldom occur with these conformations because of a large, unfavorable entropy effect. However, when the substance is an integral part of a larger, more rigid molecule, for instance a protein, it may be constrained to remain in an otherwise improbable conformation, and the common configurations of the free structure would no longer occur (Sachs et al., 1972). In effect, it becomes a new substance. Thus, "new" determinants have often been observed when a protein antigen has been denatured or has been degraded to smaller peptides. Consideration of such "frozen" conformations should enormously increase the antigen structure enumeration. In the contrary direction, one should consider that, among all possible structures, many are very closely related. Even though antibodies readily distinguish slight alterations in structure (as best shown with hapten-binding myeloma proteins), some correction for nondistinguishability should be applied. Let this correction then cancel out the frozen conformation effect (perhaps by allowing a factor of 100 or more in either direction), and one is left with 10^{16} "families" of distinguishable structures as a *lower* limit value.

Next, an upper limit to the antibody repertoire will be considered. There are roughly 2×10^8 B-type lymphocytes in a mouse which represent probably no more than about 10^7 separate clones at any given time (if one assumes a modest average of 20 cells per clone) (Klinman et al., 1976). In most instances, a mature animal will respond with at least one specific clone within a few days after immunization. Since precursor cells are somewhat stable in commitment to a given antibody combining region (i.e., pair of variable region sequences), most cells will remain unchanged in this regard during the initial inductive period. It is possible that other cells may change commitment to different variable regions as the result of somatic mutations or insertions, so that during the early stage of immunization the effective clonal repertoire may be expanded to 10^8 (let us say 10^7 cells turning over a set of surface receptors every 5 hr for 50 hr). Therefore, the *uppermost* limit of the antibody repertoire during the time required for an initial response is of the order of 10^8 to 10^9.

The paradox remains: There are *at least* 10^{16} distinguishable families of antigenic structures and *at most* 10^9 different antibody combining regions. The ratio 10^7 is a lower limit. Of course, different figures could be obtained in other ways, but it seems unlikely that the two limits will be brought closer together than a few more orders of magnitude by any reasonable process. It seems easier to regard antibodies as being generally multispecific, and to consider that a high degree of multispecificity (greater than 10^7 specificities per antibody combining region) must somehow be compatible with known facts about specificity. The exact (or "actual") degree of multispecificity is not determinable and has no useful meaning. Instead, the degree of multispecificity can be expressed as the *fraction* b of all possible antigenic structures with which an individual antibody molecule can interact with an association constant above a given value. The latter figure can be something biologically meaningful such as $1 \times 10^4\ M^{-1}$. It can be shown that the value of b for an average antibody is essentially the same as the fraction of all antibodies (in a large repertoire) that can interact with an average antigenic structure (with association constants above the same limit). The foregoing definition of the fraction b was given by Talmage (1959). This parameter has been very useful in quantitative speculations about general multispecificity.

III. MULTISPECIFIC COMBINING REGIONS

Antigens are bound by structural features of antibodies made up of the N-terminal half of the light chain and the N-terminal 115 or so amino acid residues of the heavy chain, the so-called V_L and V_H (variable) regions. Traditionally, these structures have been

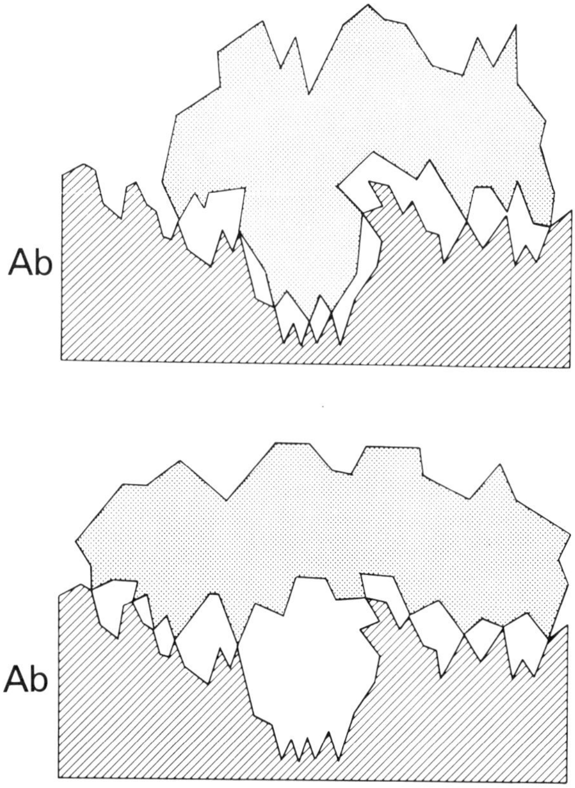

FIG. 1. A diagrammatic representation of two haptens, unrelated in structure, being bound alternatively in the same antibody combining region.

pictured as providing a depression having contours which uniquely complement the shape of the specific antigen (or some part of it). It is difficult to use such a construct in visualizing multispecific binding of a very large number of disparate structures. However, one should ask, is the notion of very close or exact fit really necessary? The requirement for an adequate association constant and corresponding free energy decrease on binding can be met by innumerable combinations of events at the atomic and molecular level. Processes contributing to free energy changes include establishing various numbers and kinds of short- and long-range interactions, removal of ligand from the solvent environment, removal of bound water and small ions from the binding surfaces, possible conformational changes in the antibody, and conformational restrictions on the antigen. Any composite event which minimizes the Gibbs' free energy of the system will be achieved quickly whether or not the shapes are right.

Multispecific binding is pictured diagrammatically in Fig. 1. Two haptens with distinctly different structures (and shapes) are shown bound by the same antibody combining region. A different set of contacts (short- and long-range interactions) are indicated. Some contacts are the same in the two cases, many are not. Portions of the combining region may be used by one hapten and not by the other. The main point is that enough interactions, or at least sufficiently energetic ones, should be established simultaneously so that an adequate free energy change results. The shape of an antibody combining region nonetheless plays a crucial role in determining specificity (which haptens bind strongly and which ones do not), but some inexactness of fit, along with incomplete filling of the potential combining region, are essential factors allowing the possibility for extensive multispecificity.

If antibodies were essentially monospecific and shape complementarity were demanded, then all cross-reacting haptens would conform to the same contours with most contacts shared. The general orientation of bound haptens would be the same. In contrast, both physical-chemical and X-ray structure studies on the binding of different haptens by homogeneous immunoglobulins strongly support the multispecific binding concept as depicted in Fig. 1. Rosenstein et al. (1972) demonstrated by selective chemical derivatization and denaturation experiments that two apparently diverse haptens, ε-dinitrophenyl-L-lysine and menadione thioglycollate, bind to mouse myeloma protein 460 in a distinctly different manner and probably in separate subsites. Manjula et al. (as cited by Richards et al., 1974) showed by energy transfer studies with nanosecond fluorimetry that the two haptens are bound in well-separated locations, although they occupy some common space which prevents their being bound simultaneously. Hsia et al. (1973), using spin-labeled hapten titration techniques with dinitrophenyl (DNP) and trinitrophenyl (TNP) groups studied changes in the thermodynamics of binding of unlabeled and spin-labeled groups to mouse myeloma protein 315. Their results strongly support the conclusion that the spatial relation between protein and bound DNP or TNP groups is quite different for the two cases, even though these polynitrophenyl ring structures are rather similar, and each often cross-reacts with antibodies raised against the other. Edmundson et al. (1974) studied a human lambda-type light chain dimer by X-ray crystallography. The two identical chains assume different conformational roles in the dimer which resembles a normal light and heavy chain. A deep cavity is formed between the chains that is comparable to the combining region of a primitive antibody. A number of disparate compounds were found to bind in the cavity. Their locations, as determined by crystallographic techniques, were often in distinctly separate subsites (as, for example, the DNP and menadione haptens). Some disparate structures were bound in the same subsite. Other haptens were bound in either of several subsites. DNP groups of bis(DNP)lysine were located simultaneously in separate subsites, as was observed by Hoffmeister and Voss (1974) in the case of certain chicken antibodies. The above research clearly points to a flexible adaptation of hapten to antibody sites, rather than restriction to the principle of unique fitting.

The nature of antibody combining regions has been explored in detail by other workers using X-ray structure analysis. Amzel et al. (1974) reported the positioning of a large ligand, vitamin K_1OH, in a shallow cleft between the V_L and V_H regions of human myeloma protein IgG *New*. Segal et al. (1974) determined the structure of mouse immunoglobulin McPC 603 showing a molecule of phosphorylcholine bound largely to one side of a deep cavity formed between the H and L chains. It was found that the individual haptens do not take up the entire space of the binding cavity. Along with the crystallographic studies of Epp et al. (1974) on the Bence-Jones protein REI, and the refinement of *New* by Poljak et al. (1974),

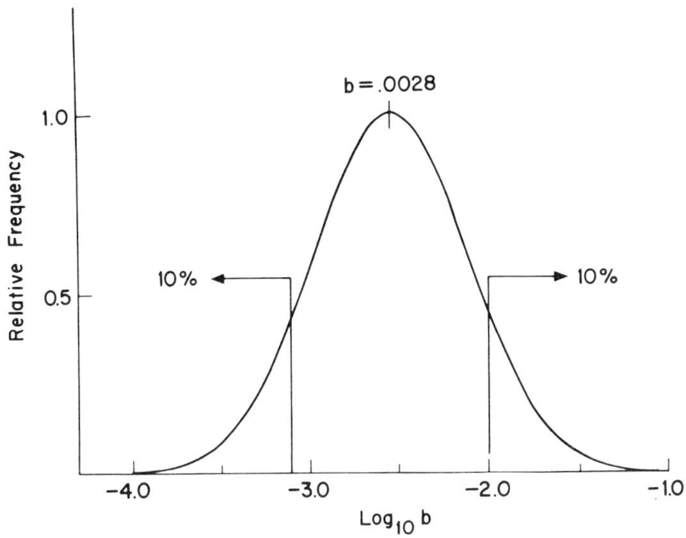

FIG. 2. A hypothetical distribution of b values among antigens and antibodies; b is defined as the fraction of all possible antigenic structures (haptens) that an individual antibody molecule can bind with an association constant equal to or greater than 1×10^4 M^{-1}. Conversely, b can be considered as the fraction of all antibodies that can similarly bind a given antigen.

the above studies lead to the general conclusion that antibody combining regions appear to vary considerably in their general shape among different immunoglobulins; some regions are shallow grooves while others are deep clefts. Commonly occurring insertions and deletions of amino acid residues in the hypervariable sequences which line the cavity walls appear to be especially important features which modulate shape (Poljak et al., 1974; Padlan and Davies, 1975).

The general shape and size of an antibody combining region may influence the degree of its multispecificity. For example, antibodies with narrow or shallow combining regions may bind well to a smaller fraction of all potential antigens than those immunoglobulins with wide and deep clefts. The latter antibodies would have the higher b values. Therefore, one might consider the likelihood that antibodies of a large repertoire may have a wide distribution in b as hypothetically represented in Fig. 2. The positioning and spread of this curve have been assigned somewhat arbitrarily, but the figure is reasonably consistent with published data on binding properties of myeloma proteins and of some normally raised antibodies. Accordingly, 10% of all antibodies would bind (with $K \geq 10^4\ M^{-1}$) 1/100 or more of all *full-sized* haptens. An average antibody may bind around 0.0028 (1/360) of all such haptens. The b values may seem high (and they may indeed be), but much of the reported screening of myeloma proteins has been carried out with haptens having less structure than can usually be accommodated by an antibody. The result would be a trend toward lower b values. On the other hand, other haptens have been deliberately selected because prior experience indicated that they bind with rather high incidence. All one can do for the present is to put the data together and assume some degree of balancing-out of bias. The purpose of Fig. 2 is to illustrate the idea of a broad distribution in the fraction b as shown by a normal distribution on a log b scale.

IV. A MODEL FOR CUMULATIVE OCCURRENCE FREQUENCIES OF ASSOCIATION CONSTANTS

Figure 1 illustrates the notion that binding of antigen by antibody is not an all-or-none phenomenon depending on an extensive complementarity in shape. Rather, it suggests that *any* substance can combine with *any* antibody molecule *to a degree*. For some pairs of randomly selected reactants, better opportunities will exist for decreasing the free energy of the system than for other pairs, and this circumstance will be a matter of chance. Accordingly, I have developed a probability-based model for describing the expected relation between association constants and their frequencies of occurrence. For simplicity, I will deal with sets of discrete interactions in describing the free energy change on binding. I will consider these interactions or "contacts" to occur independently of one another. They are comprised of the many kinds of noncovalent interactions that are known to take place between atoms or small groups of atoms (including ions). The property of independence applies simply to occurrence or nonoccurrence of a contact, rather than to freedom from various kinds of influences that neighboring atoms or groups may exert on one another. Therefore, contacts will be considered all-or-none phenomena which contribute additive increments δG to the total free energy change ΔG. Thus, $\Delta G = \Sigma\ \delta G$. The relation between the standard free energy change and the equilibrium association constant (binding constant) K, is given by

$$-\Delta G = RT \ln K = RT(\ln 10)(\log K) \quad (1)$$

where R is the universal gas constant and T is the absolute temperature. Equation (1) will be used for expressing free energy changes in terms of log K or increments thereof, $\delta \log K$. At 25°C, $\log K = 0.733\ (-\Delta G)$ for the overall binding and $\delta \log K = 0.733\ (-\delta G)$ for the component interactions or contacts. The units for G are kilocalories/mole, and for K they are liters/mole (M^{-1}).

As a further simplification, the contacts will be grouped into five uniform sets indexed 0 to 4 . If there are c_j contacts in the j'th set, then the logarithm of the binding constant becomes

$$\log K = \sum_{j=0}^{j=4} c_j (\delta \log K)_j \quad (2)$$

Table 1 gives the free energy increments which I have chosen for the five sets or groups. Group 0 (zero) contacts will be treated as van der Waals or other weak, short-range interactions. The other groups represent higher energy interactions such as weak and strong hydrogen bonds, dipole-dipole, ion-dipole, charge-transfer interactions, ionic bonds, etc. Since their free energy contributions vary and overlap considerably, I have not made any strict identification with group number. Instead, I have assigned more or less evenly spaced $(-\delta G)_j$ values which span the ranges given in physical chemistry texts for various kinds of interactions.

TABLE 1

Grouped Standard Free Energy Contributions of Interaction Units and Corresponding Log_{10} K Increments[a]

Group Index j	Unit Free Energy Contribution[b] $(-\delta G)_j$	Log K Increment $(\delta \log K)_j$
0	0.41	0.3
1	3.27	2.4
2	6.14	4.5
3	8.59	6.3
4	11.05	8.1

[a] K is the equilibrium association constant in liters/mole at 25°C. Log K increments and log K_{min} were set up as multiples of 0.3 so that solutions to Eqs. (4) and (6) would be integers.

[b] $(-\delta G)_j$ (kilocal/mole) = $(\delta \log K)_j/0.733$.

Group 0 interactions will be treated as follows. Antigenic determinants have many atoms which potentially can made van der Waals contacts with atoms of an antibody combining region. I will assume an average of 40 atoms, mostly nonskeletal, for a full-sized determinant. Two irregular surfaces can usually touch simultaneously in at least three places. Accordingly, it would be reasonable to assume that the most likely number of contacts between extended, irregular forms is slightly greater than this (say, four or five) when one surface is generally concave and the other generally convex, and both surfaces are in the configuration that provides a maximum number of contacts (corresponding to minimum free energy).

In this model the selection of any test hapten is analogous to a random drawing of v = 40 objects from an almost infinite collection. Each drawing of an object is regarded as a trial, for which the probability of success is the fraction a of the likely number of contacts (four or five), divided by the total number of potential contacts, v = 40. The probability $P_0(i)$ of obtaining i (and only i) successes in v draws is given by the binomial distribution

$$P_0(i) = \binom{v}{i} a^i (1 - a)^{v-i} \tag{3}$$

where the binomial coefficient $\binom{v}{i} = \frac{v!}{i!(v - i)!}$.

Thus, one has a means for predicting an occurrence frequency $P_0(i)$ for the number $i = c_0$ group 0 contacts corresponding to a van der Waals-type contribution $c_0(\delta \log K)_0$ to the binding constant. This frequency applies to the expected outcome of a hypothetical experiment where $i = c_0$ could be evaluated after each of many binding trials involving randomly selected immunoglobulins and haptens. An examination of these probabilities shows that the chances of achieving binding constants exceeding $10^6\ M^{-1}$ by these forces alone are excessively small. An essential role for a special, higher energy interaction is indicated.

The higher energy groups 1 through 4 are treated differently. The probability functions for the occurrence of these interactions are designated P_1, P_2, P_3, and P_4, respectively. I will consider only the events defined by i group 0 contacts taking place conjointly with zero or one interactions (totally) from groups 1 through 4. When meaningful probability values $P_j(1)$ are assigned to single group 1 through 4 contacts, the probability of two such interactions occurring becomes numerically small enough to ignore since they appear in additive terms [see Eq.(5)]. Thus, five sets of alternative binding events will be dealt with. The first set is that of i group 0 interactions occurring with none from groups 1 through 4. The probability $P(0,0,0,0)$ that no interactions from groups 1 through 4 will form is $P_1(0)P_2(0)P_3(0)P_4(0)$. Probabilities for this first set of binding events are $P(0,0,0,0)P_0(i)$. The next set of events is the conjoint occurrence of i group 0 contacts with one group 1 and zero group 2, 3, and 4 interactions. Probabilities for this set are $P_1(1)P_2(0)P_3(0)P_4(0)P_0(i) = P(1,0,0,0)P_0(i)$. Analogously, the other three sets of events have probabilities $P(0,1,0,0)P_0(i)$, $P(0,0,1,0)P_0(i)$, and $P(0,0,0,1)P_0(i)$.

For convenience, probability values will be assigned directly to the above $P(q,x,y,z)$ terms instead of separately to $P_j(0)$ and $P_j(1)$ for $j = 1$, 2, 3, and 4, and thus

$P(0,0,0,0) \approx [1 - P(1,0,0,0)][1 - P(0,1,0,0)][1 - P(0,0,1,0)][1 - P(0,0,0,1)]$ is a convenient approximation.

What is finally desired is a cumulative frequency distribution cumF as a function of $\log K_{min}$, that expresses the frequency of occurrence of bindings with log K equal to or greater than a given value $\log K_{min}$. For each of the five sets of alternative binding events discussed above, a certain minimum number t_j of group 0 contacts are required to reach the $\log K_{min}$ value according to Eq. (2). In fact we must have

$$t_0 = \frac{\log K_{min}}{(\delta \log K)_0}$$

and

$$t_j = \frac{\log K_{min} - (\delta \log K)_j}{(\delta \log K)_0} \qquad j = 1,\ldots,4 \tag{4}$$

with the proviso that $t_j = 0$ if $(\delta \log K)_j$ exceeds $\log K_{min}$, $j \geqslant 1$. For any of the five sets of binding events, the number of group 0 contacts may exceed t_j in fulfilling the condition $\log K \geqslant \log K_{min}$. The sum of probabilities for all the alternative events in all five sets gives the desired cumulative frequency

$$\begin{aligned} \text{cumF} \simeq {} & P(0,0,0,0) \sum_{i=t_0}^{i=v} P_0(i) + P(1,0,0,0) \sum_{i=t_1}^{i=v} P_0(i) \\ & + P(0,1,0,0) \sum_{i=t_2}^{i=v} P_0(i) + P(0,0,1,0) \sum_{i=t_3}^{i=v} P_0(i) \\ & + P(0,0,0,1) \sum_{i=t_4}^{i=v} P_0(i) \end{aligned} \tag{5}$$

which of course depends on $\log K_{min}$ through the values t_j.

On substituting the values in Table 1, one obtains

$$t_0 = \frac{\log K_{min}}{0.3}$$

$$t_1 = t_0 - 8$$

$$t_2 = t_0 - 15 \quad \text{or zero for all negative values} \qquad (6)$$

$$t_3 = t_0 - 21$$

$$t_4 = t_0 - 27$$

In this manner cumF = f(log K_{min}) is determined by substituting into Eq. (6) log K_{min} values which are multiples of 0.3 in order to obtain integral values for t_j. The latter in turn are entered in Eq. (5), and $P_0(i)$ terms from Eq. (3) are summed over the indicated limits.

Assignment of the probability values P(q,x,y,z) is to a degree arbitrary. A set of four such values should be chosen to yield a smooth cumF curve without peculiar inflections. Also, the curves should pass through some meaningful point or points, especially those suggested by actual data. Much of the screening data on myeloma proteins are marginally useful for this purpose, because the observations were not directly related to simple binding, and/or bias was introduced in selecting test antigens. One particularly interesting correlation was reported by Eisen et al. (1970) who presented data from about 350 myeloma proteins which had been screened against ε-dinitrophenyl-L-lysine. Binding constants were available for the strongly positive cases, and from these data a crude cumulative frequency curve with respect to log K_{min} was constructed. I found by trial four higher energy probability term values (see Table 2, curve A) that, when used in Eq. (5), nicely reproduced this curve. This curve (A), plotted in Fig. 3, passes through log K_{min} = 4.0 at cumF = 0.010; thus, the value of b is

TABLE 2

Values for the Parameters of Equations (3) and (5)
Used in Calculating Cumulative Occurrence Frequencies (cumF)

Curve[a]	v	a	va	P(0,0,0,0)[b]	P(1,0,0,0)	P(0,1,0,0)	P(0,0,1,0)	P(0,0,0,1)
A	40	0.125	5	0.9866	8.0×10^{-3}	2.5×10^{-3}	1.0×10^{-3}	2.0×10^{-3}
B	40	0.125	5	0.9959	3.6×10^{-3}	2.5×10^{-4}	1.1×10^{-4}	1.0×10^{-4}
C	40	0.100	4	0.9980	1.8×10^{-3}	1.2×10^{-4}	5.5×10^{-5}	5.0×10^{-5}
D	40	0.125	5	1.0000	0	0	0	0

[a]See Figs. 3 and 4 for graphs of resulting cumF (or log cumF) as functions of log K_{min}.

[b]Calculated by assuming
$P(0,0,0,0) \approx [1 - P(1,0,0,0)][1 - P(0,1,0,0)][1 - P(0,0,1,0)][1 - P(0,0,0,1)]$

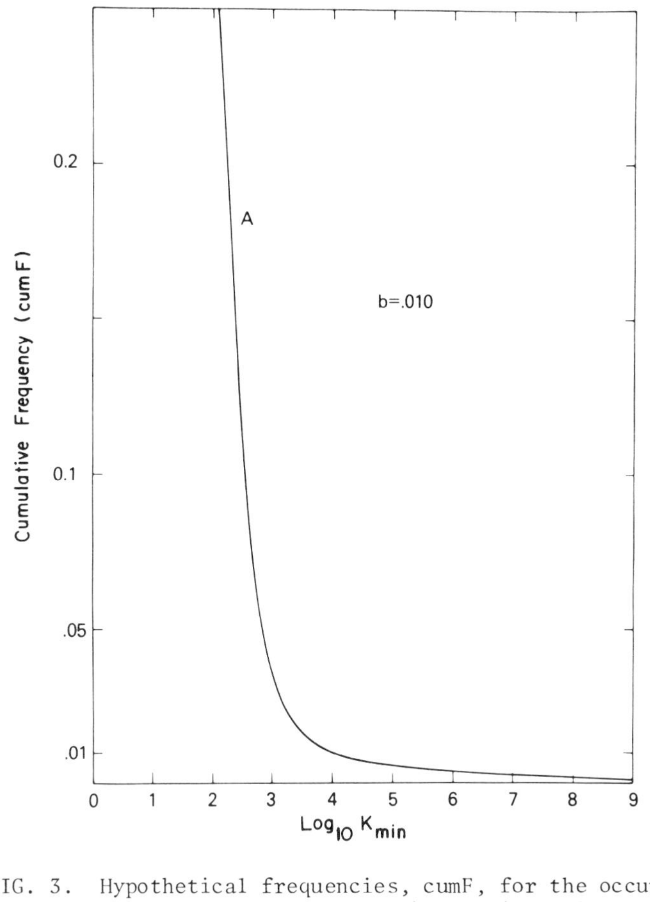

FIG. 3. Hypothetical frequencies, cumF, for the occurrence of binding constants equal to or greater than various given values, K_{min}, as a function of log K_{min}. These cumulative frequencies were calculated from the probability model developed in Section IV. Values of the model parameters were chosen so that the resulting curve (A) would be consistent with data on the screening of myeloma proteins against ε-dinitrophenyl-L-lysine as presented by Eisen et al. (1970).

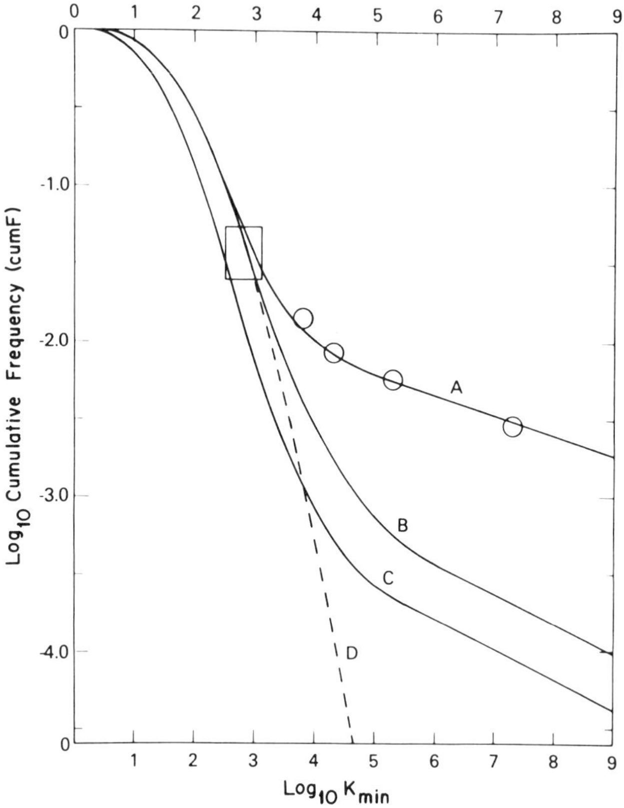

FIG. 4. Hypothetical frequencies, cumF, for the occurrence of binding constants equal to or greater than various given values, K_{min}, as a function of log K_{min}. The common logarithms of these frequencies are given on the ordinate and were calculated from the probability model in Section IV. The curves describe the expected results from testing many immunoglobulins with many disparately structured haptens. Curve A is the log form of the curve shown in Fig. 3 (see legend). Curve B represents expected results from an average (unbiased) selection of antibodies and haptens. Curve C shows expected frequencies from a selection biased toward lower b values (see Fig. 2).

0.01 (by definition) for this hapten and sample of immunoglobulins. The very steep rise in frequency below K_{min} of 10^3 M^{-1} is noteworthy. The curve is not a simple exponential form. Log cumF plotted against log K_{min} in Fig. 4 (curve A) is decidedly nonlinear. The points employed by the above authors are shown by the circles and rectangle. The rectangle also represents the experience from a screening of 10 myeloma proteins with 19 radioactive ligands by Varga et al. (1974), and from unpublished observations of Merchant et al. on inhibition of hapten-specific, hemolytic plaques with disparate compounds. Weak binding (log K approximately 2.5-3.1 and slightly higher) was observed in about 1/20 to 1/25 of the tests. When protein *New* was screened with nearly 400 compounds, two were found with K in excess of 10^5 M^{-1} (Richards et al., 1974). This result suggests a frequency of about 1/200 (log cumF = -2,3) which falls very close to curve A.

Two other curves (B and C) plotted in Fig. 4 are pitched to lower frequencies. It is generally assumed that antidinitrophenyl antibodies have a large representation in antibody repertoires, perhaps because of opportunities offered by the aromatic ring and the two nitro groups for forming strong noncovalent interactions. Curves B and C were designed to pass through log K_{min} = 4.0 at cumF equal to the b values near the peak and lower 10th percentile, respectively, in the hypothetical distribution of Fig. 2. The upper 10th percentile was placed at b = 0.01 from curve A in setting up Fig. 2. Curve B, therefore, is my present guess as to what the average situation may be. Curve D is a plot of the first term in Eq. (5), which is the frequency curve expected if only group 0 (van der Waals-type) interactions were allowed. Curve C could not be easily "bent away" from curve D by any sensible selection of P(q,x,y,z). Since curve C could represent low repertoire (low b-valued) antibodies with shallow or restricted binding regions, it seemed reasonable to reduce the expected (most likely) value in the binomial distribution (Eq. 3) from 40a = 5 to 40a = 4. Curve C was then easily constructed. The values used for the parameters of curves A, B, C, and D are listed in Table 2. Curves B and C were given a form generally similar to curve A. Taken together, the various constraints discussed above left little further latitude in assigning values to P(q,x,y,z).

The a priori reasonableness of the assigned P(q,x,y,z) values can be examined by starting with a slight modification of the above model. I will assume that among the v = 40 potential contacts in an average antigenic determinant there are a certain number of these, w_j, that can participate in either a group 0 or a j'th group higher energy interaction. The latter case will occur only if the contacting unit of the antigen interacts with a unit in the antibody of the same type but of opposite polarity. Polarity refers to the general asymmetry of these interactions, such as + or -, electron-rich or electron-poor, etc. When a higher energy contact forms, one less group 0 interaction will occur. One simply transfers the 0.3 log K increment of the usurped interaction to the $(\delta \log K)_j$ values in Table 1 for groups 1 through 4 in order to obtain the same curves shown in Figs. 3 and 4. That is the modification required. Now, the a priori chance that any of the i contacting units of the antigen will be in the j'th group (for j = 1 to 4) is $w_j/v = w_j/40$. I will assume the same likelihood $w_j/40$ that the opposing contacting structure in the antibody will be of group j type. The probability that any one interaction is in group j, because both contacting units are of the right kind *and* of opposite polarity, is $1/2(w_j/40)^2$. If there are i contacts occurring with probability $P_0(i)$ as given by Eq. (3) (where v = 40), then the chance of a j'th group interaction is approximately $1/2(w_j/40)^2 iP_0(i)$. Summing the above terms over all allowed values of i gives $P_j(1)$, the probability of having one group j interaction

$$P_j(1) \approx P(q,x,y,z) \approx \frac{1}{2}\left(\frac{w_j}{40}\right)^2 \sum_{i=0}^{i=40} iP_0(i) = \frac{1}{2}\left(\frac{w_j}{40}\right)^2 40a \qquad (7)$$

where q, x, y, *or* z is 1, and the other three indexes are 0, since

Table 3

Estimation of w_j Values from Equation (7)[a]

Curve[b]	w_1	w_2	w_3	w_4	Total = $w_1 + w_2 + w_3 + w_4$
A	2.3	1.3	0.8	1.1	5.5
B	1.5	0.4	0.25	0.25	2.4
C	1.2	0.3	0.2	0.2	1.9

[a] w_j is the average number of structural features per hapten potentially able to participate in an interaction unit of group j (Table 1) for j = 1 through 4.

[b] See Fig. 4 and Table 2.

$$\sum_{i=0}^{i=40} iP_0(i) \approx 40a \qquad (8)$$

One obtains from Eq. (7) and the figures for P(q,x,y,z) and va in Table 2 the w_j values given in Table 3 which are estimates of the average number of contacting units in an antigenic determinant potentially available for group j interactions. The resulting w_j have the right order of magnitude. If anything, they appear a little too small. The screening of ε-dinitrophenyl-L-lysine against myeloma proteins suggested the positioning of curve A of Figs. 3 and 4 as already discussed. This hapten provides potential higher energy contacts with the four oxygen atoms of the nitro groups, the π orbitals on either side of the phenyl ring plane, the ε-NH- link, and the charges of the α-carboxyl and α-amino groups. The total is nine. We have assumed that the contacting units act independently, so the nitro groups might be considered single units, and the total becomes seven. Either way, this count agrees with the value 5.5 from Table 3, curve A, within a factor of 1.6. If one imagines sampling structures of molecular weight 400 to 900 from all possibilities, which must include many diverse heteroatomic groupings, it is easy to see that the w_j totals are not too high. On the other hand, if the cumulative frequency curves were set several orders of magnitude lower than curve B, Fig. 4, as more nearly demanded by a repertoire of monospecific antibodies, let us say by using va = 4 and P(q,x,y,z) values 100 times lower than those for curve B, then one obtains $w_1 + w_2 + w_3 + w_4 = 0.27$. This result is interpreted as meaning that only about one in four possible haptens possesses a single structural feature which could interact with an energy above the van der Waals range. The result is not physically reasonable.

A description of probable interactions between protein McPC 603 and bound phosphorylcholine (Segal et al., 1974) appears not to fit the choice of binding events allowed in the model. The X-ray structure model shows that the phosphate group can participate in several hydrogen bonds and several electrostatic interactions. The positively charged choline nitrogen can interact with a negatively charged glutamic acid residue at a distance of 5 Å, and a number of van der Waals contacts are likely. The log K for binding of phosphorylcholine is close to 5.1, and it may be thought of as resulting from, say, nine van der Waals, or group 0, contacts (yielding a log K contribution of 2.7) and a single interaction *unit* from group 1 (for the remaining log K contribution of 2.4). The five long-range interactions are grouped together as a single unit because they act through relatively large distances and are correspondingly weak (average δ log K = 0.48). These interactions take place through various distances allowing for a flexibility of configuration. Thus, they lack the all-or-none character of independence as specially defined for the interaction unit of this model. The group of five interactions, as a whole, can be regarded as a unit acting independently of the van der Waals contacts. On the other hand, when a *single* electrostatic interaction or hydrogen bond contributes negative free energy sufficient for a group 1 through 4 interaction, the distance between atomic (or charge) centers must be somewhat smaller, and the allowance for variation (to stay within a given energy group) would be slight. The single interaction then would have more nearly all-or-none character in keeping with the imagery used in constructing the model.

V. A PROBABILITY MODEL OF SEROLOGICAL CROSS-REACTIONS WITH MULTISPECIFIC ANTIBODIES

Talmage (1959) first clearly proposed the hypothesis of general multispecificity and presented some lines of reasoning which explained how multispecific antibodies could populate highly specific immune sera. Later, Rosenstein et al. (1972) reiterated these ideas in terms of the clonal selection theory and specific B-cell receptors.

In brief, the explanation goes as follows. Specific antibodies populating an immune serum are derived from many cell clones each secreting uniform and structurally distinct antibodies. All of the antibodies share the ability to combine reasonably well with the eliciting antigen, and, if multispecific, they can combine with many other substances unrelated in structure to the immunogen. Because of structural differences in their variable sequences, antibodies derived from different clones may not share their alternate specificities. Therefore, cross-specificity with a given, structurally unrelated antigen will usually involve only one or two of the antibody components. Serological reactions, such as precipitation, toxin neutralization, and agglutination, have definitive thresholds which depend on antibody concentration and binding constant (Talmage, 1959). Association constants with disparate structures are likely to be low as predicted from curves in Fig. 4. Thus, with a heterogeneous antiserum, an inappropriate reaction of one or a few antibody species is likely to fall below threshold of detection; the more heterogeneous is the antibody population, the more likely this will be so. Consequently, it is possible for an antiserum to react much more specifically than can its component antibodies.

Previously I proposed a probability model for quantitatively examining the above concept (Inman, 1974). The underlying assumption of the model is that homologous and disparate specificities associate independently among different antibody species. An antiserum of h antibody species can be considered as a randomly drawn sample from a total repertoire of n variable region structures ($V_L \times V_H$ pairs). A certain number of species d among n happen to be reactive with a disparate test hapten. Since h kinds of antibodies are drawn without replacement, the probability that this sample will include k and only k species with the disparate reactivity is given by a hypergeometric distribution

$$P(k) = \frac{\binom{d}{k}\binom{n-d}{h-k}}{\binom{n}{h}} \tag{9}$$

If, for simplicity, the threshold of a serological reaction is defined by some fraction of the number of species h in the serum such as 1/10, then positive reactions will occur whenever k exceeds that level, that is, when $k \geqslant (h/10) + 1$. The probability $P(> \pm)$ of fulfilling this condition is simply

$$P(> \pm) = \text{cum}P\left(\frac{h}{10} + 1\right) = \sum_{k=h/10+1}^{k=h} P(k) \tag{10}$$

using P(k) terms from Eq. (9). These cumulative probabilities have been evaluated by computer over realistic ranges of values for the parameters of Eq. (9). The probabilities of positive serological cross-reactions with disparate structures are plotted on a logarithmic scale in Fig. 5 as a function of antiserum heterogeneity (parameter h). In most instances, the probabilities decrease rapidly and exponentially as h increases beyond approximately 10. Thus, the concept is confirmed that antisera can be more specific (in regard to disparate reactivities) than individual antibodies, and that antisera increase in specificity as they become more heterogeneous. I will refer to this concept as the heterogeneity principle.

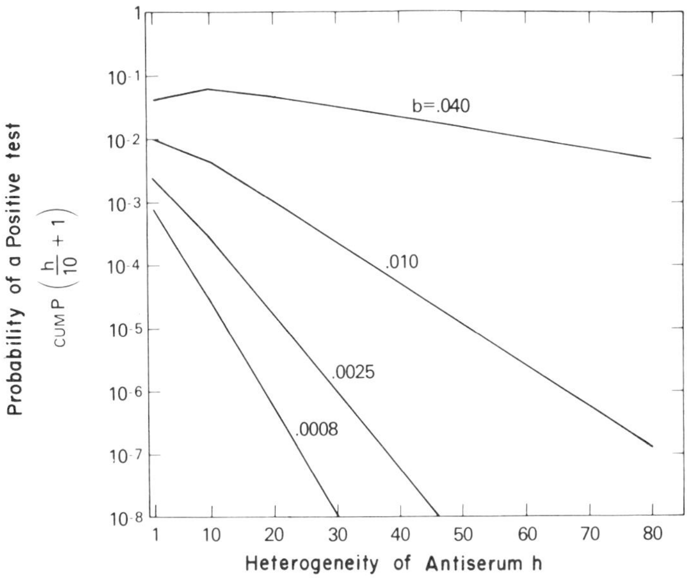

FIG. 5. Probabilities of positive serological cross-reactions with multispecific antibodies and disparately structured test haptens as a function of the number h of different antibody combining region structures ($V_H \times V_L$ pairs) represented in an antiserum. An assumed threshold (± reaction) is reached when h/10 of the species cross-react. The probabilities for (h/10) + 1 species cross-reacting were calculated from the model discussed in Section V and are given on the ordinate on a log scale. The curves were calculated with b = d/n held constant and n = 200,000. The b values used are shown above the curves (see Fig. 2).

The curves in Fig. 5 were calculated for n = 200,000 and for constant values of d/n. The latter ratio is simply the fraction b of the antibody repertoire that can bind a given disparate hapten with $k \geqslant 10^4\ M^{-1}$ as defined earlier. The corresponding b values are shown above the curves. The lower three curves correspond in descending order closely with curves A, B, and C in Fig. 4 with respect to b. The heterogeneity principle appears to break down when $b \geqslant 0.04$ (log b = -1.40). According to the hypothetical distribution of b given in Fig. 2, this circumstance should be met for only a small fraction of all haptens.

The size of the antibody repertoire n can be reduced to as low as 10,000 or increased toward infinity without appreciably affecting the plotted curves in Fig. 5. Below $n = 10{,}000$ there are simply too few antibodies (less than about 25) to populate antisera over the stipulated range of h. Because P(k) are relatively insensitive to n for $n > 10{,}000$ when b is held constant, a binomial distribution

$$P(k) \simeq \binom{h}{k} b^{k}(1 - b)^{h-k} \tag{11}$$

can be used as a satisfactory approximation for P(k) of Eq. (9) if $b < 0.04$. Equation (11) is easier to evaluate than the hypergeometric formula.

In conclusion, the model indicates that the heterogeneity principle could explain increases in specificity of several orders of magnitude for average cases. Specificity in this context refers to a low incidence of reaction with disparate structures. The power to discriminate similar antigenic determinants should be characteristic of either monospecific or multispecific antibodies. Finally, it has been noted that many antisera are either highly restricted in heterogeneity or else contain antibodies having shared variable region structural features (idiotypic determinants) which, if pronounced, could abolish much of the effect of the heterogeneity principle. Disparate structure reactivities would then be shared by many antibody components so that cross-reactions involving these components would exceed the threshold. However, in the worst cases, serological cross-reactions will not occur on the average more frequently than predicted by $P(> \pm) = b$. These probabilities are plotted at $h = 1$ in Fig. 5. Still, it would be necessary to test over 100 disparate haptens to average a single cross-reaction. There is little evidence of this kind extensive enough to test even this limiting case.

VI. ESTIMATION OF A MINIMUM ANTIBODY REPERTOIRE SIZE

In this Section I wish to consider a reasonable minimum size for an antibody repertoire in keeping with the type and degree of multi-specificity stipulated in Sections III, IV, and V. It is desired that the repertoire size n be large enough to allow antigen universality; that is, the repertoire should be capable of furnishing antibodies for an adequate response to any possible antigen. In order to meet this requirement, an antibody repertoire must provide (a) some antibodies against ($K \gtrsim 10^4\ M^{-1}$) any antigen, and (b) enough antibodies against most antigens so that a selection can be made having a good average binding constant and enough members to confer increased serological specificity in keeping with the heterogeneity principle (see Section V).

A few antigens may bind to only 0.01% of the antibody repertoire with $K \geqslant 10^4\ M^{-1}$ (Figure 2, log b = -4.0). If it is required that there be a few antibody species against any of these antigens with binding constants of around 10^5 to $10^7\ M^{-1}$, then there may need to be 20 or 30 such species in the repertoire with affinities greater than $10^4\ M^{-1}$. Therefore, a minimum repertoire size of 200,000 or 300,000 is demanded.

Another kind of estimation is made as follows. One finds from curve B, Fig. 4, the number of antibodies (per 10^5) reactive with an average antigen with log K between 8.0 and 9.0 to be 5.5, and with log K > 9.0 to be 9.6. A symmetrical distribution of affinities with average log K = 8.5 could be made with at most 5.5 + (2 × 9.6) = 24.7 antibody species per 10^5. For the heterogeneity principle to operate (see Fig. 5), there should be at least 20 species in an antiserum within the above distribution. In order to have available 20 such antibodies during an immunization period, perhaps three times as many species should be present in the all-time repertoire, or at least 60. The minimum repertoire size then becomes $(60/24.7) \times 10^5 \approx 240{,}000$. Analogous reasoning for curve C requiring a distribution of antibodies around log K = 7.5 yields an estimate of about 360,000 species.

Experimental evidence bearing on the value of n comes from the work of Kreth et al. (1973) who estimated the number of antibodies reactive with the hapten NIP (3-iodo-4-hydroxy-5-nitrophenylacetyl) in the CBA/H mouse strain. By means of limited cell transfers from immunized donors to irradiated recipients and subsequent identification of anti-NIP antibody species by isoelectric gel focusing, they determined repeat frequencies of individual species. Statistical calculations from the data indicated that something of the order of 5000 anti-NIP combining region structures were represented in the CBA/H repertoire. Pink and Askonas (1974), using the dinitrophenyl and trinitrophenyl haptens were able to show, in several strains of mice by cross-reactive stimulation and isoelectric focusing, that there are around 500 repertoire antibodies, each of which can bind both DNP or TNP (above their threshold of detection). They reasoned that those species able to bind DNP alone could number an order of magnitude larger, that is, around 5000 as in the case of anti-NIP in CBA/H. If one assumes that NIP and DNP binding frequencies follow curve A of Fig. 4, and that the isoelectric focusing visualization technique detects antibodies with $K > 10^{3.5}\ M^{-1}$, then a repertoire size of about 300,000 is obtained. Uncertainties in these figures could readily allow an estimate several times or more great.

On the whole it appears that an antibody combining region repertoire in the range of 10^5 to 10^6, perhaps around 300,000, is compatible with the requirements for general multispecificity, antigen universality, and adequate serological specificity. Finally, it may be interesting to note that about 2000 V_H and 1000 V_L sequences, pairing randomly within six independent subgroupings, could generate 300,000 combining regions according to the formula given by Inman (1974, p. 49). If antibody repertoires are in fact as small as the above estimates of minimum size, it should be feasible to account for antibody diversity by invoking a rather modest degree of somatic variation upon the minimally required germ-line repertoires of structural genes.

VII. GENERAL DISCUSSION

The concept of general multispecificity can be developed by starting with the notion that any immunoglobulin combining region will interact *to a degree* with any substance having access to it. For the most part, positive (attractive) interactions should occur, and some particular configuration of the system will result in a minimum in free energy. The system is made up not only of the two major interactants but also of other solute species and solvent (both in bulk and as bound water). The configuration of the system is properly defined in terms of the degrees of freedom allowed each component and the temperature. These parameters comprise a very complex manifold. Mainly, one should realize that a simple geometric model such as fitting jigsaw pieces together is not likely to yield an adequate understanding of how antibodies and ligands behave. The opportunities for appreciable minimization of free energy must certainly be far more abundant than the singular prescription of topological complementarity would allow.

The model presented in Section IV is an attempt to give a more general approach to understanding specificity in protein-ligand interactions by first removing the constraint of all-or-none binding for which it is difficult to attach physical (thermodynamic) meaning. The model, of course, employs a number of necessary simplifications. Although it was set up with the help of simple geometric imagery such as the contacting of atoms or groups of atoms (interaction units), the probabilistic considerations would include rather than exclude various conformational degrees of freedom of the antigen and antibody structures. The interaction units were associated with but not fully defined by discrete noncovalent interactions. Thus, the grouped free energy changes could be thought of as including apportioned contributions to free energy changes resulting from conformational adjustments, removal of ligand from bulk solvent, displacement of bound water and small ions, etc. The model describes (a) how a continuous variety of binding constants can be expected from testing many immunoglobulins with randomly selected substances,

(b) why the vast majority of interactions will occur below the normal threshold of measurement (around $K = 10^3\ M^{-1}$), and (c) how progressively higher binding constants will be observed with progressively decreasing frequency.

The cumulative frequency distributions of log K (Fig. 4) are based on realistic assignments of unit free energy changes with a probability treatment that, when put together, allows some reasonable explanation for the observed high binding frequencies of myeloma proteins, "strange" cross-reactions and the occurrence of natural antibodies. It is a direct consequence of the cumulative frequency function that, for any defined minimum binding constant K_{min}, an antibody will interact with a certain fraction of all possible antigens, or a given antigen will interact with that fraction of all antibodies, with a K equal to or greater than K_{min}. That is to say, a certain fraction of all *tests* (one antibody vs. one potential ligand) will occur with $K \geqslant K_{min}$. This principle provides a solution to the antibody repertoire paradox presented in Section II: No matter how many possible antigens there can be, any one of them can be bound well by some members of a reasonably populated repertoire of antibodies. But will most such antigen-antibody interactions be adequately specific and biologically functional?

The above question has been discussed by Richards and Konigsberg (1973) and Richards et al. (1975). I would like to comment further on the specificity issue. Specificity is usually defined as the discriminating power that an antibody (or group of antibodies) has toward antigens of similar structure, the so-called fine specificity. If each antibody species must be able to combine well with a large number of possible antigens to explain observed antigen universality, then an average monospecific antibody must combine well with that same large number of *similar* structures. From the reasoning given in Section II, this number must be very large, and the fine specificity of monospecific antibodies must be correspondingly small. Multispecific antibodies make up for the disparity between numbers of antigens and antibodies by reacting with *many* dissimilar families of similar antigens. Each family is accordingly smaller in size, and the various fine specificities are correspondingly greater. In this view, the considerable discriminating power that has been observed for antibodies toward similar substances agrees better with the multispecificity hypothesis. For the proper functioning of immune systems, it may be more essential to have a high order of fine specificity than complete freedom from disparate cross-reactions.

I am tempted to speculate that multispecificity is a general characteristic of all ligand-binding proteins, including various kinds of cell surface receptors. I call attention to the multispecific binding by enzymes reported by Glazer (1970). The action of many drugs is mediated by their being bound to certain cell surface receptors. It is possible that the structures of some drugs bear little resemblance to those of the normal effector molecules. If so, drug screening should not be drastically confined to modulations of structures with known biological activity. Thus, many questions arise from the concepts of multispecificity. Some of the answers may come from studies of antibodies which can serve as varied and highly accessible models for ligand-binding systems.

REFERENCES

Amzel, L. M., Poljak, R. J., Saul, F., Varga, J. M., and Richards, F. F. (1974). The three-dimensional structure of a combining-region-ligand complex of immunoglobulin NEW at 3.5-Å resolution. *Proc. Nat. Acad. Sci. (USA) 71:* 1427-1430.

Burnet, F. M. (1959). *The Clonal Selection Theory of Acquired Immunity.* Vanderbilt University Press, Nashville.

Cameron, D. J. and Erlanger, B. F. (1976). Nucleic acid-reactive antibodies of restricted heterogeneity. *Immunochem. 13:* 263-269.

Edmundson, A. B., Ely, K. R., Girling, R. L., Abola, E. E., Schiffer, M., Westholm, F. A., Fausch, M. D., and Deutsch, H. F. (1974). Binding of 2,4-dinitrophenyl compounds and other small molecules to a crystalline λ-type Bence-Jones dimer. *Biochemistry 13:* 3816-3827.

Eisen, H. N. (1971). Combining sites of anti-2,4-dinitrophenyl antibodies. In *Progress in Immunology* (B. Amos, ed.). Academic, New York, pp. 243-251.

Eisen, H. N., Little, J. R., Osterland, C. K., and Simms, E. S. (1967). A myeloma protein with antibody activity. In *Antibodies, Cold Spring Harbor Symposia on Quantitative Biology*, vol. 32 (L. Frisch, ed.). Cold Spring Harbor Laboratory of Quantitative Biology, Cold Spring Harbor, Long Island, New York, pp. 75-81.

Eisen, H. N., Michaelides, M. C., Underdown, B. J., Schulenburg, E. P., and Simms, E. S. (1970). Myeloma proteins with antihapten antibody activity. *Fed. Proc. 29:* 78-84.

Epp, O., Colman, P., Fehlhammer, H., Bode, W., Schiffer, M., and Huber, R. (1974). Crystal and molecular structure of a dimer composed of the variable portions of the Bence-Jones protein REI. *Eur. J. Biochem. 45:* 513-524.

Glazer, A. N. (1970). On the prevalence of "nonspecific" binding at the specific binding sites of globular proteins. *Proc. Nat. Acad. Sci. (USA) 65:* 1057-1063.

Haber, E. (1964). Recovery of antigenic specificity after denaturation and complete reduction of disulfides in a papain fragment of antibody. *Proc. Nat. Acad. Sci. (USA) 52:* 1099-1106.

Hirschfeld, J. (1974). Some notes on the concept of cross-reactivity. *Vox Sang. 27:* 254-260.

Hoffmeister, M. J. and Voss, E. W., Jr. (1974). Binding of ε-DNP-L-lysine exceeding two moles by purified chicken IgG anti-DNP antibody. *Immunochem. 11:* 641-650.

Hood, L. and Talmage, D. W. (1970). Mechanism of antibody diversity: germ line basis for variability. *Science 168:* 325-334.

Hsia, J. C., Wong, L. T. L., Pryse, K., and Little, J. R. (1973). Alteration of binding specificity of murine myeloma protein-315 to 2,4-dinitrophenyl and 2,4,6-trinitrophenyl ligands. *Immunochem. 10:* 517-520.

Inman, J. K. (1974). Multispecificity of the antibody combining region and antibody diversity. In *The Immune System: Genes, Receptors, Signals* (E. E. Sercarz, A. R. Williamson, and C. F. Fox, eds.). Academic, New York, pp. 37-52.

Jaton, J.-C., Klinman, N. R., Givol, D., and Sela, M. (1968). Recovery of antibody activity upon reoxidation of completely reduced polyalanyl heavy chain and its Fd fragment derived from anti-2,4-dinitrophenyl antibody. *Biochem. 7:* 4185-4195.

Kabat, E. A. (1976). *Structural Concepts in Immunology and Immunochemistry* 2nd ed. Holt, Rinehard and Winston, New York.

Klinman, N. R., Press, J. L., Segal, N. H., and Gearhart, P. J. (1976). The acquisition of the B cell specificity repertoire: the germ line theory of predetermined permutation of genetic information. In *The Generation of Diversity: A New Look* (A. J. Cunningham, ed.). Academic, London, pp. 127-149.

Kreth, H. W., Williamson, A. R., Wybrow, G. M., and Berryman, I. L. (1973). The extent of diversity of anti-hapten antibodies in inbred mice: Anti-NIP (4-hydroxy-5-iodo-3-nitrophenacetyl) antibodies in CBA/H mice. *Eur. J. Immunol. 3:* 141-147.

Landsteiner, K. (1945). *The Specificity of Serological Reactions*, revised ed. Harvard University Press, Cambridge, Massachusetts.

Padlan, E. A. and Davies, D. R. (1975). Variability of three-dimensional structure in immunoglobulins. *Proc. Nat. Acad. Sci. (USA) 72:* 819-823.

Pauling, L. (1940). A theory of the structure and process of formation of antibodies. *J. Am. Chem. Soc. 62:* 2643-2657.

Pink, J. R. L. and Askonas, B. A. (1974). Diversity of antibodies to cross-reacting nitrophenyl haptens in inbred mice. *Eur. J. Immunol. 4:* 426-430.

Poljak, R. J., Amzel, L. M., Chen, B. L., Phizackerley, R. P., and Saul, F. (1974). The three-dimensional structure of the Fab' fragment of a human myeloma immunoglobulin at 2.0-Å resolution. *Proc. Nat. Acad. Sci. (USA) 71:* 3440-3444.

Richards, F. F., Amzel, L. M., Konigsberg, W. H., Manjula, B. N., Poljak, R. J., Rosenstein, R. W., Saul, F., and Varga, J. M. (1974). Polyfunctional antibody combining regions. In *The Immune System: Genes, Receptors, Signals* (E. E. Sercarz, A. R. Williamson, and C. F. Fox, eds.). Academic, New York, pp. 53-67.

Richards, F. F. and Konigsberg, W. H. (1973). How specific are antibodies? *Immunochem. 10:* 545-553.

Richards, F. F., Konigsberg, W. H., Rosenstein, R. W., and Varga, J. M. (1975). On the specificity of antibodies. *Science 187:* 130-137.

Riesen, W. and Morell, A. (1972). A human myeloma protein with specificity against dinitrophenyl and nucleic acid derivatives. *Immunochem. 9:* 979-985.

Rosenstein, R. W., Musson, R. A., Armstrong, M. Y. K., Konigsberg, W. H., and Richards, F. F. (1972). Contact regions for dinitrophenyl and menadione haptens in an immunoglobulin binding more than one antigen. *Proc. Nat. Acad. Sci. (USA) 69:* 877-881.

Sachs, D. H., Schechter, A. N., Eastlake, A., and Anfinsen, C. B. (1972). An immunologic approach to the conformational equilibria of polypeptides. *Proc. Nat. Acad. Sci. (USA) 69:* 3790-3794.

Schubert, D., Roman, A., and Cohn, M. (1970). Anti-nucleic acid specificities of mouse myeloma immunoglobulins. *Nature 225:* 154-158.

Segal, D. M., Padlan, E. A., Cohen, G. H., Rudikoff, S., Potter, M., and Davies, D. R. (1974). The three-dimensional structure of phosphorylcholine-binding mouse immunoglobulin Fab and the nature of the antigen binding site. *Proc. Nat. Acad. Sci. (USA) 71:* 4298-4302.

Talmage, D. W. (1959). Immunological specificity. *Science 129:* 1643-1648.

Tolleshaug, H. and Hannestad, K. (1975). Binding of ligands to a monoclonal IgM macroglobulin with multiple specificity. *Immunochem. 12:* 173-182.

Underdown, B. J. and Eisen, H. N. (1971). Cross-reactions between 2,4-dinitrophenyl and 5-acetouracil groups. *J. Immunol. 106:* 1431-1440.

Varga, J. M., Konigsberg, W. H., and Richards, F. F. (1973). Antibodies with multiple binding functions. Induction of single immunoglobulin species by structurally dissimilar haptens. *Proc. Nat. Acad. Sci. (USA) 70:* 3269-3274.

Varga, J. M., Lande, S., and Richards, F. F. (1974). Immunoglobulins with multiple binding functions. II. The use of nylon-polyserine whisker discs in screening myeloma immunoglobulins for binding activity. *J. Immunol. 112:* 1565-1570.

Whitney, P. L. and Tanford, C. (1965). Recovery of specific activity after complete unfolding and reduction of an antibody fragment. *Proc. Nat. Acad. Sci. (USA) 53:* 524-532.

Williamson, A. R. (1972). Extent and control of antibody diversity. *Biochem. J. 130:* 325-333.

Part V

INTERACTIONS AMONG B CELLS, T CELLS, AND MACROPHAGES

Chapter 10

INDUCTION OF HUMORAL RESPONSES IN VITRO

Marc Feldmann

ICRF Tumour Immunology Unit
Department of Zoology
University College
London, England

Current knowledge of the mechanism of induction of antibody responses is reviewed. The key points are the diversity of cells involved, and their interaction by a multitude of factors.

I. INTRODUCTION

The heterogeneity of the lymphoid system has been appreciated since the principle of clonal selection was formulated (Burnet, 1959). This heterogeneity resides in the specificity of receptors for antigen on the membrane of individual lymphocytes. More recently, lymphocyte heterogeneity has been extended, first to cover two major types of lymphocytes (T, or thymus-derived lymphocytes; and B or bursal equivalent or bone marrow-derived lymphocytes), and more recently to subpopulations within these groups (e.g., Beverley, 1976). Since these subpopulations of cells, separated on the basis of cell membrane markers, correlate with distinct lymphoid functions, there is increasing evidence that the concept of lymphocyte subpopulations is both valid and important in understanding the induction and regulation of immune functions (e.g., Cantor and Boyse, 1975). Thus, despite the relative newness of much of this information, it seems essential to incorporate it.

There has been an ever-increasing mass of information pertinent to the mechanisms of induction and control of immune responses, with various antigens in various species, leading to different types of responses. It is clearly not possible, or even desirable to catalog or summarize these, and this chapter will present a highly selected and filtered view of immunology with a very marked emphasis on the work of the author and his colleagues.

Since induction of antibody responses cannot be divorced from their regulation, the induction of specific suppressor T cells is also discussed.

II. HETEROGENEITY OF THE LYMPHOID SYSTEM

It is well known that lymphocytes are the principal cells involved in immune responses. Despite the morphological homogeneity of lymphocytes within each size range (small, medium, and large), their heterogeneity by other criteria has been apparent for many years. Physical methods of cell separation, such as on the basis of size (Miller and Phillips, 1969), density (Shortman, 1968), or charge (e.g., Nordling et al., 1972), have provided evidence of heterogeneity of lymphocytes. The use of hetero- or alloantisera to lymphocytes has also provided evidence for lymphocyte heterogeneity. A list of known lymphocyte cell surface markers is illustrated in Table 1, which provides clear evidence of lymphocyte heterogeneity. A summary of T-cell subpopulations is described in Table 2. A fuller discussion of lymphocyte heterogeneity may be found in Beverley (1976).

III. OVERVIEW OF ANTIBODY PRODUCTION

It is clear that we do not yet understand much about the mechanisms regulating antibody production. Yet there is much more information available now than previously, and this has led to a variety of speculations and theories about the underlying molecular mechanisms (see *Transplantation Reviews*, Vol. 23).

Our current experimental goal is to ascertain the degree of complexity of the cellular interactions involved in antibody production and its regulation, by separating the pathway into several stages, each of which can be studied in isolation. Within each stage, there is a range of cells involved, producing various immunologically active mediators (termed factors), which interact with other cells and act to permit or facilitate lymphocyte proliferation and/or differentiation from the precursor to the activated stage. Thus, immune responses may be viewed in the same (cascade) sequence

TABLE 1
Mouse Lymphocyte Cell Surface Markers[a]

Antigens defined by	Distribution		
Heteroantisera	T	B	Plasma cells
MSLA	+	-	-
MBLA	-	+	+
MSPCA	-	-	+
Th-B	-	+	+
Alloantisera			
Thy 1	+	-	-
Ly 1	+ S[b]	-	-
2	+ S		
3	+ S	-	-
4	-	+	+
5	+ S	-	-
6	+ S	±	+
7	+ S	±	+
PC 1	-	-	+
Ala 1	Activated cells only		+
Ia	± S	+	+
H-2	+	+	+
Receptors			
Fc	+	++	-
C3	-	+	-

[a]For details, see Beverley (1976).
[b]Some (S) but not all T cells.

TABLE 2

T-Cell Subpopulations[a]

Ly Phenotype:	1^+	2^+ 3^+	2^+ 3^+
Function:	Helper cells	T Killer cells	Amplifying cells
Property:	(Both specific, nonspecific)	Suppressor cells	For helper cells
	Delayed hypersensitivity.		And suppressor cells

[a]Concept of T_1 and T_2 cells: T_1 are short-lived, nonrecirculating cells; T_2, long-lived, recirculating cells. These can be purified by these properties: T_1 by the injection of antilymphocyte serum which depletes recirculating cells, and T_2 by adult thymectomy which after a few weeks results in a depletion of short-lived T cells (T_1). Amplifiers for helper suppressor and killer cells are T_1. Precursors of helper, suppressor, and killer cells are all T_2. But it is evident that T_2 is a heterogeneous cell group.

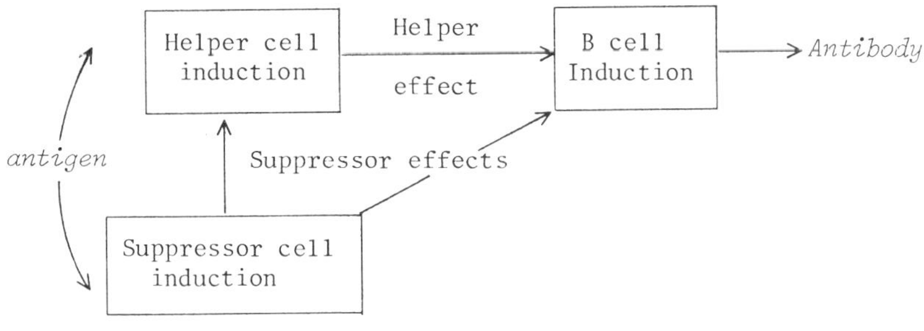

FIG. 1. Areas of cell interaction

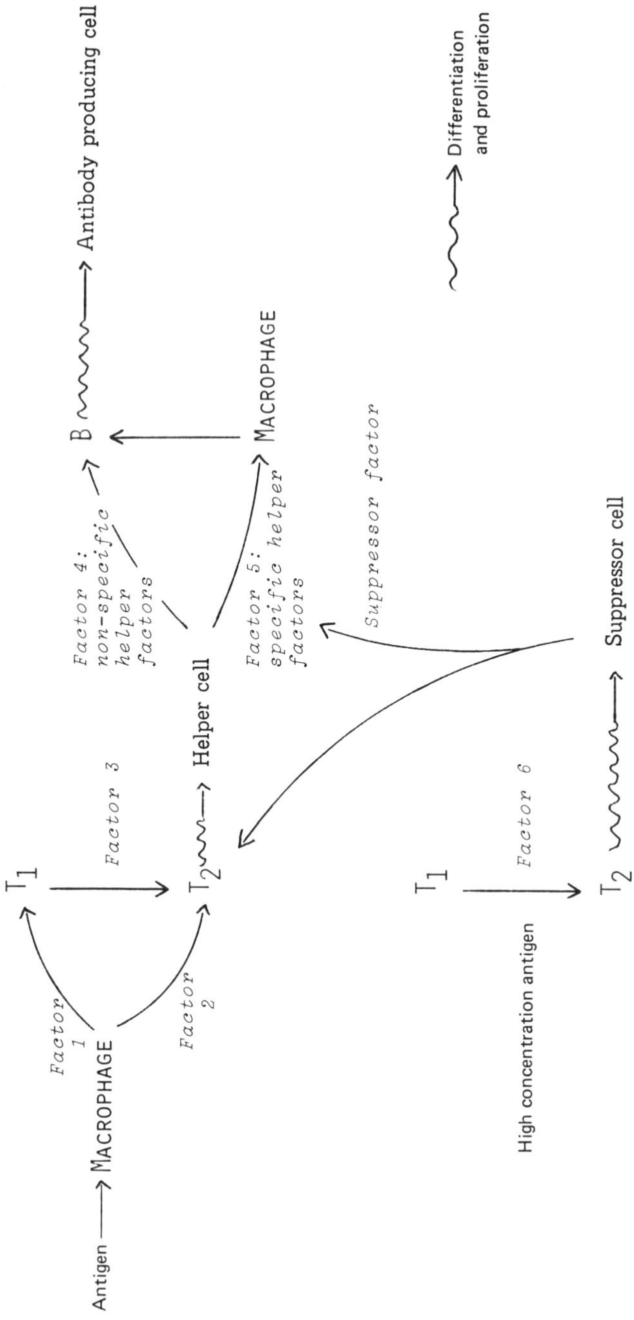

FIG. 2. Scheme of cell interaction in antibody production.

that biochemical reactions are represented, such as metabolic pathway , or the complement or blood clotting pathway. Initial experiments of this type indicated that there were three major areas of cell interactions involved in the antibody response, as shown in Fig. 1. Our current view of the cells involved, the factors, etc., are summarized in Fig. 2, which is to be viewed as a framework, rather than a completed or definite scheme. Already there are at least seven cells, and nine factors or groups of factors have been tentatively identified.

IV. MECHANISM OF ANTIBODY PRODUCTION

A. Induction of Helper Cells

Helper cells (HC) are the T cells that collaborate with B cells. Their function is measured indirectly by their "cooperative effect," assessed by measuring the antibody or antibody forming cells generated by B cells. This indirect test is unfortunate, because the relation between T cell help and antibody production is not always simple, as the helper cell antibody response titration curves are often bi- or triphasic. Thus in most experiments, helper cells must be tested (for cooperative capacity) at several cell doses.

There are two types of cell interactions involved in helper cell induction: those between T cells (as a group) and macrophage-like cells, and those between subpopulations of T cells. For simplicity these will be discussed separately.

B. Macrophage-T Cell Interaction

Depletion of macrophages from normal spleen, lymph node, or cortisone-resistant thymus cell suspensions abrogates their capacity to be induced into helper cells (Erb and Feldmann, 1975a). This is true both with soluble protein antigens and particulate antigens in which the same protein has been conjugated to surfaces, such as acrylamide or sepharose beads. However, the macrophage requirements differ somewhat. With unprimed T cells and particulate antigens, any source of mouse macrophages suffice. In contrast, with soluble antigens, macrophages derived from allogeneic donors were not effective but those from syngeneic or semisyngeneic donors were effective (Erb and Feldmann, 1975a). The genetic requirements of the macrophage-T cell interaction were studied, by using cells derived from mice of different strains, mice congenic at the H-2 complex, and recombinants within the H-2 complex. The results, using two different antigens in mice having several different H-2 haplotypes, were consistent: for effective T-macrophage interaction there must be similarity in the I-A subregion of the mouse H-2 complex (Erb and Feldmann, 1975b). Whether this genetic restriction (I-A region similarity) is true for all antigens or T cells is not yet know. It is of interest, however, that antigen-primed guinea pig peritoneal T cells require macrophage similarity at the 2 or 13 locus (equivalent to the mouse I region) to proliferate in vitro in response to the priming antigen (Rosenthal and Shevach, 1973). Experiments illustrating the genetic restrictions are shown in Fig. 3.

The mechanism of T-macrophage interaction was investigated. One of the important questions was to determine whether membrane contact was required, or whether cooperation occurred at a distance with the participation of diffusable mediators. These hypotheses may be tested in vitro by using double-chamber culture flasks, and placing the two cell types in different compartments. Such experiments, and the generation of active cell-free supernatants from antigen incubated macrophages (Erb and Feldmann, 1975c), indicated that cell contact was not essential. Fractionation of these cell-free supernatants indicated that the active component had a molecular weight of about 55,000 (as judged by Sephadex G-100 fractionation) and contained Ia antigen and a fragment of the immunizing antigen (Erb et al., 1976). These experiments do not provide information about the physiology of macrophage-T cell interaction. For example, they do not exclude that T-macrophage contact is *also* a pathway of stimulation. It is of interest that in the guinea pig antigen induced proliferation assay, supernatants have not yet been found to replace macrophages.

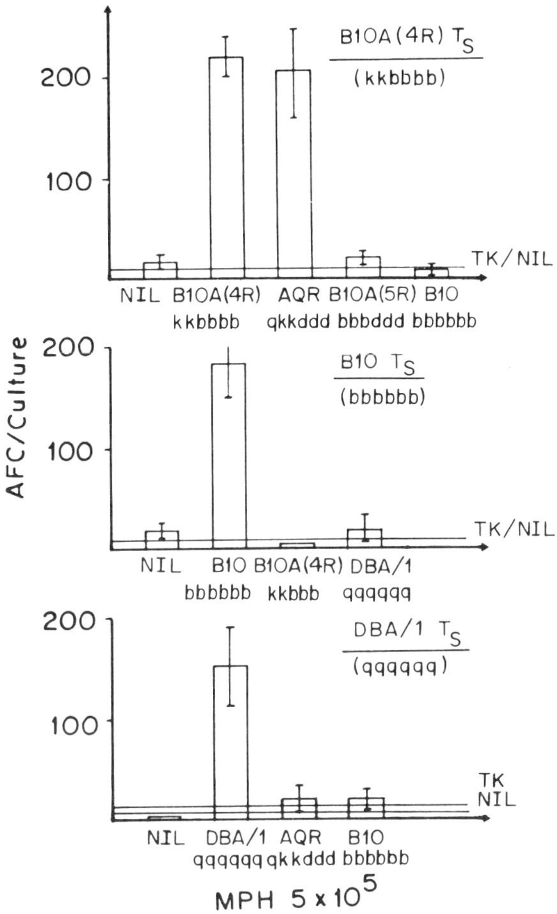

FIG. 3. Genetic mapping of the locus permitting T-macrophage interaction in the generation of helper cells to soluble antigen (KLH) in vitro. In the assay for helper-cell function, the number of antibody forming cells (AFC) per culture is determined after potential helper cells are cultured with antigen in the presence of 5 X 10^5 macrophages from the indicated donors. Gene sequences in the H-2 complex are indicated by the strings of letters, and identity at the second position is seen to be required for collaboration. Top graph: stimulation of B10.A (4R) T cells by macrophages of the B10.A (4R), AQR, but not by B10.A (5R) and B10 congenic strains. Middle graph: lack of stimulation of B10 T cells by B10.A (4R) and DBA/1 macrophages. Bottom graph: lack of stimulation of DBA/1 T cells by AQR macrophages. Together these results permit localization of the T-macrophage interaction locus in the I-A region of the mouse H-2 complex. Reprinted from *Membrane Receptors of Lymphocytes (1975)*. (M. Seligman, J. L. Preud'homme, and F. Kourilsky, eds.) North Holland, Amsterdam, pp. 305-310.

As yet little more is known of the details of this T-macrophage interaction. A schematic representation is shown in Fig. 4.

Rather different results have been obtained using particulate antigen. No genetic restrictions of macrophage source were found, and even 2-mercaptoethanol partially replaced macrophages. The reasons for this difference are not yet known in detail, although it seems that there is activation of the T_2 cell directly, without cooperation with the T_1 (Feldmann and Erb, 1977).

C. T-T Interactions in the Induction of Helper Cells

Evidence for T-T interaction was first obtained in the graft-vs.-host response (Cantor and Asofsky, 1970). Essentially similar results were obtained in the generation of killer cells in vitro (e.g., Wagner, 1973). It was thus of interest to ascertain whether T-T interaction was also needed for the generation of helper cells. The antigen-oxidized ferrodoxin (OFd), a polypeptide of molecular weight 5500 derived from *Clostridium pasteurianum*, was first used to test this concept. This antigen was used because it contained two antigenic determinants of known composition and sequence, termed the N- and C-terminal peptide determinants. These determinants can be conjugated to other proteins, for example, bovine serum albumin (BSA), and mice can be primed to each determinant separately, for example by injection of N-BSA or C-BSA. Helper-cell induction was only effective in vitro, using OFd as antigen, if spleen cells were obtained from mice primed to OFd, or if a *mixture* of N- and C-primed spleen cells were cultured (Feldmann, Kilburn and Levy, 1975). A representative experiment of this type is shown in Fig. 5.

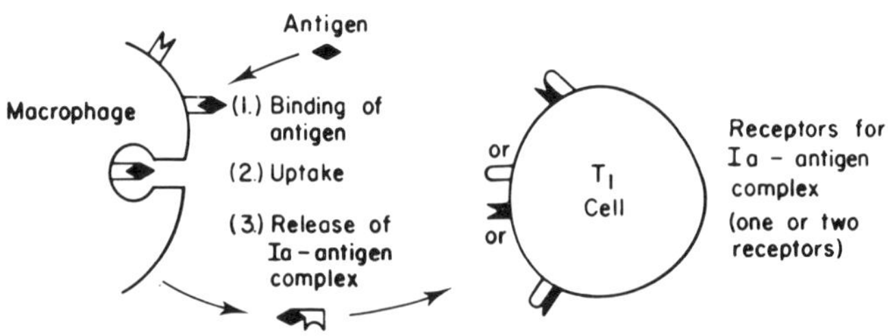

FIG. 4. Schematic representation of T-macrophage interaction.

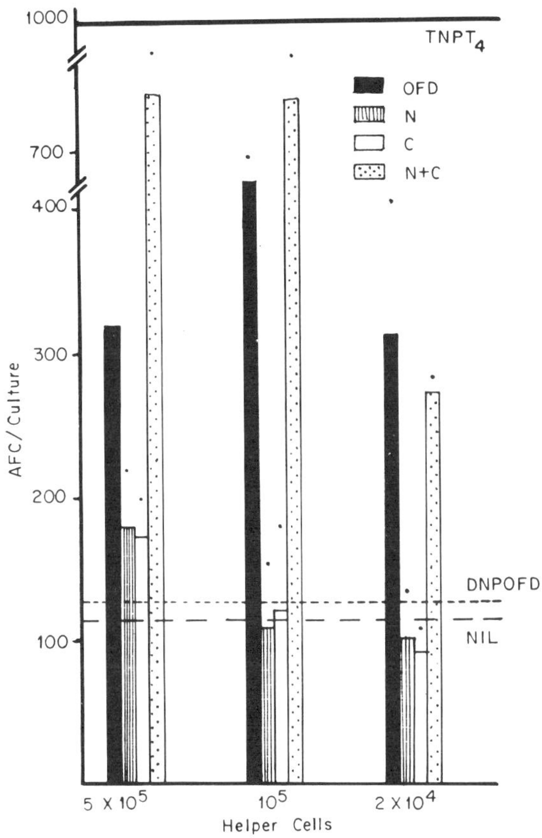

FIG. 5. Synergy between N- and C-primed T cells. Spleen T cells were obtained from mice immunized with OFd, N-BSA, or C-BSA and assayed for their ability to help B cells produce anti-DNP antibody, in the presence of the antigen OFd-DNP. Responses without antigen, without helper cells, or with a thymus-independent antigen are given by the lines nil, DNP-OFd, and $TNPT_4$, respectively. Significant helper cells for OFd were only induced provided OFd primed T cells, or a *mixture* of N- and C-BSA primed spleen cells were used in the assay for T-cell help. The dots above the bars indicate the upper limit of the standard error. (Reprinted from *Nature 256:* 741-743).

However, there are a few antigens resembling OFd. Most protein antigens have more than two antigenic determinants, and these are not of known composition or sequence. Thus it was not known whether the evidence for T-T interaction obtained with OFd was true for other antigens. Experiments were performed using T_1 cells, obtained from the spleens of mice injected with antilymphocyte serum, and T_2 cells, obtained from the spleens of adult thymectomized mice. It was found, using more conventional protein antigens like keyhole limpet hemocyanin (KLH), that a mixture of T_1 and T_2 cells were required for helper-cell induction. Cell contact was not required, as effective interaction occurred across Cell contact was not required, as effective interaction occurred across a membrane. Furthermore, since helper cells were only found in the T_2 pool, we concluded that T_2 cells are the direct precursors of the helper cells.

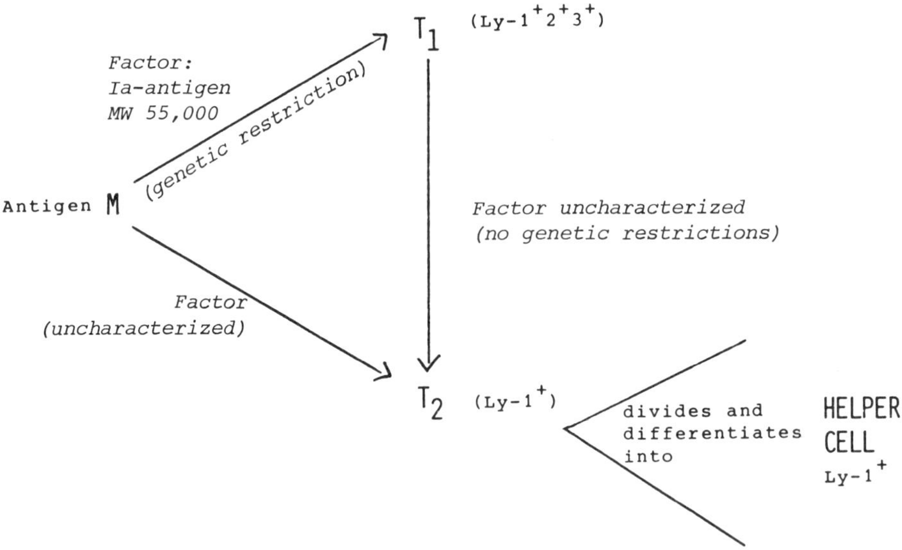

FIG. 6. Helper cell induction

The obvious question remains of how to combine the T-macrophage and T-T data into a coherent framework. To do this it was essential to determine which T cell (T_1 or T_2) interacted with macrophages. Several approaches were used, and these all indicated that the T_1 cells interact with macrophages (Erb et al., 1977). A summary of the minimal pathway for in vitro helper-cell induction is shown in Fig. 6, together with the phenotypes of the relevant cells.

D. Induction of Antigen-specific Suppressor Cells

Suppressor cells are T cells which diminish immune responses. They have been described in a variety of circumstances (reviewed by Gershon, 1973), many of which resemble the conditions for inducing tolerance. Incubation of spleen cells or T cells with high concentrations of antigen for 3 to 5 days induces a population of antigen specific suppressor cells (Kontiainen and Feldmann, 1976).

These cells act on helper cells. By serological analysis of membrane markers, T-helper cells (Ly 1^+ 2^- 3^- Ia^-) can be distinguished from T-suppressor cells (Ly 1^- 2^+ 3^+ Ia^+) activated in vitro (Feldmann et al., 1975). Tada and his colleagues have found a suppressive factor from lysed suppressor cells. This factor was of molecular weight 50,000, was antigen-specific (adhered to antigen columns), and was absorbed by columns of anti-Ia antiserum (Takemori and Tada, 1975). Our preliminary experiments, using supernatants of in vitro activated T-suppressor cells, have indicated broadly analogous results.

Since the induction of helper cells required the interaction of T cells with macrophages, it was of interest to determine whether this was also true for suppressor-cell induction. In marked contrast, there was no evidence of macrophage requirement, using adherence (to plastic, glass beads, or nylon wool), combined with phagocytosis (adherence) of carbonyl iron to eliminate macrophages (Feldmann and Kontiainen, 1976). These experiments do not prove that *no* macrophages at all are required in this reaction, but convincingly demonstrate that whatever the requirement is, it is strikingly different from the macrophage requirement for helper cell induction. The only

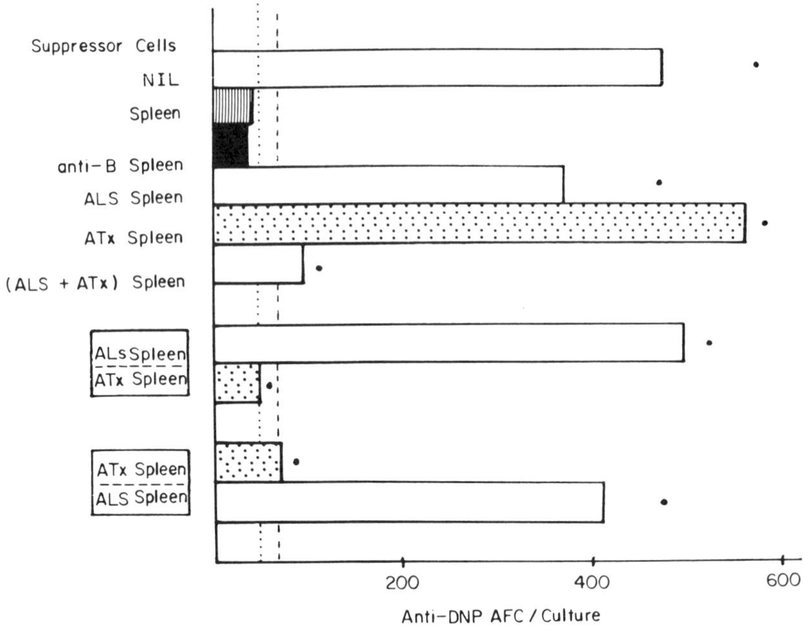

FIG. 7. Induction of KLH suppressor cells across a cell impermeable membrane. Suppressor cells were spleen cells treated as indicated. Anti-B, with an antiserum against B cells (showing that suppressors are not B cells); ATS, with anti-lymphocyte serum which eliminates T_2 cells; ATx, from adult thymectomized animals, which lack T_1 cells. Because the viability of cells in the upper compartment is not as good (about half of the lower), results with T cells from ATx spleen in the lower as well as the upper chamber are shown in the lower four bars. In both instances, suppressor cells are only found in the ATx compartment. Background responses, with no antigen, or TNP-KLH in the absence of helper cells, are shown by the dotted and dashed lines, respectively. Results are arithmetic means of three cultures. Dots indicate ± 1 standard error of the mean. (Reprinted from *Eur. J. Immunol. 6*, 302-305, 1976).

evidence suggesting that macrophages are not required comes from experiments designed to test the antigen concentration requirements for suppressor-cell induction in the absence of macrophages which are about 10-fold lower than in the presence of macrophages.

The question of T-T interaction in suppressor-cell induction was also of interest. Experiments performed using T_1 and T_2 cells (purified by antilymphocyte serum or adult thymectomy, respectively), indicated that suppressor cell induction requires T_1-T_2 interaction. By the use of double-chamber flasks, it was shown that this interaction occurs by means of subcellular factors, and that the direct precursors of suppressor cells are cells. Some of these results are illustrated in Fig. 7 (Feldmann and Kontiainen, 1976).

E. Typing of Helper Cells, Suppressor Cells, and Their Precursors

The relation between T-helper cells and suppressor cells is of importance in understanding the regulation of the antibody response. Ly antisera were used to determine whether these cells are the same. Differentiated helper and suppressor cells were found to be phenotypically distinct by four different markers:

Helper cells Ly 1^+ 2^- 3^- Ia

Suppressor cells Ly 1^- 2^+ 3^+ Ia^+

Using the same antisera, the precursors of the helper cells were also found to be different from the precursors of suppressor cells. Thus, there are present in the peripheral lymphoid tissue several distinct lines of T cells, differentiating along diverse pathways. The basic problem in understanding the regulation of the antibody response now becomes one of understanding how the various T-cell classes are selectively stimulated under different conditions.

V. INTERACTION OF HELPER T CELLS WITH B CELLS

While this was the first example of cell interactions to be identified in the immune system, there is still no universal concensus as to its mechanism. This area has been reviewed recently (Miller, 1972) and will not be extensively discussed here since there has not been much recent conceptual progress.

Current ideas revolve around helper T-cell function being mediated by factors, which are antigen-specific or nonspecific and permit the triggering of B cells. Differences of opinion rest on the chemical nature of these factors, cellular target of these factors, and the relation of histocompatibility antigens/genes in these interactions.

With respect to nonspecific factors, differences of opinion exist as to the molecular weight of these factors, and their mode of action.

A. Cooperation via IgT

Cell-free supernatants from activated T cells (helper cells induced in vivo) were found to induce thymus-dependent responses in normal or primed mouse spleen cell suspensions or T-depleted spleen cells (Feldmann and Basten, 1972). The major active component in the supernatant was inactivated or absorbed by antiimmunoglobulin antisera (either polyvalent, anti-κ or anti-μ). Since it came from viable T cells (as samples depleted of T cells did not release it) it was termed IgT (Feldmann, 1972).

Other workers have, in different systems, obtained evidence for molecules of this type. Tada and his colleagues, using lysates of rat spleen or thymus, found an antigen specific helper factor of molecular weight 150,000, which was absorbed with anti-κ and anti-μ chain antisera (Taniguchi and Tada, 1974), and which was active in transfer experiments into irradiated rats. Rieber and Riethmuller (1974) obtained helper factors from thymus cell supernatants incubated with Fab fragments of rabbit anti-mouse Ig. These factors augmented the response of T-depleted mice (in vivo) to rabbit Ig, were of molecular weight 150,000, and contained Ig determinants.

The mechanism of action of IgT is not fully known. Certain studies have clearly indicated that it acts via macrophages (Feldmann, 1972; Rieber and Riethmuller, 1974), but exactly how this results in the triggering of B cells is not known.

B. Non-Ig-specific Helper Factors

Other workers have reported the existence of specific helper factors which were not absorbed with anti Ig antisera (Taussig et al., 1975). Supernatants from T cells activated to (T,G)-A--L, a synthetic polypeptide antigen, were not absorbed by anti Ig columns but were absorbed by anti-H-2 or anti-Ia antisera. These factors were antigen specific. The immunological deficit of genetically nonresponder mice to these antigens was ascribed to either a T-cell or a B-cell defect, depending on the strain (Munro and Taussig, 1975).

At the moment it is not clear whether there are two groups of antigen-specific helper factors for all antigens, whether antigens select one type depending on the nature of the antigen, or whether the discrepancy is more apparent than real and can be attributed to contaminants in the antisera used, or to the assay techniques. For example, there is evidence that antisera to Ig may be contaminated with antimembrane antibodies, and conversely there is evidence that anti-H-2 antisera may contain anti-Ig antibody (Goding, personal communication). Experiments to clarify this issue have been performed by Howie and Feldmann (1977). Helper factors to (T,G)-A--L were induced and assayed in vitro. Properties were similar to *both* IgT and non Ig helper factors, that is, acted on macrophages, contained both Ig and Ia determinants. Since these were produced in the same nonresponder strains which made non Ig helper factor, I currently feel that there is only one class of helper factor, and reported differences are due to technical considerations I discussed (Feldmann et al., 1977).

C. Nonspecific Helper Factors

Many workers have reported the existence of factors, derived from populations containing T cells, which have helper activity to antigens unrelated to those used to elicit the factors (e.g., Schimpl and Wecker, 1972; Armerding et al., 1974; Waldmann and Munro, 1974; Dutton, 1975). Alternatively, these may be produced by T cells activated by mitogens. A number of different nonspecific factors have been described, varying in molecular weight and in serological nature.

VI. ROLE OF THE MAJOR HISTOCOMPATIBILITY COMPLEX IN CELL INTERACTION

The major histocompatability complex (MHC) is a fascinating genetic region. Within the space of 0.5 centimorgans on chromosome 17 in the mouse there are four genetic regions: coding for cell surface antigens on all cells (H-2 antigens), for antigens on some cells (Ia antigens), immune response genes, lymphocyte activating determinants, and complement components. The role of this region in cell interactions has been emphasized by Katz et al. (1973), who reported that allogeneic T and B cells could not collaborate, and concluded from their experiments that there were "cell interaction" molecules responsible for this effect. Other workers have challenged this concept (e.g., Heber-Katz and Wilson, 1975; von Boehmer et al., 1975; Waldmann, 1977) and at the moment the role of the H-2 complex in these interactions is unclear.

Another role of the MHC (the I region in fact) is in the interaction of T cells and macrophages (Rosenthal and Shevach, 1973; Erb and Feldmann, 1975b). Again it is not clear whether this I region is involved in all T-macrophage interactions. The relation of the I region to helper and suppressor factors was described earlier.

However, the clearest evidence for the involvement of the MHC in cell interactions is the existence of immune response genes within the I region. The mechanism of action of these genes in controlling the immune response is not known, but it is apparent that unraveling their mode of action will tell us a lot about cell interactions.

REFERENCES

Armerding, D., Sachs, D. H., and Katz, D. H. (1974). Activation of T and B lymphocytes in vitro. III. Presence of Ia determinants in allogeneic effect factor. *J. Exp. Med. 140:* 1717-1722.

Beverley, P. C. L. (1976). Heterogeneity of Lymphocytes. In *T and B Lymphocytes in Immune Recognition* (G. Roelants and F. Loor, eds.). John Wiley and Sons, New York.

Burnet, F. M. (1959). *The Clonal Selection Theory of Acquired Immunity.* Cambridge University Press, London.

Cantor, H. and Asofsky, R. (1970). Synergy among lymphoid cells mediating the graft versus host response. II. Synergy in graft versus host reactions produced by BALB/c lymphoid cells of different anatomic origins. *J. Exp. Med. 131:* 235-246.

Cantor, H. and Boyse, E. A. (1975). Functional subclasses of T lymphocytes bearing different Ly antigens. I. The generation of functionally distinct T-cell subclasses is a differentiative process independent of antigen. *J. Exp. Med. 141:* 1376-1389.

Dutton, R. W. (1975). Separate signals for the initiation of proliferation and differentiation in the B cell response to antigen. *Transplant. Rev. 23:* 66-77.

Erb, P. and Feldmann, M. (1975a). Role of macrophages in the generation of T helper cells. The requirement for macrophages in helper cell induction and characteristics of macrophage-T cell interaction. *Cell. Immunol. 19:* 356-367.

Erb, P. and Feldmann, M. (1975b). Role of macrophages in the generation of T helper cells. II. The genetic control of macrophage - T cell interaction for helper cell induction with soluble antigen. *J. Exp. Med. 142:* 460-472.

Erb, P. and Feldmann, M. (1975c). Role of macrophages in the generation of T helper cells. III. Influence of macrophage derived factors in helper cell induction. *Eur. J. Immunol. 5:* 766-770.

Erb, P., Feldmann, M., and Hogg, N. M. (1976). Role of macrophages in the generation of T helper cells. IV. Nature of genetically related factor derived from macrophages incubated with soluble antigen. *Eur. J. Immunol. 6:* 365-372.

Erb, P., Vogt, P., Meier, B., and Feldmann, M. (1977). Role of macrophages in generation of T helper cells. V. Evidence for differential activation of short-lived T_1 and long-lived T_2 lymphocytes by macrophage factors BRF and NMF. *J. Immunol.* (in press).

Feldmann, M. (1972). Cell interaction in the immune response in vitro. V. Specific collaboration with complexes of antigen and thymus derived cell immunoglobulin. *J. Exp. Med. 136:* 737-760.

Feldmann, M., Baltz, M., Erb, P., Howie, S., Kontiainen, S., Woody, J., and Zvaifler, N. (1977). A comparison of I-region associated factors involved in antibody production. *Proc. 3rd International Congress of Immunology* (in press).

Feldmann, M. and Basten, A. (1972). Specific collaboration between T and B lymphocytes across a cell impermeable membrane in vitro. *Nature New Biology 237:* 13-15.

Feldmann, M., Beverley, P. C. L., Dunkley, M., and Kontiainen, S. (1975). Different Ly antigen phenotypes of in vitro induced helper and suppressor cells. *Nature 258:* 614-616.

Feldmann, M. and Erb, P. (1977). Requirement for interactions between 2 subpopulations of T cells for helper cell induction in vitro. *Z. Imm. Forsch.* (in press).

Feldmann, M., Kilburn, D., and Levy, J. (1975). T-T interactions in the generation of helper cells. *Nature 256:* 741-743.

Feldmann, M. and Kontiainen, S. (1976). Suppressor cell induction in vitro. II. Cellular requirements of suppressor cell induction. *Eur. J. Immunol. 6:* 302-305.

Gershon, R. K. (1973). Suppressor T cells. *Contemp. Topics Immunobiol. 3:* 1-37.

Heber-Katz, E. and Wilson, D. B. (1975). Collaboration of allogeneic T and B lymphocytes in the primary antibody response to sheep erythocytes in vitro. *J. Exp. Med. 142:* 98-111.

Howie, S. and Feldmann, M. (1977). In vitro studies on H-2 linked unresponsiveness to synthetic polypeptides. III. Production of an antigen specific T helper cell factor to (T,G)-A--L. *Eur. J. Immunol. 7:* 417-420.

Katz, D. H., Homaoka, T., and Benacerraf, B. (1973). Cell interactions between histoincompatible T and B lymphocytes. II. Failure of physiologic cooperative interactions between T and B lymphocytes from allogeneic donor strains in humoral response to hapten-protein conjugates. *J. Exp. Med. 137:* 1405-1427.

Kontiainen, S. and Feldmann, M. (1976). Suppressor cell induction in vitro. I. Kinetics of induction of specific suppressor cells. *Eur. J. Immunol. 6:* 296-301.

Miller, J. F. A. P. (1972). Lymphocyte interactions in antibody responses. *Int. Rev. Cytology 33:* 77-102.

Miller, R. G. and Phillips, R. A. (1969). Separation of cells by velocity sedimentation. *J. Cell. Physiol. 73:* 191-201.

Munro, A. and Taussig, M. (1975). Two genes in the major histocompatibility complex control immune response. *Nature 256:* 103-107.

Nordling, S., Andersson, L., and Hayry, P. (1972). Separation of T and B lymphocytes by preparative cell electrophoresis. *Eur. J. Immunol. 2:* 405-410.

Rieber, E. P. and Riethmuller, G. (1974). Surface immunoglobulin in thymus cells. Increased immunogenicity of heterologous anti-Ig bound to thymus cells. *Z. Immun. Forsch. 147:* 262-275.

Rosenthal, A. S. and Shevach, E. M. (1973). The function of macrophages in antigen recognition by guinea pig T lymphocytes. I. Requirement or histocompatible macrophages and lymphocytes. *J. Exp. Med. 138:* 1194-1212.

Schimpl, A. and Wecker, E. (1972). Replacement of T cell function by a T cell product. *Nature New Biology 237:* 15-17.

Shortman, K. (1968). The separation of different cell classes from lymphoid organs. II. The purification and analysis of lymphocyte populations by equilibrium density gradient centrifugation. *Aust. J. Exp. Biol. Med. Sci. 36:* 375-396.

Taussig, M., Munro, A. J., David, C. S., and Staines, N. A. (1975). Antigen specific T-cell factor in cell cooperation. Mapping within the I region of the H-2 complex and ability to cooperate across alloeneic barriers. *J. Exp. Med. 142:* 694-700.

Taniguchi, M. and Tada, T. (1974). Regulation of homocytotropic antibody formation in the rat. X. IgT like molecule for the induction of homocytotropic antibody response. *J. Immunol. 113:* 1757-1769.

Takemori, T. and Tada, T. (1975). Properties of antigen specific suppressive T cell factor in the regulation of the antibody response of the mouse. I. In vivo activity and immunochemical characterization. *J. Exp. Med. 142:* 1241-1257.

von Boehmer, H., Hudson, L., and Sprent, J. (19). Collaboration between histocompatible T and B lymphocytes using cells from tetraparental bone marrow chimeras. *J. Exp. Med. 142:* 989-997.

Wagner, H. (1973). Synergy during in vitro cytotoxic allograft responses. I. Evidence for cell interaction between thymocytes and peripheral T cells. *J. Exp. Med. 138:* 1379-1397.

Waldmann, H. (1977). Conditions determining the generation and expression of T helper cells. *Immunological Reviews 35:* 121-145.

Waldmann, H. and Munro, A. (1974). T cell-dependent mediator in the immune response. II. Physical and biological properties. *Immunology 27:* 53-64.

Chapter 11

GENETIC RESTRICTIONS ON CELL INTERACTIONS IN THE IMMUNE RESPONSE

Richard W. Dutton and Susan L. Swain

Department of Biology
University of California at San Diego
La Jolla, California

In this chapter we will describe the various examples of cellular cooperation in the immune response and discuss whether there are features common to all such interactions. The relation between these studies and the nature of the dictionary of lymphocyte recognition structures for alloantigens and other antigens will also be considered.

I. INTRODUCTION

Cell-cell interactions occur in virtually all metazoan organisms and are essential for the development of any complex biological system. In essence, various specialized cell types emerge during development. They then engage in specific patterns of behavior by mutual interaction. These interactions elicit different phenotypic expressions of the total gene repertoire present in all cells. In some interactions, one cell "signals" another to turn on or turn off a particular gene or group of genes or cistrons. There is a transmitter, a gene which directs the synthesis of a message. There must be a gene coding for a receptor for this messenger molecule either in the genome of the recipient or in the periphery, usually at the cell surface, which relays the signal via a second message to the genes in the nucleus. The signal may involve a humoral factor which can act on the recipient cell at a distance, or the factor could be cell-bound, in which case, direct cell surface-cell surface contact would be required. Cell-cell interactions that do not involve gene expression in either the transmitter or receiver or both, are not considered relevant to this discussion.

The possibility of interactions between identical cells rather than between *different* cells will also be ignored.

In the immune system of the higher vertebrates there are three major cell types that may be involved in cell interactions. There are the B lymphocytes, T lymphocytes, and the macrophages.

The B lymphocytes respond to antigen by proliferation and differentiation leading to immunoglobulin synthesis and secretion. The antigen is recognized by surface immunoglobulin carrying the same specificity component (V region) that will appear in the molecules subsequently secreted. Subpopulations of B cells specialized to produce the different classes and subclasses of immunoglobulin probably exist but have not been well characterized. Different subsets may have different requirements for the triggering of their immune response. Cell-cell interactions between B cells of different subsets are conceivable but have not been described (except for antibody feedback inhibition).

T cells respond to antigen in a quite different way from B cells. They proliferate (as do B cells) but then express a variety of the effector functions that are encompassed in cell-mediated immunity. These include synthesis and release of various mediators such as migration inhibition factor (MIF), chemotactic factor, etc., and the regulation (amplification or suppression) of the activities of other lymphocytes. A number of T-cell subpopulations have been described. Originally a distinction was made between newly formed, short-lived, radiosensitive, recirculating T_1 cells and long-lived, radioresistant, recirculating T_2 cells (Raff and Cantor, 1971).

T_2 cells were considered to be derived from T_1 cells when useful members of the T-cell repertoire were selected and retained upon encounter with antigen. This subdivision was based upon the physiological state or the stage which a particular T cell had reached during its development. More recently it has been shown that T cells can be separated into three major subpopulations on the basis of the expression of the Ly cell surface antigens (Cantor and Boyse, 1975a,b). Immature cells (perhaps equatable to T_1) express Ly1, Ly2, and Ly3. These constitute about 50% of the T cell population. More mature cells express either Ly1 or Ly23, and constitute 35% and 5 to 10% of the population, respectively. Helper cells for both the humoral and cellular responses and the cells involved in delayed type hypersensitivity (DTH) are $Ly1^+$, $Ly23^-$. This appears to be true for both the precursor and the effector T-cell populations.

The third major cell type, the macrophage, appears to be involved in some way in antigen presentation to T cells or B cells, at least in some experimental models. Macrophages from different tissues, alveolar, spleen, and lymph node, or peritoneal cavity, can have markedly different properties, but no clearly separate subpopulations of macrophages relevant to their role in the immune system have so far been described.

Cell interactions between the following different pairs of cells are clearly possible: B-T_{Ly1}, B-T_{Ly23}, T_{Ly1}-T_{Ly23}, Mac-B, T_{Ly1}-Mac, and T_{Ly23}-Mac. T_{Ly123} are omitted because they are not considered to be capable of interaction.

A. How are Interactions Recognized?

Experimentally, cell interaction or cooperation is recognized by synergy between two cell populations in the carrying-out of some function. The first clear example was the demonstration of synergy between populations of thymus and bone marrow cells injected into irradiated recipients. Here the function measured was the humoral response to the subsequent challenge with sheep red blood cells (RBC) as antigen. Other studies have measured proliferation, the production of T-cell mediators, suppression of antibody formation, the development of suppressor activity, and the development of cytotoxic killing of target cells. Specific references to these studies will be found in the more detailed discussions contained in Section III.

Although conceptually simple, the actual demonstration of synergy requires that the response or suppression of the response measured when the two cell types are combined be significantly different from the sum of the responses seen with either cell type alone. Since it is seldom possible to isolate a cell subpopulation free from other cell types, it is often difficult to determine whether cell cooperation is mandatory for the effect or merely facilitates it.

After synergy has been demonstrated it is necessary to characterize the two cell types involved and the mechanism of interaction. Genetic analyses have proven very useful in this context. Two approaches have been used. (a) The two cell types have been obtained from a pair of congenic strains that differ at a limited, defined, genetic region. Failure to collaborate in the face of such a difference indicates that the products of such genes are somehow involved in the interaction. Recombinant strains can be used for a more precise mapping of the gene. (b) "Nonresponder" strains that lack a gene required to carry out a step in the interactive process can also be used to define the gene locus involved.

II. GENETIC CONSIDERATIONS

Two major classes of genes have been implicated in the antigen-specific control of the immune response. The presence or absence of an immunoglobulin V gene will directly determine whether a particular antibody can be made, as these are considered to be structural genes coding for the specificity-determining half of the heavy and light chains of the immunoglobulin molecule. It now appears that these same V genes are expressed in T cells as part of the T-cell receptor for antigen and may be involved in cooperative cell interactions. More interest has centered on the role of the histocompatibility-linked Ir genes. These do not code for polypeptides of the immunoglobulin molecule, and the gene product has not been unequivocally identified with any known molecule or antigen. In some hypotheses (see below), Ir gene products are suggested to be molecules involved in cell interactions, while in others they are presumed to be the antigen recognition molecule of the T cell.

Little attention has been paid to any other classes of genes that might regulate cell interactions, although there is some indication that such may exist. Thus Hill (1976) has shown that the F_1 hybrid of two $H\text{-}2^b$ nonresponders to hen egg white lysozyme is a

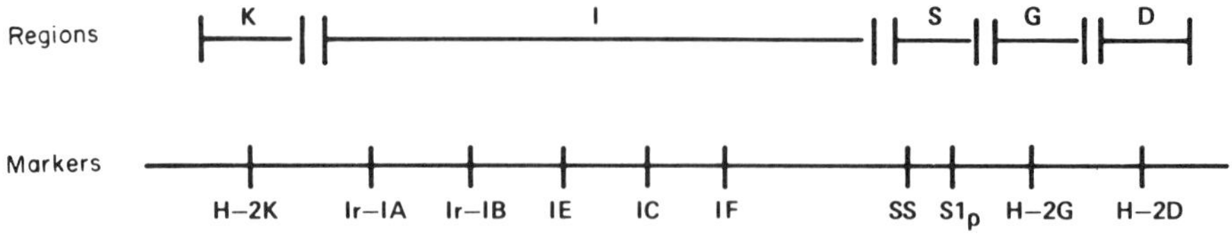

FIG. 1. The H-2 complex. The regions of the H-2 complex are indicated on the upper line and the positions of the gene loci on the lower line. The information is presented only as a rough guide to the positions of the markers described in the text since the map is constantly being revised as new information becomes available. For further references see Shreffler and David (1975) and Klein (1975, 1976).

responder suggesting complementation at some locus not in the H-2 region that reverses the negative Ir status of the H-2^b haplotype.

In this section we have summarized a number of general statements that can be made about Ir genes and the genetics of cell interactions. The H-2 complex is illustrated in Fig. 1.

1. A number of immune functions, responses, and interactions are affected by genes that have been mapped to the histocompatibility complex in guinea pig, mice, rat, chimpanzee, rhesus monkey, dog, pig, rabbit, and chicken (Frelinger and Shreffler, 1975).

2. These functions include proliferation in the mixed lymphocyte reactions (MLR), production of mediators, successful transfer of delayed hypersensitivity, allogeneic stimulation of the humoral response and T-helper activity, which are all said to map in the I region. Ir Genes have been mapped to IA, IB, IF, and IC. Some helper factors carry Ia antigens (antigens that map to the I region). Some suppressor factors also carry Ia antigens. Some T-B and T-macrophage interactions require identity at IA and a macrophage-derived, macrophage replacing factor is said to carry Ia antigens.

Cell-mediated lysis requires H-2 identity between stimulator cell and target which is said to map to H-2K and/or H-2D. It is suggested that negative allogeneic effects (allosuppression) may also map to K and/or D. The experimental evidence for these assertions will be outlined below and has been the subject of a number of recent reviews (e.g., Benacerraf and Katz, 1975; Klein, 1975; Shreffler and David, 1975; and Klein, 1976).

3. From the above statements it can be seen that in any particular interaction (or confrontation) between two cells with similar or dissimilar haplotypes the following possibilities exist:

a. There could be a *need for identity* at a locus for a *direct* positive effect (collaboration, killing).
b. There could be a difference at a locus that could lead to a *direct* positive effect (e.g., the positive "allogeneic effect").
c. There could be a difference at a locus that could lead to a *direct* negative effect (e.g, "allogeneic suppression").
d. There could be a need for identity at one locus so that collaboration in response (positive or negative) to a difference at another locus can occur.
e. There could be a need for an Ir^+ gene at one locus so that the response (positive or negative) to a difference at another locus can occur.

4. It is important not to be trapped into a simplistic view of the histocompatibility region by our systems of gene notation. Thus:

a. The difference between, say, k and b haplotypes may be much greater than the difference between, say, q and s in terms antigenic strength.
b. The degree of the difference between two haplotypes may not uniform at all loci. For example, in the combination d vs. b, the differences might be very great at IA and D while quite weak at IC and S. While on the other hand, in q vs. s, differences at IA and D may be trivial while the difference at IB might be strong.

This is because the isolation of a particular inbred strain which we then designate as x, i.e., x x x x x x, may be given only an accidental association of a set of alleles in which the allele at a particular locus is not necessarily any more related to the alleles at the other loci in the set than to alleles at other loci in another set.

5. The size of the response may be controlled by genes outside the H region. Thus, the background of the strain may influence the outcome. There are several examples where this appears to be the case (e.g., Hill, 1976).

Thus, the *actual* outcome of a particular interaction between two haplotypes will depend on a number of factors:

Identity at some loci
Differences at other loci
Possession of the appropriate Ir genes
The background of the strain

As a result of all this it seems that the gene for a particular function may sometimes appear to map in one place and sometimes map in another.

The mapping experiments conducted so far are probably too fragmentary to know whether they are absolutely reliable in identifying a function with a gene difference at a particular locus. For example, the mapping of cell interaction (CI) function to IA depends only on the use of strain combinations in which k + k at IA and IB gives a response while s + k fails (Katz and Benacerraf, 1975), and in a second study that d (at K and IA) could collaborate with d but not with b (Katz and Benacerraf, 1976).

Nevertheless, some sort of picture has emerged and can be provisionally summarized as follows.

Ir genes map in the various subregions of the I region. Where two Ir genes are required they may both map in the same subregion or in different subregions.

Cell-mediated target antigens map in general to K and D, but target antigens may also be found in the I region (H-2I), or between S and D (H-2G) (Klein, 1976).

I-region differences trigger proliferation in MLR, but it is not clear whether the same regions trigger the production of mediators of T help or T suppression.

T help and T suppression require B-cell compatibility at certain loci in the I region. By analogy with cell-mediated cytotoxicity to alloantigens, it seems possible that allosuppression might require I-region differences in its induction and K- and D-region differences as targets for suppression. There seems to be no published evidence that this is the case.

III. EXPERIMENTAL MODELS

In this section we will summarize the essential features of the relevant experimental models. No attempt will be made to present a comprehensive summary, and the experimental details will be discussed only when there is some ambiguity as to the conclusion that can be drawn from the particular experiment. The survey of the literature on which this section is based was completed in May 1976.

A. T Cell-Macrophage Interaction in Guinea Pigs

The T cell-macrophage interaction in response to antigen has been studied in two inbred strains of Hartley guinea pigs, strain 2 and strain 13. These strains are identical at the serologically defined (SD) histocompatibility locus but differ at the lymphocyte defined (LD) locus. Strain 2 carries Ia antigens 2 and 4, and strain 13 antigens 1 and 3. (For references see Schwartz et al., 1976.) This interaction leads to T-cell proliferation which can be measured by uptake of [^{3}H]-thymidine and MIF production (Ben-Sassoon et al., 1974), if antigen is presented on the macrophage surface and if the purified lymph node cells come from a previously immunized donor. The response of the T cell does not take place in the absence of the macrophage (Waldron et al., 1973). Very large numbers of macrophages are necessary, however, to restore the response of macrophage-depleted cultures, raising the possibility that it is really some other cell type that is required. It is an interesting feature of the system that the antigen can be introduced into the system by preincubation of the macrophages, but not of the lymphocytes, with antigen before combining the two cell types. The response is not seen when allogeneic combinations of macrophage and T cell are used (Rosenthal and Shevach, 1973). In addition, it would appear that F_1 hybrid macrophages are less effective than parental cells in stimulating parental T cells, and F_1 T cells respond less well to parental macrophages than they do to F_1 macrophages. Thus, completely syngeneic combinations appear to be better than semisyngeneic in *either* direction.

The stimulating interaction is blocked by alloantisera directed against the histocompatibility antigen(s) involved in the interaction (Shevach et al., 1972; Rosenthal and Shevach, 1973). Thus, 13 anti-2 will block the interactions

	Mac		T
a)	2	+	2
b)	(2 X 13) F_1	+	2
c)	2	+	(2 X 13) F_1

but will not block

d)	13	+	13
e)	(2 X 13) F_1	+	13
f)	13	+	(2 X 13) F_1

The reciprocal situation is seen with 2 anti-13. The lack of inhibition in lines (e) and (f) shows that interaction with the irrelevant histocompatibility antigen on the F_1 does not block the interaction. The activity of the antisera is not absorbable on insolubilized alloimmunoglobulin (Shevach et al., 1972), and the antiserum does not block the uptake of antigen by macrophages.

Further information comes from the use of antigens under the control of immune response (Ir) genes. The presence of the Ir gene for a particular antigen controls the development of a delayed hypersensitivity skin reaction, the development of helper T-cell activity, and the production of T-cell mediators (Benacerraf et al., 1967). Strain 2 responds to poly-L-lysine (PLL), the copolymer of L-glutamic and L-lysine (GL), the copolymer of glutamic and alanine (GA), and others, but is unresponsive to the copolymer of L-glutamic and L-tyrosine (GT), and low doses of DNP-GPA. Strain 13 are PLL^-, GL^-, and GT^+. F_1 hybrid T cells will respond to both antigens but will only do so in the presence of F_1 macrophages or parental macrophages that carry the Ir gene for that antigen (Shevach et al., 1972; Shevach and Rosenthal, 1973).

T cell		Macrophage	Response to ag	
F_1	+	2	GL^+	GT^-
		13	GL^-	GT^+
		(2 × 13) F_1	GL^+	GT^+

Thus the parental macrophage, as well as being histocompatible, must be compatible for the haplotype that is Ir^+ for the restricted antigen. This implies that, *either* two separate interactions are needed, one involving the Ia antigen and one involving the Ir gene, *or* the Ir-gene component is in some way physically or functionally linked to the Ia antigen. The antiserum inhibition data, however, favor the latter alternative. Only antisera to the "linked" Ia antigen are able to block the reaction between F_1 macrophage and F_1 T cell in an Ir-restricted response (Shevach and Rosenthal, 1973).

Interestingly, an F_1 macrophage which has the Ir gene represented only once is as effective as the appropriate parent (where the gene is represented twice) in the stimulation of the F_1 T cell. Here, complete histocompatibility is not better than semiidentity (Shevach and Rosenthal, 1973).

A number of further points have also been established. Studies with outbred populations, in which individuals are found where the Ir gene is associated with another Ia antigen (e.g., GA^+, 2^- instead of GA^+, 2^+ as in strain 2), show that it is antiserum against the histocompatibility antigen, not the Ir-gene product, that effects the inhibition (Shevach et al., 1974).

Studies on the physical interaction between macrophages and T cells show that there is a reversible, antigen-independent aggregation (Lipsky and Rosenthal, 1975a), followed by an irreversible, antigen-dependent association. The latter does not occur in allogeneic macrophage-lymphocyte combinations (Lipsky and Rosenthal, 1975b; Rosenthal et al., 1975).

It might be argued that the lack of optimal interactions and stimulation in allogeneic combinations was due to negative allogeneic interactions between the incompatible components of the interaction. This was excluded when it was shown that neither allogeneic T cells nor allogeneic macrophages could interfere with a syngeneic interaction (Rosenthal and Shevach, 1973). Thus an incompatible cell cannot block the activity of a compatible cell.

In summary, it can be stated that the following requirements must be met for antigeneic restimulation of a T cell to proliferate:

1. The antigen must be presented by a macrophage that is histocompatible (presumably at the I region).
2. The T cell must be Ir^+ for the response to a genetically restricted antigen, and the macrophage must have the haplotype that carries the Ir^+ gene.
3. (a) The interaction can be blocked by antisera directed against the *Ia antigen* involved in the compatible interaction. (b) In the case of interaction between F_1 macrophages and F_1 T cells in response to an Ir restricted antigen, only the antiserum to the Ia antigen linked to the Ir gene is effective.
4. A compatible reaction is not blocked by the presence of an incompatible Ia, either on the same cell or another cell.

   The simplest hypothesis that can be made is as follows. The event that requires Ia compatibility is in some way physically and/or functionally linked to the event that requires the presence of the antigen-specific Ir-gene product in the T cell. T-cell activation will only occur when both interaction events take place.

In this model the Ir gene *need* not be expressed in the macrophage. Very recently, however, Shevach (1976) has presented evidence which can be interpreted as indicating that the Ir gene must also be present in the collaborating macrophage. The Ia gene *need* not be expressed in the T cell if the T cell is hypothesized to have a receptor for the Ia antigen of its own strain. If the connection between the Ia receptor (or Ia antigen) and the Ir-gene product is functional rather than of close physical proximity, there is no need to invoke steric hindrance to explain antibody blocking.

B. T Cell-Macrophage Interactions in Mice

Until very recently, attempts to develop a similar experimental model in mice had met with no success. However, Schwartz et al. (1975) have been able to demonstrate that purified lymphocyte populations from the peritoneal exudate cells of previously immunized mice will proliferate in response to antigen in vitro. This system now offers the possibility of a more detailed analysis of the genetic restrictions that may exist using the congenic resistant and recombinant strains that are available.

Already, it has been shown that the proliferative response to a random polymer of L-glutamic, L-lysine, and L-phenylalanine (GLΦ) is under the same two-gene control as has been shown for this antigen in the humoral response, as will be discussed below (Schwartz and Paul, 1976). Both genes appear to be required in the T-cell response to antigen, and complementation was shown in the F_1 hybrid of certain pairs of nonresponder strains. In some cases, cis-complementation in recombinant mice was more effective than trans-complementation in the F_1 hybrids. The strain distribution of R and NR mice was identical to that described for the humoral response.

Pierce et al. (1976) have shown that mice can be primed in vivo by antigen (a terpolymer of L-glutamic, L-alanine, and L-tyrosine, GAT) bound to macrophages. Mice can be primed by antigen bound to either syngeneic or allogeneic macrophages. However, the secondary response (measured in vitro) can only be elicited by antigen bound to the macrophages of the same histocompatibility type as were used for the in vivo priming. It is a curious feature of this system that the first exposure to antigen on a macrophage of a particular haplotype preempts the subsequent response, in the sense that the "wrong" macrophage in the secondary challenge will no longer give even the primary response that it would otherwise have elicited.

Prior to this, however, Erb and Feldmann had developed a quite different model in which helper T-cell activity could be generated in cultures of cortisone-resistant thymocytes from unprimed mice (Kontiainen and Feldmann, 1975; Erb and Feldmann, 1975a,b,c). This system is dependent on the presence of adherent cells from a peritoneal exudate. The macrophages (adherent cells) must be genetically identical in the IA region for the two antigens tested, poly (Try, glu)-poly DL ala -- poly Lys [(T,G)-A--L] and keyhole limpet hemocyanin (KLH). That the requirement was not due to suppressor effects was excluded by admixture experiments. It was also claimed that the macrophages could be replaced by a supernatant factor obtained when macrophages were incubated with antigen and that the factor carried Ia determinants. It is important to note that this is the only experimental model where genetic restriction is found for cell interactions in the primary immune response.

C. Collaboration Between T Cells and B Cells in the Secondary Response in Mice

1. Response to the Hapten-Carrier Conjugates

The secondary response to hapten-carrier conjugates is dependent on the presence of carrier-primed T cells. In this system only the response of the B cells to hapten is measured. Katz and his collaborators (see Benacerraf and Katz, 1975, for a recent review) have studied the genetic restrictions on such cooperation following the original observation by Kindred and Shreffler (1972). They have established in both in vivo and in vitro models that collaboration will occur when T cells and B cells are syngeneic at the IA (and possibly IB) region. Incompatibility at K, IC, S, or D, or of the non-H-2 background, did not prevent collaboration. The number of tests, however, was limited. $H\text{-}2^a$ was shown to cooperate with $H\text{-}2^a$ or $H\text{-}2^k$, but not $H\text{-}2^b$ in vivo. In vitro the intra H-2 mapping showed only that s at IA and IB would collaborate with s but not k. Incompatibilities at K and S did not interfere when IA and IB were compatible. The response was dependent on carrier priming of the T-cell donor, and the extraneous presence of incompatible T cells did not interfere with collaboration.

In addition, it was shown that F_1 hybrid T cells of a responder X nonresponder strain were able to collaborate only with hapten-primed B cells from the responder strain when challenged with the hapten on the restricted carrier (Katz et al., 1973). This observation was recently confirmed and some additional information was provided (see below).

Katz and Benacerraf (1975) have proposed that there are cell interaction genes (CI) whose gene products are involved in T cell-B cell collaboration, and that both the T cell and the B cell must be compatible at this locus for collaboration to occur.

2. *T-Cell Replacing Factors*

Further information comes from the study of T-cell replacing factors. It has been shown that supernatants of allogeneic lymphocyte cultures contain a factor or factors that replace the requirement for T cells in the primary (Dutton et al., 1971) and secondary (Armerding et al., 1974) immune response. It was shown that the activity of such a factor obtained from $H\text{-}2^d$ cells responding to $H\text{-}2^k$ cells was absorbed on insolubilized B10.A anti-B10 serum (presumably directed against Ia-8, an Ia specificity shared between $H\text{-}2^b$ and $H\text{-}2^d$). Partial absorption was seen with (B6A) F_1 anti B10.D2. It was concluded that the factor carries Ia determinants. In a later study (Armerding et al., 1975) evidence was presented that the factor consisted of two chains of molecular weight 40,000 and 12,000, the smaller of which reacted with antiserum to β_2 microglobulin.

3. Complementation in F_1 Hybrid of Two Nonresponder Strains

In the course of their studies on the genetic control of the response to (T,G)-A--L, Munro and Taussig (1975) (Taussig et al., 1975) showed that there were two types of nonresponder strains distinguishable by whether their primed T cells were able to make a T-cell replacing factor when incubated with antigen. Further analysis showed that the B cells of the nonresponder strains that were able to make factor, were unable to respond to the factor. They suggested that there were two genes involved in the control of responsiveness and characterized the various haplotypes as indicated below. F_1 hybrids of two nonresponder strains that differed at different loci were responders.

H-2		Factor	B-cell response
b, d	high	+	+
k, j	low	+	-
f	low	-	+
s	low	-	-
$\frac{k}{f}$ F_1	high	+	+

They proposed a model in which small clusters of V genes coding for antigen recognition were operationally linked to a pair of genes, one coding for the T-cell factor and the other for the B-cell acceptor for that factor (Munro and Taussig, 1975).

There are three additional points that must be made concerning the Munro-Taussig study:

1. They use an unusual experimental model involving adoptive cell transfers in which they find (in contrast to other workers) that the IgM response to (T,G)-A--L is Ir-gene restricted.
2. In analogous studies with (Phe, G)-A--L the factor made in any of the b, d, or k haplotypes will act on B cells of b, d, and k, that is, across haplotype barriers (Taussig et al., 1975).

3. The k haplotype which can make factor specific for (T,G)-A--L in the Taussig study is unable to give T cell proliferation response to antigen stimulation in the study of Schwartz and Paul (1976). The reason for this apparent discrepancy is not clear. One possibility is that the stimulation of T-cell proliferation is macrophage-dependent while the production of T-cell factor is not. The defect would thus be expressed both in the macrophage and the B cell but not in the T cell.

A number of other cases of complementation in F_1 hybrids of two nonresponders have been reported. Some of these have been analyzed in detail and do not appear to follow the same pattern described by Taussig and Munro (i.e., one gene expressed in the T cell and the other gene in the B cell).

Dorf and Benacerraf (1975) have studied the response to GLΦ in the mouse. This response was found to be under the control of two dominant genes: one they term α, which maps in a region between IB and IC which they have called IF, and the other β, which maps in IA. Examples of all four combinations of the two genes were found. Responder mice such as $H\text{-}2^d$ or $H\text{-}2^q$ were α^+ and β^+. Complementation was observed in F_1 hybrids between certain pairs of nonresponders such as B10.A(2R) which was $\alpha^+ \beta^-$ and B10 which was $\alpha^- \beta^+$. It was found that complementation in some cases was more effective in the recombinant strains than the F_1 hybrid, suggesting an advantage of the cis arrangement of the two genes rather than the trans (Dorf and Benacerraf, 1975; Dorf et al., 1976). Strains carrying $H\text{-}2^f$ and the recombinant $H\text{-}2^{h4}$ appeared to be $\alpha^- \beta^-$.

Surprisingly F_1 mice from two strains C57BL/6 and SJL both $\alpha^- \beta^+$, were responders. This could be explained by complementation between two α genes $(\alpha_1^-, \alpha_2^+, \beta^+) \times (\alpha_1^+, \alpha_2^-, \beta^+)$, or it could conceivably represent another example of the situation suggested by Hill (1976) in which complementation at some non-H-2 locus overcomes the nonresponder status of the $H\text{-}2^b$ haplotype for hen egg white lysozyme.

A further striking feature was observed when the response to DNP-GLΦ was examined in a cell transfer model in which T cells and B cells were injected into irradiated F_1 recipients (Katz et al., 1976). In this case, in contrast to Munro and Taussig (1975), F_1 T cells of a complementing strain pair (B10 × A) were not able to collaborate with B cells of *either* parental strain, suggesting that both genes were required in the B cell. The reciprocal situation was also true in that neither parental T cell could provide help to the F_1 B cells. Thus α and β genes were both required for T-cell function (as has also been shown to be the case for GLΦ-specific stimulation of the peritoneal T cells from primed donors (Schwartz and Paul, 1976).

It was also found, however, that F_1 T cells would not collaborate with F_1 B cells but only with B cells from the recombinant (responder) strain ($B6AF_1$).

This is a somewhat surprising result that is difficult to explain satisfactorily on any model of cell collaboration. It must be remembered that in this experimental model the T-cell donor was primed with GLΦ and the B-cell donor with DNP (dinitrophenyl) coupled to fowl gamma globulin (DNP-FGG). Three interpretations can be considered. First, it could be that the α and β genes must be in the cis position in the B cell for cooperation to be effective in the transfer model, whereas, in the whole F_1 animal, the trans arrangement is effective. Second, priming with GLΦ (in the T-cell donor) selects a subset of CI molecules not selected in the DNP-FGG primed F_1 B-cell donor but which is utilized in the DNP-FGG primed recombinant B-cell donor. A third interpretation is that there is also a two-gene GLΦ suppressor system that requires a B-cell acceptor component still present in the F_1 hybrid but lost in the recombinant. This requires an ad hoc hypothesis concerning the existence of the suppressor system, and that the suppression is only seen under the conditions of the transfer model. Recent unpublished experiments (Katz, personal communication) suggest that DNP-GLΦ primed F_1 B cells will cooperate satisfactorily. This supports the second interpretation.

4. *T Cell-B Cell Collaboration Across a Haplotype Barrier*

Collaboration between T cells and B cells of different H-2 haplotypes has been demonstrated in a number of experimental models.

a. Chimeras. 1. Bechtol and her colleagues (Bechtol et al., 1974) made allophenic mice from a responder ($H\text{-}2^b$) and a nonresponder ($H\text{-}2^k$) strain to the antigen (T,G)-A--L. These mice were challenged with (T,G)-A--L and the allotype markers on the antibodies to (T,G)-A--L were determined. It was found that the antibody was made by cells of both parental types. It was concluded that $H\text{-}2^b$-responder T cells must have collaborated with $H\text{-}2^k$ B cells since the nonresponder gene defect has been shown to be expressed in the $H\text{-}2^k$ T cell in other experiments.

Chimeras of two nonresponder strains made no antibody, suggesting that positive allogeneic effects were not responsible for the nonresponder antibody in the responder × nonresponder chimeras.

2. von Boehmer et al. (1975) made chimeras by injecting anti-Θ treated bone marrow as a source of T-cell precursors into an irradiated allogeneic recipient and waited until it became repopulated with donor T (and B) cells tolerant to the host. These animals were injected with sheep RBC and their nylon passed spleen cells were used as a source of primed T cells to test for collaboration with both syngeneic or allogeneic B cells. Antibody was made in both combinations, demonstrating that carrier-primed T cells from a donor made "tolerant" to allogeneic cells could collaborate with B cells of that same allogeneic strain.

Similar experiments were carried out by Waldmann et al. (1975) using trinitrophenylated (TNP)-KLH as the antigen.

It was not demonstrated in either of these systems that the response was dependent on priming to the specific carrier and positive allogeneic effects were not totally excluded.

In both these models (allophenic mice and irradiation chimeras), allogeneic T cells, B cells, and macrophages were exposed to one another for some time before the test for collaboration. It is possible that some subpopulation of lymphocytes that could collaborate was in some way selected or adapted. Alternatively, collaboration may have occurred because the T cells were primed by exposure to antigen presented on the allogeneic macrophages, as will be discussed in Section .

b. Populations Depleted by Alloreactive Cells. Heber-Katz and Wilson (1975) have used a 24-hr passage of thoracic duct lymphocytes through an allogeneic host (in rats) to remove all cells reactive to the host and recover the remaining cells which now have no reactivity to the host alloantigens. Such cells are used as a T-cell source and can be demonstrated to collaborate with B cells from the same allogeneic strain in a primary in vitro response to sheep RBC. The titration curve of the T-cell activity is indistinguishable from that of syngeneic T cells.

In this model it is assumed that alloreactive cells capable of mediating a negative allogeneic effect are merely removed, and the remaining cells have had no chance to become adapted, or selected to cooperate with the allogeneic cells during the brief 24-hr period of exposure.

Collaboration across an allogeneic barrier was also shown for both IgM responses and IgG by Pierce and Klinman (1975) and Pierce (1976). In these experiments, hapten-primed B cells were injected into irradiated carrier-primed recipients. Single clones of B cells arose in cultured segments of the recipient's spleen.

c. T Cell Factors. As we have already discussed in an earlier section, Taussig and his colleagues have shown that T-cell factors made in one strain will cooperate with B cells from both syngeneic and certain allogeneic strains (Taussig et al., 1975). A similar lack of haplotype restriction has been shown by Waldmann et al. (1976) and is referred to by Katz as allogeneic effect factor (Benacerraf and Katz, 1975).

d. Populations Depleted of Suppressor Cells. One of us (Swain) has shown that very small numbers of allogeneic cells can suppress syngeneic collaboration between T cells and B cells (Swain et al., 1976). In these experiments it has been shown that carrier-primed T cells will collaborate with allogeneic hapten-primed B cells in an in vitro secondary response to hapten carrier conjugates if $Ly\text{-}2^+$

allosuppressor cells are removed from the T-cell population. The response is dependent on the carrier priming of the T-cell population; it does not appear to depend on a nonspecific positive allogeneic effect.

In this model there is again no possibility of selection or adaptation, as the collaborating allogeneic cells are exposed to one another for the first time at the moment when collaboration is required.

D. T Cell Mediated Suppression

It has been demonstrated in a number of experimental models that activated suppressor T cells can inhibit or suppress the activities of other lymphocytes (see *Transplantation Reviews*, Vol. 26). In the case of the humoral response it is clear that two possibilities exist for the target of suppression. The suppressor T cells could act on the responding B-cell populations indirectly by removing or suppressing the helper T-cell population. In the case of the allotype-specific suppression, the target appears to be an allotype-specific helper T cell (Herzenberg et al., 1975). The molecular nature of the target of suppression is at present unknown.

Examples of antigen-specific suppression, allotype-specific suppression, and nonspecific mitogen-induced suppression have been described. What concerns us here are studies in which genetic restrictions have been investigated.

Suppressor activity may be considered analogous to helper activity, and would thus be expected to exhibit a requirement for I-region identity in the collaborative, suppressive event. However, suppressor cells have been shown to be $Ly\text{-}1^{-}Ly\text{-}23^{+}$, and hence suppression could be seen as analogous to T cell mediated killing. In this case, the target of suppression might require K- and D-region identity with the suppressor cell. Indeed, some investigators have concluded that suppression and cytotoxicity are two manifestations of the same phenomenon. In either model the occurrence of antigen-specific immune response genes might be anticipated and have indeed been described. Debré, Kapp, and Benacerraf (1975) have shown that an H-2-linked dominant gene (termed immune suppression gene, Is) controls the suppressor T-cell response to GT. Later studies (Waltenbaugh et al., 1976) have shown that two complementing genes are involved, one to the right and one to the left of the crossovers [B10.A.(9R), B10.HTT] between IB and IC.

Antigen-specific suppression for a related polymer, GAT, was shown to be under separate Is-gene control (Debré, Kapp, Dorf, and Benacerraf, 1975). A suppressive factor could be extracted from GAT-specific suppressor cells (Kapp et al., 1976). It has a molecular weight in the range 10,000 to 40,000, possesses antigen-binding activity, and does not carry Ig determinants. In another system, Tada et al. (1975) showed that similarly prepared suppressor factors carried Ia determinants (Taniguchi et al., 1976).

Rich and Rich (1975, 1976) have looked at suppressor T cells that suppress T-cell proliferation in a mixed lymphocyte reaction. They showed that suppressive extracts isolated from T cells activated by alloantigens would suppress only T cells identical at the IC or S region. Other regions of the H-2 complex and non-H-2 background were irrelevant. The suppressor factor could be absorbed only by *activated* syngeneic T cells (Rich and Rich, 1976).

Suppressor cells can be activated by exposure to H-2 alloantigens. It is not clear which region(s) of the H-2 complex are responsible for this activation.

E. H-2 Restriction of Cell-mediated Cytotoxicity

It has been shown in a number of experimental models that cytotoxic T cells specific for non-H-2 antigens will only kill target cells that carry both non-H-2 antigen and the H-2 antigens that were present on the sensitizing cell. Thus, cells from LCM-infected hosts will kill LCM-infected syngeneic cells infected with an unrelated virus (Zinkernagel and Doherty, 1975). Neither uninfected syngeneic cells nor viral-infected allogeneic cells would block the killing of infected syngeneic cells. A similar requirement is also seen for cytotoxic responses against ectromelia virus, vaccina, and paramyxovirus-infected cells (for a review, see Zinkernagel and Doherty, 1976). Shearer (1974), Shearer et al. (1975), Forman (1975), and others have shown that the same restrictions are seen in cytotoxic reactions to TNP-modified cells. Responses to minor histocompatibility antigens (Bevan, 1975a,b) and to the male H-Y antigen (Gordon et al., 1975), are also H-2-restricted. Although there are some minor variations between systems, it would appear that this is a general phenomenon for all cell-mediated responses to non-H-2 antigens, at least in mice.

Mapping experiments (e.g., Rehn et al., 1976) have shown that the H-2 restriction is limited to the K and D regions of the H-2 complex. In the original experiments, the stimulator cell and the responding cell were K and D identical with the target cell when lysis occurred. Later experiments demonstrated that the requirement was for identity between target and stimulator cell. Spleen cells from an LCM-infected chimera of parental cells in an F_1 host killed LCM-infected cells from both parental types, even though the effector cells were of one parental type only (tolerant to the other) (Zinkernagel, 1976). In another type of experiment (Bevan, 1975), it was shown that an F_1 effector cell raised in response to background differences carried on a strain bearing one of the parental H-2 types would not kill cells carrying the same background differences carried on cells of the other parental H-2 type.

Two major types of hypotheses have been put forward to explain this phenomenon. (a) In the *dual recognition* hypothesis, it is suggested that two separate interactions must take place between effector and target cell: one is a self-self interaction between K or D structures, and the other is an interaction between the foreign antigen and a receptor for it on the effector cell. (b) In the *interaction* hypothesis, it is proposed that the T-cell receptor is specific for some antigenic structure arising out of some sort of interaction between the antigen (virus, minor histocompatibility antigen, etc.) and the K or D molecules. Suggestions for the nature of the interaction have ranged from enzymatic modification (Blanden et al., 1976) to association by mere proximity.

A third possibility favored by us represents a hybrid model. The T-cell recognition molecule has two specificity components, one directed to K or D and the other directed to the antigen. The latter could be a V-region gene drawn from the immunoglobulin pool although this is not an essential feature of the model. The advantage of this model is that association between the two recognition events necessary in any explanation is achieved at the level of the T-cell receptor and the only "interaction" required of the two antigens is that they both engage with the receptor at the same time.

The target competition experiments and the specificity of killing in the chimera argue against the dual recognition model and strongly in favor of some version of the interaction hypothesis.

Recent evidence (Zinkernagel, 1976; von Boehmer and Haas, 1976) suggests that cytotoxic responses to virus or TNP on allogeneic cells is also H-2-restricted, indicating that the necessary homology is only between the stimulator and target cells.

F. The Nature of the T-Cell Receptor for Antigen

The nature of the T-cell receptor for antigen has been hotly debated for many years, and we do not propose to review this material here. We will briefly describe the recent studies that strongly suggest that the same specificity determining structures are used in both T-cell and B-cell receptors specific for the same antigenic determinant.

In the first experimental model, Binz and Wigzell (1975) have examined the response of Lewis rats to the alloantigens of the DA strain.

F_1 rats injected with T lymphocytes from Lewis rats make antibody to the receptors on Lewis T cells that recognize the DA alloantigens. This antibody, directed against the T-cell receptor of Lewis for DA alloantigens was able to (a) block all T cell reactivity of Lewis cells against DA antigens (MLR or GVH), and (b) reacted with Lewis antibody to DA alloantigens, that is, with the B-cell product.

Extensive studies failed to separate these two activities. Further studies demonstrated that the idiotypic structure of the Lewis anti-DA recognition molecules was present on 6% of normal Lewis T cells (Binz and Wigzell, 1976a). The antiserum could be used to separate Lewis T cells reactive to DA antigens by affinity chromatography (Binz and Wigzell, 1975b, 1976b) and to show that two types of molecules carrying the idiotype determinants were present in the normal Lewis rat. One equivalent in size to 7s IgG was found in the serum, the other, molecular weight 35,000, was found in the serum and in the urine (Binz and Wigzell, 1976b). Studies in the mouse (Binz et al., 1975) demonstrated that 5 to 10% of purified CBA T cells carried the idiotype present on CBA antibody to BL/6 alloantigens.

Eichmann and Rajewsky and their colleagues have shown that if antiidiotype antisera prepared against the idiotype of immunoglobulin specific for group A streptococcal carbohydrate (A-CHO) was injected into normal mice (of the appropriate strain), the mice developed T cells specific for A-CHO and capable of acting as helper T cells in the B-cell response to TNP presented on strep A particles (Eichmann and Rajewsky, 1975). Similar findings using the phosphorylcholine idiotype system have been reported by Trenkner and Riblet (1975). Further studies (Black et al., 1976; Hämmerling et al., 1976) extended these observations and make a very strong case for the conclusion that the cell surface recognition molecules of both T cells and B cells have identical idiotypes and are coded for by the same V genes, which furthermore show genetic linkage to the immunoglobulin heavy chain markers. This is most important, since the genetic linkage implies that the whole V region is used and that the two structures are identical and not just similar.

In summary, it seems hard to escape the conclusion that T-cell receptors for both alloantigens and other antigens utilize a component which is the same as the V gene used in B-cell immunoglobulins directed against the same antigens. The nature of the remainder of the T-cell receptor is now known.

IV. DISCUSSION

A. Review

We have described a number of experimental models in which various cell interactions of immunological significance appear to be subject to a common pattern of genetic restrictions. They can be summarized as follows and their special features listed.

1. Macrophage-T Cell Interactions

In the guinea pig, the secondary proliferative response of primed T cells is dependent on the presentation of antigen on macrophages that are compatible at certain loci in the I region, and both T cell and macrophage must come from an Ir-positive strain. It is not clear whether the requirement for Ir and Ia are two separate requirements, or whether the functional marker, Ir, and the antigen marker, Ia, are two aspects of the same entity. There is no test of whether the genetic requirement is for a macrophage compatible with the T cell or with the priming macrophage (these are the Shevach, Rosenthal, and Paul studies*).

In the mouse there appears to be no genetic restriction on the macrophage in the primary humoral response to macrophage-bound antigen. In the secondary response the antigen must be presented on macrophages H-2 identical with the priming macrophage, and the animal is now unable to give even a primary response to antigen on other macrophages. This preemption suggests some form of "capture" at the time of antigen presentation rather than a selection of a preexisting association. T cells primed and secondarily challenged by antigen on allogeneic macrophages, nevertheless, collaborated with syngeneic B cells in the secondary response (these are the studies of Pierce,

---

*In this section we have resorted to listing the names of some of the authors most associated with work to identify the study under discussion. We apologize for any unfair omissions that must result from the use of this convenient shorthand.

Kapp, and Benacerraf). In contrast to the above, the Erb and Feldmann studies demonstrate a requirement for genetic identity in the I region in the *primary* response of T cells to antigen. They show a second unusual feature in that a soluble factor carrying Ia determinants could be obtained from, and would substitute for, macrophages incubated with antigen.

2. *T Cell-B Cell Interactions*

These can lead to both help and suppression of the B-cell response, and helper and suppressor T cells can regulate the activities of effector T cells in a number of experimental models. The earlier Katz, Benacerraf studies showed a requirement for genetic identity in the I region between T cell and B cell, but were not designed to distinguish between this interpretation and one in which the requirement was for identity between the T cells used in the priming and in the secondary challenge. The later experiments (Katz et al., 1976; and Katz, personal communication) argue in favor of the latter interpretation.

Bechtol, von Boehmer, and others working with chimeras appeared to show that T cells and B cells could collaborate across haplotype barriers once alloreactive cells were removed or made unresponsive. The alternative interpretation, that the T cells were primed in the presence of allogeneic macrophages and B cells and could now collaborate with either the syngeneic or the allogeneic haplotype present in the chimera, was not tested. It is important to note that if such were the case it would appear to represent a change in the B-cell requirement rather than the macrophage requirement, as shown in the Pierce experiments.

Other examples of collaboration across haplotype barriers in a primary response (the Heber-Katz and Wilson experiment), or in a secondary response (the Susan Pierce and our own experiments), take place under conditions where T cells and B cells confront one another for the first time when required to collaborate. Here there would appear to be no opportunity for prior selection or adaptation. These studies are best explained by the hypothesis that genetic "restrictions" are imposed by negative allogeneic effects, and once these are removed there are no restrictions on T cell-B cell collaboration. It is clear that there is an unresolved conflict between the experimental observations here and those of the Katz, Benacerraf and the Shevach studies, where the relevant controls failed to demonstrate any negative allogeneic effects.

The studies with suppressor T cells follow the same general pattern of genetic restriction seen in the "classic" T-B studies.

3. *H-2 Restriction in Cell-Mediated Cytoxicity*

The genetic restrictions for cytotoxic responses to viral, chemically modified, and minor histocompatibility antigens all show the same general pattern. The requirement is for K- or D-region identity between the target cell in the assay and the immunizing cell. It is not necessary for the cytotoxic effector T cell and the target cell to share H-2 antigens.

4. *Ir Genes*

An Ir gene is defined by a functional assay demonstrating an antigen-specific, H-2-linked variation in the size of the response to antigen. In many cases it is clear that two genes are involved, and complementation can be observed in F_1 hybrids or recombinants obtained from two low responders. There would appear to be two key questions concerning the role of Ir genes. The first is the cell type in which the gene or genes are expressed. In some studies it would appear to be the T cell, in others, the T cell and B cell, and in still others, the T cell and macrophage. Although all these Ir genes share the property of being histocompatibility-linked, and presumably all belong to a special class of genes, it is probable that they do act at a number of different points in cell interactions and hence can be expressed in any of the three cell types. The second question concerns the nature of the interaction between Ir genes and Ia genes for successful cell collaboration. It is not clear whether this is a requirement for a cis arrangement of the two genes on the chromosome, or whether the two gene products must be physically and/or functionally associated at the cell membrane.

B. Hypotheses

1. *T Cells Interact With Antigen Only When Presented in Association With H-2*

The same essential features are common to all three major types of collaboration, and it is hard to escape the conclusion that they represent three variations of a basic theme.

It is not clear, however, whether all the experimental observations can be fitted into a single model in view of the conflict over the evidence concerning T cell-B cell interactions noted above. If one ignores the evidence that collaboration can occur across a haplotype barrier, the remaining information can be accommodated to a common, although somewhat complex, model. There are many variants, but one such model can be presented as follows.

The T-cell receptor has two components. One component is the immunoglobulin V-gene product, and the other is a receptor for an H-2 gene product which presumably is coded for by a gene in the H-2 complex. (For Ly-23$^+$ cytotoxic cells the H-2 product it recognizes is a K- or D-region antigen, for Ly-1$^+$ helper cells the product is an I-region antigen. It is not clear to which group the suppressor cell should be assigned.) The T cell is triggered only when both components of the T-cell receptor interact with their counterparts. In other words, all antigens must be presented on a cell surface in association with an H-2 structure.

The complications are as follows:

1. There must be T cell receptors for all the allo-H-2 structures (including H-2 mutants?) to explain how responses can become restricted to allo-H-2 antigens.
2. The Ir gene product must be placed in an antigen-specific chain of events. In order to do this, different restricted

subsets of V genes must be coupled to different T-cell receptors for H-2 antigens.

3. It would appear that the association between V gene and the receptor for H-2 cannot be analogous to the variable and constant region coupling in immunoglobulin, since the former is linked to immunoglobulin C_H markers (not H-2-linked), and it seems most plausible to assume the gene for the latter is H-2-linked.

The model seems complicated and inadequate in some respects, but some variants of it might prove acceptable.

The model, however, fails to provide any good explanation of the studies which show no haplotype restriction after the removal of negative allogeneic effects.

2. Negative Allogeneic Effects Explain all H-2 Restriction

In this model it is proposed that there are no restrictions on cell collaboration per se, but that the recognition of alloantigens activates a strong suppressive response. It would appear that the suppressor cell would have to be a different cell from the collaborating cell, since reactivity to alloantigens is clonally distributed.

The first problem with such a model is that although striking negative allogeneic effects could be demonstrated in some studies (as for example, our own), the appropriate controls failed to reveal such effects in the Katz and Benacerraf or the Shevach, Rosenthal, and Paul experiments.

The second problem is to explain how priming with antigen on allogeneic cells could establish an H-2 restriction for the allogeneic cell in the secondary response.

The third and most serious problem is the difficulty of conceiving that effective alloinhibition could be generated in the short time span of the cell-mediated cytoxicity assay. It would appear that H-2 restriction in this system would have to be explained by some other means and the idea of a common mechanism would be lost.

C. Conclusion

The conclusion is regrettably brief. At the present time there would appear to be no satisfactory hypothesis free from serious problems. There remains the impression that some key point, whether it be one of fact or one of interpretation, still eludes us. We still do not understand, for instance, why the T-cell response to alloantigens is so intense. The rapid unfolding of new facts in the past 2 years has presented us with one of the most intriguing questions to date in cellular immunology. This same rapid progress, however, may well have yielded some new information or some new insights by the time this chapter is read.

ACKNOWLEDGMENTS

Dr. Susan Swain is supported by a Damon Runyon Grant (DRG-5-F) and our research is supported in part by grants from the National Institute of Health (AI 08795) and the American Cancer Society (IM-1-I).

The authors are indebted to their colleagues for helpful comment and discussion, particularly Drs. Park Trefts, Ann Feeney, and Peter Panfili; and to Kathy Wong for her most helpful assistance in the preparation of this manuscript.

REFERENCES

Armerding, D., Kubo, R. T., Grey, H. M., and Katz, D. H. (1975). Activation of T and B lymphocytes in vitro. Presence of β2-microglobulin determinants on allogeneic effect factor. *Proc. Nat. Acad. Sci. (USA) 72:* 4577-4581.

Armerding, D., Sachs, D. H., and Katz, D. H. (1974). Activation of T and B lymphocytes in vitro. III. Presence of Ia determinants on allogeneic effect factor. *J. Exp. Med. 140:* 1717-1722.

Bechtol, K. B., Freed, J. H., Herzenberg, L. A., and McDevitt, H. O. (1974). Genetic control of the antibody response to the poly-L-(try-glu)-poly-D-L-ala-poly-L-Lys in C3H ↔ CWB tetraparental mice. *J. Exp. Med. 140:* 1660-1675.

Benacerraf, B., Green, I., and Paul, W. E. (1967). The immune response of guinea pigs to hapten-poly-L-lysine conjugates as an example of the genetic control of the recognition of antigenicity. *Cold Spring Harbor Symp. Quant. Biol. 32:* 569-575.

Benacerraf, B. and Katz, D. H. (1975). The nature and function of histocompatibility linked immune response genes. In *Immunogenetics and Immunodeficiency* (B. Benacerraf, ed.). Medical and Technical Publ. Co. Ltd., London, pp. 81-116.

Ben-Sassoon, S. Z., Shevach, E., Green, I., and Paul, W. E. (1974). Alloantiserum induced inhibition of migration inhibition factor production in immune response gene-controlled immune systems. *J. Exp. Med. 140:* 383-395.

Bevan, M. J. (1975a). Interaction antigens detected by cytotoxic T cells with the major histocompatibility complex as modifier. *Nature 256:* 419-421.

Bevan, M. J. (1975b). The major histocompatibility complex determines susceptibility to cytotoxic T cells directed against minor histocompatibility antigens. *J. Exp. Med. 142:* 1349-1364.

Binz, H., Bachi, T., Wigzell, H., Ramseier, H., and Lindenmann, J. (1975). Idiotype positive T cell visualized by autoradiography and electron microscopy. *Proc. Nat. Acad. Sci. (USA) 72:* 3210-3214.

Binz, H. and Wigzell, H. (1975a). Shared idiotypic determinants on B and T lymphocytes reactive against the same antigenic determinants. I. Demonstration of similar or identical idiotypes on IgG molecules and T cell receptors with specificity for the same alloantigens. *J. Exp. Med. 142:* 197-211.

Binz, H. and Wigzell, H. (1975b). Shared idiotypic determinants on B and T lymphocytes reactive against the same antigenic determinants. IV. Isolation of two groups of naturally occurring idiotypic molecules with specific antigen-binding activity in the serum and urine of normal rats. *Scand. J. Immunol. 4:* 591-600.

Binz, H. and Wigzell, H. (1976a). Shared idiotypic determinants on B and T lymphocytes reactive against the same antigenic determinants. II. Determination of frequency and characteristics of idiotypic T and B lymphocytes in normal rats using direct visualization. *J. Exp. Med. 142:* 1218-1230.

Binz, H. and Wigzell, H. (1976b). Shared idiotypic determinants on B and T lymphocytes reactive gainst the same antigenic determinants. III. Physical fractionation of specific immunocompetent T lymphocytes by affinity chromatography using anti-idiotype antibodies. *J. Exp. Med. 142:* 1231-1240.

Black, S. J., Hämmerling, G. J., Berek, C., Rajewsky, K., and Eichmann, K. (1976). Idiotypic analysis of lymphocytes in vitro. I. Specificity and heterogeneity of B and T lymphocytes reactive with anti-idiotypic antibody. *J. Exp. Med. 143:* 846-860.

Blanden, R. V., Hapel, A. J., and Jackson, D. J. (1976). Mode of action of Ir genes and the nature of T cell receptors for antigen. *Immunochem. 13:* 179-191.

Cantor, H. and Boyse, E. A. (1975a). Functional subclasses of T lymphocytes bearing Ly antigens. I. The generation of functionally distinct T-cell subclasses is a differentiative process independent of antigen. *J. Exp. Med. 141:* 1376-1389.

Cantor, H. and Boyse, E. A. (1975b). Functional subclasses of T lymphocytes bearing Ly antigens. II. Cooperation between subclasses of Ly+ cells in the generation of killer activity. *J. Exp. Med. 141:* 1390-1399.

Debré, P., Kapp, J. A., and Benacerraf, B. (1975). Genetic control of specific immune suppression. I. Experimental conditions for the stimulation of suppressor cells by the copolymer L-glutamic acid 50-L-tyrosine 50 (GT)in nonresponder Balb/c mice. *J. Exp. Med. 142:* 1436-1446.

Debré, P., Kapp, J. A., Dorf, M. E., and Benacerraf, B. (1975). Genetic control of specific immune suppression. II. H-2-linked dominant genetic control of immune suppression by the random copolymer L-glutamic acid 50-L-tyrosine 50 (GT). *J. Exp. Med. 142:* 1447-1454.

Dorf, M. E. and Benacerraf, B. (1975). Complementation of H-2-linked Ir genes in the mouse. *Proc. Nat. Acad. Sci. (USA) 72:* 3671-3675.

Dorf, M. E., Maurer, P. H., Merryman, C. F., and Benacerraf, B. (1976). Inclusion group systems and cis-trans effects in responses controlled by the two complementing Ir-GLΦ genes. *J. Exp. Med. 143:* 889-896.

Dutton, R. W., Falkoff, R., Hirst, J. A., Hoffmann, M., Kappler, J. W., Kettman, J. R., Lesley, J. R., and Vann, D. (1971). Is there evidence for a nonantigen specific diffusable chemical mediator from the thymus-derived cell in the initiation of the immune response? In *Progress in Immunology* (B. Amos, ed.). Academic, New York, pp. 355-368.

Eichmann, K. and Rajewsky, K. (1975). Induction of T and B cell immunity by anti-idiotype antibody. *Eur. J. Immunol. 5:* 661-666.

Erb, P. and Feldmann, M. (1975a). Role of macrophages in the in vitro induction of T-helper cells. *Nature 254:* 352-354.

Erb, P. and Feldmann, M. (1975b). The role of macrophages in the generation of T-helper cells. I. Requirement for macrophages in helper cell induction and characteristics of the macrophage - T-cell interaction. *Cell. Immunol. 19:* 356-367.

Erb, P. and Feldmann, M. (1975c). The role of macrophages in the generation of T-helper cells. II. The genetic control of the macrophage - T cell interaction for helper cell induction with soluble antigens. *J. Exp. Med. 142:* 460-472.

Forman, J. (1975). On the role of the H-2 histocompatibility complex in determining the specificity by cytotoxic effector cells sensitized against syngeneic trinitrophenyl-modified targets. *J. Exp. Med. 142:* 403-418.

Frelinger, J. A. and Shreffler, D. C. (1975). The major histocompatibility complex. In *Immunogenetics and Immunodeficiency* (B. Benacerraf, ed.). Medical and Technical Publ. Co. Ltd., London, pp. 81-116.

Gordon, R. D., Simpson, E., and Samuelson, L. E. (1975). In vitro cell-mediated immune response to male specific (H-Y) antigen in mice. *J. Exp. Med. 143:* 1108-1120.

Hämmerling, G. J., Black, S. J., Berek, C., Eichmann, L., and Rajewsky, K. (1976). Idiotypic analysis of lymphocytes in vitro. II. Genetic control of T helper cell responsiveness to anti-idiotypic antibody. *J. Exp. Med. 143:* 861-869.

Heber-Katz, E. and Wilson, D. B. (1975). Collaboration of allogeneic T and B lymphocytes in the primary antibody response to sheep erythrocytes in vitro. *J. Exp. Med. 142:* 928-935.

Herzenberg, L. A., Okumura, K., and Herzenberg, L. A. (1975). Mechanism of allotype suppression. In *Suppressor Cells in Immunity* (S. R. Singhal and N. Sinclair, eds.). University of Western Ontario Press, Toronto, pp. 93-104.

Hill, S. W. (1976). Modification of an Ir-gene-controlled nonreponder phenotype by genes which segregate with H-2. *Fed. Proc. 35:* 825.

Kapp, J. A., Pierce, C. W., de La Croix, F., and Benacerraf, B. (1976). Immunosuppressive factors, extracted from lymphoid cells of non-responder mice primed with L-glutamic and 60-L-alakine-30-L-tyrosine 10 (GAT). I. Activity and antigenic specificity. *J. Immunol. 116:* 305-309.

Katz, D. H. and Benacerraf, B. (1975). The function and interrelationships of T cell receptors, Ir genes and other histocompatibility gene products. *Transplant. Rev. 22:* 175-195.

Katz, D. H. and Benacerraf, B. (1976). The role of the histocompatibility gene complex in immune responses. In *Proceedings of an Internations Conference at Brook Lodge, Michigan* (D. H. Katz and B. Benacerraf, eds.). Academic, New York.

Katz, D. H., Dorf, M. E., and Benacerraf, B. (1976). Control of T-lymphocyte and B-lymphocyte activation by two complementing Ir-GLΦ immune response genes. *J. Exp. Med. 143:* 906-918.

Katz, D. H., Hamaoka, T., Dorf, M. E., and Benacerraf, B. (1973). Cell interactions between histoincompatible T and B lymphocytes. IV. Involvement of the immune response genes in the control of lymphocyte interaction in responses controlled by the gene. *J. Exp. Med. 138:* 734-739.

Kindred, B. and Shreffler, D. C. (1972). H-2 dependence of cooperation between T and B cells in vivo. *J. Immunol. 109:* 940-943.

Klein, J. (1975). *Biology of the Mouse Histocompatibility-2 Complex* Springer-Verlag, New York.

Klein, J. (1976). An attempt at an interpretation of the mouse H-2 complex. *Contemp. Topics Immunobiol. 5:* 297-336.

Kontiainen, S. and Feldmann, M. (1975). Conditions for inducing T helper cells in vitro. *Scand. J. Immunol. 4:* 121-128.

Lipsky, P. E. and Rosenthal, A. S. (1975a). Macrophage-lymphocyte interaction: antigen independent binding of guinea pig lymph node lymphocytes by macrophages. *J. Immunol. 115:* 440-445.

Lipsky, P. E. and Rosenthal, A. S. (1975b). Macrophage-lymphocyte interaction. II. Antigen-mediated physical interaction between immune guinea pig lymph node lymphocytes and syngeneic macrophages. *J. Exp. Med. 141:* 138-154.

Munro, A. and Taussig, M. J. (1975). Two genes in the major histocompatibility complex control immune response. *Nature 256:* 103-106.

Pierce, C. W., Kapp, J. A., and Benacerraf, B. (1976). Regulation by the H-2 gene complex of macrophage-lymphoid cell interactions in secondary responses in vitro. *J. Exp. Med. 144:* 371-381.

Pierce, S. K. (1976). Allogeneic carrier specific enhancement of secondary B cell responses. *Fed. Proc. 35:* 627.

Pierce, S. K. and Klinman, N. R. (1975). The allogeneic bisection of carrier-specific enhancement of monoclonal B-cell responses. *J. Exp. Med. 142:* 1165-1179.

Raff, M. C. and Cantor, H. (1971). Subpopulations of thymus cells and thymus-derived lymphocytes. In *Progress in Immunology* (B. Amos, ed.). Academic, New York, pp. 83-93.

Rehn, T. G., Shearer, G. M., Koren, H. S., and Inman, J. K. (1976). Cell mediated lympholysis of N-(3-Nitro-4 hydroxy-5-10 dopheny L acetyl)-β alanyl lycyl-modified autologous lymphocytes controlled by the H-2K and H-2D serological regions of the murine major histocompatibility complex. *J. Exp. Med. 143:* 127-142.

Rich, S. S. and Rich, R. R. (1975). Regulatory mechanisms in cell-mediated immune responses. II. A genetically restricted suppressor of mixed lymphocyte reactions released by alloantigen activated spleen cells. *J. Exp. Med. 142:* 1391-1402.

Rich, S. S. and Rich, R. R. (1976). Regulatory mechanisms in cell-mediated immune response. III. I region control of suppressor cell interaction with responder cells in mixed lymphocyte reaction. *J. Exp. Med. 143:* 672-677.

Rosenthal, A. S., Blake, J. T., and Lipsky, P. E. (1975). Inhibition of macrophage-lymphocyte interaction by cytoclasin B during antigen recognition by T lymphocytes. *J. Immunol. 115:* 1135-1139.

Rosenthal, A. S. and Shevach, E. M. (1973). The function of macrophages in antigen recognition by guinea pig T lymphocytes. I. Requirement for histocompatible macrophages and lymphocytes. *J. Exp. Med. 138:* 1194-1212.

Schwartz, B. D., Kask, A. M., Paul, W. E., and Shevach, E. M. (1976). Structural characteristics of the alloantigens determined by the major histocompatibility complex of the guinea pig. *J. Exp. Med. 143:* 541-558.

Schwartz, R. H., Jackson, L., and Paul, W. E. (1975). T lymphocyte-enriched murine peritoneal exudate cells. I. A reliable assay for antigen-induced T lymphocyte proliferation. *J. Immunol. 115:* 1330-1338.

Schwartz, R. H. and Paul, W. E. (1976). T lymphocyte-enriched murine peritoneal exudate cells. II. Genetic control of antigen-induced T lymphocyte proliferation. *J. Exp. Med. 143:* 529-540.

Shearer, G. M. (1974). Cell-mediated cytotoxicity to trinitrophenyl-modified syngeneic lymphocytes. *Eur. J. Immunol. 4:* 527-532.

Shearer, G. M., Rehn, T. G., and Garbarino, C. A. (1975). Cell-mediated lympholysis of trinitrophenyl-modified autologous lymphocytes. Effector cell specificity to modified cell surface components controlled by the H-2K and H-2D serological regions of the major histocompatibility complex. *J. Exp. Med. 141:* 1348-1364.

Shevach, E. M. (1976). The function of macrophages in antigen recognition by guinea pig T lymphocytes. III. Genetic analysis of the antigens mediating macrophage - T lymphocyte interaction. *J. Immunol. 116:* 1482-1489.

Shevach, E. M., Green, I., and Paul, W. E. (1974). Alloantiserum-induced inhibition of immune response gene product function. II. Genetic analysis of target antigens. *J. Exp. Med. 139:* 679-695.

Shevach, E. M., Paul, W. E., and Green, I. (1972). Histocompatibility-linked immune response gene function in guinea pigs: specific inhibition of antigen-induced lymphocyte proliferation by alloantisera. *J. Exp. Med. 136:* 1207-1221.

Shevach, E. M. and Rosenthal, A. S. (1973). The function of macrophages in antigen recognition by guinea pig T lymphocytes. II. Role of the macrophage in the regulation of the immune response. *J. Exp. Med. 138:* 1213-1229.

Shreffler, D. C. and David, C. S. (1975). The major histocompatibility complex and the I immune response region in genetic variation, function and organization. *Adv. Immunol. 20:* 125-195.

Swain, S., Trefts, P., Tse, H. Y.-S., and Dutton, R. W. (1977). The significance of T-B collaboration across haplotype barriers. *Cold Spring Harbor Symp. Quant. Biol. 41:* 597-609.

Tada, T., Taniguchi, M., and Takemori, T. (1975). Properties of primed suppressor T cells and their products. *Transplant. Rev. 26:* 106-129.

Taniguchi, M., Hayakawa, K., and Tada, T. (1976). Properties of antigen specific suppressive T cell factor in the regulation of antibody response of the mouse. II. In vitro activity and evidence for I region gene product. *J. Immunol. 116:* 542-548.

Taussig, M. J., Munro, A. J., Campbell, R., David, C. S., and Staines, N. A. (1975). Antigen-specific T cell factor in cell cooperation. Mapping within the I region of the H-2 complex and ability to cooperate across allogeneic barriers. *J. Exp. Med. 142:* 694-700.

Trenkner, E. and Riblet, R. (1975). Induction of anti-phosphoryl choline antibody formation by anti-idiotype antibodies. *J. Exp. Med. 142:* 1121-1132.

von Boehmer, H. and Haas, W. (1976). Cytotoxic T lymphocytes recognize allogeneic tolerated TNP-conjugated cells. *Nature 261:* 141-142.

von Boehmer, H., Hudson, L., and Sprent, J. (1975). Collaboration of histoincompatible T and B lymphocytes using cells from tetraparental bone marrow chimeras. *J. Exp. Med. 142:* 989-997.

Waldmann, H., Pope, H., and Munro, A. J. (1975). Cooperation across the histocompatibility barrier. *Nature 258:* 728-730.

Waldmann, H., Poulton, P., and Desaymard, C. (1976). Antigen-nonspecific T cell factor in B cell activation. Origin: biological properties and failure to show a relationship to H-2. *Immunology 30:* 723-734.

Waldron, J. A., Horn, R. G., and Rosenthal, A. S. (1973). Antigen-induced proliferation of guinea pig lymphocytes in vitro: obligatory role of macrophages in the recognition of antigen by immune T-lymphocytes. *J. Immunol. 111:* 58-64.

Waltenbaugh, C. R., Debré, P., Dorf, M., and Benacerraf, B. (1976). The H-2 gene control of GT specific immune suppression. *Fed. Proc. 35:* 713.

Zinkernagel, R. (1976). Virus-specific T cell mediated cytotoxicity across the H-2 barrier to virus altered alloantigen. *Nature 261:* 139-141.

Zinkernagel, R. M. and Doherty, P. C. (1975). H-2 compatibility requirement for T cell mediated lysis of target cells infected with lymphocytic choriomeningitis virus. Different cytotoxic T cell specificities are associated with structures coded from H-2K or H-2D. *J. Exp. Med. 141:* 1427-1436.

Zinkernagel, R. M., Dunlop, B. C., and Doherty, P. C. (1975). Cytotoxic T cell activity is strain specific in outbred mice infected with lymphocytic choriomeningitis virus. *J. Immunol. 115:* 1613-1616.

Chapter 12

LYMPHOCYTE TRAFFIC PATTERNS AND CELL-CELL INTERACTIONS

George I. Bell

Theoretical Division
University of California
Los Alamos Scientific Laboratory
Los Alamos, New Mexico

Major sources and recirculation patterns of lymphocytes are reviewed. Lymphocytes born in the bone marrow and thymus seed the peripheral lymphoid organs and, at least after suitable contact with complementary antigen, give rise to a long-lived pool of immunocompetent B and T cells which recirculate throughout the body in blood and lymph. Numerical values are suggested for some of the important populations.

The source of lymphocytes from proliferation in the bone marrow and thymus far exceeds that required to maintain the recirculating pool, and possible reasons are discussed.

Approximately 20% of the lymphocytes reaching a lymph node in the blood leave the node in efferent lymph, and this percentage depends to some extent on surface properties of the particular lymphocytes. This traffic amounts to 3×10^7 lymphocytes per hour in a normal sheep node weighing 1 g and can be increased 10-fold by antigen stimulation of the node. The rate of possible distinct contacts between T and B cells in a sheep node is estimated to be $\lesssim 200$ per hour per cell, assuming interactions take place between sessile B (T) cells and recirculating T (B) cells. This rate should be sufficient to reliably initiate a T-dependent humoral response in a single sheep node (or a whole mouse) but will not be realized if both T and B cells become bound to antigen on macrophages or on reticular cells in the node.

I. INTRODUCTION

When a theorist first tries to understand the functioning of the immune system as a whole, he or she is likely to be depressed by its complexity and to start by approximating the system as a homogeneous volume containing interacting populations of lymphocytes, antigen, and antibody molecules. While such models, and several examples are presented in this volume, can be useful, there are a number of general reasons for wishing to model the system more realistically. These include: (a) it is known that for many antigens, the binding of the antigen to a lymphocyte having complementary receptors does not suffice for activation of the lymphocyte. Rather, an interaction between two or three cell types (for example T cell, B cell, and macrophage) in the presence of antigen may be required for activation. In general, interactions between cells appear important in regulating immune responses. One needs more than a uniform model for estimating interaction rates and their importance. (b) Numerous in vitro experiments have been performed on the interactions between cells and antigen, and models of interaction mechanisms have been formulated. In order to understand whether these in vitro mechanisms are important in vivo, it may be important to have a fairly detailed view of the in vivo conditions in lymphoid organs. (c) Interaction of the immune system with antigen can modulate the quantitative and probably the qualitative lymphocyte traffic patterns and cell-cell interaction rates. Such modulations may be important regulatory mechanisms in immune responses. (d) In considering the response to a localized antigen such as a subcutaneously injected insoluble antigen, or a graft or tumor, it is probably important to consider where and how the immune system encounters the antigen and what kind of a response can thereby be generated. Moreover, natural threatening antigens are most likely to gain entry to the body from the gut, the respiratory system, or through breaks in the skin, and they will first be engaged by the immune system in relatively local combat regions, specific for those paths of entry. Since the immune system must have evolved, in large part, to cope with such initially localized threats, it is likely that critical regulatory and functional features of the immune system are concerned with initially localized responses.

II. TRAFFIC PATTERNS OF RECIRCULATING LYMPHOCYTES

Lymphocytes are the cells of the immune system which have the ability to recognize specific antigens and to respond, under appropriate conditions, by proliferation, antibody secretion, cytoxicity, etc. In young and adult animals, lymphocytes are found in the bone marrow and thymus, where they are believed to arise from division of more or less multipotential stem cells, in the spleen, lymph nodes, tonsils, Peyers patches, and other peripheral lymphoid tissue, and circulating throughout the body in blood and lymph. The human lymphoid system is depicted in Fig. 1. Major organs, circulation paths, and approximate numbers of lymphocytes in a 200 g rat are indicated in Fig. 2. As will be discussed in the following, lymphocytes from the bone marrow and thymus seed the peripheral lymphoid organs and give rise to a pool of long-lived lymphocytes which recirculate from blood to lymph and back again to the blood.

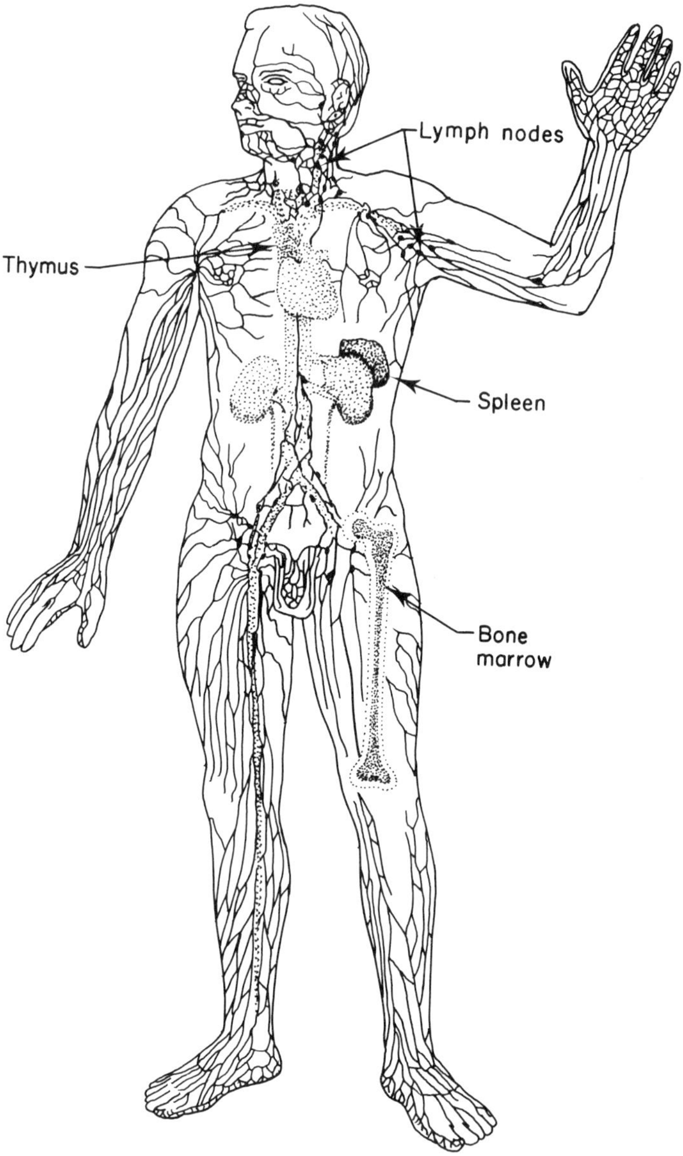

FIG. 1. The human lymphatic system. Lymphocytes arising in bone marrow and thymus seed the peripheral lymphoid organs, including the lymph nodes and spleen. Lymphocytes are carried to all parts of the body in the blood. Many lymphocytes, particularly in the lymph nodes, will pass from blood to the lymphatic circulation as detailed in the text. After Jerne (1971).

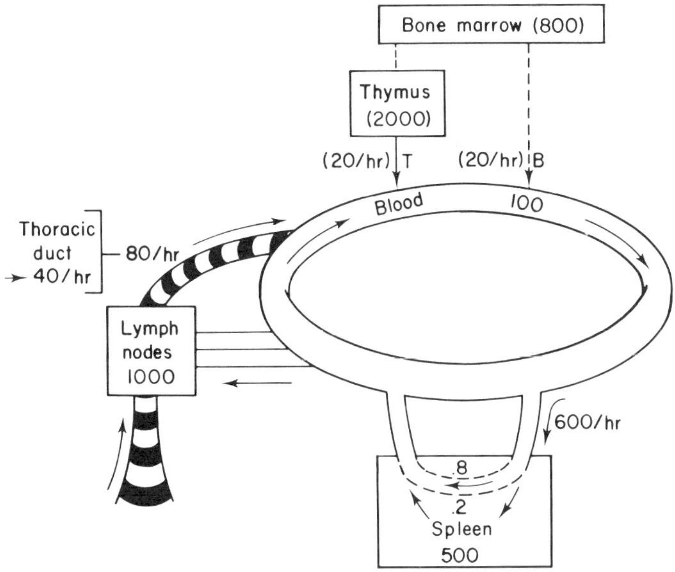

FIG. 2. Recirculating lymphocyte pool and possible sources. The numbers $\times 10^6$ are approximate for a 200 g rat. Values for blood, thoracic duct, and lymph nodes are taken from Gowans (1970), for spleen and total lymph flow from Hammond (1975), and Ford and Simmonds (1972). Eighty percent of the lymphocytes entering the spleen pass through within 5 min, while 20% have much longer residence times. Thymus values depend on animal age, are extrapolated from the P_2 population of Bryant (1972), and are in parentheses to indicate that lymphocytes in the thymus do not recirculate and that exported cells may be mostly very short-lived, or even die in the thymus. Bone marrow values are from Everett and Tyler (1967) and are in parentheses to indicate that lymphocytes in the bone marrow do not recirculate and the exported cells are probably very short-lived.

The bone marrow is a primary source of lymphocytes, in particular of the B lymphocytes which bear immunoglobulin receptors and can be stimulated to become antibody secreting cells (Osmond and Nossal, 1974). In birds, the development of mature B lymphocytes after they leave the marrow, takes place in a gut-associated lymphoid organ, the bursa of Fabricius, but in mammals, the analogous site of maturation is unknown and may not be so well localized. In any case, the bone marrow is an active center for lymphocyte proliferation. Approximately half the lymphocytes in rat bone marrow are newborn each day

(Everett and Tyler, 1967) and in steady state, which is a good approximation even in a growing animal, approximately half must therefore be exported or die each day. From the numbers given in Fig. 2, it is apparent that the rate of lymphocyte birth in the bone marrow ($\sim 2 \times 10^7$/hr) is sufficient to replace the entire recirculating pool of lymphocytes ($\sim 1.6 \times 10^9$) in only a few days. This potential source vastly exceeds that required to maintain most of the pool, for thymidine labeling experiments have shown that the majority of the recirculating lymphocytes ($\sim$ 90% in thoracic duct lymph and two-thirds in blood, Everett and Tyler, 1967) are long-lived, with lifetimes on the order of months, rather than days. The remainder of the small recirculating lymphocytes have lifetimes of a few days or weeks and recirculate poorly from blood to lymph; it is possible that this population arises from freshly exported bone marrow (and thymus) lymphocytes, as will be discussed later. It is not known how many cell divisions or maturation steps are involved in going from a stem cell to a mature recirculating lymphocyte. Estimates of a typical clone size of mature but unstimulated B cells (Klinman and Press, 1975) range from 10 to 3×10^3, and if each clone is assumed to arise from a single stem cell, then a minimum of 3 to 12 cell divisions would be required. One of the central unresolved problems in immunology lies in understanding the continuous proliferation of lymphocytes in bone marrow (and thymus), to no apparent useful end. I shall return to this point in the discussion.

The thymus is an important intermediate organ in the generation of lymphocytes, being the proximate source of T cells (thymus-derived lymphocytes) which are the most abundant class of recirculating lymphocytes (Metcalf, 1966; Bryant, 1972,1974). In a young or adult animal the thymus is a more or less autonomous center of cell proliferation and lymphocyte export.* It does not seem to receive many

---

*Thymus activity declines with age of the animal, and the reader is referred to the literature cited for details. Numbers in Fig. 2 are intended to represent young adult animals.

cells from the bone marrow, although restoration of an irradiated thymus may require the immigration of bone marrow derived stem cells (Kadish and Basch, 1975). Cell kinetics in the thymus have been studied experimentally in rodents (Metcalf, 1966; Miller and Osoba, 1967; Bryant, 1972) and mathematically (Lumb, 1975; Prothero and Tyler, 1975). The rate at which lymphocytes are produced by cell division in the thymus is comparable to the rate in bone marrow and is much larger than the rate at which such cells are found to appear in the lymphoid tissues. Therefore, most of the lymphocytes which arise from proliferation within the thymus must either die in the thymus (Metcalf, 1966; Miller and Osoba, 1967) or have very short lifetimes on export. Relatively few dying, pycnotic cells are seen in the thymus (Miller and Osoba, 1967; Bryant, 1974). Moreover, the net lymphocyte output in thymic blood has been measured to be about 10^6 cells/day per gram body weight (Williams et al., 1971; Pearson et al., 1976). For a 200 g rat this would yield $\sim 10^7$ thymocytes/hr, which is one-half the production rate estimated in Fig. 2. Additional thymocytes could emigrate in lymph directly to the thoracic duct. From these numbers it appears that most of the lymphocytes which are derived from proliferation within the thymus may be exported. Only a small fraction of these cells, however, can survive to join the recirculating pool of long-lived lymphocytes. The fate and function of the bulk of the exported and necessarily short-lived cells is unknown.

Lymphocytes arise not only from mitoses in thymus and bone marrow, but, at least in any animal subject to normal antigenic exposure, throughout the lymphoid tissue. I have not attempted to quantitate these sources. Thymidine labeling data and mitotic indices are available (e.g., Everett and Tyler, 1967; Metcalf, 1966) but their interpretation is obscured by uncertainties of lymphocyte traffic. This could be a fruitful field for mathematical modeling.

Lymphocytes are to be found circulating with blood and lymph, and are a major cell population in the spleen, the lymph nodes, and other lymphoid organs such as the gut-associated Peyers patches and appendix. Typical concentrations are 2×10^3 cells/mm^3 in blood and $10^4/mm^3$ in lymph from a lymph node (Morris, 1968). All cells enumerated in Fig. 2 (except for those in and exported from the thymus and bone marrow) are to be viewed as continuously recirculating from blood to lymph and back to blood in the following manner. First, the recirculation is established during fetal life, in the absence of antigen stimulation or competence (Pearson et al., 1976). Lymphocytes in the blood are carried to all parts of the body. In particular, around 1% of the cardiac output will pass through lymph nodes (Hall, 1967). From small blood vessels in each node, namely post-capillary venules, lymphocytes are specifically able to escape from the blood. The far more numerous red blood cells do not escape. At one time it was believed from electron micrographs that the lymphocytes often escape by penetrating through and not between the endothelial cells which line the blood vessel (Marchesi and Gowans, 1964). More recent investigators have concluded that the lymphocytes usually escape by insinuating themselves between the endothelial cells (Schoefl, 1972; Anderson et al., 1975). Scanning electron micrographs have suggested that the microvilli on recirculating lymphocytes first interact with specific receptor sites on the endothelial cell surfaces and that this attachment phase is followed by active migration between the endothelial cells (Anderson and Anderson, 1976). Escape is affected by surface properties of the lymphocyte. For example, lymphocytes from intestinal lymph having surface IgA preferentially pass from blood to gut-associated lymphoid tissue (Guy-Grand et al., 1974; Williams and Gowans, 1975; Scollay et al., 1976; Hall et al., 1972; Hopkins and Hall, 1976). Treatment of the lymphocytes with neuraminidase, trypsin, or mitogens alters their migration properties (Berney and Gesner, 1970; Woodruff, 1974), but it appears that the effects of neuraminidase and mitogens, at least, are primarily to enhance lymphocyte retention in lungs, liver, and spleen, rather than to directly alter the migration across venule walls (Freitas and de Sousa, 1975, 1976; Hall et al., 1972; Ford et al., 1976). Moreover, antigen stimulation of a node can enhance the flux of lymphocytes by an order of magnitude. As will be seen, this enhancement is accompanied by an increase in blood flow, but in addition it is possible that the flux of antigen reactive cells is specifically favored. Thus, the rate at which lymphocytes leave the blood, in a lymph node, can be modulated by a variety of factors, some of which are doubtless important in regulating immune responses.

Lymphocyte traffic in a node will be discussed in a later section of this paper, but it should be noted that it takes many hours, $\sim$ 30 in sheep, for the average lymphocyte to traverse a node. After leaving a node, in the efferent lymph, a lymphocyte will pass through a series of valves and possibly other nodes of the lymphatic system to be collected in one of several large ducts through which the lymph and lymphocytes are discharged into the venous circulation, thereby completing the migration from blood to lymph to blood. Most important is the thoracic duct which collects around half the lymph in a rat principally from intestinal lymphoid tissue (Ford and Simmonds, 1972; Hopkins and Hall, 1976). This duct is a convenient source for the collection of recirculating lymphocytes and, in addition, the response of the system to chronic drainage of the thoracic duct is an interesting observable.

The spleen is an important lymphoid organ traversed by lymphocytes. Lymphocyte circulation through an isolated rat spleen has been studied in perfusion experiments (Ford, 1969), and a compartmental analysis has been made of the results (Hammond, 1975). It was concluded that approximately 80% of the lymphocytes pass through the spleen within 5 min and that the remaining 20% are about equally divided between those which pass through the "marginal zone" and "white pulp," having a transit time $\sim$ 5.5 hr, and those passing through the red pulp with a transit time $\sim$ 2.3 hr. It was estimated that about half the lymphocytes in the spleen are nonrecirculating (Ford, 1969), though it is possible that they could be mobilized to recirculate by treatments such as chronic thoracic duct drainage. In addition, there are efferent lymphatics from the spleen which presumably form a pathway for lymphocyte recirculation (Anderson and Weiss, 1976).

III. T AND B LYMPHOCYTES

The abundance of T and B lymphocytes in lymphoid organs have been measured in Lewis rats and Balb/c and CBA mice (Goldschneider and McGregor, 1973; Raff and Owen, 1971), with results tabulated in Table 1. These measurements were performed by staining the lymphocytes with antisera which are more or less specific for T-cell antigens. In the rat it was also found that most of the remaining lymphocytes were B cells, for they could be stained with anti B-cell (largely anti-Ig) sera.

Many other investigators have measured the proportion of rodent lymphocytes with surface Ig, which are presumably B cells. Results are found to vary somewhat between different animal strains, so that the values in Table 1 should not be accepted as universally valid. In particular, the proportion of T cells in rat thoracic duct is usually found to be lower than the 90% suggested in Table 1 with values of 50 to 80% being found by others (Ford, private communication).

From the data in Table 1, it appears that B and T cells do not recirculate identically. In particular, since the relative abundance of T cells is higher in the thoracic duct than in lymphoid organs, T cells must be relatively mobile and B cells relatively sessile. This conclusion has been reinforced by other measurements, for example, the observation that during chronic thoracic duct drainage, the proportion of T cells in the lymph drops to around 50% (Sprent, 1973).

In addition, it has been found that T and B cells are concentrated in different regions of the lymph nodes and, to a lesser extent, spleen (Sprent, 1973; Howard et al., 1972; Goldschneider and McGregor, 1973) and that they have different lifetimes (Howard, 1972; Sprent and Basten, 1973). However, neither T nor B cells constitute a homogeneous population. For example, helper and killer T cells are antigenically distinct (Cantor and Boyce, 1975b) and may have distinct patterns of circulation. Moreover, there is considerable evidence

TABLE 1

Percentages of Lymphocytes Which Are T Cells

	Mouse	Rat
Thymus	100	100
Thoracic duct	80-85	90
Lymph nodes	65-70	80
Blood	70	60
Spleen	30-35	50
Peritoneum	30-35	
Peyers patches	20-25	
Marrow		10

that the migratory patterns and lifetimes of both T and B cells are decisively affected by exposure to antigen. We shall return to this important topic in a succeeding section.

In principle it would be possible to construct a compartmental model of the immune system using data such as are given in Fig. 2, Table 1, and kinetic data to be discussed later. At the present time such a model would have to be arbitrary in many details, but I believe that it would be useful for the interpretation of existing data and for planning new experiments. Moreover, it is apparent that the quantity and quality of relevant data are increasing rapidly.

IV. RESPONSE TO ANTIGEN

The adaptability of the immune system in response to an antigen challenge is not confined to clonal selection and cellular activation/suppresion as might be described in a uniform model. In addition, the traffic patterns change. A particularly dramatic example is afforded by the response to a subcutaneous injection of antigen in Freund's incomplete adjuvant (largely mineral oil). This establishes a chronic center of inflammation (granuloma) which with time comes to resemble a lymph node, complete with circulation and efferent lymphatic, assembled de novo to meet the challenge (Smith, McIntosh and Morris, 1970). Further examples to be discussed in some detail are the activation of a lymph node and alterations in T- and B-lymphocyte lifetime and recirculation properties.

A. Activation of a Lymph Node

Morris and others have collected the efferent lymph from individual sheep lymph nodes and analyzed the cells therein and the ways in which cellular traffic is influenced by antigen in the node. In the efferent lymph from a typical unstimulated node, weighing roughly 1 g, approximately 3×10^7 cells per hour are emerging (Hall, 1967; Smith, Pedersen, and Morris, 1970; Hay, Cahill, and Trnka, 1974). The vast majority are small recirculating lymphocytes which have entered the lymph node from the blood. In addition, there may be small percentages of large lymphocytes, which have arisen from cell division in the node, and of macrophages and monocytes, which are believed to have entered the node in the afferent lymph.

It is of interest to compare this throughput of lymphocytes with the total number of lymphocytes which are brought to the node by the circulating blood. The difference, if large, would presumably be mostly lymphocytes which are carried through the node in the blood stream. Two measurements of the blood flow to individual lymph nodes have been carried out. In the first, Hall (1967) cannulated the vein from the prefemoral lymph node in a merino ewe and was able to measure venous outflow for about 15 min prior to clotting. He obtained an average flow rate of 1 mℓ/min g^{-1} node weight for eight nodes. The mean lymphocyte count of jugular venous blood was 3.5×10^6 cells/mℓ, so that about 2.1×10^8 lymphocytes per hour would reach a 1 g node in the blood. The number of lymphocytes leaving the node in efferent lymph (3×10^7/hr) is thus about 14% of the number arriving in afferent blood. More recently Hay and Hobbs (private communication) measured blood flow by determining the percentage of injected labeled microspheres which lodge in a node.

Per gram of node, 0.012% of the microspheres were collected and it was assumed that this represents the fraction of the cardiac output (3.3 liters/min) passing through the the node, namely 0.40 mℓ/min. These sheep had a mean lymphocyte count of 4.7×10^6 cells/mℓ, so that $0.40 \times 4.7 \times 10^6 \times 60 = 1.12 \times 10^8$ lymphocytes per hour would reach the 1 g node per hour. This is about half of Hall's value. In this case, the efferent lymphatic would export about 27% of the incoming blood lymphocytes. In either case, a small fraction (∿ 5%) of the lymphocytes in efferent lymph are derived from the afferent lymph.

I conclude that approximately 20% of the lymphocytes which reach an unstimulated lymph node will escape through the postcapillary venule to emerge in efferent lymph. Since, as noted earlier (e.g., Hopkins and Hall, 1976), there is selectivity in the escape, some fraction of the lymphocyte population must escape to a greater extent than 20%.

The average time for recirculating sheep lymphocytes to traverse a node has been measured to be about 30 hr (Frost et al., 1975; Scollay et al., 1976). Using this time, I estimate that a typical node will contain around 10^9 (∿ 30 hr × 3 10^7/hr) recirculating lymphocytes. Since these cells have an average diameter of about 7 μm, the mass of 10^9 cells is about 0.2 g (Hall, 1967), which must be a large fraction of the lymphocytes in a 1 g node (Everett and Tyler, 1967). These estimates for a sheep may be compared with those in Fig. 2 for a rat; there a lymph-blood throughput of 8×10^7 cells/hr was associated with a node population of 10^9 recirculating lymphocytes, so that the average transit time through nodes and lymphatic system would be about 12.5 hr. Since a rat weighs only about 5×10^{-3} as much as a sheep, so that lymphocytes have only to travel about $0.17=[(5 \times 10^{-3})^{1/3}]$ as far, it is perhaps surprising that these transit times are so similar. However, the figures are not very precise, and it should be noted that the transit time (30 hr) for a single sheep node was being compared with a transit time (12.5 hr) for complete recirculation in a rat. By injecting labeled

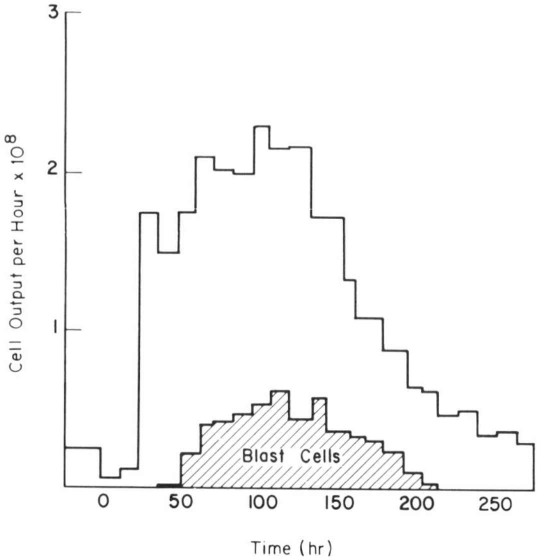

FIG. 3. Cell changes in efferent lymph. The output of white cells in the efferent lymph from the popliteal node of a sheep during an immune response to killed salmonella organisms. The organisms were injected under the skin of the leg at zero time. The open area represents the total white cell output, the shaded area the output of blast cells. After Smith, Pedersen, and Morris (1970).

lymphocytes in the blood of CBA mice and collecting them in thoracic duct lymph, Sprent (1973) determined recirculation times to be $\sim$ 20 hr. This suggests that a simple scaling of recirculation times with linear animal dimensions may be unreliable and that relative recirculation times may be much longer in mice.

When a lymph node is exposed to a bacterial, viral, protein, or cellular antigen, either by direct injection or by subcutaneous injection into the node drainage area, dramatic changes in the lymphocyte output ensue (Smith, Pedersen, and Morris, 1970; Hall et al., 1976; Hay, Cahill, and Trnka, 1974; Cahill et al., 1976). Some typical results are shown in Fig. 3. Shortly after antigen arrival, the lymphocyte output usually falls for a period of about 24 hr. This "shutdown" phase, however, appears rather variable in amplitude and duration and lymphocyte *input* to the node is increasing during this phase (Cahill et al., 1976). Beginning around 30 hr after exposure, a marked increase in lymphocyte output is observed. As is seen from Fig. 3, during this "recruitment" phase the cell output may increase by an order of magnitude and remain elevated for around a week. Initially, nearly all of the enhanced output consists of small lymphocytes from the recirculating pool which are found to enter the node at an increased rate (Dresser et al., 1970; Cahill et al., 1976) and the weight of the lymph node may be correspondingly increased by a factor of 2 or more. The transit time across the node does not change much during recruitment (Cahill et al., 1976; Hall et al., 1976), so that the increased weight may be largely in recirculating lymphocytes. It appears that the rate of blood flow to the the node is increased in order to accommodate such a large increase in cell supply (Hay and Hobbs, private communication), and dilation of the capillaries and venules is observed in the inflamed node (Smith, Pedersen, and Morris, 1970). In rat nodes draining tissue allografts, a prompt increase (70% in 12 hr) in the number of migrating lymphocytes per endothelial cell was observed (Anderson et al., 1975). This was followed by the localized proliferation of endothelial cells, leading to an increased vascularization and blood flow. In addition, the endothelial cells showed phagocytic activity.

For the first day or two after antigen injection, specific antigen-reactive cells are deficient in the exported population (Hay, Cahill, and Trnka, 1974; Hay and Morris, 1976). There does not appear to be any evidence that antigen-specific cells preferentially leave the postcapillary venules, but data on this very important point leave much to be desired.

After the enhanced output has continued for a day or so, blast cells begin to be prominent in the efferent lymph. These are large lymphocytes which have arisen from cell division in the node, and many are synthesizing antibodies which are specific for the immunizing antigen (Hay et al., 1972; Frost et al., 1976). In addition, the cells in the efferent lymph carry the basis for immunological memory which is required in order to mount a secondary response on later challenge with the antigen, anywhere except in the original node.

That is, if cells in the efferent lymph are collected and discarded, the sheep will retain no general immunological memory. If, however, the collected cells are reinjected, they will first of all seed the lymphoid tissues (Hopkins and Hall, 1976) to establish a systemic and normal primary immune response, and subsequently establish the immunological memory required to give a secondary response (Morris, 1968). Only a small fraction ($\lesssim$ 5%) of the exported lymphoblasts ever contribute, either themselves or their progeny, to the recirculating pool (Hall, 1974). Most of the cells probably reach the bloodstream wherein they are widely distributed to lymphoid tissue, but a few regain the lymphatic circulation. It is nevertheless possible that this minority recirculating population is a major component of immunological memory, as will be discussed later. There is so great a proliferation of antigen-specific cells, that even a few percent can represent an enormous amplification of responsiveness.

Frost et al. (1976) have observed antibody production and blast export from a single sheep node stimulated with 2.5 μg of streptococcal polysaccharide. The peak antibody production rate, 800 μg/hr, was reached around 100 hr after injection and had a strong monoclonal IgG component. If the cells involved were secreting IgG at the rate 2,000 molecules/sec (= 7.2×10^6 molecules/hr = 1.8×10^{-12} g/hr), about 4×10^8 cells would be required to give the observed antibody production rate. The total output of cells in the lymph was around 2×10^8/hr for many hours, but specific plaque forming cells only reached a peak output of 10^6/hr and a total output of $\sim 3 \times 10^7$ during 11 days of observation. From these numbers we conclude that cells responsible for antibody production *in the node* are mostly not exported or exported at only a very slow rate. The total number of cells exported far exceeds the number required for antibody production in the node.

It is not known whether the observed response is more properly characterized as primary or secondary since the sheep may have had prior exposure to cross-reacting antigens. It is tempting to wonder if the monoclonal component could have arisen from a single stimulated

B cell in the node. If so, to reach 10^8 cells in 100 hr would require 27 cell divisions or a mean time between divisions of about 3.8 hr. This average interdivision time seems remarkably small and suggests to me that many cells from the dominant clone were present in the node and circulation prior to immunization. For example, starting from 10^4 cells, only 14 cell divisions and a mean interdivision time of 7.6 hr, would be required to reach 10^8 cells in 100 hr. The dominance of a single clone is, of course, of great interest and not uncommon for bacterial polysaccharide antigens.

The general picture which emerges from all those studies is that soon after antigen is accumulated in a node, an inflammatory process initiates a much increased but nonspecific throughput of recirculating lymphocytes. Antigen-specific and perhaps other lymphocytes begin to proliferate and to secrete antibodies, and the recirculation of such cells to other lymphoid tissues will establish a normal primary response and make possible a systemic secondary response. Far more surprising have been observations of diminished antigen-specific reactivity of cells in the efferent lymph from unstimulated nodes (Hay, Cahill, and Trnka, 1974) and in thoracic duct lymph (Rowley et al., 1972). When, for example, allogeneic lymphocytes are injected into the drainage area of a particular node, the output of cells from that node, capable of giving a mixed lymphocyte reaction, declines to near zero in around 30 hr, but, in addition, the output of antigen-reactive cells in a control node on the opposite side of the animal declines to zero in about 60 hr. This occurs even though all efferent lymph and cells from the stimulated node are collected and discarded so that very few, if any, cells would be expected to get from the stimulated node to the control node.

One possibility to consider is that all antigen-sensitive recirculating lymphocytes could reach and be trapped in the single sensitized lymph node within $\sim$ 60 hr. However within this time only around 10^{10} cells were collected in the efferent lymph from the stimulated node (Hay, Cahill, and Trnka, 1974) and presumably no more than five (or possibly ten) times this number have been brought to the node in the blood. The recirculating pool in a sheep must contain $\sim 3 \times 10^{11}$ lymphocytes, so that only 15% (or possibly a third) of the recirculating pool could reach the sensitized node in 60 hr. Even if each antigen-specific cell entering a node were removed from circulation, it would appear to take many days or weeks before all of these cells would be removed from the recirculating pool. While one could imagine a more rapid depletion of a critical minority population which recirculated with great rapidity ($\sim$ 10 times faster than the bulk of the pool), this seems to me an unattractive ad hoc hypothesis.

It may be noted that when antigen is present in the *spleen*, it does have a good chance of trapping most sensitive lymphocytes in the recirculating pool within a few days. For example in the rat, we see from Fig. 2 that all lymphocytes in the pool ($\sim 1.6 \times 10^9$) could circulate through tortuous routes in the spleen (rate $\sim 0.2 \times 600 \times 10^8$/hr $= 1.2 \times 10^8$/hr) in around 13 hr which is also similar to the recirculation time through the nodes and lymphatic system. Intravenously injected particulate or cellular antigens are likely to become localized in the spleen and there to efficiently trap sensitive recirculating lymphocytes (Rowley et al., 1972; Ford, 1972).

I therefore believe that it is not possible for most of the lymphocytes specific for any antigen to be trapped in a single node within a few days. Alternative mechanisms must thus be sought for the general disappearance of sensitive lymphocytes due to a localized antigen. One possibility may be that fragments of antigen, for example surface antigens from lysed cells, can escape from the inflamed node into venules to reach and be trapped in other lymphoid tissues. In addition, soluble suppressive factors might leave the node, possibly in combination with antigen fragments.

It has also been reported that if efferent lymphocytes are collected from a cannulated antigen-stimulated sheep node for more than 3 weeks, the animal becomes specifically unresponsive to the antigen used (McConnell et al., 1974). In particular, helper T cells were depleted. During such a prolonged collection, it appears that most of the antigen-sensitive recirculating lymphocytes could enter the stimulated node and be diverted into the cannula. However, other investigators have been unable to similarly induce tolerance (Hay and Morris, 1976). In the interpretation of such experiments, it may be important to keep in mind that the thymus and bone marrow are presumably producing large numbers of lymphocytes during the experiment, which are potentially responsive to the antigen. Depending on the antigen and prior exposure of the animal, such lymphocytes might be able to generate immunocompetence which would override effects of pool depletion.

Qualitatively, the alterations in cell traffic within a node seem similar in primary and secondary responses. We presume that this is because the qualitative features, such as recruitment, are dominated by an inflammatory reaction, and that when details of the antigen-specific cells are studied, such as their kinetics and class of secreted antibodies, marked differences between primary and secondary responses will be seen. Since many popular antigens cross-react with environmental antigens, there is a possibility of obtaining a secondary response from a first immunization.

B. Frequency of Cell-Cell Interactions

Using numbers discussed in the preceeding section, I will now develop a simple model for estimating an upper limit to the frequency of encounters between antigen-specific lymphocytes in a node. I have in mind, for example, the possibility that in order to initiate a humoral response, an antigen-specific B cell may have to encounter an antigen specific T helper cell in the presence of antigen and possibly of other nonspecific accessory cells.

In a lymph node there are, in addition to recirculating and possibly sessile lymphocytes, large numbers of cells, especially the macrophages and reticular (or dendritic) cells, which are able to trap many antigens, particularly large multivalent antigens including bacteria, virus, foreign cells, and probably some immunogenic polymers (Nossal and Ada, 1971). The macrophages are mobile but do not follow the same migration paths as the recirculating lymphocytes, while the reticular cells are sessile. The mechanisms whereby macrophages and reticular cells recognize and trap antigen are unclear. If antibodies to the antigen are present and bound to the antigen, the macrophages can recognize the bound antibodies, via their Fc portions, and thereby be stimulated to phagocytose the antigen. Reticular cells may similarly recognize bound antibodies and bind antigen-antibody complexes on their surfaces. It is likely that natural antibodies are present to many pathogenic microorganisms and assist as opsonins in recognition and destruction of the microorganisms by macrophages. It is also reasonable that macrophages, which evolved prior to lymphocytes and antibodies, have other and more primitive mechanisms for recognizing microorganisms, and that such mechanisms are responsible for trapping antigen as well as for phagocytosis (Unanue and Calderon, 1975). The dendritic cells may share such recognition mechanisms even though they do not engage in much phagocytosis (Nossal and Ada, 1971).

In vitro experiments have suggested that antigen bound to macrophages is highly immunogenic (Unanue and Calderon, 1975; Rosenthal et al., 1975), and that macrophages are required for the initiation of any T-cell function (Erb and Feldmann, 1975; Rosenstreich et al., 1976; Lipsky et al., 1976). A role of reticular cells is less clear since they are not available for in vitro experiments, but they are intermingled with lymphocytes in a node and are effective trappers of antigen (Nossal and Ada, 1971).

The essence of our model is that a high and near-maximum rate of cell-cell encounters (at least neglecting chemotactic effects) will be obtained if one of the reactive partners is fixed, for example to a macrophage or to a reticular cell, while past it streams the migration of recirculating lymphocytes which includes other potential partners. For example, we may imagine that an antigen-sensitive B cell becomes stuck to antigen which it encounters bound to a reticular cell or macrophage, or that alternatively the B cell first binds antigen and is thereupon recognized by any macrophage as an object worthy of attention and immobilization. We assume that the bulk of the recirculating lymphocytes migrate past the immobilized cell with a velocity v such that each cell covers a distance comparable to the node diameter (∿ 1 cm for a sheep) in the transit time (∿ 30 hr). Thus for a sheep, v ∿ 0.3 mm/hr. If the migrating cells are closely packed, then a stationary cell can encounter ∿ 2 v/r recirculating cells per unit time, where r is a cell radius, ∿ 3.5 μm. Hence, a stationary cell could encounter ∿ 200 recirculating cells per hour (or vice versa). While recirculation patterns could be imagined which would increase encounter frequencies, I suspect that in an actual lymph node it is difficult to exceed such rates over more than a small fraction of the node, especially since the T cells, B cells, and macrophages tend to be concentrated in different regions of a node (Nossal and Ada, 1971: Goldschneider and McGregor, 1973: Sprent, 1973).

In an unimmunized mouse, the fraction of B cells which can be activated by exposure to a simple antigen is ∿ 10^{-4}, while the fraction of cells capable of binding the antigen may be ∿ 10^{-3} (Klinman and Press, 1975). If we assume these same frequencies for a sheep, and that a lymph node contains ∿ 2×10^8 B cells, these will include ∿ 2×10^4 antigen-specific (activatable) B cells and 2×10^5 antigen binding B cells. Confining our attention to the former, we estimate ∿ 4×10^6 encounters per hour would be possible between immobilized antigen-specific B cells and recirculating lymphocytes. If the latter include antigen-specific T cells with a frequency ∿ 10^{-4} (Hoffmann and Kappler, 1973), we could obtain ∿ 400 antigen-specific T-B encounters per hour. This should be an adequate number of encounters to reliably initiate a response to a T-dependent antigen in a single lymph node of a sheep. In a mouse the situation is somewhat more marginal. While a whole adult mouse may contain ∿ 2×10^8 B cells, and hence an encounter frequency similar to that for a single sheep node, an individual mouse node would have $\lesssim 1$ specific B-T encounter per hour.

In the above arguments we considered a single sessile cell interacting with a migrating population. However, even in the absence of antigen stimulation, the various classes of lymphocytes migrate through nodes at different rates (Sprent, 1973), so that, in a sheep node, relative velocities between cells ∿ 0.3 mm/hr are probably common. Thus, in a population of 10^9 more or less migratory lymphocytes, we could expect ∿ 10^{11} distinct cell-cell encounters per hour. We also considered a stuck B cell interacting with migrating T cells. However antigen-specific T cells also stick to antigen on macrophages (Rosenthal et al., 1975; Nieuwenhuis and Ford, 1976), so that a sessile T cell could be considered as interacting with migratory B cells, which had perhaps capped and lost many of their receptors. In fact, both antigen-specific T and B cells may stick to the reticular cells and macrophages and be unable to make contact with each other. In this case the cells could communicate with each other using antigen specific diffusable factors (Feldmann, 1972; see also Chap. 10; Taussig et al., 1974) or nonspecific factors (Marrack and Kappler, 1975; Dutton and Swain, Chap. 11) which are capable of activating lymphocytes which have bound antigen.

The actual interactions of cells with antigen and with each other will strongly depend on the antigen. In many of the experiments on lymphocyte traffic in nodes, cellular or viral antigens have been used at rather high doses. These antigens may be efficiently trapped by macrophages and thereby initiate a general inflammatory reaction, independent of interactions with antigen-specific lymphocytes. Presumably both T and B cells would then be likely to encounter antigen bound to macrophages or reticular cells. If, however, a protein carrier with hapten were the immunogen, this molecule might not by itself interact with macrophages or reticular cells but first bind to antigen-specific lymphocytes. Such lymphocytes, altered by antigen binding, could then interact with macrophages.

The foregoing discussion has not taken into account the detailed architecture of a lymph node (Nossal and Ada, 1971), nor the various types of lymphocytes, except the T/B division, which may be interacting. There has been recent progress in delineating the recirculation patterns of lymphocytes, both B and T, at various stages of maturity. For example, virgin and memory lymphocytes differ widely in lifetime and ability to recirculate. To these topics we now turn our attention.

C. The Recirculation of Virgin and Memory Lymphocytes

Recirculating lymphocytes are heterogeneous in several respects. First, there are the B cells and T cells, and among at least the latter, different classes are distinguishable by surface antigens and by function (Cantor and Boyce, 1975a,b). In addition, a multitude of clones are represented with receptors specific for diverse antigens. Finally, the cells will differ in their stage of maturation and history of exposure to antigen.

As noted earlier, the recirculating lymphocytes are predominantly long-lived T cells. In addition, short-lived T cells and long- and short-lived B cells have been identified as minority populations (Howard, 1972; Sprent and Basten, 1973), although the short-lived cells do not recirculate very effectively and are more abundant in blood than lymph (Everett and Tyler, 1967).

Raff and Cantor (1971) proposed that the short-lived, poorly recirculating T cells (found predominantly in spleen and thymus), and long-lived recirculating T cells (called T_1 and T_2, respectively), represent sequential stages in the maturation of T cells. In particular, they proposed that freshly exported thymocytes are, or become, T_1 cells which shortly die, unless they encounter antigen and are thereby induced to become T_2 cells which can give rise to primary or, later on, secondary T-cell responses. Relatively pure populations of T_1 and T_2 cells are readily available in mice. After adult thymectomy, the T_1 population is found to decay with a half life $\sim$ 2 weeks (Raff and Cantor, 1971; Kappler et al., 1974; Simpson and Cantor, 1975). Conversely, certain antisera can be used specifically to deplete the T_2 population in vivo (Raff and Cantor, 1971; Araneo et al., 1975). In addition, the T_1 cells have substantially more Thy 1.2 (theta) surface antigens and can be separated from T_2 cells on this basis (Cantor et al., 1975).

Using such purified populations, evidence has been obtained which tends to confirm the Raff and Cantor model. However, there are complications which arise from functional heterogeneity of T cells (Cantor and Boyce, 1975a; Simpson and Cantor, 1975), including suppressor T cells (Burns et al., 1975). In addition, it is difficult to determine if T_1 cells can transform to T_2 cells in the absence of antigen. For example, it has been found that T-helper activity for a primary in vitro response to the thymus-dependent antigen sheep red cells, resides primarily in the T_2 population, in that it is undiminished by thymectomy prior to priming. Moreover, priming is found to promote effectively T_1 cells into the T_2 class (Araneo and Kappler, private communication). These results may be interpreted by assuming that only the T_2 cells are effective helpers, but that antigen can promote T_1 cells into the T_2 class within a few days. Natural antigens, which are known to cross-react with sheep cells, may be postulated to have induced T_1 cells to become T_2 cells, but it is also possible that some T_1 cells might graduate to T_2 without antigen intervention. Whether T_1 to T_2 transformation requires cell division is unknown, but some proliferation might well be expected.

Somewhat analagous results have been reported for B cells in rats (Strober, 1975). Populations of long-lived B cells may be obtained by subjecting the short-lived cells to radioactive thymidine suicide, and populations of recirculating lymphocytes are obtained by passaging from blood to lymph in an intermediate irradiated host. That is, in the latter case, donor cells of interest are injected intravenously and collected from the thoracic duct of the intermediate host. Such experiments (Strober, 1972; Strober and Dilley, 1973a,b) have shown that "memory" B cells, whether obtained from spleen or thoracic duct, are predominantly long-lived recirculating small lymphocytes. Memory B cells were defined by the ability to transfer specific responsiveness to adoptive irradiated hosts 4 to 8 weeks after immunization of the donor, subcutaneously and sometimes also intraperitoneally, and with helper T cells in excess. In addition, "virgin" B cells were obtained from unimmunized donors and tested for their abilities to confer responsiveness on irradiated hosts. The properties of virgin B cells were found to depend on the antigen used for testing. For dinitrophenyl (DNP) containing antigens, virgin B cells were obtained from spleen or thoracic duct, and found to recirculate poorly and to be relatively long-lived (Strober and Dilley, 1973b). The virgin B cells for horse spleen ferritin as antigen recirculated poorly and were short-lived (Strober, 1972), while for sheep red cells they were long-lived and recirculating (Strober, 1975). It is suggested (Strober and Dilley, 1973b) that these differences reflect the extent to which natural antigens cross-react with those used in immunization, with cross-reactivity being large, moderate, and slight for the three antigens, sheep red cells, DNP, and ferritin, respectively. It would then be concluded that a B cell which had never been exposed to complementary antigen would be short-lived and sessile, but that on encountering antigen, in spleen, lymph nodes, or elsewhere, it could be transformed to give rise to long-lived and recirculating memory B cells which were found for all of the antigens tested. It remains difficult to rule out some degree of antigen-independent transformation. In sheep nodes it has been found that antilymphocyte serum can block recirculation of small lymphocytes without affecting the export of blast or plaque forming cells in a primary response to salmonella antigens (Hay, Yamashita, and Morris, 1974). This is in accord with the picture that virgin B cells are sessile.

In addition, the number and class of immunoglobulin receptors on B lymphocytes change during maturation (Strober, 1975; Klinman and Press, 1975; Vitteta and Uhr, 1975), and such changes may be partly responsible for the altered recirculation patterns of memory B cells.

D. Trapping

In our earlier discussion of lymphocyte traffic through a sheep lymph node, it was observed that localized antigen can substantially increase the flux of cells into the node. In animals such as rodents, where it is not feasible to collect the efferent lymph from single nodes, related information may be obtained by observing the effects of antigen on migration patterns of responsive cells, or by injecting labeled lymphocytes and following their accumulation in spleen and other lymphoid organs or their abundance in the circulation. Rodents have the advantage that their several classes of lymphocytes are better understood and manipulable.

The results of such "trapping" experiments (e.g., Zatz and Lance, 1971; Rowley et al., 1972; Zatz and Gershon, 1975) depend on the antigen, dose, route of immunization, and whether the animal has prior exposure to the antigen. Antigen which concentrates in the spleen (e.g., high molecular weight antigens, injected intravenously) will tend to trap transiently lymphocytes therein (Zatz and Lance, 1971), although diminished localization has also been observed (Zatz and Gershon, 1975). Correspondingly, the thoracic duct lymph becomes depleted of responsive cells (Rowley et al., 1972). Similar results were found for soluble DNP-protein conjugates which may trap lymphocytes both in the spleen and in nodes. With sheep cells as antigen, a prior injection of specific anti-sheep-cell antibodies abolishes the trapping effect (Rowley et al., 1972). Subcutaneous injection of sheep red cells results in a diminished supply of responsive thoracic duct cells (Rowley et al., 1972), which again we must view as a rather mysterious result, inasmuch as it seems impossible for the affected lymph nodes to be traversed by the bulk of the responsive cells in the required short time ($\lesssim$ 1 day). However, in these experiments, efferent lymph and lymphocytes could circulate freely throughout the animal and affect the immune system in many ways.

In the secondary response, smaller antigen doses suffice to induce trapping (Zatz and Lance, 1971). Such a result might be explained in various ways, but in view of the many differences between virgin and memory lymphocytes noted earlier, we hesitate to advance any particular model.

V. DISCUSSION

In this brief review, I have attempted to sketch some of the principle experimental findings and theoretical models concerning lymphocyte circulation and how it is affected by exposure to antigen. The general picture which has emerged may be characterized as follows. In the young or adult animal, lymphocytes are being continuously generated at a high rate by cell division in the bone marrow and thymus. Some uncertain but perhaps large fractions of these cells are exported to peripheral lymphoid organs as relatively short-lived T or B cells. As a result of suitable exposure to antigen, these virgin T_1 and B_1 cells give rise to long-lived memory T_2 and B_2 cells, which recirculate freely from blood to lymph to blood. When the system is exposed to a localized concentration of antigen, as in a lymph node, an inflammatory reaction can give rise to greatly increased lymphocyte traffic in that area. It was noted, however, that lymphocyte recirculation is taking place even in the immunologically incompetent and unstimulated fetus.

Numerical values were presented for some of the population components, and I developed some simple models for relating the values. Approximately 20% of the lymphocytes incident on a lymph node in afferent blood will exit in efferent lymph. In addition, I estimated that within a lymph node, distinct cell-cell contacts are made at a rate which is unlikely to exceed 200/hour per cell, and that this rate might be approached for a cell stuck by antigen to a macrophage or reticular cell in the midst of the migration of recirculating lymphocytes. Whether such contacts are in fact important probably depends on the nature of the antigen, its mode of presentation, and the experimental animal. I suggest that it will be fruitful to compare the postulated conditions in a node with in vitro experimental results.

It appears to me that there are two major puzzles concerning lymphocyte traffic and its regulation. The first concerns the mechanisms by which antigen in a single lymph node is able, within a day or two, to systematically deplete the whole animal of antigen-specific recirculating cells. Whether the animal has been rendered tolerant in any usual sense, and if so how, are particularly important questions.

The second puzzle I noted earlier, namely that the rate of lymphocyte proliferation in the bone marrow and thymus far exceeds that required to maintain the pool of long-lived recirculating lymphocytes. To what end does an animal devote so much of its resources to this proliferation? There are at least four possibilities for explaining why an animal should generate far more cells than are apparently needed in order to stock its immune system. (a) A large fraction of these nascent lymphocytes may have receptors for self antigens and must be eliminated by contact with self antigens at an early sensitive stage. Indeed, it does appear that young bone marrow lymphocytes are sensitive and would be eliminated by premature contact with complementary antigens (Nossal and Pike, 1975). Jerne (1971) has pointed out that the proliferation of self-reactive cells followed by their elimination would be an efficient mechanism for the selection of somatic mutants having slightly different from self receptors. (b) If somatic mutation is an important mechanism for the generation of diversity, proliferation may be required, at least in the newborn, in order to generate rapidly an adequate repertoire, and the proliferation cannot then be shut off rapidly. Such models are described by Adam in Chap. 21. Moreover, many nonfunctional receptors may be generated, and cells expressing them should be eliminated promptly, for example by failing to find a complementary antigen within some short life span. Similar arguments could be made for other random generators of diversity, for example, in which variable regions of light and heavy chains are randomly expressed from a larger germ line dictionary. (c) Newly generated lymphocytes may be multipotential, and depending on the conditions which they encounter, able to differentiate accordingly. The simplest possibility would seem to be if the cells were not altogether committed to expression of a single receptor specificity. However, they might also have functional flexibility. For example, if there were an infection in the gut, B lymphocytes trapped in Peyers patches, etc., might differentiate to secrete IgA rather than IgM and IgG. Since T cells have so many functions, the one chosen might be determined by the detailed circumstances of antigen encounter. Against this possibility is evidence that peripheral T cells have already decided whether to become helper or cytotoxic T cells prior to contact with antigen (Cantor and Boyce, 1975a). However, freshly exported thymocytes might be more adaptable. (d) Newborn lymphocytes may simply represent a reserve capacity which is ordinarily unused but can be called into action in case of a life threatening confrontation with antigen. While many mammalian systems have reserve capacity, it would seem surprising if the lymphocyte system could not turn down its proliferative capacity when unneeded.

Perhaps all four possibilities are partially realized, or a further explanation may be the correct one. At present the truth is hidden.

ACKNOWLEDGMENTS

I am indebted to Drs. B. Bryant, W. Ford, J. Hall, H. Hay, and J. Kappler for helpful comments and for communication of results prior to publication.

REFERENCES

Anderson, A. O. and Anderson, N. D. (1976). Lymphocyte emigration from high endothelial venules in rat lymph nodes. *Immunol. 31:* 731-748.

Anderson, N. D., Anderson, A. O., and Wyllie, R. G. (1975). Microvascular changes in lymph nodes draining skin allografts. *Am. J. Pathol. 81:* 131-153.

Anderson, N. D. and Weiss, L. (1976). Lymphocyte traffic in the spleen. *Fed. Proc. 35:* 608.

Araneo, B. A., Marrack, P. C., and Kappler, J. W. (1975). Functional heterogeneity among T-derived lymphocytes of the mouse. II. Sensitivity of subpopulations to anti-thymocyte serum. *J. Immunol. 114:* 747-751.

Berney, S. N. and Gesner, B. M. (1970). The circulatory behavior of normal and enzyme altered thymocytes in rats. *Immunology 18:* 681-691.

Bryant, B. J. (1972). Renewal and fate in the mammalian thymus; mechanisms and inferences of thymocytokinetics. *Eur. J. Immunol. 2:* 38-45.

Bryant, B. J. (1974). Thymic and bursal microenvironments in the context of alternative pathways of immunogenesis, II. In *Progress in Immunology,* Vol. 3. North Holland Publ. Co., Amsterdam, pp. 5-14.

Burns, F. D., Marrack, P. C., Kappler, J. W., and Janeway, C. A., Jr. (1975). Functional heterogeneity among T-derived lymphocytes of the mouse. IV. Nature of spontaneously induced suppressor cells. *J. Immunol. 114:*1345-1347.

Cahill, R. N. P., Frost, H., and Trnka, Z. (1976). The effects of antigen on the migration of recirculating lymphocytes through single lymph nodes. *J. Exp. Med. 143:* 870-888.

Cantor, H. and Boyce, E. A. (1975a). Functional subclasses of T lymphocytes bearing different ly antigens. I. The generation of functionally distinct T-cell subclasses is a differentiative process independent of antigen. *J. Exp. Med. 141:* 1376-1389.

Cantor, H. and Boyce, E. A. (1975b). Functional subclasses of T lymphocytes bearing different ly antigens. II. Cooperation between subclasses of ly^+ cells in generation of killer activity. *J. Exp. Med. 141:* 1390-1399.

Cantor, H., Simpson, E., Sato, V. L., Fathman, C. G., and Herzenberg, L. A. (1975). Characterization of subpopulations of lymphocytes. I. Separation and functional studies of peripheral T-cells binding different amounts of fluorescent anti-thy 1.2 (theta) antibody using a fluorescence-activated cell sorter. *Cell. Immunol. 15:* 180-196.

Dresser, D. W., Taub, R. N., and Krantz, H. R. (1970). The effect of localized injection of adjuvant material on the draining lymph node. *Immunology 18:* 663-670.

Erb, P. and Feldmann, M. (1975). The role of macrophages in the generation of T helper cells. III. Influence of macrophage-derived factors in helper cell induction. *Eur. J. Immunol. 5:* 759-766.

Everett, N. B. and Tyler (Caffrey), R. W. (1967). Lymphopoiesis in the thymus and other tissues: functional importance. *Int. Rev. Cytol. 22:* 205-237.

Feldmann, M. (1972). Cell interactions in the immune response in vitro. V. Specific collaboration by complexes of antigen and thymus-derived immunoglobulin. *J. Exp. Med. 136:* 737-760.

Ford, W. L. (1969). The kinetics of lymphocyte circulation within the rat spleen. *Cell Tissue Kinet. 2:* 171-191.

Ford, W. L. (1972). The recruitment of recirculating lymphocytes in the antigenically stimulated spleen. *Clin. Exp. Immunol. 12:* 243-254.

Ford, W. L., Sedgley, M. Sparshott, S. M., and Smith, M. E. (1976). The migration of lymphocytes across specialized vascular endothelium. II. The contrasting consequences of treating lymphocytes with trypsin or neuro minidoes. *Cell Tissue Kinet. 9:* 351-361.

Ford, W. L. and Simmonds, S. J. (1972). The tempo of lymphocyte recirculation from blood to lymph in the rat. *Cell Tissue Kinet. 5:* 175-189.

Freitas, A. A. and de Sousa, M. (1975). Control mechanisms of lymphocyte traffic. Modification of the traffic of ^{51}Cr-labeled mouse lymph node cells by treatment with plant lectins in intact and splenectomized hosts. *Eur. J. Immunol. 5:* 831-833.

Freitas, A. A. and de Sousa, M. (1976). The role of cell interactions in the control of lymphocyte traffic. *Cell. Immunol. 22:* 345-350.

Frost, H., Braun, D. G., Poshitt, D., Cahill, R. N. P., and Trnka, Z. (1976). Antipolysaccharide antibodies of restricted heterogeneity secreted by a single lymph node. *J. Exp. Med. 143:* 707-711.

Frost, H., Cahill, R. N. P., and Trnka, Z. (1975). The migration of recirculating autologous and allogeneic lymphocytes through single lymph nodes. *Eur. J. Immunol. 5:* 839-843.

Goldschneider, I. and McGregor, D. D. (1973). Anatomical distribution of T and B lymphocytes in the rat. *J. Exp. Med. 138:* 1443-1465.

Gowans, J. L. (1970). Lymphocytes. *Harvey Lectures 64:* 87-119.

Guy-Grand, D., Griscella, C., and Vassali, C. (1974). The gut-associated lymphoid system: nature and properties of the large dividing cells. *Eur. J. Immunol. 4:* 435.

Hall, J. G. (1967). Quantitative aspects of the recirculation of lymphocytes; an analysis of data from experiments on sheep. *Q. J. Exp. Physiol. 52:* 76-85.

Hall, J. G. (1974). Observations on the migration and localization of lymphoid cells, II. In *Progress in Immunology*, Vol. 3 (L. Brent and J. Holborow, eds.). North Holland Publ. Co., Amsterdam, pp. 15-24.

Hall, J. G., Parry, D. M., and Smith, M. E. (1972). The distribution and differentiation of lymph-borne immunoblasts after intravenous injection into syngeneic recipients. *Cell Tissue Kinet. 5:* 269-281.

Hall, J. G., Scollay, R., and Smith, M. (1976). Studies on the lymphocytes of sheep. I. Recirculation of lymphocytes through peripheral lymph nodes and tissues. *Eur. J. Immunol. 6:* 117-120.

Hammond, B. J. (1975). A compartmental analysis of circulatory lymphocytes in the spleen. *Cell Tissue Kinet. 8:* 153-169.

Hay, J. B., Cahill, R. N. P., and Trnka, Z. (1974). The kinetics of antigen-reactive cells during lymphocyte recruitment. *Cell. Immunol. 10:* 145-153.

Hay, J. B. and Morris, B. (1976). The generation and selection of specific reactive cells by antigen. *Br. Med. Bull. 32:* 2.

Hay, J. B., Murphy, M. J., Morris, B., and Bessis, M. C. (1972). Quantitative studies on the proliferation and differentiation of antibody-forming cells in lymph. *Am. J. Pathol. 66:* 1-24.

Hay, J. B., Yamashita, A., and Morris, B. (1974). Effects of anti-lymphocyte serum on the traffic of cells through the popliteal lymph node and on antibody-forming cells produced within the node. *Lab. Invest. 31:* 276-285.

Hoffmann, M. and Kappler, J. W. (1973). Regulation of the immune response. II. Qualitative and quantitative differences between thymus and bone marrow derived lymphocytes in the recognition of antigen. *J. Exp. Med. 137:* 721-739.

Hopkins, J. and Hall, J. G. (1976). Selective entry of immunoblasts into gut from intestinal lymph. *Nature 259:* 308-309.

Howard, J. C. (1972). The life-span and recirculation of marrow-derived small lymphocytes from the rat thoracic duct. *J. Exp. Med. 135:* 185-199.

Howard, J. C., Hunt, S. V., and Gowans, J. L. (1972). Identification of marrow-derived and thymus-derived small lymphocytes in the lymphoid tissue and thoracic duct lymph of normal rats. *J. Exp. Med. 135:* 200-219.

Jerne, N. K. (1971). The somatic generation of immune recognition. *Eur. J. Immunol. 1:* 1-9.

Jerne, N. K. (1973). The immune system. *Scientific American 229/1:* 52-60.

Kadish, J. L. and Basch, R. S. (1975). Thymic regeneration after lethal irradiation: evidence for an intrathymic T-cell precursor. *J. Immunol. 114:* 452-458.

Kappler, J. W., Hunter, P. C., Jacobs, D., and Lord, E. (1974). Functional heterogeneity among the T-derived lymphocytes of the mouse. I. Analysis by adult thymectomy. *J. Immunol. 113:* 27-38.

Klinman, N. R. and Press, J. L. (1975). The B cell specificity repertoire: its relationship to definable subpopulations. *Transplant. Rev. 24:* 41-83.

Lipsky, P. E., Ellner, J. J., and Rosenthal, A. S. (1976). Phyto-hemaglutinin-induced proliferation of guinea pig thymus-derived lymphocytes. I. Accessory cell dependence. *J. Immunol. 116:* 868-875.

Lumb, J. R. (1975). A regenerating computer model of the thymus. *Comp. Biomed. Res. 8:* 379-392.

Marchesi, V. T. and Gowans, J. L. (1964). The migration of lymphocytes through the endothelium of venules in lymph nodes. *Proc. Roy. Soc. B 159:* 283.

Marrack, P. C. and Kappler, J. W. (1975). Antigen specific and nonspecific mediators of T cell/B cell cooperation. I. Evidence for production by different T-cells. *J. Immunol. 114:* 1116-1125.

McConnell, I., Lachmann, P. J., and Hobart, M. J. (1974). Restoration of specific immunological virginity. *Nature 250:* 113-116.

Metcalf, D. (1966). *The Thymus*. Springer-Verlag, New York.

Miller, J. F. A. P. and Osoba, D. (1967). Current concepts of the immunological function of the thymus. *Physiol. Rev. 47:* 437-520.

Morris, B. (1968). The lymphatic system and the immune response. *Austr. J. Sci. 31:* 13-18.

Nieuwenhuis, P. and Ford, W. L. (1976). Comparative migration of B and T lymphocytes in the rat spleen and lymph nodes. *Cell. Immunol. 23:* 254-267.

Nossal, G. J. V. and Ada, G. L. (1971). *Antigens, Lymphoid Cells, and the Immune Response*. Academic, New York.

Nossal, G. J. V. and Pike, B. L. (1975). Evidence for the clonal abortion theory of B-lymphocyte tolerance. *J. Exp. Med. 141:* 904-917.

Osmond, D. G. and Nossal, G. J. V. (1974). Differentiation of lymphocytes in mouse bone marrow. II. Kinetics of maturation and renewal of antiglobulin-binding cells studied by double labeling. *Cell. Immunol. 13:* 132-145.

Pearson, L. D., Simpson-Morgan, M. W., and Morris, B. (1976). Lymphopoiesis and lymphocyte recirculation in the sheep fetus. *J. Exp. Med. 143:* 167-186.

Prothero, J. W. and Tyler, R. W. (1975). A model of thymocyte proliferation. *J. Theor. Biol. 51:* 357-382.

Raff, M. C. and Cantor, H. (1971). Subpopulations of thymus cells and thymus-derived lymphocytes. In *Progress in Immunology* (B. Amos, ed.). Academic, New York. pp. 83-93.

Raff, M. C. and Owen, J. J. T. (1971). Thymus-derived lymphocytes: their distribution and role in the development of peripheral lymphoid tissues of the mouse. *Eur. J. Immunol. 1:* 27-30.

Rosenstreich, D. L., Farrar, J. J., and Dougherty, S. (1976). Absolute macrophage dependency of T lymphocyte activation by mitogens. *J. Immunol. 116:* 131-139.

Rosenthal, A. S., Lipsky, P. E., and Shevach, E. M. (1975). Macrophage-lymphocyte interaction and antigen recognition. *Fed. Proc. 34:* 1743-1748.

Rowley, D. A., Gowans, J. L., Atkins, R. C., Ford, W. L., and Smith, M. E. (1972). The specific selection of recirculating lymphocytes by antigen in normal and preimmunized rats. *J. Exp. Med. 136:* 499-513.

Schoefl, G. I. (1972). The migration of lymphocytes across the vascular endothelium in lymphoid tissue. *J. Exp. Med. 136:* 568-588.

Scollay, R., Hopkins, J., and Hall, J. (1976). Possible role of surface Ig in non-random recirculation of small lymphocytes. *Nature 260:* 528-529.

Simpson, E. and Cantor, H. (1975). Regulation of the immune response by subclasses of T lymphocytes. II. Effect of adult thymectomy on humoral and cellular responses in mice. *Eur. J. Immunol. 5:* 337-343.

Smith, J. B., McIntosh, G. H., and Morris, B. (1970). The migration of cells through chronically inflamed tissues. *J. Pathol. 100:* 21-29.

Smith, J. B., Pedersen, N. C., and Morris, B. (1970). The role of the lymphatic system in inflammatory responses. *Ser. Haemat. III, 2:* 17-61.

Sprent, J. (1973). Circulating T and B lymphocytes of the mouse. I. Migratory properties. *Cell. Immunol. 7:* 10-39.

Sprent, J. and Basten, A. (1973). Circulating T and B lymphocytes of the mouse. II. Lifespan. *Cell. Immunol. 7:* 40-59.

Strober, S. (1972). Initiation of antibody responses in different classes of lymphocytes. V. Fundamental changes in physiological characteristics of virgin B lymphocytes and B memory cells. *J. Exp. Med. 136:* 851-871.

Strober, S. (1975). Immune function cell surface characteristics and maturation of B cell subpopulations. *Transplant. Rev. 24:* 84-112.

Strober, S. and Dilley, J. (1973a). Biological characteristics of T and B memory lymphocytes in the rat. *J. Exp. Med. 137:* 1275-1292.

Strober, S. and Dilley, J. (1973b). Maturation of B lymphocytes in the rat. I. Migration pattern, tissue distribution, and turnover rate of unprimed and primed B lymphocytes involved in adoptive anti DNP response. *J. Exp. Med. 138:* 1331-1344.

Taussig, M. J., Mozes, E., and Isac, R. (1974). Antigen-specific thymus cell factors in the genetic control of the immune response to poly (T,G)-A-L. *J. Exp. Med. 140:* 301-312.

Unanue, E. R. and Calderon, J. (1975). Evaluation of the role of macrophages in immune induction. *Fed. Proc. 34:* 1737-1742.

Vitetta, E. S. and Uhr, J. W. (1975). Immunoglobulin-receptors revisited. *Science 189:* 964-969.

Williams, A. F. and Gowans, J. L. (1975). The presence of IgA on the surface of rat thoracic duct lymphocytes which contain internal IgA. *J. Exp. Med. 14:* 335-345.

Williams, R. M., Chanana, A. D., Cronkite, E. P., and Waksman, B. H. (1971). Antigenic markers on cells leaving calf thymus by way of the efferent lymph and venous blood. *J. Immunol. 106:* 1143-1146.

Woodruff, J. J. (1974). Role of lymphocyte surface determinants in lymph node homing. *Cell. Immunol. 13:* 378-384.

Zatz, M. M. and Gershon, R. K. (1975). Regulation of lymphocyte trapping: the negative trap. *J. Immunol.* *115:* 450-453.

Zatz, M. M. and Lance, E. M. (1971). The distribution of ^{51}Cr-labeled lymphocytes into antigen-stimulated mice. *J. Exp. Med.* *134:* 224-241.

Part VI

MODELS OF CELL POPULATION DYNAMICS

Chapter 13

MODELING OF THE IMMUNE RESPONSE: A SYSTEM APPROACH

Carlo Bruni

Istituto di Automatica
University of Rome
Rome, Italy

Maria Adelaide Giovenco

Centro Studi Sistemi
Controllo e Calcolo Automatici
C.N.R.
Rome, Italy

Giorgio Koch*

Istituto di Automatica
University of Rome
Rome, Italy

Roberto Strom

Istituto di Chimica Biologica
University of Rome
Rome, Italy

*Present affiliation: Istituto di Matematica, University of Lecce, Lecce, Italy

After an introduction to the system approach to modeling problems, attention is focused on mathematical models for the humoral immune response. A number of assumptions are introduced to describe mathematically the different interacting cell populations and the basic phenomena involved. Thus a model is arrived at in the form of a system of nonlinear integro-differential equations. The model is then situated within the class of bounded rate systems, which leads to a suitable analysis of its structural properties, with interesting results on existence, uniqueness, and stability of solutions. The model was simulated on a computer and its validation, using experimental results available in the literature, is discussed. Finally, the model is critically analyzed and some comments are made on future developments, with specific attention to multivalency of the antigen, cellular cooperation, and switchover phenomena.

I. INTRODUCTION

A system theory approach to the analysis of the behavior of a given natural or artificial process is characterized by the attention focused on the mutual functional relations among the variables of the process itself, rather than on their physical nature. In this approach the first step is therefore the elaboration of a mathematical model, that is, a formal representation of the above-mentioned functional relations.

Such a model can be arrived at through a detailed description of the basic phenomena which occur in the process, as well as through a "black box" approach which takes into account only input and output experimental data. In fact, only through a mutual interaction of both approaches is it possible to build a model simple enough to allow the development of a structural analysis (controllability, stability, etc.), and complex enough to adhere to experimental data and adequately describe the physical phenomena. A mathematical model having well-defined structural properties, and which adequately describes experimental facts, is indeed an extremely useful tool for a better comprehension of a process and for the evaluation of and discrimination among different mechanisms. Besides, it is essential for the simulation and prediction of the process behavior, as well as to the designing of suitable control policies.

The aim of this work is to present a mathematical model for the humoral immune response from the point of view of system theory. The humoral immune response is a typical example of a system in which the input function (dependent on injected antigen dose and on inoculation procedure), and several output variables (antibody concentration, antibody affinity distribution, number of antibody forming cells) may be known with good accuracy. However, the detailed knowledge of single steps in the process is often inadequate.

Our model (Bruni et al., 1975a) which owes much to previous contributions by different authors (Bell, 1970, 1071a,b; Jilek, 1971a,b; Jilek and Ursjnyova, 1970; Hege and Cole, 1966), is built of a number of interconnected blocks which correspond to the basic biological phenomena and which lend themselves to a suitable mathematical description. Simplifying assumptions were introduced to account for the incomplete knowledge of some of the above-mentioned basic phenomena, and to reconcile the needed tractability of the model with its fitness to the biological facts.

Indeed, a simulation of the model was made to validate it against available experimental data and the agreement obtained was satisfactory. It was also possible to place the model in the framework of a more general class of systems (i.e., bounded rate systems); this led to a thorough investigation of some of its structural properties, like existence, uniqueness, and stability of its solutions.

As will be discussed in the following, the authors are convinced that the model may be substantially improved by discarding some oversimplifying hypotheses and exploiting further experimental results. Also, a deeper investigation of its general properties is recommended.

Research work is currently in progress along these directions.

II. BASIC ASSUMPTIONS AND CONSTRUCTION OF THE MODEL

According to the general approach indicated in the introduction, the immune response process is represented by the block diagram shown in Fig. 1, which outlines the elementary phenomena of the process. The basic mathematic notation is summarized in Appendixes A and B.

1. We assume that, before any stimulation, there is already a population of immunocompetent cells. The *original distribution* of the association constant K of the cell receptors, for the particular antigenic determinant considered, is indicated by $\bar{p}_c(K)$. Throughout the whole mathematical development, we shall postulate that K is a continuous variable which can assume any value in some interval (K_1, K_2), although such a hypothesis is not essential for the validity of the model.

Independent of the immune process, there is a continuous production of these cells from the stem cells. This production occurs with a rate β, and the distribution of the new immunocompetent cells is

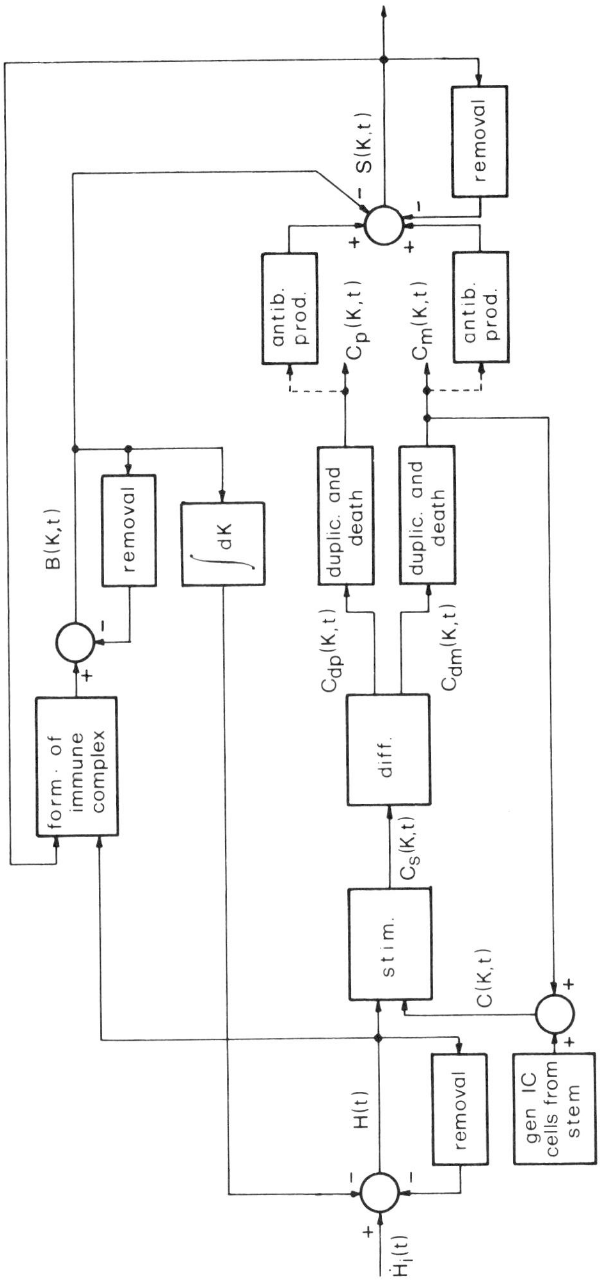

FIG. 1. Block diagram of the immune response.

similar to the original one. Therefore, the contribution of this process to the variation of the immunocompetent cell population in the interval (t, t + dt) is given by

$$\beta \bar{p}_c(K)\, dt \tag{1}$$

2. In the course of the immune response, that is, upon stimulation by the antigen, *different types of immunocompetent cells* are generated. In the models described in the literature, these cells have been named in different ways. In Jilek's model (Jilek, 1971a,b; Jilek and Ursjnyova, 1970), which follows essentially a scheme put forward by Sercarz and Coons (1962), there are three classes of immunocompetent cells indicated as X, Y and Z: X cells, upon contact with antigen, differentiate into Y cells, which begin to proliferate. These proliferating cells, which are the basis for the immunological memory, can differentiate, upon a second contact with the antigen, into Z cells (plasma cells), which produce antibodies without undergoing further mitosis. In Bell's model (Bell, 1970; 1971a,b), there are four classes of immunocompetent cells. *Target cells* are the virgin cells, which may bind the antigen. Upon stimulation they become *proliferating cells* which duplicate and produce antibodies as long as the stimulus is present. These proliferating cells then differentiate into two classes of cells: *plasma cells*, which produce antibodies and cannot undergo further mitosis, and *memory cells*, which do not produce antibodies, have a long lifespan, and are the basis for the immunological memory.

In our model, these different types of cells are reduced, according to their role, to two classes: memory cells and plasma cells. The memory cells are essentially similar to the immunocompetent cells from which they derive, as far as the responsiveness to antigenic stimulation is concerned; by this term we shall therefore indicate both the original population of immunocompetent cells and those cells which, formed upon antigenic stimulation, are still able to be triggered by the antigen and to undergo division. The plasma cells, which also derive from stimulated immunocompetent cells through a duplication and differentiation process, are instead unable to undergo further division, have a relatively short life, and are the major producers of antibodies.

3. *Stimulation* occurs only when the fraction of receptors which is occupied by the antigen, according to an instantaneous and reversible mass action law (Möller, 1970), falls, as suggested by some experimental results, between two values σ_1 and σ_2.

Let R(K, t) and L(K, t) be, respectively, the number of free and bound receptors on the cell surface per unit volume. For each value of K we have at a given concentration of identical free antigenic determinants H(t), and assuming each determinant to be independent from the others,

$$\frac{L(K, t)}{R(K, t)H(t)} = K \tag{2}$$

The probability that a receptor of affinity K is occupied is

$$p(KH) = \frac{L(K, t)}{R(K, t) + L(K, t)} = \frac{KH(t)}{1 + KH(t)} \tag{3}$$

The probability that exactly n receptors, out of a total number m per cell, are occupied is expressed by Bernoulli's distribution

$$p^{(n)}(KH) \equiv \binom{m}{n} p^n(KH)[1 - p(KH)]^{m-n} \tag{4}$$

The probability that a cell with affinity K is stimulated is therefore

$$p_s(KH) = \sum_{n=n_1}^{n_2} p^{(n)}(KH) = \frac{\sum_{n=n_1}^{n_2} \binom{m}{n} (KH)^n}{(1 + KH)^m} \tag{5}$$

where n_1 is the smallest integer such that $n_1 \geqslant m\sigma_1$, and n_2 is the largest integer such that $n_2 \leqslant m\sigma_2$. The distribution in Eq. (5)

can be approximated by the simple two-valued function*

$$p_s(KH) \simeq \begin{cases} 1 & \text{if } \dfrac{\sigma_1}{1-\sigma_1} \leqslant KH \leqslant \dfrac{\sigma_2}{1-\sigma_2} \\ 0 & \text{otherwise} \end{cases} \tag{6}$$

Denoting by $C(K, t)$ the concentration density of immunocompetent cells, the number of stimulated cells per unit volume is therefore

$$C_s(K, t) = p_s(KH)C(K, t) \tag{7}$$

4. *Duplication* occurs as a consequence of stimulation, with a time constant $1/\alpha_c$.

5. *Differentiation* is an instantaneous process which again depends on the fraction of mother cell receptors which are occupied. Since it is known that the number of plasma cells increases with the antigen dose (Levi et al., 1973; Sterzl, 1966), the probability of differentiation into plasma cells is assumed to be proportional to that fraction of occupancy. The probability that a cell of affinity K with n occupied receptors generates plasma cells has been taken equal to the n/m ratio, and therefore the probability that any cell of affinity K gives rise to plasma cells is

$$p_d(KH) = \sum_{n=0}^{m} \frac{n}{m} p^{(n)}(KH) = \frac{KH}{1 + KH} \tag{8}$$

The number of stimulated cells which differentiate, respectively, into plasma cells and memory cells is therefore

$$C_{dp}(K, t) = p_d(KH)C_s(K, t) = \frac{KH}{1 + KH} p_s(KH)C(K, t) \tag{9}$$

---

*Indeed, the mean value and the variance of Eq. (5) are respectively

$$E\{n\} = \frac{mKH}{1 + KH} \qquad \text{Var}\{n\} = \frac{mKH}{(1 + KH)^2}$$

Because of the high value of m, and assuming for σ_1 and σ_2 the values given in Table 2, when stimulation occurs Var{n} turns out to be at least one order of magnitude less than E{n}.

$$C_{dm}(K, t) = [1 - p_d(KH)]C_s(K, t) = \frac{p_s(KH)}{1 + KH} C(K, t) \qquad (10)$$

The stimulated cells $C_s(K, t)$ disappear and become $2C_{dm}(K, t)$ memory cells and $2C_{dp}(K, t)$ plasma cells. Therefore, the contribution of the stimulation, duplication, and differentiation process to the variation of $C(K, t)$ in the interval $(t, t + dt)$ is given by:

$$2\alpha_c C_{dm}(K, t)\ dt - \alpha_c C_s(K, t)\ dt = \alpha_c \frac{1 - KH}{1 + KH} p_s(KH)C(K, t)\ dt \qquad (11)$$

Similarly, the same contribution to the plasma cell population density $C_p(K, t)$ in the same interval is

$$2\alpha_c C_{dp}(K, t)\ dt = 2\alpha_c \frac{KH}{1 + KH} p_s(KH)C(K, t)\ dt \qquad (12)$$

6. *Cell death* can be described as occurring with time constants τ_c and τ_p for immunocompetent and plasma cells respectively.

7. *Antibodies* are considered as being divalent, each site, however, being independent of the other. Binding of antigenic determinants to antibody sites occurs according to the mass action law. It is assumed that all antibodies, as well as the antigen, are uniformly distributed in the circulating fluid.

The dynamics of antibodies, considered as isolated sites $S(K, t)$, are due to four phenomena:

a. Production by plasma cells: the variation of $S(K, t)$ due to plasma cells in the interval $(t, t + dt)$ is given by

$$\alpha_s C_p(K, t)\ dt \qquad (13)$$

where α_s is the rate constant of antibody production by plasma cells.

b. Production by memory cells: in the model proposed, under the name of memory cells are included all cells which have been stimulated, but which have not differentiated into plasma cells. The situation, as far as antibody production by these cells is concerned, is likely to be different immediately after stimulation as compared to longer times after it. It was therefore assumed that these cells are always able to secrete antibodies, but that, during an interval T_0 following their generation, the intensity of production is higher. No distinction is made, in our model, between true antibody secretion and the possible generation and shedding of antibody-like receptors.

Let us denote by α'_s the rate constant of the basal antibody production by memory cells, and by I(K, t) the intensity at time t of the initial additional production, extended to all memory cells with a given affinity K. The variation of S(K, t) due to the production by memory cells in the interval (t, t + dt) is then given by

$$I(K, t)\ dt + \alpha'_s C(K, t)\ dt \tag{14}$$

I(K, t) can be expressed by

$$I(K, t) = \int_{-\infty}^{t} i(t - \theta) 2\alpha_c \frac{p_s(KH)}{1 + KH}\ C(K, \theta)\ d\theta \tag{15}$$

where i(t), which is zero for $t > T_0$, is the intensity of the initial additional production by a single memory cell generated at time zero.

c. The binding of antibody sites to antigenic determinants: if the dissociation and association rate constants are respectively c(K) and $c_1(K) = Kc(K)$, the contribution of this phenomenon to the variation of S(K, t) in the interval (t, t + dt) is expressed by the term

$$-Kc(K)S(K, t)H(t)\ dt + c(K)B(K, t)\ dt \tag{16}$$

where B(K, t) is the concentration density of bound antibody sites.

d. The decrease, due to metabolic turnover of antibodies, contributes the term

$$-\frac{1}{\tau_s} S(K, t)\ dt \tag{17}$$

where τ_s is the time constant of the disappearance of the free antibody sites.

8. The *antigen* is introduced into the organism with a given time dependent law. It is assumed that each antigenic determinant behaves independently from all the others. The variation of the concentration of the free antigen, considered as a single determinant H(t), can be reduced to three phenomena:

a. Inoculation of the antigen, which is the fundamental step triggering the immune response. Denoting by $H_i(t)$ the total amount of the injected antigen up to time t, assuming this function to be almost everywhere differentiable, the variations of antigen concentration due to this input in the interval (t, t + dt) is described by the term

$$dH_i(t) = \dot{H}_i(t)\ dt \tag{18}$$

b. Formation of immune complexes described by a term similar to Eq. (16), but extended over the whole range (K_1, K_2) of the association constants of antibodies

$$-H(t)\int_{K_1}^{K_2} Kc(K)S(K, t)\ dK\ dt + \int_{K_1}^{K_2} c(K)B(K, t)\ dK\ dt \tag{19}$$

c. Catabolism of the free antigen, contributing the term

$$-\frac{1}{\tau_H} H(t)\ dt \tag{20}$$

where τ_H is the time constant of the disappearance of the free antigen.

9. The *concentration of immune complexes*, measured as bound sites and indicated by B(K, t) varies according to two phenomena:

a. Formation of the complex, expressed by the term

$$Kc(K)S(K, t)H(t)\ dt - c(K)B(K, t)\ dt \tag{21}$$

b. Its catabolism, contributing the term

$$-\frac{1}{\tau_B} B(K, t)\ dt \tag{22}$$

where τ_B is the time constant of the disappearance of the immune complex.

On the bases of the above mentioned considerations, the set of differential equations describing the *dynamics of the immune response* is therefore:

immunocompetent cells

$$\frac{\partial C(K, t)}{\partial t} = \alpha_c \frac{1 - KH}{1 + KH} p_s(KH)C(K, t) - \frac{1}{\tau_c} C(K, t) + \beta \bar{p}_c(K) \tag{23}$$

plasma cells

$$\frac{\partial C_p(K, t)}{\partial t} = 2\alpha_c \frac{KH}{1 + KH} p_s(KH)C(K, t) - \frac{1}{\tau_p} C_p(K, t) \tag{24}$$

antibody sites

$$\frac{\partial S(K, t)}{\partial t} = \alpha_s C_p(K, t) + 2\alpha_c \int_{-\infty}^{t} i(t - \theta) \frac{p_s(KH)}{1 + KH} C(K, \theta)\, d\theta$$
$$+ \alpha_s' C(K, t) - Kc(K)S(K, t)H(t) + c(K)B(K, t)$$
$$- \frac{1}{\tau_s} S(K, t) \tag{25}$$

immune complexes

$$\frac{\partial B(K, t)}{\partial t} = Kc(K)S(K, t)H(t) - c(K)B(K, t) - \frac{1}{\tau_B} B(K, t) \tag{26}$$

antigenic determinants

$$\frac{dH(t)}{dt} = -H(t)\int_{K_1}^{K_2} Kc(K)S(K, t)\, dK + \int_{K_1}^{K_2} c(K)B(K, t)\, dK - \frac{1}{\tau_H} H(t) + \dot{H}_i(t) \tag{27}$$

Equations (23) to (27) clearly form a nonlinear integro-differential model distributed with respect to K. The two independent variables $\bar{p}_c(K)$ and $\dot{H}_i(t)$ may be considered as input variables. The former is a time invariant reference input while the latter is controllable from outside.

III. THE IMMUNE RESPONSE AS A BOUNDED RATE SYSTEM

To investigate the immune response model in the framework of system theory, it is worthwhile to introduce a suitable class of systems.

The class should be broad enough, so as to include models for several significant processes in different fields, but at the same time not so broad that one is unable to carry out successfully the analytical study of its properties.

Indeed, an interesting class of nonlinear systems suitable to that purpose was recently introduced (Bruni et al., 1975), that is, the so-called *bounded rate systems*.

A bounded rate system can be thought of as a dynamical *bilinear system* (Bruni et al., 1974; Mohler, 1974; Mohler and Ruberti, 1972; Ruberti and Mohler, 1975)* in which the free response parameters are allowed to depend, within a bounded range, on the state variables themselves, through a nonlinear instantaneous feedback loop. It has been shown that such a class plays an important role in modeling fundamental processes in biology (e.g., enzyme kinetics, bacterial growth, interacting populations), as well as in physiology, engineering, and socioeconomics. In order to give a formal definition of bounded rate systems, let Ω be an open subset in the state space X, and let U be the control space. Both X and U may be taken as Banach spaces. Denoting, for each time t, the state by $x(t) \in X$ and the control by $u(t) \in U$, a bounded rate system is defined by the following equation:

$$\dot{x}(t) = \Phi(x) + Nxu + Bu \qquad (28)$$

---

*Bilinear systems are nonlinear systems whose dynamical equation contains products between input and state variables. They are far more general than linear systems, and have been extensively investigated recently both from theoretical and applied points of view.

where the operator Φ: $\Omega \to X$ is assumed to be locally Lipschitzian (i.e., Lipschitzian within any bounded closed set in Ω) with at most a linear growth with respect to x, that is,

$$\|\Phi(x)\| \leq \gamma_1 \|x\| + \gamma_2 \tag{29}$$

with γ_1 and γ_2 nonnegative constants; the operators N: $\Omega \times U \to X$ and B: $U \to X$ are, respectively, bilinear and linear bounded operators.

This class lies between the classes of linear-in-control and bilinear systems. Indeed Eq. (28) is clearly *linear-in-control* with the restrictions that the free response (u = 0) has a bounded growth rate and the u-dependent term is at most linear in x. On the other hand, it can be proven* that the assumptions on Φ are equivalent to assuming

$$\Phi(x) = F(x)x + f(x) \tag{30}$$

where the operators F: $\Omega \to L(X, X)$ and f: $\Omega \to X$ are locally Lipschitzian with bounded range.

This elucidates the structure of Φ and at the same time shows that Eq. (28) may be also considered as a bilinear system with an instantaneous locally Lipschitzian and uniformly bounded state feedback h (Fig. 2), as soon as one defines

$$F(x) = A + N'h(x) \tag{31}$$

$$f(x) = Bh(x) \tag{32}$$

Because of the assumption, Eq. (30), the class of systems considered may also be represented by the general form

$$\dot{x}(t) = F(x)x + f(x) + Nxu + Bu \tag{33}$$

It is interesting to point out that the u-dependent part of Eq. (33) has essentially the same behavior as in linear-in-control and bilinear

---

*In Bruni et al. (1975) the proof is given for the case in which X is the n-dimensional Euclidean space R^n; following the same line, the proof may be extended to the general infinite dimensional case (Bruni and Koch, 1976).

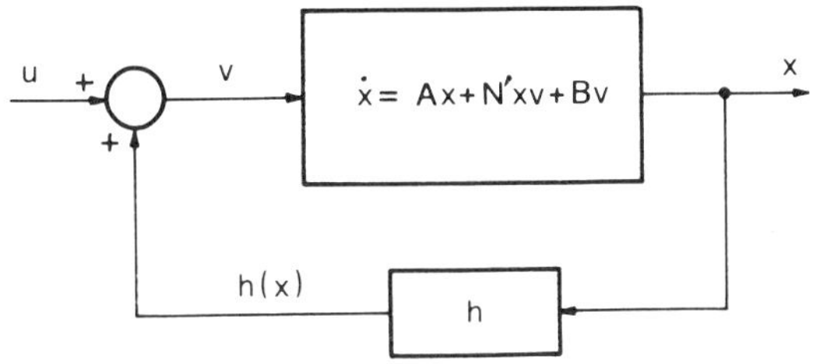

FIG. 2. Bounded rate system block diagram.

systems while the free response dynamics is indeed characteristic of the new class of systems. In fact, it is neither linear as in bilinear systems nor a general nonlinear function as in linear-in-control systems, but it is allowed to have at most a linear growth with x.

For this reason we have proposed the name "bounded rate" for this class of systems. Because of the structure of bounded rate systems, half-way between linear-in-control and bilinear systems, important *theoretical results* could be achieved for such a class of systems, both exploiting known results for linear-in-control systems and suitably extending bilinear systems properties.

These results would be relevant from a practical standpoint in that they would allow one to analyze in a unified framework the behavior of a number of important processes in different applied fields, as already mentioned above.

Coming back to the proposed model for the immune response, the set of Eqs. (23) to (27) defines a *nonlinear dynamic model* which is *distributed* with respect to K. We may stress the fact that even though the model is *infinite-dimensional*, there are no derivatives with respect to K. To show how this model may be given a state space description as a bounded rate system, it is convenient to first transform the integral relation in Eq. (15) which appears in Eq. (25). I(K, t) is actually for each K the output of a linear, time-invariant, asymptotically stable system. For the sake of simplicity, assuming that, for $t > T_0$, i(t) goes to zero with an extremely fast exponential decay rather than with an abrupt step, the state x(K, t) of such a system belongs to a space of finite dimension ν. This system may be modeled by the following input-state-output equations:

$$\frac{\partial \tilde{x}(K, t)}{\partial t} = \tilde{A}\tilde{x}(K, t) + \tilde{B}2\alpha_c \frac{p_s(KH)}{1 + KH} C(K, t) \quad (34)$$

$$I(K, t) = \tilde{D}\tilde{x}(K, t) \quad (35)$$

with suitable initial conditions, where $\tilde{A}$, $\tilde{B}$, and $\tilde{D}$ are constant matrices of suitable dimensions. Let us now define a state vector x, such that for each t, $x(t) \in X \triangleq C^{4+\nu}(K_1, K_2)xR^1$:

$$x(t) = \left[x_1(t)\ x_2(t)\ x_3(t)\ x_4(t)\ x_5^T(t)\ x_6(t)\right]^T$$

$$\triangleq \left[C(\cdot, t)\ C_p(\cdot, t)\ S(\cdot, t)\ B(\cdot, t)\ \tilde{x}^T(\cdot, t)\ H(t)\right]^T \quad (36)$$

We also define an input vector u, such that, for each t, $u(t) \in U \triangleq C^1(K_1, K_2)xR^1$:

$$u(t) = \left[u_1(t)\ u_2(t)\right]^T \triangleq \left[\bar{p}_c(\cdot)\ \dot{H}_i(t)\right]^T \quad (37)$$

and the set of admissible input functions

$$U = \left\{u: R^+ \to U: u(t) \geqslant 0,\ u \text{ continuous}, \int_0^\infty u_2(\tau)\, d\tau < \infty\right\} \quad (38)$$

which is quite natural to assume owing to the physical meaning of the input variables. From Eqs. (23) to (27) we see that the u-dependent part is linear in u and independent of x, while the free response part includes products of state variables by suitable functions of x. Thus the set of equations may be given the form

$$\dot{x}(t) = F[x(t)]x(t) + Bu(t) \quad (39)$$

$$F(x) = \begin{bmatrix} \left[\alpha_c \dfrac{1 - Kx_6}{1 + Kx_6} p_s(Kx_6) - \dfrac{1}{\tau_c}\right]E & 0 & 0 & 0 & 0 & 0 \\ 2\alpha_c \dfrac{Kx_6}{1 + Kx_6} p_s(Kx_6)E & -\dfrac{1}{\tau_p}E & 0 & 0 & 0 & 0 \\ \alpha_s' E & \alpha_s I & -x_6\Gamma_1 - \dfrac{1}{\tau_s}E & \Gamma_2 & \tilde{D}E & 0 \\ 0 & 0 & x_6\Gamma_1 & -\Gamma_2 - \dfrac{1}{\tau_B}E & 0 & 0 \\ 2\alpha_c \dfrac{p_s(Kx_6)}{1 + Kx_6}\tilde{B}E & 0 & 0 & 0 & \tilde{A}E & 0 \\ 0 & 0 & -x_6 J\Gamma_1 & J\Gamma_2 & 0 & -\dfrac{1}{\tau_H} \end{bmatrix}$$

$$B = \begin{bmatrix} \beta E & 0 \\ 0 & 0 \\ 0 & 0 \\ 0 & 0 \\ 0 & 0 \\ 0 & 1 \end{bmatrix} \qquad (40)$$

In Eq. (40) the following linear bounded operators have been introduced:

$$\begin{aligned} &E : \text{identity operator} \\ &\Gamma_1 : C^1(K_1, K_2) \to C^1(K_1, K_2), \quad (\Gamma_1\xi)(K) = Kc(K)\xi(K) \\ &\Gamma_2 : C^1(K_1, K_2) \to C^1(K_1, K_2), \quad (\Gamma_2\xi)(K) = c(K)\xi(K) \\ &J : C^1(K_1, K_2) \to R^1 \quad , \quad J\xi = \int_{K_1}^{K_2} \xi(K)\, dK \end{aligned} \qquad (41)$$

We now observe that Eq. (39) is a particular form of Eq. (33); thus the immune response model may be considered as a bounded rate system as soon as we verify that there exists a suitable open subset $\Omega \subset X$ such that the operator $F: \Omega \to L(X, X)$ defined in Eq. (40) is locally Lipschitzian with a bounded range.

The following lemma can be proved:

Lemma 1. *Let us define the open subset* $\Omega \subset X$:

$$\Omega = \left\{ x \in X: -\frac{1}{2K_2} < x_6 < \infty \right\} \tag{42}$$

Then for each $x(0) \in \Omega$ *and each* $u \in U$, $F: \Omega \to L(X, X)$ *is locally Lipschitzian with a bounded range.*

Proof: For a detailed proof, see Bruni et al. (1975). The proof is based on the following facts:

1. As may be seen in Eq. (40), F depends only on x_6, through the functions $[(1 - Kx_6)/(1 + Kx_6)]p_s(Kx_6)$, $[Kx_6/(1 + Kx_6)]p_s(Kx_6)$, $[1/(1 + Kx_6)]p_s(Kx_6)$, x_6 .

2. Each one of these functions may be proved to be bounded in Ω. This is directly checked for the first three of them, noting that due to the definition Eq. (5), $0 \leqslant p_s(Kx_6) \leqslant 1$, and due to the choice of Ω, $0 < 1/(1 + Kx_6) \leqslant 2$. As far as x_6 is concerned, from Eqs. (26) and (27) the following inequality may be derived:

$$x_6(t) \leqslant x_6(0) + \int_{K_1}^{K_2} x_4(K, 0)\, dK + \int_0^\infty u_2(\tau)\, d\tau \tag{43}$$

and the right side of Eq. (43) is bounded because of the assumptions introduced on x_4, u_2. This clearly means that x_6 is bounded above by the concentration of all previously injected antigen, as should be from a physical point of view.

3. The local Lipschitzness of the functions in (1) may be checked directly.

As usual in systems theory, we define some output variables which correspond to physically measurable quantities and whose behavior is worth observation. Thus we define an output vector y:

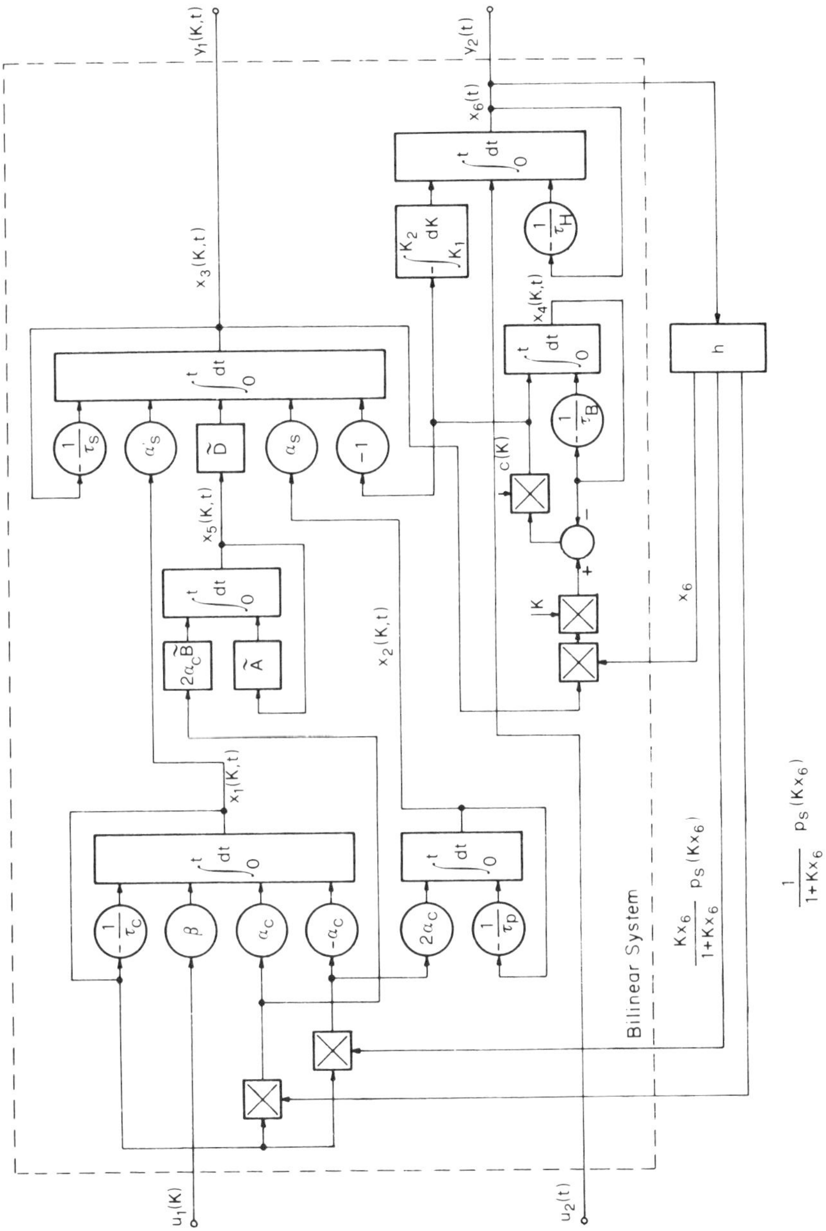

FIG. 3. Simulation scheme of the mathematical model of the immune response as a bilinear system with a nonlinear instantaneous bounded state feedback.

$$y(t) = \left[y_1(t)\ y_2(t)\right]^T \triangleq \left[S(\cdot,t)\ H(t)\right]^T \tag{44}$$

A block diagram of the above defined state space model is given in Fig. 3, where the bilinear system with nonlinear bounded state feedback structure is displayed.

IV. STRUCTURAL PROPERTIES OF THE MODEL

In this section we present some important properties of the immune response model, that is, existence and uniqueness of solutions and free evolution stability.

In order to prove them, a fundamental step is the description of the model as a state space model and in particular its formulation in terms of bounded rate systems. A convenient extensive analysis of such a class will hopefully cast more light on the structural properties and control policies of the model.

A. Existence and Uniqueness of Solutions

Let us define the closed subset $Z \subset \Omega$:

$$Z = \left\{x \in \Omega:\ x_i(K) \geqslant 0,\ i = 1, 2, 3, 4,\ \ \tilde{D}x_5(K) \geqslant 0, \forall K \in (K_1, K_2),\ x_6 \geqslant 0\right\}$$

Due to the physical meaning of the state variables, this is the set in which we may naturally expect all the possible solutions of the model equations to evolve. Indeed, the following Lemma has been proved (Bruni et al., 1975):

Lemma 2. *For each* $u \in U$ *and for each given* $x(0) \in Z$, *the solution* $x(t)$ *of Eqs. (39) and (40), if it exists, turns out to be confined in* Z *for each* $t \in R^+$.

The above mentioned Lemmas may be usefully exploited to prove the following Theorem.

Theorem 1* *For each initial state* $x(0) \in Z$, *and each* $u \in U$, *there exists a unique solution* $x(t)$ *of Eqs. (39) and (40) for* $t \in R^+$.

Proof: The theorem may be easily proved along these lines:

1. Recalling Lemma 1, for each $u \in U$, the right side of Eq. (39) may be seen to be locally uniformly bounded and continuous with respect to t, within a suitable neighborhood of each $x(0) \in Z$. Moreover, in the same neighborhood, the same quantity is locally uniformly Lipschitzian. Consequently (see, e.g., Ladas and Lakshmikantham, 1972, Theorem 5.1.1), local existence and uniqueness of solutions of Eqs. (39) and (40) is guaranteed.
2. Due to Lemma 2, such a solution always lies in Z.
3. Again recalling Lemma 1, global existence of the solutions in Z easily follows (see, e.g., Ladas and Lakshmikantham, 1972, Theorem 5.6.1).

This conclusion is in agreement with the physical behavior of the natural process.

B. Stability

To investigate the stability properties of the model Eqs. (39) and (40), in this section we assume the input variables $u_1(t) = \beta\bar{p}_c(\cdot)$, $u_2 = 0$, and we look at the response for any given $x(0) \in Z$.

The analysis of such a solution is highly simplified if we take for c(K) a constant value

$$c(K) = \chi, \quad K \in (K_1, K_2) \tag{45}$$

and this will be assumed throughout this section.

The assumption, Eq. (45), has no actual biological basis: indeed, very little is known about the link between the dissociation reaction

---

*In Bruni et al. (1975) the validity of the result of this theorem is proved for the general class of bounded rate systems.

rate constant of the immune complex and its affinity K. This hypothesis is here introduced only for mathematical convenience; the authors are strongly inclined to conjecture that the validity of the results proved below shall hold even without it.

We now proceed to investigate the equilibrium points.

Remark 1: With the above-mentioned choice of u, Eqs. (39) and (40) admit in Z a unique equilibrium point x^e:

$$x^e = \left[x_1^e \; x_2^e \; x_3^e \; x_4^{e} \; x_5^{e^T} \; x_6^e\right]^T$$

$$= \left[\tau_c \beta \bar{p}_c(\cdot) \;\; 0 \;\; \tau_s \alpha_s' \tau_c \beta \bar{p}_c(\cdot) \;\; 0 \;\; 0^T \;\; 0\right]^T \tag{46}$$

Indeed, from Eqs. (26) and (27) and recalling Eq. (36), it follows:

$$\dot{x}_6(t) + \int_{K_1}^{K_2} \dot{x}_4(K, t)\, dK = -\frac{1}{\tau_B}\int_{K_1}^{K_2} x_4(K, t)\, dK - \frac{1}{\tau_H} x_6(t) + u_2(t) \tag{47}$$

which shows that for any equilibrium point in Z we must have $x_4^e = 0$, $x_6^e = 0$.

Recalling Eq. (5) and the stability property of Eq. (34), Eq. (46) easily follows. Possible equilibrium points out of Z are not of interest, owing to the results of Theorem 1.

At this point we can prove a stability theorem for the immune response model.

Theorem 2 *Let us assume* $\tau_c > \max(\tau_B, \tau_H)$. *Then for* $u_1(t) = \beta\bar{p}_c(\cdot)$ *and* $u_2(t) = 0$, *the equilibrium point (46) of Eqs. (39) and (40), unique in Z, is globally asymptotically stable in Z.*

Proof: Recalling the block diagram of Fig. 3, the system, Eqs. (39) and (40), may be thought of as a bilinear system in a nonlinear instantaneous feedback loop. Thus, stability of the closed loop system may be investigated by looking at stability properties of the open loop (bilinear) system and at suitable decay properties of the feedback signal $h(x_6)$. To be more specific, the proof of the theorem goes along the following lines (Bruni et al., 1975b):

1. Due to the assumption on τ_c, the asymptotic stability of the bilinear system free response is established. This assumption corresponds to the widely admitted fact that immunocompetent and memory cells have a death rate constant much smaller than the rate constant for removal of antigen or of antibody sites (Bruni et al., 1975b).
2. For each $x(0) \in Z$, and for the assumed input, and from Eq. (47), it is possible to prove that

$$x_6(t) \leqslant \left[x_6(0) + \int_{K_1}^{K_2} x_4(K, 0)\, dK\right] \exp\left(-\frac{t}{\tau_c}\right), \quad t \in R^+ \qquad (48)$$

   due to the Lipschitzian property of h, a similar inequality holds for $\|h(x_6)\|$.
3. By exploiting a general result for bilinear systems (Bruni et al., 1975b), two positive constants μ_1, μ_2 may be found such that for the closed loop solution x(t):

$$\|x(t) - x^e\| \leqslant \mu_1 \exp -t\mu_2 \qquad (49)$$

The inequality, Eq. (49), amounts to saying that x^e is globally asymptotically stable for the system, Eqs. (39) and (40).

V. SIMULATION AND VALIDATION OF THE MODEL

The model described by Eqs. (23) to (27) was simulated and its validity tested by comparing its output with sets of data reported in the literature (Eisen and Siskind, 1964; Siskind et al., 1968; Werblin and Siskind, 1972; Werblin et al., 1973). These experimental data refer to white New Zealand rabbits immunized with a single inoculation of dinitrophenylated bovine gamma globulin (DNP-BGG) emulsified in Freund's complete adjuvant.

1. In order to simulate the injection in Freund's adjuvant, the input variable of the model $\dot{H}_i(t)$ was assumed to be the sum of two functions: an exponential (with time constant τ_u) which accounts for one third of the total antigen inoculated Q, and a function which is constant for the time interval $[0, T_u]$ which accounts for the remaining two-thirds of Q. Thus

$$\dot{H}_i(t) = \frac{Q}{3\tau_u V} \exp\left(-\frac{t}{\tau_u}\right) + \frac{2}{3}\frac{Q}{\tau_u V} \delta_{-1}(T_u - t) \qquad (50)$$

where V is the volume of the circulating fluids of the animal in which the antigen distributes itself, and $\delta_{-1}(t)$ is the unit step function.

Such a choice differs from Bell's (Bell, 1970, 1971a,b), where the antigen input was assumed to follow a linear ramp. The exponential part should account for the relatively fast onset of the immune response following inoculation, while the linear ramp should simulate the slow release at a constant rate of the fraction of the total antigen segregated in a separate compartment.

2. The initial conditions assumed for testing the model implied that no stimulation had previously occurred. In particular, C(K, 0) and S(K, 0) were taken proportional to $\bar{p}_c(K)$, while all other variables were initialized with zero values.

The *initial affinity distribution* of immunocompetent cells in the virgin animal, $\bar{p}_c(K)$, was assumed to be Gaussian with respect to the binding free energy ΔG_0, with zero mean and variance σ_G.

Since

$$\Delta G_o = -RT \ln K \qquad (51)$$

the distribution in ln K is

$$\bar{p}_c(\ln K) = \frac{1}{\sqrt{2\pi}} \frac{RT}{\sigma_G} \exp\left[-\frac{1}{2}\left(\frac{RT}{\sigma_G} \ln K\right)^2\right] \qquad (52)$$

3. As mentioned above, it seemed reasonable to assume that there is a burst of antibody synthesis just after stimulation and duplication of immunocompetent and memory cells, as described by an

intensity function i(t). This high intensity function was taken to be equal to α_s'' in the interval $(0, T_0)$ and equal to zero outside this interval.

Since this assumption, together with the short lifetime of plasma cells, led to a rapid decay of the immune response, a low basal antibody production by all immunocompetent and memory cells was added; this basal production was assumed to occur with a constant rate α_s'.

4. Other assumptions for simulation of the model were that the reaction between antigen and antibody sites is instantaneous, and that each DNP-BGG molecule bears a single DNP determinant.

The *numerical values* adopted for all the parameters of the model are listed in Appendix C.

The *computed values* of log S(t) and log K(t), are reported in Figs. 4 and 5, together with the *experimentally determined values* of antibody titers and of the mean association constants obtained by different authors for Q = 5 mg (Eisen and Siskind, 1964; Siskind et al., 1968; Werblin et al., 1973).

Figure 6 reports the affinity distribution of antibodies at day 40, as derived from simulation of the present model with Q = 0.5 mg, and the bimodal distribution which can be derived (Bruni et al., 1974; Bruni et al., 1976) from the binding data obtained by Werblin et al. (1973) at day 42 under the same conditions.

A fairly good agreement with the data can be obtained over a relatively wide range of Q (Bruni et al., 1975a), although it must be said that some discrepancies come out when large doses of antigen (Q = 50 mg) are considered, especially with respect to the decay of antibody production at long times ($\geqslant$ 180 days). So far, the model is unable to account for high-dose paralysis, since the inhibition postulated upon occupancy of too many cell receptors is, in our model, fully reversible and therefore unable to cause a prolonged state of immunological unresponsiveness.

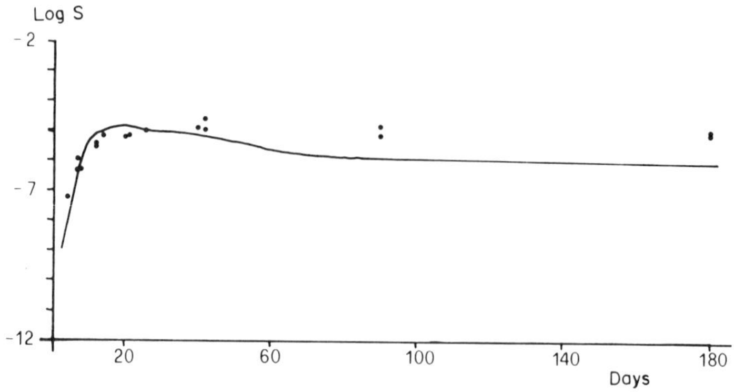

FIG. 4. Symbols represent anti-DNP levels taken from Siskind et al. (1968) and Werblin et al. (1973), after injection of 5 mg of DNP-BGG. The full line was obtained by simulation of the model.

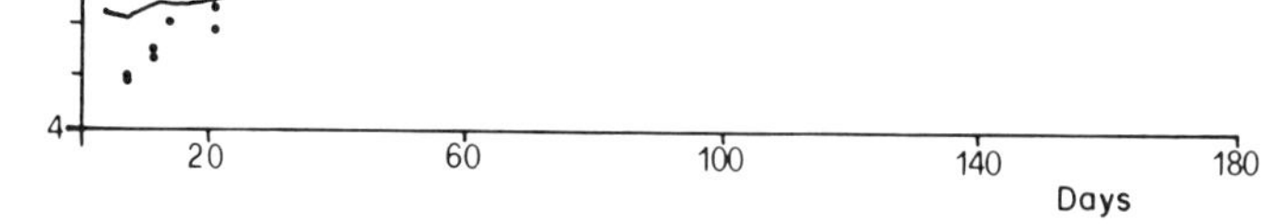

FIG. 5. Symbols represent the mean intrinsic association constant of anti-DNP antibodies taken from Eisen and Siskind (1964), Siskind et al. (1968), and Werblin et al. (1973), after injection of 5 mg of DNP-BGG. The full line was obtained by simulation of the model.

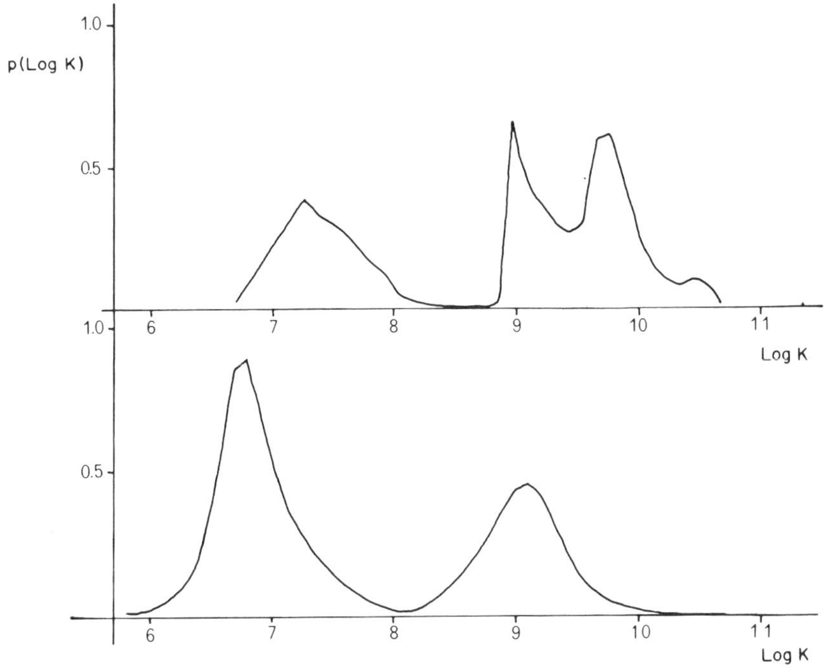

FIG. 6. The lower part of the figure shows the affinity distribution of anti-DNP antibodies which can be derived (Bruni et al., 1974; Bruni et al., 1976) from the experimental results in Werblin et al. (1973), 42 days after injection of 0.5 mg DNP-BGG. The upper part of the figure shows the affinity distribution obtained by simulation of the model, 40 days after injection of 0.5 mg DNP-labeled antigen.

VI. CRITICAL ANALYSIS AND FUTURE DEVELOPMENTS OF THE MODEL

As already mentioned, in order to build a model simple enough to allow the simulation of the immune response process and the study of the structural properties, some simplifying assumptions were introduced. This is also justified by the controversial interpretation of some experimental results in the context of the different theories. It is sometimes difficult indeed to compare the experiments in vivo to those in vitro. In vivo the preexisting conditions are not always well defined; in vitro, it is difficult to ascertain the physiological meaning of the events studied.

With a view to future developments of the model a reconsideration of some oversimplified assumptions, related mainly to the mechanisms of immunocompetent cell stimulation and differentiation, will be needed. The following aspects appear particularly worthy of reappraisal.

A. Multivalency of the Antigen

Multivalency of the antigen raises two types of questions:

1. Binding of antigen with antibody which, rather than being expressed by a simple mass-action law, is better described in terms of interactions within a lattice, that is, according to the equations put forth by Goldberg (1952), Flory (1941), and DeLisi, Chap. 8.

2. Triggering of immunocompetent cells through either multipoint binding of the antigen with cell receptors or lattice formation at the cell surface (Bell, 1975). In the former case, occupancy of neighboring membrane sites is regulated by the mass action laws, but the sites cannot be considered independent from each other. In the latter case, where a more complex description of the binding process is required (Flory, 1941; Goldberg, 1952), B lymphocytes are activated through a cross-linking of their receptors by multivalent antigen to form a receptor-ligand lattice which perturbs the lymphocyte surface (Edelman et al., 1973; Taylor, et al., 1971; Perelson, Chap. 7).

B. Cooperation Between B Lymphocytes and Other Types of Cells; Necessity of More Than One Signal

The problem of cellular cooperation in the immune response to thymus-dependent antigens is still a controversial question. It seems that, at least in some cases, three different kinds of cells are involved in the process: B lymphocytes, T lymphocytes, and macrophages.

A future development of the present model might, for example, follow the hypothesis put forward by Dutton (1975), of cellular cooperation with separate signals for proliferation and differentiation as far as humoral immune response to T-dependent antigens is concerned. The proliferation signal for B lymphocytes would be given by a multipoint binding to the cell receptors of the multivalent antigen; this population of "proliferating cells" requires, for differentiation into plasma cells, a second signal, arising from the interaction with a monovalent nonspecific substance produced by T lymphocytes.

Activation of T cells to produce this second signal can also be assumed to occur upon a multipoint binding of their receptors to the antigen, either directly or through presentation by macrophages. Differentiation of proliferating cells into plasma cells would then be regulated by the level of binding to the B-proliferating cells of the T-cell factor. Memory cells would be those B lymphocytes which, after proliferation, fail to differentiate into plasma cells.

The increasing complexity of such a model suggests that one should simulate in vitro conditions so as to obtain clarification of single steps. In modeling an in vivo situation, the existence of several populations leads to problems of compartmentation and diffusion of the antigen, and of the various cells and their products.

C. Switchover Phenomenon

That is, different types of immunoglobulin secreted during the maturation of the activated B lymphocytes. The problem of different types of immunoglobulins secreted can be treated by assuming either of the following two hypotheses:

1. There are *two separate and independent* B-lymphocyte subpopulations, each one producing a class of Ig. These two subpopulations may differ in that only the IgG producing cells require a T-cell cooperative factor. Therefore, the relative amount of different types of Ig would not depend on a switchover phenomenon but on the relative numbers of corresponding cells.
2. There is only *one type* of B-lymphocyte precursor, which under proliferation and differentiation signals generates IgM plasma cells. If during their maturation process they

receive a suitable T cell dependent *switchover signal*, they differentiate into IgG plasma cells. Here the relative amount of IgM and IgG secreted depends on an intracellular switchover phenomenon.

VII. FINAL REMARKS

The model described in the present work is based on the theory of clonal selection (Burnet, 1959; Jerne, 1955), that is, it assumes that the immunocompetent cells have a random initial distribution of their antigen binding capacity, that memory cells are identical to the immunocompetent cells from which they originate, and that stimulation by antigen occurs according to the mass action law.

As compared to the theory of Sercarz and Coons (1962), where three cell populations X, Y, and Z are considered, our model differs by assuming that differentiation is determined by the site occupancy on the mother cell. As a consequence, while the plasma cells of our model coincide with the Z cells of Sercarz and Coons (1962), our population of immunocompetent and memory cells comprise both the X and Y families.

As compared to the model proposed by Bell (1970, 1971a,b), we propose that the affinity K continuously ranges in a given interval (K_1, K_2). Although the finite number of cells prevents K from assuming all possible values, this hypothesis offers the advantage of mathematical tractability and appears to be sounder (Siskind and Benacerraf, 1969) than the arbitrary assumption (Bell, 1970, 1971a,b) of a finite and relatively low number of possible values of K.

Furthermore, the probability of differentiation into plasma cells was, in our model, related to the occupancy of sites, while in Bell's model, the fraction of newly formed plasma cells was arbitrarily fixed.

As far as the antibody production by immunocompetent and memory cells is concerned, it seemed reasonable to assume that there is a burst of antibody synthesis just after stimulation and duplication, as described by i(t). However, it was noticed that this assumption, together with the short lifetime of plasma cells, led to a rapid decay of the immune response. A low basal antibody production from any immunocompetent cell was therefore added. This assumption, together with the choice of a composite input function, is probably responsible for the multimodal affinity distribution of antibodies shown in Fig. 6. A bimodal affinity distribution had been found by Werblin et al. (1973), and confirmed by ourselves both on a theoretical basis (Bruni et al., 1976) and experimentally (unpublished results).

As mentioned in a previous section, in our model several simplifying assumptions were made. Nevertheless it was found to behave quite satisfactorily as far as the description of a prolonged primary response is concerned.

It should, however, be checked for the behavior in the case of a fast injection of a very high antigen dose which should lead to immunological unresponsiveness (Landy and Braun, 1969; Sercarz and Coons, 1962).

As far as the fundamental structural properties of the model are concerned, especially about existence, uniqueness, and stability of the equations, we established existence in the large, and uniqueness of such a solution for any physically meaningful choice of input variable and initial conditions; furthermore, the solution is always nonnegative.

The model equations admit a unique equilibrium point within the physically admissible state set, and this equilibrium point has been proved to be globally, asymptotically stable.

Future development will proceed along three different lines:

1. Further investigation of the model from a theoretical standpoint (controllability and observability properties, filtering of the output data, optimal control)
2. Parameter identification and validation of the model against sets of data obtained through ad hoc designed experiments
3. Introduction of phenomena so far disregarded, as mentioned in a previous section

APPENDIX A: LIST OF SYMBOLS

$H_i(t)$	Concentration of antigen sites introduced, per unit volume of circulating fluids, up to time t
$H(t)$	Concentration of free antigen sites
$C(K, t)$	Concentration density, with respect to K, of immunocompetent and memory cells
$C_s(K, t)$	Concentration density of stimulated immunocompetent cells
$C_{dp}(K, t)$ and $C_{dm}(K, t)$	Concentration density of stimulated immunocompetent cells which, upon duplication and differentiation, give rise, respectively, to plasma cells and to memory cells
$C_p(K, t)$	Concentration density of plasma cells
$\bar{p}_c(K)$	Original distribution of immunocompetent cells
$S(K, t)$	Concentration density of free antibody sites
$B(K, t)$	Concentration density of bound antibody sites

APPENDIX B: LIST OF MATHEMATICAL NOTATIONS

$a \in A$	a is an element of the set A
$T: A_1 \to A_2$	T is an operator which takes elements of A_1 into elements of A_2
$\Vert \quad \Vert$	Norm
$A_1 \times A_2$	Cartesian product of A_1, A_2, i.e., the set of pairs (a_1, a_2), $a_1 \in A_1$, $a_2 \in A_2$
R^n	n-dimensional Euclidean space
$L(A_1, A_2)$	Set of linear bounded operators which take elements of A_1 into elements of A_2
T'	Adjoint operator of the operator T
$\triangleq$	Equal by definition
$\mathcal{C}^n(K_1, K_2)$	Space of n-dimensional real continuous functions on the interval (K_1, K_2)

a^T	Transposed vector of the vector a
$a(\cdot)$	The whole function a with respect to the argument replaced by the dot
R^+	Set of nonnegative real numbers
$A_1 \subset A_2$	The set A_1 is contained in the set A_2
$A = \{a: P(a)\}$	A is the set of all elements a which satisfy the property P(a)
$\forall$	For any

APPENDIX C: NUMERICAL VALUES OF PARAMETERS EMPLOYED IN THE SIMULATION

Initial total number of immunocompetent cells	$C(0) = 5 \times 10^8$ cells liter^{-1} $= 0.8 \times 10^{-15}$ M*
Volume of circulating fluids	$V = 0.2$ liter
Standard deviation of the original distribution of affinities of immunocompetent cells	$\frac{\sigma_G}{RT} = \frac{\ln 10^5}{3}$
Interval of association constants	$\begin{cases} K_1 = 1.69 \times 10^5\ M^{-1} \\ K_2 = 6.47 \times 10^{10}\ M^{-1} \end{cases}$
Interval of occupancy of receptor sites causing stimulation	$\begin{cases} \sigma_1 = 0.01 \\ \sigma_2 = 0.9 \end{cases}$
Rate of production of new immunocompetent cells from stem cells	$\beta = 7 \times 10^4$ cells liter^{-1} hr^{-1}
Proliferation rate constant of stimulated immunocompetent cells	$\alpha_c = 57.8 \times 10^{-3}$ hr^{-1}
Mean lifetime of immunocompetent cells	$\tau_c = 7140$ hr

*In order to express the number of cells and the concentration of soluble macromolecules in a homogeneous manner, the value of C(0) is reported as number of cells per unit volume divided by Avogadro's number.

Mean lifetime of plasma cells	τ_p = 71 hr
Rate constant of antibody production by plasma cells	$\alpha_s = 10^8$ molecules $cell^{-1}$ hr^{-1}
Rate constant of basal antibody production by immunocompetent cells	$\alpha'_s = 2 \times 10^6$ molecules $cell^{-1}$ hr^{-1}
Rate constant of extra antibody production by newly formed memory cells, in the interval $[0,T_0]$	$\alpha''_s = 2 \times 10^7$ molecules $cell^{-1}$ hr^{-1}
Duration of the interval of extra antibody production by newly formed memory cells	T_0 = 300 hr
Mean lifetime of antibody sites	τ_s = 200 hr
Mean lifetime of the immune complex	τ_B = 50 hr
Mean lifetime of antigenic determinants	τ_H = 100 hr
Time constant of the exponential portion of the antigen input function Eq. (50)	τ_u = 100 hr
Time interval during which the constant portion of the antigen input function is nonzero	T_u = 1000 hr

ACKNOWLEDGMENTS

This work was partially supported by C. N. R., Italy.

REFERENCES

Bell, G. I. (1970). Mathematical model of clonal selection and antibody production, I. *J. Theor. Biol. 29:* 191-232.

Bell, G. I. (1971a). Mathematical model of clonal selection and antibody production, II. *J. Theor. Biol. 33:* 339-378.

Bell, G. I. (1971b). Mathematical model of clonal selection and antibody production, III. The cellular basis of immunological paralysis. *J. Theor. Biol. 33:* 379-398.

Bell, G. I. (1975). B lymphocyte activation and lattice formation. *Transplant. Rev. 23:* 23-36.

Bruni, C., Di Pillo, G., and Koch, G. (1974). Bilinear systems: an appealing class of "nearly linear" systems in theory and applications. *IEEE Trans. Automatic Control AC-19:* 334-348

Bruni, C., Germani, A., and Koch, G. (1974). On the distribution of antibody affinities in the immune response. *Boll. Soc. It. Biol. Sper. 50:* 1057-1069.

Bruni, C., Germani, A., and Koch, G. (1975). An introduction to bounded rate systems. *VII IFIP Conference on Optimization.* Nice, France.

Bruni, C., Germani, A., Koch, G., and Strom R. (1976). Derivation of antibody distribution from experimental data. *J. Theor. Biol. 61:* 143-170.

Bruni, C., Giovenco, M. A., Koch, G., and Strom, R. (1975a). A dynamical model of humoral immune response. *Math. Biosciences 27:* 191-211.

Bruni, C., Giovenco, M. A., Koch, G., and Strom, R. (1975b). The immune response as a variable structure system. In *Variable Structure Systems with Application to Economics and Biology* (A. Ruberti and R. R. Mohler, eds.). Springer-Verlag, New York, pp. 244-264.

Bruni, C. and Koch, G. (1976). A degenerate (bounded rate) class of distributed parameter systems. *IFIP Working Conference on Distributed Parameter Systems Modeling and Identification,* Rome.

Burnet, R. M. (1959). *The Clonal Selection Theory of Immunity.* Vanderbilt and Cambridge University Presses, London and New York.

Dutton, R. W. (1975). Separate signals for thc initiation of proliferation and differentiation in the B cell response to antigen. *Transplant. Rev. 23:* 66-77.

Edelman, G. M., Yamara, I., and Wang, J. L. (1973). Receptor mobility and receptor - cytoplasmic interactions in lymphocytes. *Proc. Nat. Acad. Sci. (USA) 70:* 1442-1446.

Eisen, H. N. and Siskind, G. W. (1964). Variations in affinities of antibody during the immune response. *Biochem. 3:* 996-1008.

Flory, P. J. (1941). Molecular size distribution in three dimensional polymers. I. Gelation. *J. Am. Chem. Soc. 63:* 3083-3090.

Goldberg, R. J. (1952). A theory of antibody-antigen reactions. I. Theory for reactions of multivalent antigen with bivalent or univalent antibody. *J. Am. Chem. Soc. 74:* 5715-5725.

Hege, J. S. and Cole, L. J. (1966). A mathematical model relating circulating antibody and antibody forming cells. *J. Immunol. 97:* 34-40.

Jerne, N. (1955). The natural-selection theory of antibody formation. *Proc. Nat. Acad. Sci. (USA) 41:* 849-857.

Jilek, M. (1971a). The number of immunologically activated cells after repeated immunization (a mathematical model). *Folia Microbiol. Praha 16:* 12-23.

Jilek, M. (1971b). On contacts of immunocompetent cells with antigens (note on a probability model). *Folia Microbiol. Praha 16:* 83-87.

Jilek, M. and Ursjnyova, Z. (1970). On the distribution of the epoch of the first contact of immunocompetent cell with antigen. *Folia Microbiol. Praha 15:* 492-499.

Ladas, G. E. and Lakshmikantham, V. (1972). *Differential Equations in Abstract Spaces.* Academic, New York.

Landy, M. and Braun, W. (Eds.) (1969). *Immunological Tolerance.* Academic, New York.

Levi, M. I., Durikhin, K. H., Besova, N. N., and Famenco, G. A. (1973). Cyclic kinetics and mathematical expression of the primary response to soluble antigen. *Folia Microbiol. Praha 18:* 237-241.

Mohler, R. R. (1974). *Bilinear Control Processes with Application to Engineering, Ecology and Medicine.* Academic, New York.

Mohler, R. R. and Ruberti, A. (1972). *Theory and Applications of Variable Structure Systems.* Academic, New York.

Möller, G. (1970). Induction of DNA synthesis in human lymphocytes: interaction between non-specific mitogens and antigens. *Immunology 19:* 583-598.

Ruberti, A. and Mohler, R. R. (1975). *Variable Structure Systems with Applications to Economics and Biology.* Springer-Verlag, New York.

Sercarz, E. and Coons, A. H. (1962). The exhaustion of specific antibody producing capacity during a secondary response. In *Mechanism of Immunological Tolerance* (M. Hesek, A. Langerova, and M. Vojtiskova, eds.). Academic, New York.

Siskind, G. W. and Benacerraf, B. (1969). Cell selection by antigen in the immune response. *Adv. Immunol. 10:* 1-50.

Siskind, G. W., Dunn, P., and Walker, J. G. (1968). Studies on the control of antibody synthesis. III. Effect of antigen dose and of suppression by passive antibody on the affinity of antibody synthesized. *J. Exp. Med. 127:* 55-66.

Sterzl, J. (1966). Immunological tolerance as a result of terminal differentiation of immunologically competent cells. *Nature 209:* 416-417.

Taylor, R. B., Duffus, W. P. H., Raff, M. D., and de Petris, S. (1971). Redistribution and pinocytosis of lymphocyte surface immunoglobulin molecules induced by anti-immunoglobulin antibody. *Nature New Biology 233:* 225-229.

Werblin, T. P. and Siskind, G. W. (1972). Distribution of antibody affinities. Technique of measurement. *Immunochem. 9:* 987-1011. 987-1011.

Werblin, T. P., Young Tai Kim, Quagliata, F., and Siskind, G. W. (1973). Changes in heterogeneity of antibody during the course of the immune response. *Immunology 24:* 473-492.

Chapter 14

T AND B CELLS IN THE IMMUNE SYSTEM

R. R. Mohler, Claude F. Barton, and Chin-Shung Hsu

Department of Electrical and Computer Engineering
Oregon State University
Corvallis, Oregon

Two mathematical models of B-cell and T-cell kinetics are presented to explain the complex dynamic behavior of the humoral immune process and cell-mediated immune responses. Both models are based on clonal selection theory, classical birth-death cell population balances, and an average fixed antibody-antigen affinity constant. The system dynamics are linear with respect to the state variables (cell population densities) and the control variables (probabilities of stimulation and differentiation of cells), but not jointly linear as is frequently assumed for biological systems. The first model describes the differentiation of B cells into plasma cells after stimulation by a thymus-independent hapten and the subsequent production of antibody. A fairly good agreement of the model simulation with experimental data (Werblin et al., 1973) is obtained, and the system behavior agrees with the results of Bell (1970). The second model analyzes the cooperation effect of T cells with B cells. Stimulation and inhibition effects of T cells are based on the assumption formulated by Greaves et al. (1974) that T complexes of T antibody and antigen are released from their T-cell binding to bind to macrophages. The macrophage-bound T complexes bind through antigen with B-cell receptors. Experiments are in progress to verify this model.

I. INTRODUCTION

The purpose of this paper is to present a basic mathematical model to explain the complex dynamic behavior of the humoral immune process and cell-mediated immune responses. The potential role of mathematical modeling in long-range systematic planning of immunological experimentation is presented. Although the major contribution of mathematical modeling and computer simulation of immunological mechanisms may be in providing direction to a sometimes scattered experimental program, they could lead to a more effective synthesis of immunotherapy.

II. BACKGROUND

In comparing the relative role of experimentation and mathematical models, Jerne (1974) states that "as long as the quantitation of the immune response remains elusive, immunology will remain a phenomenology, an ever accumulating catalogue of such phenomena as are at present our daily bread."

An early preliminary model of the immune process was presented by Hege and Cole (1966). Then, Jilek (1973; Jilek and Sterzl, 1971) developed a probability model of different cell types undergoing repeated contacts with specific antigens. He assumed a process of Poisson form and considered a Monte Carlo simulation. The most complete studies of mathematical models in immunology have been presented by Bell (1970, 1971a,b), which included binding of antigen to antibodies according to their specificities and binding constants. More recently, Bell (1974) and Bell and DeLisi (1974) derived simple mathematical models for specific binding of multivalent antigen to immune cell receptors when competition exists, with nonspecific binding of antigen to cell surfaces, and with binding of hapten to receptors. Effectively, such competition reduces the binding constant.

The network topology of the immune system arises from the antigenic properties of each antibody molecule which interacts with lymphocytes. Jerne (1974) and Richter (1974, 1975; see also Chap. 19) provide some basis for a network model. The latter gives a general modeling approach to activation and suppression of antibody production of different classes, with each class suppressing the class from which it was activated and stimulating production of the following class. While this model lacks precise experimental verification, it does simulate the essence of low zone and high zone tolerance, along with primary and secondary responses. T cell dependent factors are considered in a recent study by Hoffmann (1975; see also Chap. 20). Hoffman suggests a model which includes antigen-binding ("positive") T cells and antiidiotypic ("negative") T cells.

None of the aforementioned models include modes of spatial distribution, such as arise from circulation of antigen, cells, and antibodies through humoral fluid, blood, and tissue, including thymus, spleen, and other distributed organs. Bystryn et al. (1971) presented a nonmathematical compartmental model consisting of functional compartments for immunogen and antibody secretion. A more recent compartmental model of circulating lymphocytes in the spleen was analyzed by Hammond (1975). The model is compartmented by marginal zones and red and white pulp zones with the usual fluxes (lymphocytes) between compartments.

III. MODEL USE IN EXPERIMENTAL PLANNING

The success of mathematical modeling and computer simulation will depend on the ability to integrate this development with an experimental program, and the success of an experimental program may be enhanced greatly by such a development. An effective model and simulation might resolve conflicting hypotheses, it might duplicate particular experimental conditions, and it may point the direction of future experiments while bringing focus to the relevant issues.

Figure 1 gives a functional description of the interrelations of experimentation, immune theory, modeling, and simulation. In contrast to the conventional approach, the "systems approach" requires formulation of a mathematical model based upon assumptions and immunological phenomena which clearly illustrate the interacting subsystems. With the aid of computer simulation and control theory, an effective experimental plan may be designed to provide time-series data for identifying the parameters upon which the understanding of the homeostatic mechanisms of the immune system faithfully depends.

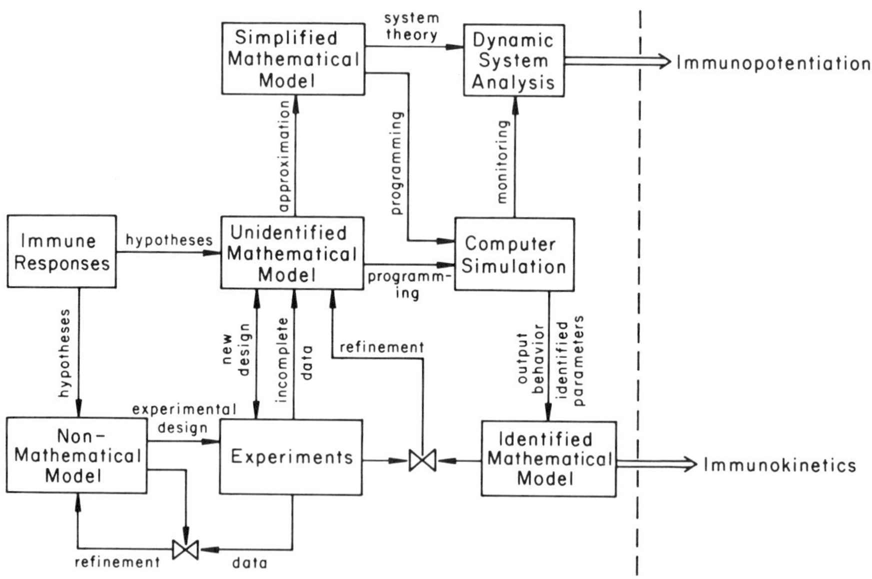

FIG. 1. Role of model in experimental planning.

As presented in this paper, the kinetic mathematical model is able to deal with both B-cell and/or T-cell population dynamics in the regulation of immune response. It is very possible that the manipulation and control realized by such a model will have significant clinical implications with respect to immunopotentiation and synthetic therapies.

IV. B-CELL MODEL

The development here follows the recent model of Bruni et al. (1975a,b; see also Chap. 13) which was generated in conjunction with our joint United States-Italy cooperative program. Clonal selection theory, along with classical birth-death cell population balances, forms the basis of the model. In the initial model, the effect of T cells, multivalent antigens, cell-mediated immunity, antibody switchover, mutual interaction of receptors, dependence of parameters (such as cell lifetimes) on cell populations, and the existence of various classes of antibodies and cells and complement are all neglected.

The process is described by the following variables with the arguments (t, time and k, association constant) omitted for brevity:

x_1 Population density of immunocompetent cells (ICC), which are sensitized lymphocyte cells with particular surface receptors having association constant k for antigen. They may differentiate into plasma cells and divide into memory cells. The latter may further divide and enter the pool of immunocompetent cells.

x_2 Population density of plasma cells which are nonreproducing offspring of stimulated immunocompetent cells.

x_3 Population density of "antibody sites," unbound to antigen.

x_4 Population density of immune complexes, which individually include antibody sites and antigen.

$h(t)$ Antigen concentration, unbound to antibody, which triggers the response mechanism.

Consideration of immunocompetent cells first leads to a change of population density, Δx_1, on an interval Δt due to mitosis, given by

$$[2\alpha(1 - p_d)\, p_s x_1 - \alpha p_s x_1]\, \Delta t$$

where α is the birth-rate constant of stimulated immunocompetent cells, p_d is the probability that an immunocompetent cell differentiates into a plasma cell (h, k dependent), and p_s is the probability that antigen stimulates a cell (h, k dependent).

To this must be added the source of new stem cells $\beta_k \Delta t$, and the death of cells $x_1\ \Delta t/\tau_1$, where β_k is the rate of generation of new immunocompetent cells (from bone marrow), and τ_1 is the mean lifetime of immunocompetent cells. In the limit, the process is described by an ordinary differential equation of form

$$\frac{dx_1}{dt} = \alpha u_1 x_1 - \frac{x_1}{\tau_1} + \beta_k \qquad (1)$$

where $u_1 = p_s(1 - 2p_d)$. Similarly, plasma cells, antibody sites, and immune complex generation for each k may be approximated by birth-rate minus death-rate equations as follows:

$$\frac{dx_2}{dt} = 2\alpha u_2 x_1 - \frac{x_2}{\tau_2} \qquad (2)$$

$$\frac{dx_3}{dt} = -c_k khx_3 - \frac{x_3}{\tau_3} + \alpha' x_2 + c_k x_4 + \alpha'' x_1 \qquad (3)$$

$$\frac{dx_4}{dt} = c_k khx_3 - \left(c_k + \frac{1}{\tau_4}\right) x_4 \qquad (4)$$

where τ_2, τ_3, and τ_4 are appropriate lifetimes,

$$u_2 = p_s p_d$$

α' is plasma-cell antibody production rate, α'' is ICC antibody production rate, and c_k and kc_k are dissociation rate and association rate coefficients, respecitvely, of immune complex (k-dependent).

By comparison of response times, however, the dynamics of Eq. (4) may be approximated by

$$x_4 \simeq khx_3 \tag{5}$$

for most purposes; that is, the complex and antigen reach equilibrium instantly.

An interesting structural feature of this system is that the system is linear in control (u_1, u_2), linear in state (x_1, x_2, x_3, x_4), but not jointly linear. Since product terms of state and control variables appear in the dynamics, the system is not linear as is so frequently assumed for systems studies. Mohler (1973, 1974), Mohler and Ruberti (1972), and Ruberti and Mohler (1975) provide a summary of significant theoretical developments of bilinear systems and their application to biological processes.

The free antigen population density appears as an input to which the immune control system responds. The antibodies secreted after inoculation of the antigen population $dh_i(t) = \dot{h}_i(t)dt$ include a distribution of association constants which would require a summation over the appropriate values of k in the model. The rate of generation of a free antigen density may be approximated by the inoculation rate minus rate of catabolism minus net complex association rate,

$$\frac{dh}{dt} = \dot{h}_i - \frac{h}{\tau_h} - \sum_k kc_k hx_3 + \sum_k c_k x_4 \simeq \dot{h}_i - \frac{h}{\tau_h} - \sum_k \frac{x_4}{\tau_4} \tag{6}$$

where τ_h is the average lifetime. While x_4/τ_4 may be small compared to the other terms as assumed in Eq. (5), here a summation over k [last term in Eq. (6)] might be appreciable.

With $r_b(t, k)$ and $r_f(t, k)$ the number of bound and free receptors on B-cell surfaces per unit volume, the affinity k and probability p_r that a receptor of affinity k is occupied, are

$$k = \frac{r_b}{r_f h} \tag{7}$$

and

$$p_r = \frac{r_b}{r_b + r_f} = \frac{kh}{1 + kh} \tag{8}$$

Then, it is reasonable to assume (see Bruni et al., 1975) that

$$p_d = \frac{kh}{1 + kh} \tag{9}$$

and

$$p_s \simeq \begin{cases} 1 & \text{for some sensitive interval, } \gamma_1 \leqslant kh \leqslant \gamma_2 \\ 0 & \text{for other } kh \end{cases} \tag{10}$$

The model was simulated on a digital computer (Cyber-system) with a program based on a Runge-Kutta fourth-order method of integration. The parameters used in the simulation are listed in Table 1. They represent typical observed values to simulate the injection of antigen in Freund's adjuvant; the antigen inoculation rate was represented by the sum of two functions; a step function δ_{-1} accounting for two-thirds of the total amount of antigen injected and an exponential function accounting for the remaining one-third. See Bruni, et al (1975b). Consequently, it is assumed that

$$\dot{h}_i(t) = \frac{Q}{3\tau_u V} \exp -\frac{t}{\tau_u} + \frac{2}{3} \frac{Q}{T_u V} \delta_{-1} (T_u - t)$$

where Q is the total inoculation of antigen, V is the estimated volume of circulating animal fluids in which the antigen distributes itself, and T_u is the interval of time for which the constant level of antigen is diffused from Freund's adjuvant.

The results of the simulation are shown in Fig. 2. The kinetics of the cell and antibody-molecule populations is consistent with known immunological phenomena.

From the graph of antibody production vs. time in Fig. 2, it is observed that the model predicts very accurately the experimental concentration of antibody published by Siskind et al. (1968) and Werblin et al. (1973). While consistent experimental data on the other variables have not been obtained, their graphs seem reasonable

TABLE 1

Parameters Used in the Simulation

α	5.780×10^{-2}	hr^{-1}
β_k	1.627×10^{-22}	mole/hr
τ_1	7140	hr
τ_2	71	hr
k	10^6	$mole^{-1}$
c_k	3.5×10^3	hr^{-1}
α'	10^8	hr^{-1}
α''	0.2×10^7	hr^{-1}
τ_3	200	hr
τ_4	50	hr
τ_h	100	hr
Q	3.33×10^{-8}	mole
V	0.2	liter
T_u	1000	hr
τ_u	100	hr
γ_1	0.01	
γ_2	0.10	
$x_I(0)$	0.8262×10^{-20}	mole/liter

and are similar to those presented by Bell (1970). An experimental plan has been made and preliminary experiments conducted which should proceed hand-in-hand with model development.

The object of the immune system would seem to be to eliminate antigen in some optimal manner (see Chap. 7). The quality of such biocontrol processes, however, can be very difficult to ascertain since it may involve so many considerations. For example, they may include minimum response time, minimum control effort, and minimum likelihood of failure, as well as other criteria. It should be noted that the removal rate for antigen, as shown by Fig. 2, is quite sensitive to experimental estimates of complex life and removal time, τ_4, and antigen lifetime, τ_h, neither of which is well established.

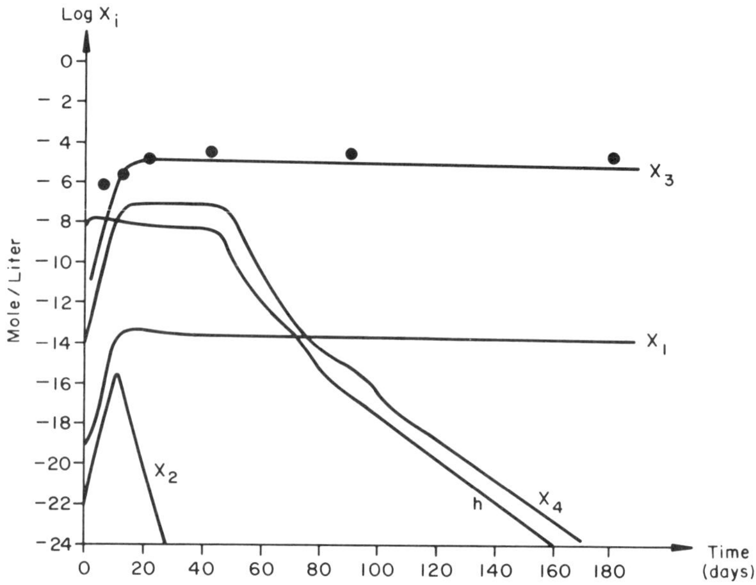

FIG. 2. Simulation response of B-cell model. Data from rabbit immunized with 5.0 mg DNP-BGG in complete Freund's adjuvant. The antibody concentration expressed in mg/mℓ by Werblin is converted in mole/liter (MW of antibody equal to 150,000 with two antibody sites per molecule).

While the simulation model assumes an average fixed affinity k, with state variables equal to total population densities (all k), it is not too difficult, in concept at least, to solve the state equations for each value of k. In this case, the stem-cell generator β_k and the initial ICC population density $x_1(0, k)$ are assumed to be normally-distributed as functions of k. From experimental results, it is also possible to approximate the dynamics by computation of state variables for a time-variant average affinity k(t). This approach is used by Bruni et al. (1975). In any case, experimental results have been so inconsistent in estimating distributions according to affinity that the assumption of an average affinity does not seem unreasonable for simulation purposes.

This model may be used to simulate a secondary response as well as a primary response, with the main difference being a much larger initial value of the ICC population density x_1 at the start of the secondary response. For this mode, however, it is more accurate to define the memory cell population as a new state variable since it is this increased population which, as a new initial condition, really causes the magnified secondary response. The memory cell population density, $x_{1m}(t, k)$, may be defined by

$$\frac{dx_{1m}}{dt} = 2\alpha p_s p_m x_1 - \frac{x_{1m}}{\tau_{1m}} \tag{11}$$

where τ_{1m} is the memory cell lifetime, and p_m is the probability that a stimulated ICC generates a memory cell. u_1 in Eq. (1) needs to be corrected so that

$$u_1 = p_s(1 - 2p_d - 2p_m)$$

V. T-B CELL MODEL

The existence of a second class of lymphocytes, called T lymphocytes, has been well established for some time. Recently, Greaves et al. (1974) provided an excellent review of T-cell properties and their role in immune control, as far as was known at that time. It should be noted, however, that this is a rapidly changing field as a consequence of a large experimental research program. Certainly, a model can be no more accurate than the theory and the experiments from which it is derived. But by proper integration of all these most important phases of research, a mathematical model and its computer simulation can lead to a more systematic program of immunological research.

Several important publications by Feldmann (1974), Dutton (1974), Herzenberg and Metzler (1974), Cantor and Boyse (1975), Dutton et al. (1974), and McCluskey and Cohen (1974) provide a theoretical and experimental base (though not entirely consistent) for the T-B model. Here it is assumed that T cells, like B cells, have subclasses such as T_x, T_y, and T_z which are referred to here as T-ICC, T-memory

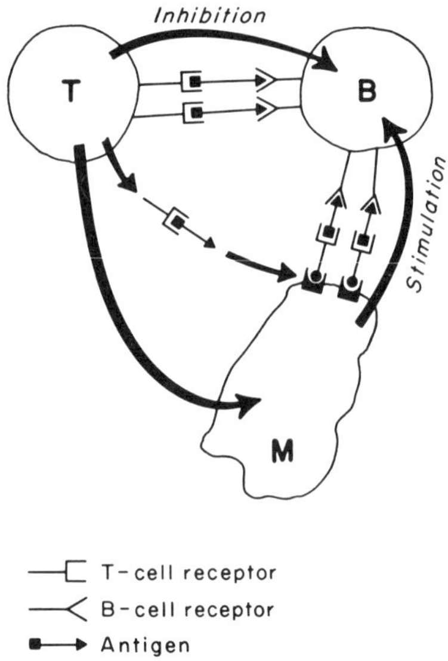

FIG. 3. T-B cell collaboration by means of antigen-antibody bridge with a macrophage, M.

cells, and T-plasma cells. Further, it is assumed that T-plasma cells do not reproduce to form other cells, but that they do generate a form of antibody-like molecules (7S IgM or so-called IgT or T-Ab).

According to the model formulated here, immune complex molecules (T complexes) of T antibody and antigen are released from their T-cell binding to bind via their Fc regions to a third-party cell such as a macrophage. The macrophage-bound T complexes in turn bind, through antigen, with B-cell receptors. Thereby, they indirectly *stimulate* antibody production. Those T complexes which bind directly with B-cell receptors have almost negligible stimulatory effect but do cause *inhibition*, by capping of B-cell receptors, from further stimulation. See Greaves et al. (1974, pp. 154-164). Figure 3 shows a schematic representation of T-B cell interaction by means of the antigen-antibody bridge with macrophage cooperation.

It is assumed in the model here that macrophages are available for instant binding with the T complexes, but that they have limited area (or receptor sites) available. This limitation results in inhibition by further direct capping of B-cell receptors as discussed above. While T-Ab does lead to removal of antigen, it should be noted that all evidence indicates the major T-Ab role is in stimulation of B-Ab production, which in turn is the major binding agent leading eventually to Ag removal.

It is interesting that stimulation and inhibition arise naturally by macrophage coupling and B-cell capping, respectively, in this model. Thus it does not require a definition of separate T-helper cells for these two functions. Further assumptions implicitly assumed here include the neglect of null cells, spatial distribution and circulation times, any dependence of lifetimes on densities or concentration of cells or molecules, any coupling between cell receptors, and the role of complement.

The following development shows that the B-cell component of the T-B cell model is essentially as given above by Eqs. (1) to (6). The major addition to this submodel includes specific stimulation and inhibition in the stochastic coefficients (p_s, p_d). Consequently, the rate of change of B-ICC population is

$$\frac{dx_1}{dt} = \alpha p_s(1 - 2p_d)x_1 - \frac{x_1}{\tau_1} + \beta_k \tag{12}$$

where consideration of added T-complex density, $x_{4T}(t, k, k')$, for B-cell binding yields

$$p_s = \begin{cases} 1 & \gamma_1' \leqslant kh + \gamma_T \dfrac{x_{4T}}{x_3} \leqslant \gamma_2', \; x_3 > 0 \\ 0 & \text{elsewhere} \end{cases}$$

and

$$p_d = \begin{cases} \dfrac{kh + \gamma_T(x_{4T}/x_3)}{1 + kh + \gamma_T(x_{4T}/x_3)} & x_{4T} \leqslant x_{4M} \quad x_3 > 0 \\[2ex] \dfrac{kh + \gamma_T[(2x_{4M} - x_{4T})/x_3]}{1 + kh + \gamma_T(x_{4T}/x_3)} & x_{4T} \geqslant x_{4M} \quad x_3 > 0 \end{cases}$$

k' is affinity of T-Ab for antigen

γ_1', γ_2' are limits of distribution of p_s

γ_T is a T-B coupling coefficient to account for T-complexes lost to bridging, and for increased stimulation of B-cell activity relative to that from simple antigen binding

x_{4M} represents the finite limitation of bindings that can be made with available macrophage surface.

These are analogous to Eqs. (9) and (10), except that kh [which was, according to Eq. (5), equal to the ratio of bound to free receptor sites] has been replaced by the ratio of the number of receptors bound to antigen and to T-Ab antigen complexes divided by number of free receptors. In addition, the parameters γ_T and x_{4M} have been introduced.

As for the previous model,

$$\frac{dx_2}{dt} = 2\alpha p_s p_d x_1 - \frac{x_2}{\tau_2} \tag{13}$$

$$\frac{dx_3}{dt} = \alpha' x_2 - \frac{x_3}{\tau_3} + c_k x_4 - kc_k hx_3 + \alpha'' x_1 \tag{14}$$

$$\frac{dx_4}{dt} = kc_k hx_3 - c_k x_4 - \frac{x_4}{\tau_4} \tag{15}$$

or

$$x_4 \simeq khx_3$$

Similar to the B-cell subsystem, the rate of generation of T-ICC population density $x_{1T}(t, k')$ is

$$\frac{dx_{1T}}{dt} = \alpha_T p_{sT}(1 - 2p_{dT})\, x_{1T} - \frac{x_{1T}}{\tau_{1T}} + \beta_{k'} \tag{16}$$

where τ_{1T} is T-ICC mean lifetime, α_T is T-ICC birth-rate constant, $\beta_{k'}$ is the rate of generation of new T-ICC (from bone marrow through thymus),

$$p_{sT} = \begin{cases} 1 & \gamma_{1T} \leqslant k'h \leqslant \gamma_{2T} \\ 0 & \text{elsewhere} \end{cases}$$

$$p_{dT} = \frac{k'h}{1 + k'h}$$

and γ_{1T} and γ_{2T} are limits of distribution.

Then it is assumed that T-plasma cells of population density $x_{2T}(t, k')$, T-Ab of molecular density $x_{3T}(t, k, k')$ and T-complexes of density $x_{4T}(t, k, k')$ are generated similarly to the way that B clones are generated, so that

$$\frac{dx_{2T}}{dt} = 2\alpha_T p_{sT} p_{dT} x_{1T} - \frac{x_{2T}}{\tau_{2T}} \tag{17}$$

$$\frac{dx_{3T}}{dt} = \alpha'_T x_{2T} - \frac{x_{3T}}{\tau_{3T}} + c_{k'} x_{4T} - k' c_{k'} h x_{3T} + \alpha''_T x_{1T} \tag{18}$$

$$\frac{dx_{4T}}{dt} = k' c_{k'} h x_{3T} - c_{k'} x_{4T} - \frac{x_{4T}}{\tau_{4T}} \tag{19}$$

or

$$x_{4T} \simeq k' h x_{3T}$$

Here, τ_{2T}, τ_{3T}, and τ_{4T} are appropriate lifetimes, α'_T is the T-plasma cell Ab production rate, α''_T is the T-ICC-Ab production rate, and $c_{k'}$ and $k'c_{k'}$ are dissociation rate and association rate coefficients, respectively, of T-complex.

With the added (though smaller) removal of antigen by T-complex, the rate of generation of free-antigen density is

$$\frac{dh}{dt} = \dot{h}_i - \frac{h}{\tau_h} - \sum_k k c_k h x_3 + \sum_k c_k x_4 - \sum_{k'} k' c_{k'} h x_{3T} + \sum_{k'} c_{k'} x_{4T} \tag{20}$$

or

$$\frac{dh}{dt} \simeq \dot{h}_i - \frac{h}{\tau_h} - \sum_k \frac{x_4}{\tau_4} - \sum_{k'} \frac{x_{4T}}{\tau_{4T}}$$

The solution of these equations for T-B dynamic control, along with experiments for appropriate parameter estimates, is in progress at this time.

VI. EXPERIMENTAL PROGRAM

In order to validate the mathematical models as presented here, two sets of experiments are in progress, one with a T-independent antigen and another with T-dependent antigen. The T-independent antigen is DNP_{60}-dextran with 60 DNP groups per molecule of dextran. This antigen has been shown to be T independent in mice by Rude et al. (1976).

Two groups of 10 animals (guinea pigs, strain 13) each were injected with (dinitrophenylated) DNP_{60}-dextran. The amounts of antigen used for both groups were 0.1 mg and 2 mg. The first group was injected intraperitoneally in saline solution for primary and secondary responses according to the following schedule: (a) first injection followed by four bleedings, one every 7 days, and (b) second injection followed again by weekly bleedings for 4 weeks. The second group was injected subcutaneously in complete Freund's adjuvant (CFA) only one time for the primary response. By radioimmunoassay, every serum was tested for the antigen-binding capacity at different times, with several dilutions of $[^3H]$-DNP-Lys and with different dilutions of the sera.

The antigen-binding capacity of every serum was very low in both groups, and it was not even possible to determine the affinities of the antibody population by the Farr technique. The same lack of response was observed also with guinea pigs when injected with a similar type of antigen such as DNP-levan as shown by Del Guercio et al. (1975). The antigen DNP_{60}-dextran does not appear to be more immunogenic with rabbits even with three repeated injections at 1-week intervals.

Two other types of experiments are planned for the antibody response of guinea pigs to DNP-dextran. DNP_6-dextran with six groups per molecule of dextran is expected to be more immunogenic, according to a pattern observed in mice with DNP-levan where the antigen with three haptens per mole of levan is more immunogenic than with 6 or 13 groups per molecule of carrier.

As suggested by studies of Del Guercio et al. (1975), the avidity of sera with very low antibody titer could be determined with the use of a multivalent antigen. For this purpose it is planned to repeat the radioimmunoassays using DNP-BSA with 6.4 DNP groups per molecule of BSA. The antigen is then labeled with Iodine-125.

The T-dependent antigen used is DNP-RNAse prepared by the method of Hirs (1962). For this experiment, 22 animals were injected with two doses of antigen (0.1 mg and 1.0 mg) in CFA for the primary and secondary response, or only for the primary response, with the same time schedule as for DNP-dextran. The first radioimmunoassays indicated a good response after 14 days from the first injection (about 80% of binding with 10^{-8} M [^{3}H]-DNP-lys).

At this time, the progress of the experiments as described above does not provide enough data to verify the computer simulation. But the plan is reported here as part of a continued development of improved models coordinated with experimentation.

VII. CONCLUSIONS

The humoral immune system is modeled here by ordinary nonlinear differential equations which may be decomposed into combinations of bilinear systems. While the model involves stochastic parameters, these may be represented by nonlinear operations and approximated by bilinear operations on state and control variables.

Even the simple model (with an average constant affinity representing the total populations of cells, and of antibody molecules) shows the kind of response expected from the humoral response to

T-independent antigens. It appears from the simulated response that the model structure is certainly as accurate as parameter resolution and published experimental data.

A dynamical T-cell component, with structure analogous to that for B-cell dynamics, is added to the model. The T-B model shows T-cell stimulation and inhibition of B-cell antibody production which is consistent with hypothesized "theories" in recent immunological developments. This model shows the role of macrophages in the regulation of antibody production. The macrophage provides a mediating role for stimulation of B-cell activity by means of more effective binding via T complexes (i.e., T-Ab and Ag), and for inhibition by limited availability of macrophage receptors. The latter leads to capping of B receptors from further excitation by T complexes without causing stimulation itself.

The model neglects numerous mechanisms which are being investigated for further analysis. For example, these include the roles of complement and nonspecific activation. Circulation of cells and antibodies throughout the body, and their delay times in recirculation back to a point in the body, have been neglected. Compartmental modeling and tracer experimentation are planned to refine the model in this respect.

Certainly, an integrated program of experimentation, modeling, and simulation is essential to the long-range success of such research.

ACKNOWLEDGMENTS

The authors wish to acknowledge the expert advice of Drs. Art Malley and Marv Rittenberg of the Oregon Regional Primate Research Center and the Oregon University Medical School in conducting this research. The work was supported in part by NSF Grant No. ENG74-15530, and related experiments were conducted by Ardvino Oratore in cooperation with the University of Rome and the Oregon Regional Primate Research Center.

REFERENCES

Bell, G. I. (1970). Mathematical model of clonal selection and antibody production. *J. Theor. Biol. 29:* 191-232.

Bell, G. I. (1971a). Mathematical model of clonal selection and antibody production, II. *J. Theor. Biol. 33:* 339-378

Bell, G. I. (1971b). Mathematical model of clonal selection and antibody production. III. The cellular basis of immunological paralysis. *J. Theor. Biol. 33:* 379-398.

Bell, G. I. (1974). Model for the binding of multivalent antigen to cells. *Nature 248:* 430-431.

Bell, G. I. and DeLisi, C. P. (1974). Antigen binding to receptors on immunocompetent cells. I. Simple models and interpretation of experiments. *Cell. Immunol. 10:* 415-431.

Bruni, C., Giovenco, M. A., Koch, G., and Strom, R. (1975a). The immune response as a variable structure system. In *Variable Structure Systems with Application to Economics and Biology* (A. Ruperti and R. R. Mohler, eds.). Springer-Verlag, New York.

Bruni, C., Giovenco, M. A., Koch, G., and Strom, R. (1975b). A dynamical model of immune response. In *Variable Structure Systems with Application to Biology and Economics* (A. Ruberti and R. R. Mohler, eds.) Springer-Verlag, New York.

Bystryn, J. C., Schenkein, I., and Uhr, J. (1971). A model for the regulation of antibody synthesis by serum antibody. In *Progress in Immunology* (B. Amos, ed.). Academic, New York, pp. 627-636.

Cantor, H. and Boyse, E. A. (1975). Functional subclasses of T lymphocytes bearing different Ly antigens. I. The generation of functionally distinct T-cell subclasses is a differentiative process independent of antigen. *J. Exp. Med. 141:* 1376-1399.

Del Guercio, P., Poirier, M. F., and Thobie, N. (1975). Immune response in mice and lack of response in guinea pigs and in rabbits to DNP on polysaccharide. *Ann. Immunol. Inst. Pasteur 126C:* 605-614.

Dutton, R. W. (1974). T-cell factors in the regulation of the B-cell response. In *The Immune System* (Sercarz, Williams, and Fox, eds.). Academic, New York, pp. 485-495.

Dutton, R. W., Falkoff, R., Hirst, J. A., Hoffman, M., Kappler, J. W., Kettman, J. R., Lesley, J. F., and Van, D. (1971). Is there evidence for a non-antigen specific diffusable chemical mediator from the thymus-derived cell in the initiation of the immune response? In *Progress in Immunology* (B. Amos, ed.). Academic, New York, pp. 355-368.

Feldmann, M. (1974). Antigen specific T-cell factors and their role in the regulation of T-B interaction. In *The Immune Response* (Sercarz, Williams, and Fox, eds). Academic, New York, pp. 497-510.

Greaves, M. F., Owen, J. J. T., and Raff, M. C. (1974). *T and B Lymphocytes: Origins, Properties and Roles in Immune Responses.* Excepta Medica, Elsevier, New York.

Hammond, B. J. (1975). A compartmental analysis of circulatory lymphocytes in the spleen. *Cell Tissue Kinet. 8:* 153-169.

Hege, J. S. and Cole, L. J. (1966). Mathematical model relating circulating antibody and antibody forming cells. *J. Immunol. 94:* 34-40.

Herzenberg, L. A. and Metzler, C. M. (1974). Antibody induced suppressors on T-cells. In *The Immune System* (Sercarz, Williams, and Fox, eds.). Academic, New York, pp. 455-470.

Hirs, C. H. W. (1962). Dinitrophenylribonucleases. *Brookhaven Symposia in Biology 15:* 154-183.

Hoffmann, G. W. (1975). A theory of regulation and self-nonself discrimination in an immune network. *Eur. J. Immunol. 5:* 638-647.

Jerne, N. K. (1974). Clonal selection in a lymphocyte network. In *Cellular Selection and Regulation in the Immune Response* (Edelman, ed.). Raven, New York.

Jilek, M. (1973). Immune response and its stochastic theory. In *Proceedings IFAC Symposium on System Identification.* The Hague, pp. 209-212.

Jilek, M. and Sterzl, J. (1971). Modeling of the immune response. In *Morphological and Functional Aspects of Immunity,* Plenum, New York, pp. 333-349.

McCluskey, R. T. and Cohen, S. (eds.) (1974). *Mechanisms of Cell Mediated Immunity,* John Wiley and Sons, New York.

Mohler, R. R. (1973). *Bilinear Control Processes.* Academic, New York.

Mohler, R. R. (1974). Biological modeling with variable compartmental structures. *IEEE Trans. Automatic Control AC 19:* 922-926.

Mohler, R. R. and Ruberti, A. (eds.) (1972). *Theory and Application of Variable Structure Systems.* Academic, New York.

Richter, P. H. (1974). Die phanomenologic der immunantwort-modell einer system theorie der evolution. In *Contribution to an Essay Competition of the Bavarian Academy of Sciences,* Göttingen.

Richter, P. H. (1975). A network theory of the immune system. *Eur. J. Immunol. 5:* 350-354.

Ruberti, A. and Mohler, R. R. (eds.) (1975). *Variable Structure Systems with Application to Biology and Economics.* Springer-Verlag, New York.

Rude, E., Wrede, J., and Gundelach, M. L. (1976). Production of IgG antibodies and enhanced response of nude mice to DNP-AE-dextran. *J. Immunol. 116:* 527-533.

Siskind, G. W., Dunn, P., and Walker, J. G. (1968). Effect of antigen dose and of suppression by passive antibody on the affinity of antibody synthesized. *J. Exp. Med. 127:* 55-66.

Werblin, T. P., Kim, Y. T., Quagliata, F., and Siskind, G. W. (1973). Changes in heterogeneity of antibody affinity during the course of the immune response. *Immunology 24:* 477-492.

Chapter 15

A THRESHOLD MODEL OF ANTIGEN-STIMULATED ANTIBODY PRODUCTION

Paul Waltman

Department of Mathematics
The University of Iowa
Iowa City, Iowa

A system of functional differential equations is derived as a model of the antibody response to antigen challenge. The delays are generated by threshold considerations in a manner suggested by the theory of epidemics. Existence theorems are derived and computability in one case is illustrated by a numerical example.

I. INTRODUCTION

As the variety of papers in this collection illustrate, the immune system's response to antigen challenge is very complex. Many facets of the mechanism are not understood and many theories are still controversial. One part of the process which does appear sufficiently well understood to profit by mathematical models is the production of antibody in response to antigen challenge. Indeed, as surveyed in the Harvey lecture of Jerne (1975), several mathematical models have been proposed. The basic, and simplest, is that of Bell (1970, 1971a,b), who is able to obtain a great deal of information from a system of ordinary differential equations. Models based on similarities to the network phenomena of neurophysiology have been given by Jerne (1975a), Richter (1975; see also Chap. 19), and Hoffmann (1975; see also Chap. 20). Models using the ideas of predator-prey dynamics with a growing antigen can be found in Bell (1973) and Pimbley (1974a,b). For a survey of these models, see Merrill (1976).

The focus here is not so much on the model as on technical problems associated with modeling the threshold inherent in such a system, and in dealing with the mathematical problems which arise from such assumptions. For example, when a sufficiently low concentration of the antigen is presented, no immune reaction may occur, while a slightly larger stimulus will produce a response. This immediately suggests a threshold phenomenon. The point of this paper is to discuss recent efforts to model thresholds in the immunological context and to deal with the mathematical difficulties which arise as consequences. The model itself will be based on a relatively simplistic view of the immune system, but this way of viewing the threshold could be incorporated into any of the abovementioned models, at the expense of increased mathematical difficulties.

Before discussing the specific model we turn first to a general view of modeling.

II. PRELIMINARIES

In the very use of the term model, a simplification is implied. This simplification can take place on various levels and it is important to distinguish them. First of all the major simplification takes place in reducing the number of variables to a conceptually manageable level. One strives to use as few variables as possible. For example, in the model presented here, target, proliferating, and plasma cells are lumped together. This simplification appears allowable if one wants only qualitative behavior of the end product (antibody). Other simplifications occur when we do not include variables which could be inserted in the model. These simplifications are not serious since if another "modeler" thinks them to be important he can put them back in. For example, equilibration time and catabolism of the antigen are not part of the model here, although it would be trivial to include them. The net effect of these two phenomena is to reduce the actual amount of antigen presented in the challenge and to delay the time of presentation. Altering the initial conditions would appear to have the same effect. The model presented here does not keep track of antigen bound to antibody, but this dependent variable could be included at the expense of another equation or could be recovered from the model's output. Antigen bound to lymphocyte receptors is included so that we may make use of it as a threshold variable.

More serious simplifications are those where factors are ignored because they are not sufficiently well understood to be modeled. For example, macrophage interaction and T-cell presence is known to be required in some cases, although the form of this interaction is not known. We skirt this by saying that our antigen is "sufficiently processed," meaning that we do not begin the model until this action — whatever it is — has taken place.

Finally, there are simplifications made for mathematical and computational reasons. For example, antibodies occur with different affinities and in different types. We assume one antibody type and affinity. This is sufficient to illustrate the basic idea for modeling thresholds, but a serious description of the immune system would have to use a system of equations, one set for each antibody type and each affinity.

III. DERIVATION

The basic driving force in the model is the rate at which antibody molecules combine with the receptor sites, and we focus on this rate throughout the derivation. If $s(t)$ denotes the concentration of unbound antigen molecules and $y(t)$ the concentration of unbound receptor molecules, then this rate is expressed by the law of mass action as

$$\begin{aligned} \dot{x} &= -rxy \qquad x(0) = x_0 \\ \dot{y} &= -rxy \qquad y(0) = y_0 \end{aligned} \tag{1}$$

where x_0 and y_0 are the initial number of each. As expressed by Eq. (1), the action is irreversible and while this is not in fact the case, we accept Eq. (1) as an approximation, assuming that the disassociation constant is small as compared with the forward rate constant. More complete discussions are given by DeLisi (Chap. 3) and Perelson (Chap. 7). It will also be convenient to include, for later use, $w(t)$, the concentration of antigen molecules bound to receptors. This reaction is given by

$$\dot{w} = rxy \qquad w(0) = 0 \tag{2}$$

Equations (1) and (2) express the state of the system until the onset of proliferation. A modeling difficulty, and a mathematical difficulty, is to express this transition in a smooth way without a loss of information for the system.

The way in which this threshold is modeled is suggested here by the theory of epidemics where a similar problem is to be found. Infectious individuals may be sustained in a population without a large outbreak of the disease if certain thresholds are not exceeded. For example, the threshold theorem of Kermack and McKendrick (1927) is of this nature. More recently, a functional integral constraint was introduced by Cooke (1967) and used by Hoppensteadt and Waltman (1970,1971) to model a threshold condition where exceeding the threshold leads to an outbreak of the disease. Here, rather than a change of form, massive growth is initiated by the lymphocytes when the threshold is triggered.

First define a time t_0 (which corresponds to the onset of lymphocyte proliferation) by

$$\int_0^{t_0} f_1(x(s),y(s),w(s))\, ds = m_1$$

where $f_1: R^3 \to R$ is a (given) positive, continuous function (positive when its arguments are in the positive octant) and m_1 is a suitably chosen threshold constant. The selection of the function f_1 corresponds to a biological hypothesis specifying the weight of the factors which initiate proliferation.

For time longer than t_0, the basic equations (1) and (2) should be modified to account for the generation of new receptor molecules on dividing cells. We take the equations to be of the form

$$\begin{aligned} \dot{x} &= -rxy \\ \dot{y} &= -rxy + \alpha r x(\tau_1(t)) y(\tau_1(t)) H(t - t_0) \\ \dot{w} &= rxy \end{aligned} \tag{3}$$

where α is an amplification factor, $\tau_1(t) \leqslant t$ and represents a delay [the rate of the reaction at time $\tau_1(t)$ is manifested as amplification at time t]. For example, $t - \tau_1(t)$, may represent the time between stimulation of a lymphocyte and subsequent mitosis. The function H(t) is given by

$$H(t) = \begin{cases} 0 & t < 0 \\ 1 & t \geqslant 0 \end{cases}$$

the usual Heavyside function. Note that Eq. (3) reduces to Eqs. (1) and (2) for $t < t_0$.

The function $\tau_1(t)$ makes the amplification depend on the rate reaction at some past time [although $\tau_1(t) = t$ is not excluded]. It is fundamental to the model presented here that $\tau_1(t)$ is to be an adaptive parameter. We tie the threshold and the delay together by defining $\tau_1(t)$ by

$$\int_{\tau_1(t)}^{t} f(x(s), y(s), w(s))\, ds = m_1 \qquad t \geqslant t_0 \tag{4}$$

We digress from the model's derivation to consider some special choices of the function f_1 in order to make its roles clearer. Before doing so we note that setting $m_1 = 0$ makes $\tau_1(t) = t$ regardless of f_1. This provides a perfectly acceptable model, but one without a time delay or threshold effect. The choice $f_1 = c$, a constant, results in $\tau_1(t) = t - m_1/c$, a constant delay, that is, Eq. (3) is a difference differential equation. A reasonable interpretation of this would be that m_1/c is the cell cycle time, although that would not give a low dose threshold. The choice $f_1(x, y, w) = w$ is biologically attractive in that it makes initiation of the proliferation phase of development dependent on the amount of antigen bound to the receptors on the cell surface over a period of time. It seems a perfectly reasonable possibility that when an appropriate fraction of the receptors on the cell surface have been bound, the cell initiates proliferation. (Note, however that this choice will assure an eventual proliferative response to even the smallest antigen dose, since w is always positive for $t > 0$.) It will turn out that this case leads to an apparently singular functional differential equation and a mathematically interesting (and previously unconsidered) question. It also produces complications in the numerical solution of the problem.

The choice $f_1(x, y, w) = k_1xy + k_2w$, where $k_1 > 0$ and $k_2 > 0$, allows the initiation of growth to depend, as above, on the proportion of surface receptors bound and on the rate of binding ($xy = \dot{w}/r$). The latter assumes some sort of biological rate meter in the cell. k_1 and k_2 represent weights assigned to each factor. The resulting mathematical problem is not singular, as we will see, so computational difficulties are avoided. Moreover, k_1 could be very small. The existence of such a "rate meter" in this situation is not suggested by any particular evidence. However, in another context, that of chemoreceptors on the surface of bacteria, rate dependence has been postulated, Brown and Berg (1974). (The author is indebted to Alan Perelson for this reference.)

With an appropriate choice of f_1, Eqs. (3) and (4) describe the system in the proliferating phase. At the end of this phase, the lymphocytes are assumed to differentiate into plasma cells which are taken to be the only antibody secreting cells in this model. To mark the first appearance of plasma cells we use another integral threshold

$$\int_0^{t_1} f_2(y(s),w(s))\,ds = m_2$$

where f_2: $R^2 \to R$ is continuous and positive in the first quadrant. We define a function $\tau_2(t)$ (another delay) by

$$\int_{\tau_2(t)}^{t} f_2(y(s),w(s))\,ds = m_2 \tag{5}$$

Evidently f_2 and m_2 must be chosen with careful reference to f_1 and m_1 in order to obtain a biologically reasonable response. Poor choices could lead to a massive production of antibody with no proliferation, for example.

The rate equation for unbound antibody is taken to be

$$\begin{aligned} \dot{z}(t) &= -sx(t)z(t) - \gamma z(t) + \beta rx(\tau_2(t))y(\tau_2(t))H(t - t_1) \\ z(0) &= 0 \end{aligned} \tag{6}$$

where the first terms represent disappearance by combination (assumed irreversible) with antigen and catabolism and the last term represents antibody secretion by plasma cells, and β is an amplication factor. Note that $z(t) = 0$ for $t \leqslant t_1$, by the uniqueness theorem for initial value problems for ordinary differential equations. Finally, the fact that antibody molecules combine with antigen changes the unbound antigen equation to

$$\dot{x} = -rxy - sxz$$

We are implicitly assuming that the number of receptors per cell does not change as the cells proliferate, so that we may convert from receptors to cells by multiplying by the appropriate constant. There is evidence that this is not strictly true, but the change may be sufficiently slight as to not modify the results of the model.

Note the integral conditions for the time delays, $t - \tau_1$ and $t - \tau_2$ may be written in differential form. For example by differentiating Eq. (5) with respect to t we get

$$f_2(y(t),w(t)) = f_2(y(\tau_2(t)),w(\tau_2(t))) \frac{d\tau_2(t)}{dt}$$

We summarize the model as follows:

$$\begin{aligned}
&\dot{x}(t) = -rx(t)y(t) - sx(t)z(t) \\
&\dot{y}(t) = -rx(t)y(t) + \alpha rx(\tau_1(t))y(\tau_1(t))H(t - t_0) \\
&\dot{w}(t) = rx(t)y(t) \\
&f_1(x(\tau_1(t)),y(\tau_1(t)),w(\tau_1(t)))\dot{\tau}_1(t) = f_1(x(t),y(t),w(t)) \\
&f_2(y(\tau_2(t)),w(\tau_2(t)))\tau_2(t) = f_2(y(t),w(t)) \qquad (7) \\
&\dot{z}(t) = -sx(t)z(t) - \gamma z(t) + \beta rx(\tau_2(t))y(\tau_2(t))H(t - t_1) \\
&x(0) = x_0 \quad y(0) = y_0 \quad w(0) = z(0) = 0 \\
&\tau_1(t) = 0 \quad 0 \leqslant t \leqslant t_0 \\
&\tau_2(t) = 0 \quad 0 \leqslant t \leqslant t_1
\end{aligned}$$

where t_0 and t_1 are defined by

$$\int_0^{t_0} f_1(x(s),y(s),w(s))\, ds = m_1$$

$$\int_0^{t_1} f_2(y(s),w(s))\, ds = m_2$$

if such exist, or by $+\infty$ if no such t_i are defined by the above integrals.

IV. BASIC EXISTENCE THEOREMS

The delays in the system in Eq. (7) are such that standard theorems for functional differential equations do not directly apply. We distinguish two cases depending on the behavior of the function f_1. For simplicity we assume $f_2(y, w) = f_2(y + w)$, that is, f_2 is a function of the total number of receptors. (While this does not give a threshold in antibody production, since y + w can never decrease, it is hoped that a reasonable response may be simulated by a large value of m_2.)

Theorem *Let* $r, s, \alpha, \beta, \gamma, \delta, m_1$, *and* m_2 *be nonnegative constants. Let* $R^+ = [0, \infty)$, $f_1: R^+ \times R^+ \times R^+ \to R^+$ *be continuous, locally Lipschitzian, and* $f_1(x, y, w) > 0$ *if* $x > 0$ *and* $y > 0$. *Let* $f_2: R^+ \to R^+$ *be continuous, locally Lipschitzian, and* $f_2(\zeta) > 0$ *if* $\zeta > 0$. *Then there exists a unique solution of Eq. (7) which depends continuously on the initial conditions and parameters.*

The proof of this theorem is given in Waltman and Butz (1975). We sketch the first part of that proof in order to make the computation of solutions more meaningful.

Let x(t), y(t), and w(t) be the unique solution of the initial value problem

$$\dot{x} = -rxy$$
$$\dot{y} = -rxy \qquad (8)$$
$$\dot{w} = rxy$$
$$x(0) = x_0 > 0, \ y(0) = y_0 > 0, \quad w(0) = 0$$

valid for $t \geqslant 0$. x(t) and y(t) are positive and monotone decreasing. $w(t) > 0$, $t > 0$, and $\dot{w}(t) \leqslant M$, for some M, so solutions of Eq. (8) extend to R^+. Since for such functions $f_1(x(t),y(t),w(t)) > 0$, $\int_0^t f_1(x(s),y(s),w(s))\,ds$ is strictly monotone increasing, the limit as $t \to \infty$ of the integral exists or properly diverges to $+\infty$. If $\int_0^\infty f_1(x(s),y(s),w(s))\,ds < m_1$, then the above functions and $\tau_1(t) = \tau_2(t) = z(t) = 0$, form a solution of the system in Eq. (7) on $[0, \infty)$. Suppose there exists a number t_0 such that

$$\int_0^{t_0} f_1((x(s),y(s),w(s))\,ds = m_1$$

Then the above functions are a solution of the system on $[0, t_0]$.

We now seek a solution defined on an interval $t_0 \leq t \leq t_0 + h$ with h to be determined.

Let $\Gamma = \{(x, y, w) | x(t_0)/2 < x < 2x_0 \quad y(t_0)/2 < y < 2y(0)$ $0 < w < 2w(t_0)\}$ and a priori restrict $h < m_1/\gamma^*$ where $\gamma^* = \sup_\Gamma f_1 \times (x, y, w) > 0$.

Consider the system

$$\begin{aligned} \dot{x} &= -rxy \\ \dot{y} &= -rxy + \alpha rx(\tau_1)y(\tau_1) \\ \dot{w} &= rxy \\ \dot{\tau}_1 &= \frac{f_1(w, y, w)}{f_1(x(\tau_1), y(\tau_1), w(\tau_1))} \end{aligned} \tag{9}$$

with initial data

$$\tau_1(t) = 0 \qquad 0 \leq t \leq t_0$$

$$\left.\begin{matrix} x(t) \\ y(t) \\ w(t) \end{matrix}\right\} = \text{solution of (4.1)} \qquad 0 \leq t \leq t_0$$

The right side of Eq. (9) with $(x, y, w) \in \Gamma$, and the initial data satisfy all of the hypotheses of Driver (1963), Theorem 3 (the requisite Lipschitz condition on the initial data is satisfied since x(t), y(t), and w(t) are all solutions of an ordinary differential equation). Note that $\inf_{\bar{\Gamma}} f_1(x, y, z) = \gamma^* > 0$ where $\bar{\Gamma}$ is the closure of Γ. Thus there exists a solution of Eq. (9) defined on $[0, t_0 + h]$ for some $0 < h < m, \gamma^*$. For this solution $(x(t), y(t), w(t)) \in \Gamma$, $0 \leq t \leq t_0 + h$ and hence

$$\tau_1(t) \leq \frac{t - m_1}{\gamma^*} < t_1 \tag{10}$$

Let $t_2 = t_0 + h$. Since $x(t_2)$ and $y(t_2)$ are positive, the above procedure may be repeated with t_0 replaced by t_2 to generate a solution on $[0, t_3]$. That this procedure may be continued to $[0, \infty)$ or to a point t_1 where

$$\int_0^{t_1} f_2(y(\zeta) + w(\zeta))\, d\zeta = m_2$$

is the major technical point in the argument and is omitted here. For $t \geqslant t_1$, Driver's theorem may again be applied. The reader is referred to Waltman and Butz (1975) for details.

The hypothesis $f_1(x, y, w) > 0$ when $x > 0$ and $y > 0$ restrict the allowable speculations as to the onset of differentiation by the lymphocytes. For example, an attractive hypothesis is that the fraction of receptors bound by antigen triggers proliferation. This could be modeled by taking $f_1(x, y, w) = w$, an example of a choice of f_1 which does not satisfy the hypothesis of the theorem. The difficulty becomes apparent when one attempts to go from the solution of Eq. (8) on $[0, t_0]$ to a solution of Eq. (9). One of the equations is of the form

$$\begin{aligned} w(\tau)\dot{\tau} &= w(t) \\ \tau(t_0) &= 0 \end{aligned} \tag{11}$$

Since $w(0) = 0$, if Eq. (11) is to make sense it must be the case that $\lim_{t \to t_0^+} \dot{\tau}(t) = +\infty$. This is an example of a singular problem. This special case was treated by Gatica and Waltman (1976).

Theorem *Let* $f_1(x, y, w) = g(w)$ *where* $g(0) = 0$, $\dot{g}(w) > 0$, *and* $\ddot{g}(w) \leqslant 0$. *Let* $r, s, \alpha, \beta, \gamma, \delta, m_1$, *and* m_2 *be nonnegative constants. Let* $f_2\colon R^+ \to R^+$ *be continuous and Lipschitzian with* $f_2(\zeta) > 0$ *if* $\zeta > 0$. *Then there exists a unique solution of Eq. (7) which depends continuously on the initial conditions and parameters.*

Again we sketch a portion of the proof. The proof proceeds as above on $[0, t_0]$. The major difficulty is to take the first step for Eq. (9) with the last equation in the form of Eq. (11). The proof of existence and uniqueness will be by the contraction mapping theorem. We consider the case when $f_1(x, y, w) = w$. The reader can supply the additional details in the more general case.

Define

$M = \{\phi | \phi \in C[0, t_0 + h], \phi(t) = w(t) \quad t \in [0, t_0] \quad 0 \leqslant \phi(t) \leqslant x_0$

$\phi(t)$ nondecreasing$\}$

where C[a, b] denotes the continuous functions on [a, b] with uniform norm (abbreviated hereafter by C when the domain is clear) and a priori take $h < m_1/x_0$. (Further restrictions on the size of h will be encountered as the proof proceeds.)

Define U: $M \to C$ by

$$U(\phi)(t) = \begin{cases} 0 \quad t \in [0, t_0] \\ \text{the unique number } \eta \text{ such that} \\ \displaystyle\int_\eta^t \phi(s)\, ds = m_1 \quad t > t_0 \end{cases}$$

(Note that η exists since $\phi(t) = w(t)$ on $0 \leqslant t \leqslant t_0$.) Let $\phi_1, \phi_2 \in M$. Then for each $t \in [t_0, t_0 + h]$,

$$\int_{U\phi_1(t)}^{t} \phi_1(s)\, ds = \int_{U\phi_2(t)}^{\tau} \phi_2(s)\, ds$$

or

$$\int_{t_0}^{t} (\phi_1(s) - \phi_2(s))\, ds = \int_{U\phi_2(t)}^{U\phi_1(t)} w(s)\, ds$$

since if $h < m_1/x_0$, $(U\phi)(t) < t_0$ for every $t \in M$ and every $t \in [t_0, t_0 + h]$. Note that $\dot{w}(t) > 0$ and

$$\ddot{w}(t) = r(\dot{x}(t)y(t) + x(t)\dot{y}(t)) < 0 \quad t \in (0, t_1)$$

so $\dot{w}(t)$ is monotone decreasing. Further, from Taylor's theorem,

$$w(t) = w(0) + \dot{w}(ct)t \geqslant \dot{w}(t_1)t \qquad 0 < c < 1$$

These estimates may be used to obtain

$$(t - t_0)\|\phi_1 - \phi_2\| \geq \frac{\dot{w}(t_0)}{2} |U\phi_1(t) - U\phi_2(t)||U\phi_1(t) + U\phi_2(t)|$$

If $t > t_0$, $U\phi$ is differentiable at t, and

$$(U\phi)_t(t) = \frac{\phi(t)}{w(U\phi(t))} \geq 1$$

Since $U\phi(t) < t$ and w is increasing and nonnegative. Hence

$$U\phi(t) \geq U\phi(t_0) + t - t_0 = t - t_0$$

for $\phi \in M$. It follows that

$$\|U\phi_1 - U\phi_2\| \leq L\|\phi_1 - \phi_2\|$$

where $L = 1/\dot{w}(t_0)$.

Now on the range of U, denoted RU, define a mapping $V: RU \to C \times C$ by $V(\phi) = (\psi_1, \psi_2)$ where in $C \times C$ we use $\max(\|\psi_1\|, \|\psi_2\|)$ as norm and where (ψ_1, ψ_2) is given by $(\psi_1(t), \psi_2(t)) = (x(t), y(t))$, $t \in [0, t_0]$, and on $[t_0, t_0 + h]$ by the unique solution of

$$\dot{u} = -ruv$$

$$\dot{v} = -ruv + \alpha ru(\phi(t))v(\phi(t))$$

$$u(t_0) = x(t_0)$$

$$v(t_0) = y(t_0)$$

Straightforward estimation yields for sufficiently small h,

$$\|u_1 - u_2\| \leq \frac{rx_0 h}{1 - \delta(h)hr} \|v_1 - v_2\|$$

where $\delta(h) = \alpha rx_0 y_0(t_0 + h) + y_0$ and

$$\|v_1 - v_2\| \leq \frac{\alpha r^2 x_0 y_0 (x_0 + y_0)h}{1 - h\rho(h)} \|\phi_1 - \phi_2\|$$

where $\rho(h) = \dfrac{r\,\delta x_0 h}{1 - \delta h} + x_0 r$. Thus

$$\|V\phi_1 - V\phi_2\| \leqslant Mh\|\phi_1 - \phi_2\|$$

On the range of V define W: $RV \to C$ by

$$W(\psi_1, \psi_2)(t) = x_0 - \psi_1(t)$$

Clearly W is Lipschitzian with Lipschitz constant one.

Define T: $M \to C$ by

$$T\phi = W(V(U\phi))$$

We have

$$\begin{aligned} \|T\phi - T\phi\| &\leqslant \|V(U\phi_1) - V(U\phi_2)\| \\ &\leqslant Mh\|U\phi_1 - U\phi_2\| \\ &\leqslant LMh\|\phi_1 - \phi_2\| \end{aligned}$$

Thus for h so small that $LMh = \alpha < 1$, T is a contraction. It is easy to show that T: $M \to M$.

By the contraction mapping theorem, T has a unique fixed point in M. We denote this fixed point by w. Let $\tau - Uw$ and $(x, y) = V(\tau)$. The quadruple (x, y, w, τ) satisfies the system of Eq. (9). Further, it is unique since the fixed point is unique and the mappings U and V single-valued.

The problem on $[t_0, + h, \infty]$ is no longer singular and the proof may proceed as above. The interested reader should consult Gatica and Waltman (1976) for details and omitted estimates.

V. SAMPLE COMPUTATION

Inequality in Eq. (10), and a similar inequality for the second delay $\tau_2(t)$, make the numerical solution of the system in Eq. (7) possible by techniques for the numerical solution of ordinary differential equations. For sufficiently small stepsize, the functional part may be treated as an ordinary forcing term. This was done for a set of realistic parameters and initial conditions. A standard fourth-order Runge-Kutta with stepsize control and error control was

TABLE 1

Threshold Times and Time of Antigen Elimination For Various Antigen Doses[a]

Ag_0	t_0	t_1	T	Ab_f
0.75×10^{-4}	32	119	120	0.57×10^{-5}
0.5×10^{-4}	32	111	113	0.24×10^{-4}
0.1×10^{-4}	33	145	159	0.33×10^{-5}
0.75×10^{5}	34	163	176	0.26×10^{-5}
0.5×10^{-5}	35	197	216	0.19×10^{-5}
0.1×10^{-5}	50	None		

[a]Threshold times are t_0 and t_1. Times are in hours and concentrations in moles per liter.

used, although after the simulation was begun, it was apparent that a program suitable for "stiff" systems would have been more convenient.

The basic parameters used were $\alpha = 1.8$, $\beta = 20$, $\gamma = 0.002\ hr^{-1}$, $r = 5 \times 10^4\ M^{-1}\ hr^{-1}$, $s = 1.0 \times 10^5\ M^{-1}\ hr^{-1}$, $m_1 = 0.3 \times 10^{-13}$, $m_2 = 1.1 \times 10^{-7}\ M^{-1}\ hr^{-1}$, and $y_0 = 1.0 \times 10^{-15}$ M. The functions were chosen as $f_1(x, y, w) = xy + w$ and $f_2(y + w) = 1.0 \times 10^{-12}\ M + y + w$. The constant term in f_2 was an artifact to avoid use of a small stepsize in the computation of $\dot{\tau}_2$.

The results are shown for some sample problems in Table 1. Ag_0 is the initial antigen dose, t_0 is the time the first threshold triggered and proliferation began, t_1 the time the second threshold triggered and antibody is first produced, T is the time when free antigen is equal to free antibody, Ab_f is antibody concentration at the terminal time. This time is either 300 hr or the time at which antigen concentration passed through 10^{-60} M. All times are given to the nearest integer.

ACKNOWLEDGMENTS

This investigation was supported by grant number R01-CA18639-02, awarded by the National Cancer Institute, DHEW.

REFERENCES

Bell, G. I. (1970). Mathematical model of clonal selection and antibody production. *J. Theor. Biol. 29:* 191-232.

Bell, G. I. (1971a). Mathematical model of clonal selection and antibody production, II. *J. Theor. Biol. 33:* 339-378.

Bell, G. I. (1971b). Mathematical model of clonal selection and antibody production, III. *J. Theor. Biol. 33:* 379-398.

Bell, G. I. (1973). Predator-prey equations simulating an immune response. *Math. Biosciences 16:* 291-314.

Brown, D. A. and Berg, H. C. (1974). Temporal stimulation of chemotaxis in *Eschericha coli*. *Proc. Nat. Acad. Sci. (USA) 71:* 1388-1392.

Cooke, K. L. (1967). Functional-differential equations: some models and perturbation problems. In *Differential Equations and Dynamical Systems*, (J. K. Hale and J. P. LaSalle, eds.). Academic, New York.

Driver, R. (1963). Existence theory for a delay-differential system. *Contributions to Differential Equations 1:* 317-336.

Gatica, J. A. and Waltman, P. (1976). A singular functional differential equation arising in an immunological model. In *Ordinary and Partial Differential Equations* (W. N. Everitt and B. D. Sleeman, eds.). Springer-Verlag, Berlin.

Hoffmann, G. W. (1975). A theory of regulation and self-nonself discrimination in an immune network. *Eur. J. Immunol. 5:* 638-647.

Hoppensteadt, F. and Waltman, P. (1970). A problem in the theory of epidemics. *Math. Biosciences 9:* 71-91.

Hoppensteadt, F. and Waltman, P. (1971). A problem in the theory of epidemics, II. *Math. Biosciences 12:* 133-145.

Jerne, N. K. (1975a). Towards a network theory of the immune system. *Ann. Immunol. Inst. Pasteur 125C:* 373-389.

Jerne, N. K. (1975b). The immune system. *Harvey Lectures*, in press.

Kermack, W. D. and McKendrick, A. G. (1927). A contribution to the mathematical theory of epidemics. *J. Roy. Statist. Soc. Ser. A 115:* 700-721.

Merrill, S. (1976). Mathematical models of humoral immune response. *Technical Report IM76-1,* University of Iowa Department of Mathematics, Iowa City.

Pimbley, G. H., Jr. (1974a). Periodic solutions of third order predator-prey equations simulating an immune response. *Arch. Rat. Mech. Anal. 55:* 93-123.

Pimbley, G. H., Jr. (1974b). Periodic solutions of predator-prey equations simulating an immune response I and II. *Math. Biosciences 20:* 27-51; *21:* 251-277.

Richter, P. H. (1975). A network theory of the immune system. *Eur. J. Immunol. 5:* 350.

Waltman, P. and Butz, E. (1975). A threshold model of antigen antibody dynamics. *J. Theor. Biol. 65*: 499-512.

Chapter 16

SIMPLE TIME-EVOLUTION EQUATIONS SIMULATING AN IMMUNE RESPONSE: THEIR DERIVATION, TREATMENT, AND INTERPRETATION

George. H. Pimbley, Jr.*

Theoretical Division
University of California
Los Alamos Scientific Laboratory
Los Alamos, New Mexico

**Present affiliation:* National Science Foundation, Washington, D.C.

The third-order model suggested by Bell consists of three coupled first-order rate equations which to some approximation describe the interaction between antigens and antibodies of the immune response. I first developed the theory of the stationary solutions of these equations, and then that of the families of periodic solutions using the Hopf Bifurcation Theorem. Next, a simpler alternate second-order model, originated by Bell, is introduced, with two coupled rate equations. This is a rougher model, but we can develop the large amplitude theory of periodic solution families, using the Andronov-Leontovich theorem on bifurcation from a closed separatix. This large amplitude family, and the small amplitude family bifurcating from a stationary solution, may join or not. If not, interesting possibilities of turning point and secondary bifurcation behavior arise, but have not yet been understood in terms of the geometry of the six-dimensional parameter space. Prospects for similarly extending the third-order model theory are discussed. The one stable stationary solution is put forward as the ground state in the health of an organism. Bifurcations therefrom are viewed as an abnormal condition, a malady.

I. INTRODUCTION

In this chapter I present a very simple mathematical model of the immune response produced when an organism is invaded by self-replicating antigens. Then I proceed to discuss the model to the extent now possible. This model was originated by Bell (1973), first in a two-population form, namely those of antigens and antibodies. Later Bell proposed the three-population version contained herein (1972), in which a population of antibody-producing cells is added to the mathematical description. The reader is also referred to papers by the author (1974a,c).

An organism is invaded by active self-replicating antigens such as viruses, bacteria, foreign cells, etc. A substance manufactured in the organism to fight this invasion is called antibody. In this model the antibody units are produced by cells that have been stimulated to do so by binding antibody, with n receptors per cell for receiving this stimulation. The antibody molecules thus produced bind with the antigen under conditions of chemical equilibrium. In this bound state the antigen is easily eliminated from the system, for example, by phagocytosis. The binding of antigen with the receptors of the antibody-producing cells also stimulates the production of more cells.

For simplicity it is assumed that each unit of antigen has only a single site for binding antibody, and that each antibody can bind only a single antigen site. This is not true for most antigens, but by treating binding sites as the fundamental units, a fairly reasonable and simple representation is obtained (see Bell, 1973).

In a more complicated model, one could have several populations of antibody-producing cells, each with receptors capable of binding a distinct type of antigen. Also, one could include additional kinds of cells capable of destroying antigens without antibody formation.

The "organism" involved in this chapter is treated as a fixed volume within which all concentrations are uniform. One could introduce compartments into a model labeled blood, lymph, etc., at the price of complicating the system. Likewise with diffusion effects.

I do take into account, however, that there is a limit to the ability of the organism to manufacture these antibody-producing cells. A saturation factor is introduced.

II. THE THIRD-ORDER MATHEMATICAL MODEL

Let $A_g(t)$ denote the concentration of antigen, $A_b(t)$ the concentration of antibody, and $C(t)$ the concentration of antibody-producing cells in the organism at time t. It is assumed that in the ab·ence of antibody, antigens multiply with rate constant λ_1, but that if antigen is bound to antibody, it is eliminated with rate constant α_1. If $(A_b)_b(t)$ denotes the concentration of bound antibody at time t, the first equation is

$$\frac{dA_g}{dt} = \lambda_1 A_g - \alpha_1 (A_b)_b \tag{1a}$$

It is assumed that in the absence of antigen, the antibody concentration decays with rate constant λ_2. In the presence of antigen it is assumed that antibodies are expended in binding antigen with rate constant α_2. On the other hand, if C_b/C denotes the average fraction of receptors of a cell bound to antigen, and that therefore $C_b(t) = [C_b(t)/C(t)]C(t)$ denotes a mean concentration of cells with receptors bound to antigen, then it is assumed that the production of antibody by these cells is stimulated with rate constant γ. There results the second equation:

$$\frac{dA_b}{dt} = -\lambda_2 A_b - \alpha_2 (A_b)_b + \gamma C_b \tag{1b}$$

Finally, it is assumed that in the absence of antigen, the concentration of antibody-producing cells decays with rate constant λ_3, while binding of antigen to the receptors of these cells stimulates the production of cells with rate constant α_3. To account for the inability of the organism to exceed a maximum concentration of antibody-producing cells, the factor $1 - (C/\theta)$ is introduced, where θ is the maximum concentration. There results the third equation:

$$\frac{dC}{dt} = -\lambda_3 C + \alpha_3 C_b \left(1 - \frac{\theta}{C}\right) + S \tag{1c}$$

where S is a possible source term.

Let $n[C_b(t)/C(t)]C(t)$ be a mean concentration of receptors bound with antigen. If we assume chemical equilibrium between bound and free antigen and antibodies on the one hand, and bound and free antigen and receptors on the other hand, and that the two forms of binding have, respectively, the association constants k and k', the laws of mass action give the following expressions:

$$(A_b)_b = k[A_b - (A_b)_b][A_g - (A_b)_b - nC_b] \tag{2a}$$

and

$$nC_b = k'[nC - nC_b][A_g - (A_b)_b - nC_b] \tag{2b}$$

where $A_b - (A_b)_b$ is the concentration of unbound antibody, $A_g - (A_b)_b - nC_b$ is the concentration of unbound antigen, and $nC - nC_b$ is the concentration of unbound receptors of antibody-producing cells.

Assuming that k = k' in Eq. (2), there results a pair of simultaneous quadratic equations to be solved for $(A_b)_b$ and C_b. Since we wish to have concrete results from our theory, I use the following rational approximations to that solution of Eq. (2) (with k = k') nearest the origin:

$$\begin{aligned} (A_b)_b &= \frac{kA_gA_b}{1 + k(A_g + A_b + nC)} \\ C_b &= \frac{kA_gC}{1 + k(A_g + A_b + nC)} \end{aligned} \tag{3}$$

[see Bell, 1973, p. 294, Eq. (4)] as well as Pimbley (1974a, p. 29; 1974c, p. 75]). The lower of the two positive solutions of Eq. (2) is needed since $(A_b)_b$ (respectively C_b) must be bounded by A_b (respectively C). We note that upon substitution of Eqs. (3), Eqs. (1) now form a closed system of differential equations (DEs).

Now we adopt a more convenient notation, letting

$$\begin{aligned} u &= A_g \\ v &= A_b \\ w &= C \end{aligned} \tag{4}$$

With a change of independent variable:

$$s = \int_0^t \{1 + k[u(t') + v(t') + nw(t')]\}^{-1}\, dt' \tag{5}$$

I reduce Eqs. (1), [with Eqs. (3) substituted], to the system of DEs that we now wish to study:

$$\frac{du}{ds} = u[\lambda_1 + k\lambda_1 u - k(\alpha_1 - \lambda_1)v + kn\lambda_1 w] \tag{6a}$$

$$\frac{dv}{ds} = \beta\{v[-\lambda_2 - k(\alpha_2 + \lambda_2)u - k\lambda_2 v - kn\lambda_2 w] + k\gamma uw\} \tag{6b}$$

$$\frac{dw}{ds} = w\left[-\lambda_3 + k(\alpha_3 - \lambda_3)u - k\lambda_3 v - kn\lambda_3 w - \frac{k\alpha_3}{\theta}uw\right] \tag{6c}$$

where I have neglected the source term S. Also I have introduced an artificial parameter $\beta > 0$ on the right side of Eq. (6b) to facilitate the later analysis. Thus we have the 10 positive "natural" parameters,

$$\lambda_1 \quad \alpha_1 \quad n \quad \lambda_2 \quad \alpha_2 \quad \gamma \quad \lambda_3 \quad \alpha_3 \quad \theta \quad k$$

and the "artificial" parameter β.

Equations (6) comprise our third order mathematical model.

III. NULL SURFACES, STATIONARY SOLUTIONS, AND LINEARIZATION

The stationary solutions of the system, Eqs. (6), occur at the intersections of the three null surfaces obtained by setting each right side equal to zero:

$$\text{I.} \quad w = \frac{-\lambda_1 - k\lambda_1 u + k(\alpha_1 - \lambda_1)v}{kn\lambda_1} \quad \text{and } u = 0 \tag{7a}$$

$$\text{II.} \quad w = \frac{v[\lambda_2 + k(\alpha_2 + \lambda_2)u + k\lambda_2 v]}{k[\gamma u - n\lambda_2 v]} \tag{7b}$$

$$\text{III.} \quad w = \frac{-\lambda_3 + k(\alpha_3 - \lambda_3)u - k\lambda_3 v}{kn\lambda_3 + k\frac{\alpha_3}{\theta}u} \quad \text{and } w = 0 \tag{7c}$$

These three null surfaces are plotted in Fig. 1. Surfaces II and III always intersect as shown in a locus of points L in the positive octant of three-space. Then it is a question of so adjusting surface I, which is a plane, so that it intersects line L. In general there are no intersections, one intersection, or two inter-

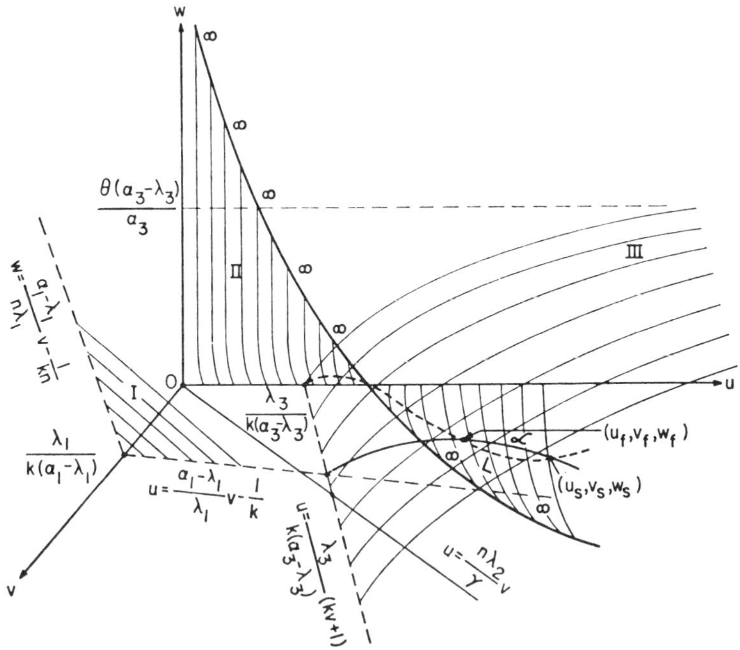

FIG. 1. Null surfaces in the positive octant.

sections. A necessary condition for two intersections, namely (u_f, v_f, w_f) and (u_s, v_s, w_s), is that:

$$\frac{\alpha_1 - \lambda_1}{\lambda_1} > \frac{\lambda_3}{\alpha_3 - \lambda_3} > 0$$

and (8)

$$\frac{\alpha_1 - \lambda_1}{\lambda_1} > \frac{n\lambda_2}{\gamma}$$

Let α_{1T} be that value of α_1 such that plane I is tangent to line L in Fig. 1. The value α_{1T} of course satisfies the condition, inequality (8). Then for $\alpha_1 > \alpha_{1T}$, the null surfaces, Eqs. (7), intersect in the two distinct points (u_f, v_f, w_f) and (u_s, v_s, w_s). In Fig. 1, line $\mathcal{L}$ represents the intersection of plane I and surface III. Thus the stationary solutions (u_f, v_f, w_f) and (u_s, v_s, w_s) occur also at the two intersections of lines L and $\mathcal{L}$.

IV. THE USE OF HOPF'S THEOREM; PERIODIC SOLUTIONS

We proceed to study the stationary solution (u_f, v_f, w_f) of Eqs. (6) nearest the origin of Fig. 1, and we linearize the DEs about this point. There results a system of three linear autonomous DEs [see Pimbley, 1974c, p. 99, Eqs. (10)]. The matrix of this linear system is given as follows:

$$A_\beta = \begin{pmatrix} k\lambda_1 u_f & -k(\alpha_1 - \lambda_1)u_f & kn\lambda_1 u_f \\ \beta k[\gamma w_f - (\alpha_2 + \lambda_2)v_f] & -\beta k\left[\lambda_2 v_f + \gamma \dfrac{u_f w_f}{v_f}\right] & \beta k[\gamma u_f - n\lambda_2 v_f] \\ kw_f[(\alpha_3 - \lambda_3) - \dfrac{\alpha_3}{\theta} w_f] & -k\lambda_3 w_f & -kw_f[n\lambda_3 + \dfrac{\alpha_3}{\theta} u_f] \end{pmatrix} \tag{9}$$

Following the usual procedures [see for example Poincaré, (1951, pp. 167-181)], the characteristic equation of the matrix, Eq. (9), is

$$F_\beta(\nu) = \nu^3 - (\text{trace } A_\beta)\nu^2 + (\text{trace } A_\beta^c)\nu - \det A_\beta = 0 \tag{10}$$

where A_β^c represents the first compound of the matrix, (9), and thus trace A_β^c is the sum of the second-order principal minors of matrix (9).

By inspection of matrix (9), we see that trace A_β, trace A_β^c, and det A_β are all linear functions of the parameter β. For $\beta > 0$ as we suppose, trace $A_\beta < 0$ and det $A_\beta < 0$, (see Pimbley, 1974c, p. 103). Moreover for

$$0 \leqslant \lambda_3 \leqslant \frac{(\alpha_3 - \lambda_1)\lambda_1\lambda_2 n}{\alpha_1\gamma + \lambda_1\lambda_2 n} \tag{11}$$

trace A_β^c is an increasing linear function of β with a positive zero intercept. Actually, the interval, inequality (11), can be extended to the interval $0 \leqslant \lambda_3 \leqslant \lambda_3^T$, where λ_3^T is the λ_3 value at a degenerate intersection of surfaces I, II, and III, (see Pimbley, 1974c, pp. 103, 104).

Being cubic with real coefficients, Eq. (10) has at least one real root ν_0. Knowing this, factorization gives

$$F_\beta(\nu) = (\nu - \nu_0)\Big[\nu^2 + (\nu_0 - \text{trace } A_\beta)\nu + (\nu_0^2 - \text{trace } A_\beta \, \nu_0 + \text{trace } A_\beta^c)\Big] \qquad (12)$$

from which we can tell that Eq. (10) has a pair of purely imaginary conjugate roots if and only if $\nu_0 = \text{trace } A_\beta$.

The occurrence of a pair of conjugate purely imaginary roots for Eq. (10) is of interest in connection with Eqs. (6) because it defines a situation where the theorem of Hopf might be applicable (see Hopf's original paper, 1942, or a review paper by Poore, 1976). Hopf's theorem asserts the existence under certain conditions of a family of stable periodic solutions of Eqs. (6), which could thereby represent a possible biological behavior.

Note that such a pair of roots occurs when $\beta = \beta_c$, where β_c is the positive root of the following equation, quadratic in β:

$$F_\beta(\text{trace } A_\beta) = (\text{trace } A_\beta)(\text{trace } A_\beta^c) - \det A_\beta = 0 \qquad (13)$$

[We may check that Eq. (13) has just one positive root by evaluating the left side at $\beta = 0$ and $\beta = \infty$, using what we have learned about trace A_β, trace A_β^c, and det A_β.]

It may be seen that the discriminant of the quadratic factor in Eq. (12) is negative in a neighborhood of $\beta = \beta_c$, and hence that there exist conjugate complex roots of Eq. (10) in the neighborhood. Let these be ν_1 and $\bar{\nu}_1$. The consideration set forth by the author (1974c, p. 106) shows clearly that for $\beta > \beta_c$ there results $\text{Re}\nu_1 < 0$, but that for $\beta < \beta_c$, $\text{Re}\nu_1 > 0$. Hence as β is increased through β_c, $\text{Re}\nu_1$ is *decreased* through zero. The author (1975), moreover, has shown that $\frac{d}{d\beta} \text{Re}\nu_1 < 0$ at $\beta = \beta_c$, so that the crossing of the conjugate roots at the imaginary axis of the ν-spectral plane takes place with transversality.

These facts now set the stage for using Hopf's theorem, according to which Eqs. (6) (with analytic right sides) have a unique family of nondegenerate periodic solutions, parametrized by β, bifurcating from the stationary solution (u_f, v_f, w_f) at the critical value $\beta = \beta_c$, with initial period $2\pi/\left|\text{trace } A^c_{\beta_c}\right|$.

The question of the direction of bifurcation is usually very difficult to settle with a set of DEs such as Eqs. (6). Cumbersome formulas have been derived in the general case which force one to resort to computation. With Eqs. (6), however, the author (1976a,b) has been successful in devising a conveniently expressed criterion. Namely, there exists a dividing value $\beta_{cc} > 0$. If the positive root β_c of Eq. (13) is such that $\beta_c > \beta_{cc}$, then the bifurcation of periodic solutions at β_c resulting by Hopf's theorem is to the left (in the direction of decreasing values of β), and the resulting family consists of stable periodic solutions. Thus if $\beta_c > \beta_{cc}$, we have the subcritical case. This is in line with our previous determination that the roots of Eq. (10) have negative real parts when $\beta > \beta_c$, for $\beta > \beta_c$ the stationary solution (u_f, v_f, w_f) is stable. There is an exchange of stabilities at $\beta = \beta_c$ when $\beta_c > \beta_{cc}$. On the other hand, if we find from Eq. (13) that $\beta_c < \beta_{cc}$, then the bifurcation of periodic solutions at β_c is to the right (in the direction of increasing values of β). The bifurcated periodic solutions are unstable and there is no exchange of stabilities at $\beta = \beta_c$.

The actual calculation of β_{cc} can be carried out using the formulation of the author (1976a,b) but it is tedious and the numerical expedience would have to be employed. From the actual formulation, however, one can discover that $\beta_{cc} > 0$ can be decreased below unity by sufficiently raising $\alpha_2 > 0$, leaving the other nine natural parameters invariant. Then with this raised α_2 (raising it higher if required), there exist values of the constants λ_1, θ, λ_2, n, α_3, $\lambda_3 > 0$, γ, and k such that $\alpha_1 > 0$ can be raised sufficiently high to raise β_c through unity. (See Pimbley, 1976b, sections 5 and 6.) By adjusting α_1 and α_2 therefore, we can arrange to have $\beta_{cc} < \beta_c$, with the consequence that bifurcation at β_c is left supercritical. Stable periodic solutions result.

V. BIFURCATION IN TERMS OF NATURAL PARAMETERS

The bifurcation of a family of periodic solutions from the stationary solution (u_f, v_f, w_f) discussed above is in terms of the real positive parameter β introduced into Eq. (6b) as an artificial parameter.

Variation of β is effectively a variation of the substitute "natural" parameters λ_2', α_2', and γ', if we define these substitute parameters as follows: $\lambda_2' = \lambda_2\beta$, $\alpha_2' = \alpha_2\beta$, and $\gamma' = \gamma\beta$, and regard the original α_2, λ_2, and γ as fixed constants [see Eq. (6b); this view of β variation was suggested by Kazarinoff].

Otherwise, recalling that $\beta_{cc} > 0$ can be depressed below unity by sufficiently raising $\alpha_2 > 0$, and that then there exist values of λ_1, θ, λ_2, n, α_3, $\lambda_3 > 0$, γ, and k such that β_c can be passed through unity by raising α_1, we can interpret β bifurcation as α_1 bifurcation. Namely, having put $\alpha_2 > 0$ high enough to have $\beta_{cc} < 1$, in raising β_c through unity by increasing α_1 we carry the entire left-facing bifurcated continuous family of periodic solutions with it. Thus is defined a critical value $\alpha_{1c} > 0$ where $\beta_c = 1$. For $\alpha_1 < \alpha_{1c}$ we have $\beta_c < 1$; then there are no periodic solutions defined in a neighborhood of (u_f, v_f, w_f). For $\alpha_1 > \alpha_{1c}$, however, $\beta_c > 1$; if β_c is not appreciably greater than unity, there are periodic solutions defined in a nighborhood of (u_f, v_f, w_f). Under these circumstances we have right supercritical bifurcation of a family of stable periodic solutions at $\alpha_1 = \alpha_{1c}$.

What does bifurcation in terms of natural parameters mean biologically?

The stationary solution (u_f, v_f, w_f) itself represents, if stable, a coexistence of antigen with antibody and antibody-producing cells.

In the first case above where we have bifurcation in terms of natural parameters, namely parameters λ_2', α_2', and γ' proportional to β, and where we vary β, we have supercritical bifurcation of stable periodic solutions from (u_f, v_f, w_f) as we decrease λ_2', α_2', and γ' through some critical values formed with $\beta_c > \beta_{cc}$. It seems reasonable that as we decrease the rate constant α_2' for expenditure of antibody in binding antigen, and at the same time decrease the rate constant γ' for production of antibody, this is a destabilizing influence. Ultimately, a critical condition is reached wherein the system breaks into oscillations which, though asymptotically orbitally stable, represent a less stable state than does the stable stationary point (u_f, v_f, w_f). The simultaneous decrease of λ_2' might be thought to be a restabilizing influence. If so, its effect must be minor compared with that of α_2' and γ'.

Let us now consider the other situation mentioned. If α_2 is sufficiently high, in Eqs. (6) with $\beta \equiv 1$, we have supercritical α_1 bifurcation of stable periodic solutions at a critical value α_{1c}. Thus, if the rate constant α_2 for expenditure of antibody in binding antigen is high, and if we increase the rate constant α_1 for elimination of bound antigen (but do nothing to increase the production of antibody), this is destabilizing for the stationary solution (u_f, v_f, w_f). Soon a critical stage is reached, at a critical value α_{1c}, where the system breaks into oscillation which, though stable, represents a less stable situation than the previous stability of the stationary solution (u_f, v_f, w_f).

It may well be possible to interpret β bifurcation of periodic solutions in terms of other natural parameters, with plausible biological meanings.

VI. AN ALTERNATIVE SECOND-ORDER DESCRIPTION OF THE SYSTEM

Presently, the above represents, to the author's knowledge, the only substantial progress that has been made in the mathematical description of the immune response by a third-order system of DEs. In Section X, I present some speculation. Numerical simulations for particular choices of parameters might be feasible and helpful. If we consider an alternate simpler second-order description, however, the mathematical theory can be extended.

In the second-order system we drop Eq. (6c) for the population of antibody-producing cells with concentration C (= w). This compels us to modify Eqs. (1b) and (6b). Namely, it is assumed that in the absence of antigen, the antibody concentration decays with rate constant λ_2. In the presence of antigen it is assumed that binding of antigen with antibody stimulates the production of antibody with rate constant $\hat{\alpha}_2$. Account is now taken that the capacity of an organism to produce antibody is limited; the saturation factor $(1 - A_b/\hat{\theta})$ is introduced, where now $\hat{\theta}$ is an *antibody* concentration which cannot be exceeded by the organism. There results a new second equation:

$$\frac{dA_b}{dt} = -\lambda_2 A_b + \hat{\alpha}_2 (A_b)_b \left(1 - \frac{A_b}{\hat{\theta}}\right) \tag{14b}$$

Equation (14a), if we were to write it, would be the same as Eq. (1a).

The law of mass action now applies only to the reaction between bound and free antigen and antibodies. Therefore, we have only Eq. (2a) with $C_b \equiv 0$. There results a rational approximation for the concentration $(A_b)_b$ of bound antibody:

$$(A_b)_b = \frac{kA_g A_b}{1 + k(A_g + A_b)} \tag{15}$$

which closes the system of DE consisting of Eqs. (1a) and (14b).

Again let $u = A_g$ and $v = A_b$. With the change of independent variable: $s = \int_0^t \{1 + k[u(t') + v(t')]\}^{-1}\, dt'$, we have the reduced system

$$\frac{du}{ds} = u[\lambda_1 + k\lambda_1 u - k(\alpha_1 - \lambda_1)v] \tag{16a}$$

$$\frac{dv}{ds} = \beta v \left[-\lambda_1 + k(\hat{\alpha}_2 - \lambda_2)u - k\lambda_2 v - \frac{k\hat{\alpha}_2}{\hat{\theta}} uv\right] \tag{16b}$$

The stationary solutions of system Eqs. (16) are the intersections of the following two null lines:

$$\text{I.} \quad u = \frac{1}{k\lambda_1}[-\lambda_1 + k(\alpha_1 - \lambda_1)v] \quad \text{and } u = 0 \tag{17a}$$

$$\text{II.} \quad u = \frac{\lambda_2}{k} \frac{1 + kv}{\hat{\alpha}_2 - \lambda_2 - (\hat{\alpha}_2/\hat{\theta})v} \quad \text{and } v = 0 \tag{17b}$$

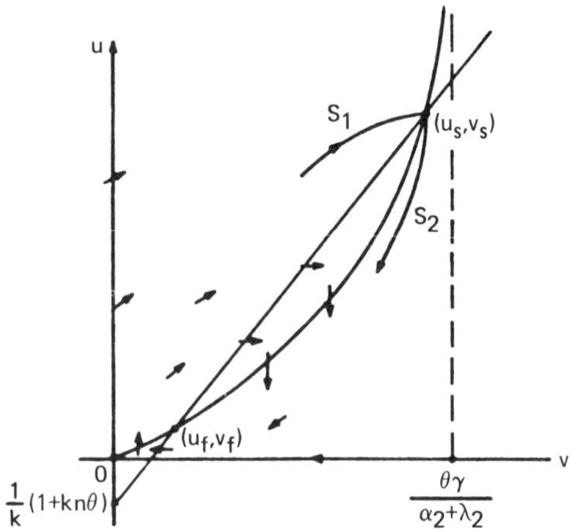

FIG. 2. Phase plane.

obtained by setting each right side equal to zero in Eqs. (16). The two null configurations intersect as shown in Fig. 2, provided $\alpha_1 > 0$ is sufficiently great. For $\alpha_1 > \alpha_{1T}$, where α_{1T} is the value at tangency, there are two intersections (u_f, v_f) and (u_s, v_s), [excluding (0,0)].

I indicate in Fig. 2 the nature of the direction field around (u_f, v_f) by arrows, and also two separatrices: S_1 approaching (u_s, v_s) as $s \to \infty$, and S_2 leaving (u_s, v_s) as s increases from $-\infty$.

As with the third-order model, we linearize Eqs. (16) about (u_f, v_f), whence we get a matrix of linearization

$$A_\beta^{(2)} = \begin{pmatrix} k\lambda_1 u_f & -k(\alpha_1 - \lambda_1)u_f \\ \beta k v_f\left[\hat{\alpha}_2 - \lambda_2 - \dfrac{\hat{\alpha}_2}{\hat{\theta}} v_f\right] & -\beta k v_f\left[\lambda_2 + \dfrac{\hat{\alpha}_2}{\hat{\theta}} u_f\right] \end{pmatrix} \tag{18}$$

The characteristic equation is now

$$\nu^2 - \left(\text{trace } A_\beta^{(2)}\right)\nu + \det A_\beta^{(2)} = 0 \tag{19}$$

where $\det A_\beta^{(2)} > 0$, [see Pimbley, 1974a, p. 34, Eq. (12)]. Equation (19) has pure imaginary roots if trace $A_\beta^{(2)} = 0$. This gives the following expression for the critical value:

$$\beta_c = \frac{\lambda_1 u_f}{v_f[\lambda_2 + (\hat{\alpha}_2/\hat{\theta})u_f]} \tag{20}$$

In this second-order case there is an explicit expression for the dividing value (see Pimbley, 1974a, p. 33)

$$\beta_{cc} = 1 - \frac{\hat{\alpha}_2 - \lambda_1 - \lambda_2}{\hat{\alpha}_2 - \lambda_2} \tag{21}$$

One can again apply Hopf's theorem, with conclusions analogous to those obtained in the third-order case. The geometric picture is much more complete here, which helps our further considerations.

VII. CONSIDERATION OF (u_s, v_s); LARGE AMPLITUDE PERIODIC SOLUTIONS

Equation (20) gives the critical value of β where Eq. (19) has conjugate pure imaginary roots. Of course, such a critical value lies in the interval, say (β_1, β_2), where Eq. (19) has conjugate complex roots. In this interval, the point (u_f, v_f) is said to have focal character, (see Lefschetz, 1957, pp. 175,176). The two values β_1 and β_2 are the (positive) roots of the discriminant of Eq. (19):

$$\left(\text{trace } A_\beta^{(2)}\right)^2 - 4 \det A_\beta^{(2)} = 0 \tag{22}$$

which is quadratic in β because the functions trace $A_\beta^{(2)}$, and det $A_\beta^{(2)}$ are linear in β.

As shown in Fig. 2, the second intersection (u_s, v_s) of the null lines, Eqs. (17), also merits attention. One can easily linearize Eqs. (16) about (u_s, v_s), obtaining the following matrix of linearization:

$$A_{\beta s}^{(2)} = \begin{pmatrix} k\lambda_1 u_s & -k(\alpha_1 - \lambda_1)u_s \\ \beta k v_s\left[\hat{\alpha}_2 - \lambda_2 - \frac{\hat{\alpha}_2}{\hat{\theta}} v_s\right] & -\beta k v_s\left[\lambda_2 + \frac{\hat{\alpha}_2}{\hat{\theta}} u_s\right] \end{pmatrix} \tag{23}$$

which is similar to the matrix, Eq. (18), but with negative determinant. In fact, (u_s, v_s) is a saddle point independent of β. Both eigenvalues of Eq. (23) are real, one being positive, the other negative. The associated eigenvectors define two real characteristic directions at the point (u_s, v_s) in Fig. 2. Along that direction associated with the negative eigenvalue, a trajectory approaches (u_s, v_s), while along the other direction associated with the positive eignevalue, a trajectory leaves (u_s, v_s); no other trajectories enter or leave (u_s, v_s). These two exceptional trajectories are known as separatrices (see Lefschetz, 1957, p. 212) and are shown in Fig. 2, respectively, as S_1 and S_2.

Using elementary arguments it was shown by the author (see 1974b, pp. 257-260) that at β_1, [the lowest of the positive roots of Eq. (22)], the separatrix S_1 connects (u_s, v_s) with (u_f, v_f), and that the separatrix S_2 lies outside the separatrix S_1. On the other hand, at β_2 [the upper root of Eq. (22)], it is the separatrix S_2 that connects (u_s, v_s) with (u_f, v_f), and the separatrix S_1 lies outside the separatrix S_2. Two illustrative drawings are given by the author (1974b, pp. 258, 260). Also, an elementary fixed point argument was made (see Pimbley, 1974b, pp. 260-262) to show that there is at least one value β^*, with $\beta_1 < \beta^* < \beta_2$, such that S_1 and S_2 unite to form a closed separatrix. We illustrate separatrices near $\beta = \beta^*$ in Fig. 3.

It is assumed for convenience that β^* is isolated from other values of β that might yield a closed separatrix. The contrary case can be handled.

The theorems of Andronov and Leontovich (1963, pp. 309-315; 1971, pp. 218-222) relative to the bifurcation of periodic solutions from a closed separatrix, now become useful. It is interesting to note that this material, as well as the Hopf result, was originally devised for mechanical systems.

First, let us define the saddle-point indicator β^{**} as that value of β for which trace $A^{(2)}_{\beta s}$ vanishes. Thus

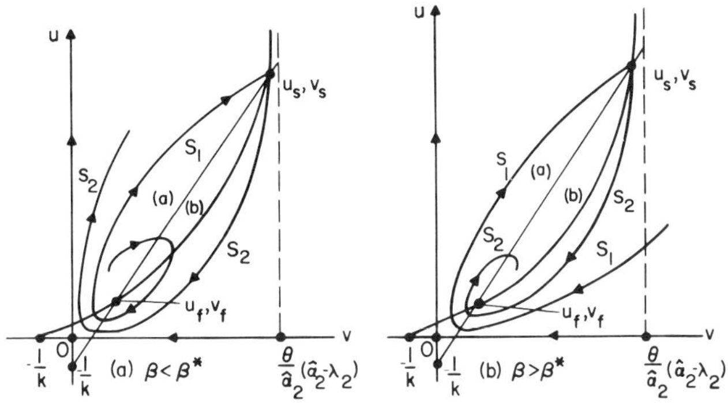

FIG. 3. Separatrices near $\beta = \beta^*$.

$$\beta^{**} = \frac{\lambda_1 u_s}{v_s[\lambda_2 + (\hat{\alpha}_2/\hat{\theta})u_s]} \tag{24}$$

According to Andronov and Leontovich (1963, p. 304; 1971, p. 214), if $\beta^* > \beta^{**}$, the closed separatrix defined for $\beta = \beta^*$ is stable in the sense that trajectories inside, but sufficiently near, the closed separatrix converge to the latter. On the other hand, if $\beta^* < \beta^{**}$, then the closed separatrix is unstable.

Again, according to Andronov and Leontovich (1963, pp. 309-315; 1971, pp. 218-223) if $\beta^* \neq \beta^{**}$, there exists a unique continuous family of periodic solutions parametrized by β, bifurcating from the closed separatrix S at β^*. If $\beta^* > \beta^{**}$, the family bifurcates to the right, and the closed separatrix disappears as soon as $\beta > \beta^*$. Moreover, the bifurcated family consists of asymptotically orbitally stable periodic solutions. On the other hand, if $\beta^* < \beta^{**}$, the family bifurcates to the left, and the solutions are unstable.

Figure 4 serves to illustrate both the small amplitude family near (u_f, v_f) and the large amplitude family near S, where S is the closed separatrix.

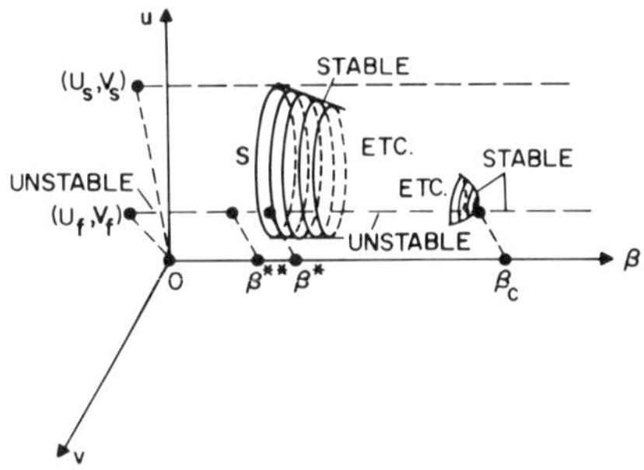

FIG. 4. Phase plane vs. β. Closed separatrix at $\beta^{*} > \beta^{**}$.

VIII. MAXIMAL FAMILIES OF PERIODIC SOLUTIONS

Both families of solutions depicted in Fig. 4 can be maximally extended by a process of "marching" in which one makes repeated application of a result given by Coddington and Levinson (1955, p. 252, see also p. 253). Let there be given a periodic solution $u_p(s)$ and $v_p(s)$ of period T_p at a parameter value $\beta_p > 0$ for Eqs. (16). Consider the following linear variational equations formed with $u_p(s)$ and $v_p(s)$:

$$\frac{dx}{ds} = [\lambda_1 + 2k\lambda_1 u_p(s) - k(\alpha_1 - \lambda_1)v_p(s)]x - k(\alpha_1 - \lambda_1)u_p(s)y$$

$$\frac{dy}{ds} = \beta_p k v_p(s)\left[(\hat{\alpha}_2 - \lambda_2) - \frac{\hat{\alpha}_2}{\hat{\theta}} v_p(s)\right]x + \beta_p\left[-\lambda_2 + k(\hat{\alpha}_2 - \lambda_2)u_p(s) - 2k\lambda_2 v_p(s) - \frac{2k\hat{\alpha}_2}{\hat{\theta}} u_p(s)v_p(s)\right]y \qquad (25)$$

Then form that matrix of linearly independent solutions of Eqs. (25):

$$\begin{pmatrix} x_1(s) & x_2(s) \\ y_1(s) & y_2(s) \end{pmatrix} \qquad (26)$$

such that $x_1(0) = 1$, $y_1(0) = 0$, $x_2(0) = 0$, and $y_2(0) = 1$. The matrix, (26), evaluated for $s = T_p$ is sometimes called the "fundamental matrix." This fundamental matrix always has the eigenvalue "one", since $x \equiv du_p/ds$, $y \equiv dv_p/ds$ is always a solution of Eqs. (25). We assume now that "one" is an eigenvalue of unit multiplicity for the fundamental matrix. Periodic solutions $u_p(s)$ and $v_p(s)$ of Eqs. (16) for which the fundamental matrix has this property are called "regular."

The result mentioned above states that there exists a neighborhood $\beta_p - \delta < \beta < \beta_p + \delta$ such that Eqs. (16) have a solution $u(s, \beta)$, $v(s, \beta)$, period $T(\beta)$, (all continuous in β), such that $u(s, 0) \equiv u_p(s)$, $v(s, 0) \equiv v_p(s)$, $T(0) = T_p$, provided that $u_p(s)$ and $v_p(s)$ are regular. The determination of $u(s, \beta)$, $v(s, \beta)$, and $T(\beta)$ is unique. Further, by the continuity of the eigenvalues of the fundamental matrix, $\delta_p > 0$ can be taken small enough that $u(s, \beta)$, $v(s, \beta)$ is regular on $\beta_p - \delta_p \leqslant \beta \leqslant \beta_p + \delta_p$.

The process of "marching" is defined as follows: starting at a regular periodic solution $u_1(s)$, $v_1(s)$, T_1 at β_1, we extend to a family of regular periodic solutions $u(s, \beta)$, $v(s, \beta)$, and $T(\beta)$ defined on the interval $\beta_1 - \delta_1 \leqslant \beta \leqslant \beta_1 + \delta_1$. Now put $u_2(s) \equiv u(s, \beta_1 + \delta_1)$, $v_2(s) \equiv v(s, \beta_1 + \delta_1)$, and $T_2 = T(\beta_1 + \delta_1)$; these are regular solutions of Eqs. (16) defined at $\beta_2 = \beta_1 + \delta_1$. Then one extends again to a family of regular periodic solutions defined on a partially overlapping interval $\beta_2 - \delta_2 \leqslant \beta \leqslant \beta_2 + \delta_2$. Now we define $u_3(s)$, $v_3(s)$, and T_3 anew at $\beta_3 = \beta_2 + \delta_2$, and perform the same process again, and repeatedly, continually extending to the right a step at a time. Performing the process ad infinitum, marching to both left and right, we attain a so-called maximal family of periodic solutions.

The author has shown (1974b, pp. 264-269) that a maximal family of periodic solutions of Eqs. (16) must terminate either in a closed separatrix S, (see Fig. 4), in the stationary solution (u_f, v_f), or in a periodic solution $u_0(s)$, $v_0(s)$, and T_0, for which the fundamental matrix, (26), has "one" as a eigenvalue of multiplicity two. (We shall denote the corresponding "terminating locus" in Fig. 4 by L_0.)

For example, in Fig. 4, the large amplitude family terminates on the left in a closed separatrix, while the small amplitude family terminates on the right in the stationary solution (u_f, v_f). On the left, the small amplitude family could actually join the large amplitude family to form one continuous family from (u_f, v_f) to S. Or, each of these families may terminate, respectively on the left and right, in separate loci L_0 of "higher multiplicity". We are as yet unable to judge from the values of the parameter set λ_1, α_1, λ_2, $\hat{\alpha}_2$, $\hat{\theta}$, k which of these phenomena should hold. The methodology is not yet sufficient for this.

Much less is understood on the question of how the parameter set λ_1, α_1, λ_2, $\hat{\alpha}_2$, $\hat{\theta}$, k governs what actually happens at a terminating locus L_0 corresponding to a higher multiplicity periodic solution $u_0(s)$, $v_0(s)$, T_0, should one exist. We do have a good idea of what *could* happen at a terminating locus L_0 of higher multiplicity as β is varied in a neighborhood of β_0, where β_0 is the value of β where L_0 would occur in Fig. 4.

Andronov and Leontovich speak of a "succession function" (1963, pp. 104-110; Andronov et al., 1971, p. 297) which could be defined on the segment of line (a) in Fig. 2 running from the horizontal v axis to the point (u_f, v_f); any locus transverse to the trajectories of Eqs. (16) would do however. This succession function seems to be a one-dimensional form of the Poincaré map. Let us measure distance along the segment from the v axis by the variable μ. For trajectories of Eqs. (16) that make the circuit around the point (u_f, v_f), the succession function maps an intersection of a trajectory with the segment (at μ) into the succeeding intersection with the segment [at $f(\mu)$]. Obviously, periodic orbits result in fixed points of the succession function $f(\mu)$.

Andronov et al. (1971, p. 398, lemmas 3 and 4) are able to discuss what can happen in the neighborhood of a periodic locus L_0 of higher multiplicity defined at β_0, as β is varied in a neighborhood of β_0, by the nature of the zero μ_0 of the function $d(\mu) \equiv f(\mu) - \mu$ which occurs because of L_0. In general it can be said that if such a zero is of even order, then there occurs a one-sided bifurcation of two families of regular periodic orbits from L_0; thus, two regular periodic solutions of Eqs. (16) exist for a β such that $\beta < \beta_0$ (or such that $\beta > \beta_0$, but not for both sides) which are members of families continuous in β, and which families approach L_0 uniformly as $\beta \to \beta_0$. On the other hand, if the zero μ_0 is of odd order, a two-sided bifurcation takes place. There can be either one family of solutions of Eqs. (16) existing on either side of β_0, or one solution family on one side and three solution families on the other side, (see Pimbley, 1974b, pp. 269-271).

This means that if μ_0 is an even-order zero of $d(\mu)$, a terminating locus L_0 is geometrically a sort of turning locus; the approaching maximal family of regular stable (say) periodic solutions reaches its terminus L_0, and another maximal family of regular unstable periodic solutions begins evolving back from L_0 in the β direction from which the approaching stable family came. Or in case μ_0 is an odd order zero of $d(\mu)$, L_0 could be a place where a pair of new families of periodic solutions are generated, that is, a forking with or without an exchange of stabilities.

If the two families shown in Fig. 4 do not join and if the large amplitude family overlaps, containing in its interior the small amplitude family for some β interval (clearly a possible situation), then simple fixed point arguments show that there exist asymptotically orbitally unstable periodic solutions between them in the phase plane. These must be members of the maximal family of unstable periodic solutions which connects the two families shown in Fig. 4. This would be in line with the first part of the last paragraph. One expects that in the second-order model, the turning type of behavior would be the rule at a terminating locus and that the forking behavior would be the exception. But again, we have as yet no hold on this question.

IX. POSSIBLE BIOLOGICAL CONSEQUENCES

At the end of Section V, possible interpretations of the transition from a stationary solution to periodic oscillatory solutions were mentioned. Evidently, according to our model, the triple (u_f, v_f, w_f) represents a "ground state", that is, a state of general health and well-being of the organism. There is antigen present, but there is also sufficient antibody that the matter is well in hand. The ground state is a stable state when $\beta > \beta_c$ (or when $\alpha_1 < \alpha_{1c}$ presuming that α_{1c} exists). With $\lambda_2' = \beta\lambda_2$, $\alpha_2' = \beta\alpha_2$, and $\gamma' = \beta\gamma$ as new parameters in Eq. (6b) representing, respectively, the rate constants for decay of the antibody level, for expenditure of antibody in binding antigen, and for stimulation of the production of more antibody, the simultaneous decrease of α_2' and γ' below critical values occasioned by the lowering of β below β_c (assuming that $\beta_c > \beta_{cc}$) evidently represents the onset of some sort of malady wherein the antigen and antibody populations perform periodic oscillations. If $\beta_c < \beta_{cc}$, on the other hand, bifurcation would be rightward and bifurcating solutions would be unstable with no biological interpretation. In this case the antigen and antibody populations could only spiral off to some more distant state, or to infinity, when criticality is reached. The malady that sets in at criticality must be sudden, intense, and uncontrollable, with death as a reasonable interpretation.

The magnitude of periods of oscillations in these biological problems may be varied. With malaria, syphilis, certain helminthic diseases, etc., observed cycles have periods in terms of months or years. On the other hand, the microscopic competition between antigens and antibodies may involve cycles, with very short periods. In our model, the length of a period seems to depend on how far β is from β_c. For large amplitude oscillations approaching a separatrix in the second-order description (see Fig. 4), periods are necessarily large. A closed separatrix itself has infinite period.

In the second-order description, we have $\beta_{cc} < 1$ by (21). Hence, when we describe bifurcation in terms of α_1 as shown in

Section V, the bifurcated solutions are always stable; likewise in the third-order description, if α_2 is raised high enough to have $\beta_{cc} < 1$.

In Section VIII, a couple of different types of behavior for a maximal family of stable periodic solutions at a terminating locus L_0 were mentioned. A turning type of behavior was described where in effect the family "turns around" at L_0, and begins evolving unstably back in the other direction in β. Thus the malady, represented by the successive stable but nontrivial periodic solutions of the maximal family, reaches a critical stage represented by the locus L_0. There being no stability at L_0, the antigen and antibody populations now spiral off to a more distant state, or the antigen population may go to infinity. Also mentioned was a possible forking behavior at L_0. If this forking were to take place with an exchange of stabilities, it could represent an onset of complications at the critical stage given by the terminating cycle L_0.

I emphasize that these interpretations are made subject to the limitations of our model. Also, there is much left to be proven about the global behavior of families of periodic solutions, as was explained in Section VIII, and as will be evident in the next section.

X. PROBLEMS OF EXTENDING THE GLOBAL THEORY TO THE THIRD-ORDER CASE

First it should be stated that, starting with the periodic solutions obtained in Section IV for the third-order description, there is no problem in defining a maximal family of periodic solutions using a marching process based on the result of Coddington and Levinson (1955, p. 352). There would be few problems in doing this, whatever the finite order of the differential equations. There would be considerable complication, however, in the matter of how such a maximal family would be terminated. It could terminate, of course, in a stationary solution (u_f, v_f, w_f). Indeed, the family arising from Hopf's theorem terminates in this way on one side. It could terminate presumably in a periodic orbit L_0 for which the fundamental matrix based on the variational equations [see Coddington and Levinson, 1955, p. 352, Eq. (2.3)] no longer has a one-dimensional eigenspace for the eigenvalue "one." Probably the alternatives available for behavior of periodic (or almost periodic) solutions in a neighborhood of such a terminating locus L_0 are more diverse than those outlined in Section VIII for the second-order description. For example, toroidal bifurcation would be geometrically possible in the third-order case.

The stationary solution (u_s, v_s, w_s) turns out to be a nodal-saddle in Poincaré's lexicon (1951, pp. 160, 167-181), with a single pair of exceptional trajectories leading away, and a separatrix surface ruled out by trajectories converging to the point. The nature of (u_s, v_s, w_s) of course does not change with the value of $\beta > 0$. Also, the nature of (u_s, v_s, w_s) is the same whatever the positive parameters in Eqs. (6), such that surfaces I, II, and III form the two points of intersection.

As yet we can only speculate whether there can exist some value β^* such that a trajectory leading away from (u_s, v_s, w_s) along an exceptional direction can globally join in some way with the trajectories making up the separatrix surface [whose component trajectories lead towards (u_s, v_s, w_s)], so as to form a closed surface surrounding (u_f, v_f, w_f). If so, could there be bifurcation of some periodic entities from such a closed separatrix surface, in a fashion reminiscent of Andronov and Leontovich in the second-order description, as β is made to differ from β^*? It would seem that such matters must be settled before further progress can be made in understanding this model!

ACKNOWLEDGMENTS

Work performed under the auspices of the U. S. Energy Research and Development Administration.

REFERENCES

Andronov, A. A. and Leontovich, E. A. (1963). Generation of limit cycles from a separatrix forming a loop and from the separatrix of an equilibrium state of saddle-node type. *AMS Transl.* Series 2, *33:* 189-231.

Andronov, A. A., Leontovich, E. A., Gordon, I. I., and Maier, A. G. (1971) *Theory of Bifurcations of Dynamic Systems on a Plane* (transl. from the Russian). U.S. Dept. Commerce, NTIS, Springfield, Virginia.

Bell, G. I. (1972). Private communication.

Bell, G. I. (1973). Predator-prey equations simulating an immune response. *Math Biosciences 16:* 291-314.

Coddington, E. A. and Levinson, N. (1955). *Theory of Ordinary Differential Equations.* McGraw-Hill, New York.

Hopf, E. (1942). Abzweigung einer periodischen Lösung eines differential systems. *Berichten der Mathematische-Physicalischen Klasse der Sachsischen Akademie der Wissenchaften zu Leipzig 94:* 3-22.

Lefshetz, S. (1957). *Differential Equations; Geometric Theory.* Interscience, New York.

Pimbley, G. H., Jr. (1974a). Periodic solutions of predator-prey equations simulating an immune response, I. *Math. Biosciences 20:* 27-51.

Pimbley, G. H., Jr. (1974b). Periodic solutions of predator-prey equations simulating an immune response, II. *Math. Biosciences 21:* 251-277.

Pimbley, G. H., Jr. (1974c). Periodic solutions of third order predator-prey equations simulating an immune response. *Arch. Rat. Mech. Anal. 55:* 43-123.

Pimbley, G. H., Jr. (1975). On the generation of periodic solutions in a third order model of the immune response. Unpublished note.

Pimbley, G. H., Jr. (1976a). A direction of bifurcation formula in the theory of the immune response. *Bull. AMS 82:* 56-58.

Pimbley, G. H., Jr. (1976b). Bifurcation behavior of periodic solutions of the third order simulated immune response problem. *Arch. Rat. Mech. Anal. 64:* 169-192.

Poincaré, H. (1951). *Collected Works* Vol. 1. Gauthier-Villus, Paris.

Poore, A. B. (1976). On the theory and application of the Hopf-Friedrichs bifurcation theory. *Arch. Rat. Mech. Anal. 60:* 371-393.

Chapter 17

A MATHEMATICAL MODEL OF THE IMMUNE SURVEILLANCE AGAINST CANCER

René Lefever and Ricardo Garay

Chimie Physique II, Faculté des Sciences
Université Libre de Bruxelles
Brussels, Belgium

We first review the salient points of the Thomas-Burnet theory of immunological surveillance against cancer and some important experiments which have tested the main predictions of this theory. This discussion provides us with a set of well-established facts. On this basis, a phenomenological model is set up which permits us to define three domains in which the normal state of a tissue is either stable, metastable, or unstable. The relation between cytotoxic cell motion and these stability properties is analyzed. A stochastic description of the model, incorporating the local character of fluctuations, is presented. It provides a way of calculating the critical size of the smallest fluctuations able to initiate tumor growth. This stochastic analysis also demonstrates that in some cases, the size of critical fluctuations may exhibit an *upper* bound.

I. INTRODUCTION

Our present understanding of the cancer problem suggests that the cancerous transformation of a normal tissue could broadly be described as follows (Ehrlich, 1957; Thomas, 1959; Burnet, 1964, 1967, 1971; Salomon, 1975; Calvin, 1975; Cairns, 1975):

1. In normal tissues, the pattern of organization is determined by a complex interplay of short- and long-range interactions between cells. These interactions control the mechanism of cellular replication.
2. Various proteins which are genetically coded mediate these interactions.
3. Any disturbance in this genetic control, either "spontaneous" or due to the action of environmental factors (physical, chemical, or biological), could yield a cell with an

abnormally coded pattern of proteins. Subsequently, these cells may exhibit a different capacity of response to the cellular interactions with normal cells. In the case of the malignant transformation, the cells are characterized by a high proliferative advantage.

4. The normal mechanisms of defense tend to destroy the abnormal cells or to damp down their rate of proliferation. It seems that one of the most important mechanisms of defense involves the immune system. The immune cells recognize the abnormal proteins and destroy the cells which bear them. This means that the immune system exerts some sort of "surveillance" on the very small population of transformed cells ("microcancer population").

The exact nature and properties of the processes mentioned in (1) to (3), are still largely hypothetical. This is mainly due to the fact that these processes correspond to subtle molecular changes taking place at the level of one cell. On the contrary, in respect to point (4), even if the underlying molecular events are not known in detail, at least there exist excellent data on the kinetics of tumor growth and on the competition of this process with the immune surveillance. Our purpose will be to show that this information can be used to build up a mathematical model which permits us to study and characterize the phenomenon of immune surveillance against cancer from a general physical point of view.

In Section II, we first summarize the Thomas-Burnet theory of immunological surveillance as it was formulated originally. Thereafter, in Section III, the basic assumptions and predictions of the theory are discussed in more detail in the light of recent experimental observations. In this way we introduce the minimum well-established information which is necessary to set up our phenomenological model. The results obtained with this model in Sections IV and V tend to demonstrate the metastable character of the normal microcancer state of tissues. The role of the highly particular kind of motion of the cytotoxic cells is analyzed. The last Section

(VI) is entirely devoted to the importance of spontaneous statistical fluctuations in the onset of cancer growth. Our results show that in order to understand completely this phenomenon it is necessary to supplement the usual average kinetic description with a more refined treatment in which fluctuations appear explicitly: in this way, features which would not be found or accounted for otherwise can be established.

II. THE THOMAS-BURNET THEORY OF IMMUNOLOGICAL SURVEILLANCE OF CANCER

The increasing knowledge of the immune processes associated with transplantation phenomena accumulated in the 1950s lead Thomas to develop an earlier suggestion of Ehrlich. He postulated that "the phenomena of homograft rejection will turn out to represent a primary mechanism of natural defense against neoplasia" (Thomas, 1959; Ehrlich, 1957). Some years later, Burnet developed this idea in a series of papers (Burnet, 1964, 1967, 1971). Schematically this theory can be stated as follows:

1. Spontaneous somatic mutations represent a continuous source of cellular transformation.
2. Most of the transformed cells have antigenic qualities different from those of the original cells from which they are derived.
3. These antigenic differences are recognized as foreign and an immune response is developed. This immune response is mediated by the T lymphocytes and is equivalent to homograft rejection.

It was in the context of this theory that Burnet claimed that the thymus-dependent immune system "is more primitive than the antibody producing (B) system and must have evolved for a function related to the structural and chemical integrity of the body rather than for better protection against invasive microorganisms" (Burnet, 1971).

As a natural consequence of all these developments Burnet is led to predict that cancer arises:

1. Under all conditions that correspond to a depression of the immune system (in the ante- and perinatal period, in old age, upon the action of some chemicals, radiations, etc.).
2. When transformed cells lack antigenicity.
3. When the growth potentiality of the transformed cells is capable of overriding any immunological control.

Together with this theory, Burnet reported an experimental basis which is consistent with the concept of immunological surveillance (see, for example, Burnet, 1964). In the following years further experimental and clinical evidence has accumulated on the subject. Although in the beginning this evidence seemed to confirm Burnet's hypotheses, in the last few years some of the postulates have been seriously questioned. Our objective in the following section is not to consider in detail all the experimental and clinical data relevant to the Thomas-Burnet theory, or to take part in the polemics generated by this subject (see, for example: Prehn and Lappé, 1971; Prehn, 1976; Salomon, 1975; Möller and Möller, 1976; Rygaard and Povlsen, 1976). Rather, we shall take the framework of the Thomas-Burnet theory as a starting point; it furnishes the appropriate basis to introduce and discuss the biologically plausible information which is necessary to make possible the analysis of the phenomenon of cancer onset in mathematical terms.

III. EXPERIMENTAL OBSERVATIONS RELATED TO THE MECHANISM OF CANCER ONSET

A. Source of Transformed Cells

As we have seen before, one of the main hypotheses made by Burnet was that transformed cells continuously appear in the organism as a result of spontaneous somatic mutations. At the time it was enunciated, this hypothesis seemed supported by the high incidence of spontaneous point mutations which are of the order of 10^6 to 10^7 mutations/gene day^{-1} in the human being (Burnet, 1967). This high value led Burnet to think that spontaneous somatic mutations were the natural source of malignant clones; during the course of evolution this process would constitute the selective pressure maintaining cell-mediated immunity (Burnet, 1971). However, in the last few years conclusive evidence has accumulated against the existence of a relation between spontaneous somatic mutations and carcinogenesis, in particular from the very precise and long experiments made with the nude mouse (Rygaard and Povlsen, 1976). The nude mouse is a mutant which lacks the thymus-dependent immune system. Under germ-free conditions, *no spontaneous malignant tumors have been observed* on 15,700 nude mice studied for a total of approximately 5600 years of mouse life. On the contrary, the nude mice have been found to be much more sensitive to some oncogenic viruses.

Thus, although it is still admitted that the primary event in the transformation of normal cells into cancerous ones is some sort of genetic damage, the point of view generally prevailing now is that this transformation needs the presence of environmental physical, chemical, or biological agents (Ames, 1973; Calvin, 1975). The nature of the alteration induced by these agents is unknown; it has been suggested that it could be "some accumulation of errors" during DNA replication or repair (a minimum number of five was suggested by Cairns, 1975). These errors could also consist of abnormal recombinations, deletions, interpositions of nucleotide sequences, or insertions of viral genetic material into the DNA of the host, etc. For the purpose of our theory, mechanisms of carcinogenesis need not be precisely defined; we only have to retain the essential fact that there exists in the tissue considered a continuous source of abnormal cells; in the kinetic equations it will simply enter through a pheonomenological constant. The value of this coefficient should depend strongly on environmental factors and will usually be very small. Then, we can expect the population of transformed cells in tissues normally to be extremely low and hardly detectable. However, indirect evidence suggests that for some malignant cells this population is probably higher than expected; they are more frequently diagnosed histologically in random pathological material than they are found clinically in comparable populations (Burnet, 1967).

B. The Antigenicity of Transformed Cells

It was clearly seen many years ago that induced tumors, either by chemicals (Foley, 1953; Prehn and Main, 1957) or by viruses (Habel, 1961; Sjögren et al., 1961) were capable of manifesting antigenicity in the strain of origin. Antigenic changes consist in the loss of some normal antigens and/or in the appearance of new antigens on the tumor cell surface (Zilber, 1958; Baldwin and Moore, 1968; Burnet, 1971). It was found later that the tumor cell surface is also immunogenic to the primary host (Haughton and Whitmore, 1976). As the Thomas-Burnet theory requires, this response is based in the thymus-dependent system. However only in certain rare cases can it lead to the destruction of the tumor.

C. Nature of the Effector Cell

As required by Burnet's formulation, a cytotoxic acitvity of T lymphocytes was demonstrated against a great variety of cancer cells either in vitro or in vivo (Brunner et al., 1968; Cerottini and Brunner, 1974; Hellström and Hellström, 1971, 1973, 1974). The properties of this reaction can be summarized as follows: it is specific against the antigens to which the T lymphocytes were sensitized; it has an extremely high lytic efficiency; and it does not need the presence of helper cells (Wagner et al., 1972; Lohmann-Matthes and Fischer, 1973). However, in spite of the high cytotoxic activity commonly observed in vitro, the immune response elicited against tumor cells in vivo is very frequently inappropriate for tumor rejection in syngeneic animals (Baldwin, 1976) and in the primary host (Haughton and Whitmore, 1976). This failure was assigned to some inhibitory mechanism operating in vivo. It seems that at least in some cases this failure is due to the presence of blocking factors which interact with the antigens of the tumor cell surface, the sensitized lymphocytes (Hellström and Hellström, 1974), or to some other kind of immunosuppressive agents probably operating in vivo (Plescia et al., 1975; Baldwin, 1976).

Besides the questioned efficiency of the surveillance exerted by the T lymphocytes, it was found that other cellular species have a cytotoxic activity. The role of macrophages in tumor immunity has been firmly established. It was seen that macrophages infiltrate developing tumors and that their population may, in some cases, be up to 56% of the total number of cells present (Evans, 1972); furthermore, the percentage of infiltration is proportional to the tumor resistance in syngeneically transplanted rats (Baldwin, 1976). This cytotoxic activity of macrophages was demonstrated in vitro and in vivo (Evans and Alexander, 1970; Lohmann-Matthes and Fischer, 1973; Pimm and Baldwin, 1975; Moore et al., 1975); it depends on activation factors, some of which, like BCG and phytohemagglutinin, are "nonspecific" while others are specific and are released by the T lymphocytes in contact with cancerous cells.

It is possible that other cellular species or subpopulations of the species mentioned (from the immune system or not) have a cytotoxic activity against cancerous cells. As far as we are concerned, we do not need to define the exact nature of the cytotoxic cellular species involved, we shall simply assume that there exists in the organism a population of cytotoxic cells (certainly formed by different cellular species) which can interact with and destroy the cancerous cells.

D. Properties of the Reaction Between Cytotoxic and Cancerous Cells

It has been established that for obtaining a cytotoxic effect, a "cellular contact" between T lymphocytes or macrophages and the cancerous cells is needed (Evans and Alexander, 1970; Lohmann-Matthes and Fischer, 1973; Henkart and Blumenthal, 1975). This fact allows us to assume that cytotoxic cells have at least two states: without cancerous cells bound to their surface (M_0) or with cancerous cells bound (M_1).

T lymphocytes in contact with transformed cells emit chemical signals usually called lymphokines (Dumonde et al., 1969). The lymphokines enhance the cytotoxic activity by the cooperation of several effects:

1. The lymphokines may modify the motion of the cytotoxic cells and induce their accumulation in the regions where the malignant cells are present.
2. The lymphokines may increase the cytotoxic activity of cytotoxic cells.
3. They may stimulate the replication of cytotoxic cells.

The best characterized lymphokine, usually called MIF (migration inhibition factor), mediates at least the first of these effects (Bloom and Bennet, 1966; Svejcar et al., 1967; Bernstein et al., 1971; Hochova et al., 1975; Nossal, Chap. 5). It is a very well established fact that MIF inhibits the diffusion of macrophages, and some recent data indicate that it can also inhibit the migration of other cells (Weisbart et al., 1975). Thus, in order to study the local effect of MIF, we will assume that the motility of cytotoxic cells is reduced in the regions where malignant cells are present.

E. The Stochastic Character of Cancer Onset

The results summarized above show that there exists an abundance of kinetic data and observations on the phenomenology of the cancerous transformation. The picture which emerges at that level is fairly coherent, and we can derive from it the ingredients of a mathematical description. To some extent the underlying molecular events were satisfactorily predicted by the Thomas-Burnet theory [see, for example, points (2) and (3) in Section II]; other aspects, like the source of malignant cells [point (1)], need to be reformulated. Below, five dimensionless parameters will be derived which characterize completely the average stability properties of tissues. However, in the case of carcinogenesis it is particularly true that the mathematical analysis needs to be pursued beyond a description of average behaviors. As Huebner points out, carcinogenesis needs to be handled in stochastic terms (Huebner et al., 1970). This is so because the emergence of a cancer is a rare and random process which in most cases *seems to arise from a single cell.* The monoclonal origin of some cancers is indeed very well documented (Burnet, 1971; Linder and Gartler, 1965; Prehn, 1970; Potter et al., 1973; Friedman and Fialkow, 1976). There are also other reasons which lead us to think that the cancer population is extremely small and thus undergoes appreciable fluctuations. The importance of fluctuations is further supported by the absence of a strict correlation, as assumed by Burnet (see above), between the occurrence of cancer and the immunological state of the host (Möller and Möller, 1976). An approach to these probabilistic aspects is reported in Section VI.

IV. A MODEL OF THE IMMUNE SURVEILLANCE AGAINST CANCER

Let us consider a volume element (ΔV) containing N cells of a given tissue (normal + malignant cells). The three cellular populations of interest are the normal cells of the tissue, the malignant cells (X), and the cytotoxic cells. Cytotoxic cells may exist under two states: not bound (M_0) and bound (M_1) to transformed cells.

As discussed above, the actual experimental knowledge of the onset of cancer permits us to formulate the following general hypotheses.

A. Hypotheses of the Model

1. Some normal cells are continuously transformed into cancerous ones at a very small rate (A) which may depend on a great number of systemic and environmental parameters.

2. The transformed cells have a high proliferative advantage, and the exponential growth of their population is characterized by the constant λ.

3. The role of cytotoxic cells is to limit the size of the population of transformed cells by recognizing and destroying them.

This yields the following simplified kinetic scheme:

$$
\begin{aligned}
\text{Normal cells} &\xrightarrow{A} X \\
X &\xrightarrow{\lambda} 2X \\
X + M_0 &\xrightarrow{k_1} M_1 \xrightarrow{k_2} M_0 + P
\end{aligned}
\tag{1}
$$

In this scheme P stands for the products of degradation of X, and the kinetic constants k_1 and k_2 characterize the binding and the destruction of the malignant cells by the cytotoxic cells. These constants, k_1 and k_2, can be greatly enhanced through the previous sensitization of T lymphocytes by the transformed cells or can be depressed either by the presence of blocking factors which prevent the recognition of malignant cells or by the action of immunosuppressive agents.

Finally we will take into account the mobility of cytotoxic cells inside the tissue.

4. In the absence of transformed cells, we assume that the local fluxes of cytotoxic cells are Fickian with diffusion coefficient μ. In the presence of a sufficient number of transformed cells, the T lymphocytes become sensitized and release lymphokines (MIF) which slow down the motion of M_0 and M_1. It must be stressed that although this effect may create important local accumulations of cytotoxic cells, it cannot be compared with a chemotactic type of attraction. The latter would orient the motion of cytotoxic cells into some particular direction. Here, rather, we have a *sticky barrier* effect which decreases the diffusion coefficient of cytotoxic cells and tends to immobilize them once they enter a domain where transformed cells are present. Therefore, we have introduced a modified diffusion law in which the effect of lymphokines appears through a phenomenological constant K (Lefever and Garay, 1977). For further discussion of the effect of MIF, see Chap. 5.

B. General Kinetic Equations

We describe the evolution in time and space of the (X, M_0, M_1) cellular populations by the following set of kinetic equations:

$$\frac{\partial X}{\partial t} = (N - X)(A + \lambda X) - k_1 M_0 X \tag{2}$$

$$\frac{\partial M_0}{\partial t} = -k_1 M_0 X + k_2 M_1 + \tilde{\mu} \frac{\partial^2}{\partial r^2}\left(\frac{M_0}{1 + KX}\right) \tag{3}$$

$$\frac{\partial M_1}{\partial t} = k_1 M_0 X - k_2 M_1 + \tilde{\mu} \frac{\partial^2}{\partial r^2}\left(\frac{M_1}{1 + KX}\right) \tag{4}$$

In Eq. (2) the multiplicative factor (N - X) expresses the constancy of N, the total number of normal plus malignant cells contained in the (ΔV). The constant K in Eqs. (3) and (4) measures the intensity of the effect of MIF. For simplicity, we have not included the synthesis of cytotoxic cells by the immune system. However, in a more detailed analysis the effect of certain lymphokines which induce cytotoxic cell replication could be taken into account without much difficulty.

In regard to the validity of our assumptions we also wish to make the following points.

1. At least for certain well known in vitro systems, as the activated peritoneal macrophages vs. lymphoma cells (Evans and Alexander, 1970), there exist precise kinetic data which can easily be interpreted on the basis of Eqs. (2) to (4) (Garay and Lefever, 1977a,b). In these experiments, the production term A and diffusion effects can be neglected. Moreover, a quasi steady-state regime may be assumed for Eqs. (3) to (4). Accordingly, the initial growth of the X cell population is simply given by:

$$\frac{dX}{dt} = \lambda NX - \frac{k_1 \sigma_0 X}{[1 + (k_1/k_2)X]} \tag{5}$$

where $\sigma_0 = M_0 + M_1$ = constant (experimentally controlled). This equation fits the experimental data very well and was used to evaluate the values of k_1 and k_2 for this particular system (Garay and Lefever, 1977a,b and see below).

2. The phenomenological law proposed to describe the local fluxes of cytotoxic cells is rather particular and has never been considered, to our knowledge, in usual physiochemical systems. Nevertheless, we have demonstrated that it could be derived rigorously from a complex mechanism which represents the sensitization of T lymphocytes by transformed cells and the release of MIF. The interaction between MIF and cytotoxic cells then decreases the mobility of the latter to a negligible value.

V. ANALYSIS OF A SIMPLIFIED VERSION OF EQUATIONS (2) TO (4)

A. Phenomenological Parameters

The analytic study of Eqs. (2) to (4) is a problem of great mathematical complexity. However, most properties and predictions of our model can conveniently be discussed by considering the following simplified situation: inside a mass of tissue of volume (V) we isolate a small subvolume element (ΔV). The state of (V - ΔV) is time invariant and plays the role of fixed boundary condition to (ΔV). Both volumes are assumed homogeneous, but their cellular population densities may become different due to cancer induction processes taking place inside (ΔV), or because of the exchange of cytotoxic cells between (ΔV) and (V - ΔV). To describe these cellular exchanges, the continuous diffusion law considered above may be replaced by a discrete two "box" approximation. Equations (2) to (4), as applied to (ΔV), can then be transformed into a set of ordinary differential equations:*

---

*To derive Eqs. (7) and (8) from Eqs. (3) and (4) we may approximate

$$\begin{aligned}\tilde{\mu}\frac{\partial^2}{\partial r^2}(\cdot) &\simeq \frac{\tilde{\mu}}{\Delta r^2}\left[(\cdot)_{V+\Delta V} - 2(\cdot)_{\Delta V} + (\cdot)_{V-\Delta V}\right]\\ &= \frac{2\tilde{\mu}}{\Delta r^2}\left[(\cdot)_{V-\Delta V} - (\cdot)_{\Delta V}\right]\\ &\triangleq \left[(\cdot)_{V-\Delta V} - (\cdot)_{\Delta V}\right]\end{aligned}$$

$$\frac{dX}{dt} = (N - X)(A + \lambda X) - k_1 M_0 X \tag{6}$$

$$\frac{dM_0}{dt} = -k_1 M_0 X + k_2 M_1 + \mu\left[\left(\frac{M_0}{1 + KX}\right)_{V-\Delta V} - \left(\frac{M_0}{1 + KX}\right)_{\Delta V}\right] \tag{7}$$

$$\frac{dM_1}{dt} = k_1 M_0 X - k_2 M_1 + \mu\left[\left(\frac{M_1}{1 + KX}\right)_{V-\Delta V} - \left(\frac{M_1}{1 + KX}\right)_{\Delta V}\right] \tag{8}$$

where the subscripts in the diffusion terms denote evaluation inside (ΔV) or ($V - \Delta V$). Furthermore, as suggested in our previous discussion of numerical data (Section IV), we shall assume that Eqs. (7) and (8) can be considered to be in a quasi steady state. Setting the left sides of Eqs. (7) and (8) to zero and adding the equations, one finds

$$M_1 = \sigma_0 \frac{1 + KX}{1 + KX_1} - M_0 \tag{9}$$

where $\sigma_0 = (M_0 + M_1)_{V-\Delta V}$ is a constant in $V - \Delta V$ and $X_1 = X_{V-\Delta V}$. In $V - \Delta V$ the effect of transport is negligible, and hence in the quasi steady state

$$k_1 M_0\Big|_{V-\Delta V} X_1 = k_2\left(\sigma_0 - M_0\Big|_{V-\Delta V}\right)$$

or

$$M_0\Big|_{V-\Delta V} = \frac{k_2 \sigma_0}{k_2 + k_1 X_1} \tag{10}$$

Substituting Eqs. (9) and (10) into the steady-state form of Eq. (7) and solving for M_0, and then substituting into Eq. (6) yields

$$\frac{dx}{d\tau} = \alpha + (1 - \theta x)x - \beta x \frac{(1 + \gamma x)[(1 + x_1)(1 + \gamma x) + D]}{(1 + \gamma x_1)(1 + x_1)[(1 + x)(1 + \gamma x) + D]} \tag{11}$$

where

$$\tau = (\lambda N - A)t \quad L = \frac{-k_1}{k_2} \quad \alpha = \frac{ANk_1}{k_2(\lambda N - A)} \quad \beta = \frac{k_1 \sigma_0}{\lambda N - A}$$
$$\gamma = \frac{k_2 K}{k_1} \quad \theta = \frac{k_2}{k_1} \frac{\lambda}{\lambda N - A} \quad D = \frac{\mu}{k_2} \quad x = LX \tag{12}$$

We see that the eight constants of the model can be combined into five dimensionless parameters α, β, θ, γ, and D whose values entirely determine the behavior of the reduced x population. The positivity of these parameters is insured by the inequality $\lambda N \gg A$ which certainly always holds. The value of x_1 is constant and represents the concentration of malignant cells in the environment of (ΔV); it will always correspond to the value of a normal tissue, as predicted by our model, which as we shall see later is extremely low. Therefore we shall use the term *microcancer* when we refer to this very small population of transformed cells (see below).

Let us now briefly summarize some representative orders of magnitude for the constants in our model.

1. *Numerical Values of Constants*

The constants appearing in Eqs. (1) to (4) have been estimated from the very precise curves of tumor growth obtained in vivo and in vitro and from in vitro experiments on the diffusion of cytotoxic cells and their interaction with malignant cells. It is hoped that the predictions which can be derived on the basis of these data are of quantitative value, at least for in vitro experiments.

2. *Cellular Populations*

The total number of cells per volume element N is the simplest constant to evaluate. A typical order of magnitude is 10^6 cells/mm^3 (Simpson-Herren and Lloyd, 1970). The number of cytotoxic cells σ_0 is variable and depends very much on the tissue considered. In the case of macrophages, σ_0 is well known and ranges between 1% and 50% of the total number of cells (Greaves et al., 1975; Evans, 1972; Eccles and Alexander, 1975), the upper value being only found in tumors.

3. *Replication constant* λN

A variety of 16 tumors have been considered (Garay and Lefever, 1977b). In all cases the values found for λN lie in the range (units: day^{-1}): $0.2 < \lambda N < 1.35$, the average being at about 0.68.

4. Rate of Carcinogenesis AN

This is the most difficult constant to determine because it is not accessible to direct measurements. For some tumors an estimate can be obtained by indirect arguments. For example, this is the case with multiple myelomatosis. Burnet (1967) reported that the probability of a plasmoblast being transformed and escaping immunological surveillance is on the order of 10^{-16} to 10^{-17}. Using this value, and assuming that all transformed cells produce a tumor, we can estimate the minimal rate of carcinogenesis. For an ideal tissue of 10^6 cells/mm^3, with a generation time of 10 days, the rate of carcinogenesis is of the order of 10^{-11} to 10^{-12} cancer cell/day and mm^3.

5. Cytotoxic Constants k_1 *and* k_2

In the case of lymphoma cells interacting with syngeneic macrophages, these constants can be calculated accurately from the in vitro experiments of Evans and Alexander (1970). One finds $k_1 = 1.56 \times 10^{-6}$ mm^3/macrophage day^{-1} and $k_2 = 0.22$ cancerous cells/macrophage day^{-1}.

6. Mobility Coefficients

$\tilde{\mu}$ has been calculated for macrophages on the basis of the rates of migration reported by several authors using different techniques (Lefever and Garay, 1977). All values lie in the range (units: mm^2 sec^{-1}): $10^{-9} \lesssim \tilde{\mu} < 10^{-8}$. The phenomenological constant K which takes into account the effect of lymphokines cannot be estimated from the data which we have found, even in the case of MIF. A value could easily be determined by measuring the migration areas of cytotoxic cells as a function of the MIF concentration. Below, we shall analyze in detail the role of this parameter.

Using the numerical values $AN \simeq 10^{-11}$, $k_1 \simeq 2 \times 10^{-6}$, $k_2 \simeq 0.2$, $\sigma_0 \simeq 7 \times 10^4$, and $\lambda N \simeq 0.7$ yields

$$\alpha \simeq 1.4 \times 10^{-16} \qquad \beta \simeq 2 \times 10^{-1} \qquad \theta \simeq 0.1 \tag{13}$$

Clearly these values are only approximate and may be expected to vary appreciably from one system to the other or under in vivo conditions. The uncertainty is mainly due to AN and to k_1 and k_2. Maximal (but less realistic) estimations of AN which we reported elsewhere (Garay and Lefever, 1977b) are in the range 10^{-4} to 10. Accordingly, the value of α could vary at least over 12 orders of magnitude. On the other hand, it would be extremely interesting to possess values for k_1 and k_2 corresponding to a choice of different tumor cells and conditions; as we show below this is fundamental in order to understand the physical nature of microcancer states.

B. Properties of the Homogeneous Steady-state Solutions of Equation (11)

We consider the time-independent solutions of Eq. (11) obtained by neglecting cytotoxic cell motion ($D = \gamma = 0$).

In that case the relation between β and the steady-state value of x can be written in the simple form

$$\beta = [\alpha + (1 - \theta x)x] \frac{1 + x}{x} \tag{14}$$

The extrema of this function (such that $d\beta/dx = 0$) are solutions of the polynomial equation

$$2\theta x^3 - (1 - \theta)x^2 + \alpha = 0 \tag{15}$$

Two physically acceptable solutions of Eq. (15) exist (i.e., correspond to real and positive values of x) provided the condition:

$$\alpha < \frac{(1 - \theta)^3}{27\theta^2} \qquad \theta < 1 \tag{16}$$

is satisfied.

Generally, α is extremely small and since θ is also smaller than one [cf Eq. (13), for example] we expect that the inequality, Eq. (16), always holds. In first approximation the extremal values of x are $\sqrt{\alpha}$ and $1/2\theta$. The corresponding values of β are respectively,

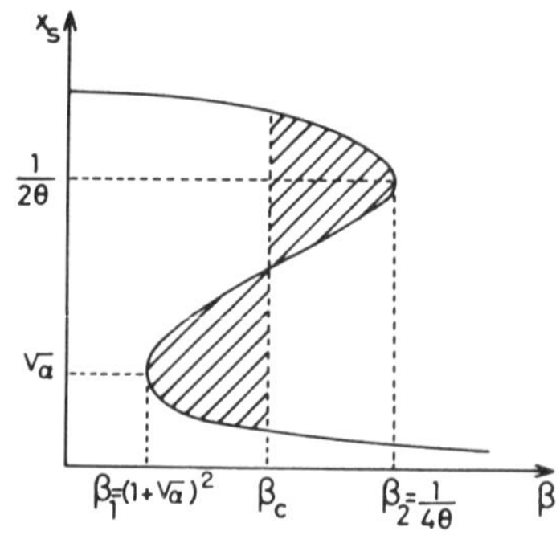

FIG. 1. Sketch of the steady-state curves for x as a function of β. The critical value β_c marks the transition between stability and metastability on the upper and lower parts of the curve ($\theta \ll 1$).

$\beta_1 = (1 + \sqrt{\alpha})^2$ and $\beta_2 = 1/4\theta$. These results are summarized in Fig. 1 and establish the following remarkable properties.

1. Within the domain of values of constants which conforms to our present knowledge, the steady-state curve of x as a function of β is sigmoidal (S-shaped). Accordingly it may be decomposed into three parts. First, for $0 \leqslant \beta \lesssim 1/4\theta$ there exists an upper branch of solutions which we shall call x_3; it is stable and since its number of malignant cells is close to N, we may say that it corresponds to the *cancerous state* of the tissue. The value of x_3 is approximately

$$x_3 \simeq \frac{1 - \theta + [(1 - \theta)^2 - 4\theta(\beta - 1 - \alpha)]^{1/2}}{2\theta} \tag{17}$$

Second, for $(1 + \sqrt{\alpha})^2 \lesssim \beta$ the lower branch of solutions x_1 is stable; in first approximation its value is given by

$$x_1 \simeq \frac{\alpha}{\beta - 1} \tag{18}$$

and corresponds to the population of transformed cells present in a normal tissue (*microcancer state*). With values for the constants of the same order of magnitude as reported above, and using Eq. (18), we find at most one transformed cell for a total number of cells of the order of that of a human being (Garay and Lefever, 1977). This extremely low value agrees with the well-known monoclonal origin of tumors (i.e., that most cancers seem to arise from a single cell) (Friedman and Fialkow, 1976). Third, for

$$\beta_1 = (1 + \sqrt{\alpha})^2 \lesssim \beta \lesssim \frac{1}{4\theta} = \beta_2 \tag{19}$$

there exists an unstable branch of steady-state solutions x_2 which plays the role of a threshold between x_1 and x_3. This threshold, beyond which no immune surveillance is ensured, arises because the population of cytotoxic cells have a saturable capacity for destroying the transformed cells.

2. Cancer induction is excluded in tissues for which β is greater than β_2. In other words, only the x_1 microcancer steady-state solution exists when the condition

$$\sigma_0 > \frac{\lambda N}{4k_2} \tag{20}$$

is satisfied. For most tissues the population of cytotoxic cells is less than 10% of the total cell population. With the numerical values presently at our disposal, the ratio $\lambda N/4k_2$ in most cases is larger or close to one, and thus the inequality, Eq. (20), is unlikely to be fulfilled. Alternatively, we could also say that it is impossible for the immune system, once the x_3 branch has been reached, to reverse the tissue back to the microcancer state x_1 simply by increasing the cytotoxic population. The variations required are far too large. From a therapeutic point of view, this suggests that the kinetic factors on which one should primarily try to act are λ and k_2. With the values considered here, the ratio $\lambda N/4k_2$ must vary at least by one order of magnitude to make a reversal from the tumor state possible.

3. As in the case of equilibrium first-order phase transitions, one must distinguish between the metastable and stable parts of the x_1 and x_3 branches of solution. A thermodynamic transition point β_c can be calculated and corresponds approximately to

$$\beta_c \simeq \frac{\exp -2}{\theta} \quad \text{for } \lim \alpha \to 0; \quad \lim \theta \to 0 \tag{21}$$

Thus, in the interval $\beta_1 < \beta < \beta_c$, the branch of solutions x_1 is metastable and has properties analogous to a supersaturated vapor in the liquid-gas equilibrium phase transition. In the interval $\beta_c < \beta < \beta_2$ it is the x_3 branch of solutions which presents these properties. For $\beta > \beta_c$, the steady states x_1 are, in the thermodynamic sense, stable with respect to any kind of perturbation, whatever its size or amplitude; while on the contrary, for $\beta < \beta_c$ it is the x_3 branch which possesses these stability properties. This analysis will be confirmed by the results which we report in Section VI. On the other hand, β_c being smaller than β_2 only by a factor of about one-half, still corresponds to a very large cytotoxic population. Therefore, it appears likely that the microcancer state of many tissues will be found to be metastable. From a physical point of view this implies that there exists a critical nucleus or critical microtumor size which must be reached before the growth process can develop. This critical nucleus may be reached as the result of a spontaneous statistical fluctuation, or it may be introduced artificially (like a seed in a supercooled liquid). It must be stressed, as we will show explicitly below, that the evaluation of this critical nucleus depends not so much on the problem of defining a critical number of cancerous cells as on the problem of defining the minimal size of a volume element in which the growth process can start by spontaneous fluctuation.

C. Role of Diffusion (D) and of Lymphokines (γ)

Up to now we have neglected the role of cellular motion in our stability considerations. This is, however, one of the key processes which favors the maintenance of the microcancer state. We shall now consider this aspect of the problem.

We first rewrite the general steady-state condition of Eq. (11) in the form

$$(1 + x_1)(1 + \gamma x_1)\left\{(1 + \gamma x)\left[-\theta x^3 + \left(1 - \theta - \frac{\beta\gamma}{1 + \gamma x_1}\right)x^2 + \left(1 + \alpha - \frac{\beta}{1 + \gamma x_1}\right)x + \alpha\right] + D\left[-\left(\theta + \frac{\beta\gamma}{(1 + x_1)(1 + \gamma x_1)}\right)x^2 + \left(1 - \frac{\beta}{(1 + x_1)(1 + \gamma x_1)}\right)x + \alpha\right]\right\} = 0 \tag{22}$$

Dividing through $(1 + x_1)(1 + \gamma x_1)(x - x_1)$ and taking into account that x_1 is a solution of the homogeneous steady-state relation, Eq (14), this expression becomes

$$(x - x_1)\left\{(1 + \gamma x)\left[-\theta x^2 + \left(1 - \theta - \theta x_1 - \frac{\beta\gamma}{1 + \gamma x_1}\right)x + \alpha + 1 + x_1 - \theta x_1 \times (1 + x_1) - \beta\right] + D\left[-\left(\theta + \frac{\beta\gamma}{(1 + \gamma x_1)(1 + x_1)}\right)x + 1 - \theta x_1 - \frac{\beta}{1 + x_1}\right]\right\} = 0 \tag{23}$$

In Fig. 2, we have plotted, for a given value of D and various values of γ, the steady state curves of x as a function of β in the domain $\beta > \beta_1 = (1 + \sqrt{\alpha})^2$; x_1 being put equal to its homogeneous micro-cancer steady-state solution, as defined above. We see that when γ increases, the sigmoid character of the curves diminishes; the value $\beta_2(\gamma)$ progressively shifts to lower β values. There exists a critical $\gamma = \gamma_c$ (in the case of the figure its value lies in the range $0.1 < \gamma_c < 1$) beyond which the sigmoid character is completely abolished. A similar behavior can be demonstrated for increasing values of D. Thus, both for $\gamma \to \infty$ and $D \to \infty$ the transition necessarily occurs at $\beta = \beta_1$; for all $\beta > \beta_1$ only the x_1 solution exists and is stable, while for $\beta < \beta_1$, it is x_3 which is the only stable steady-state solution possible. In this deterministic approach, D and γ seem to produce rather similar effects: when their value increases, the domain of metastability tends to disappear. This point

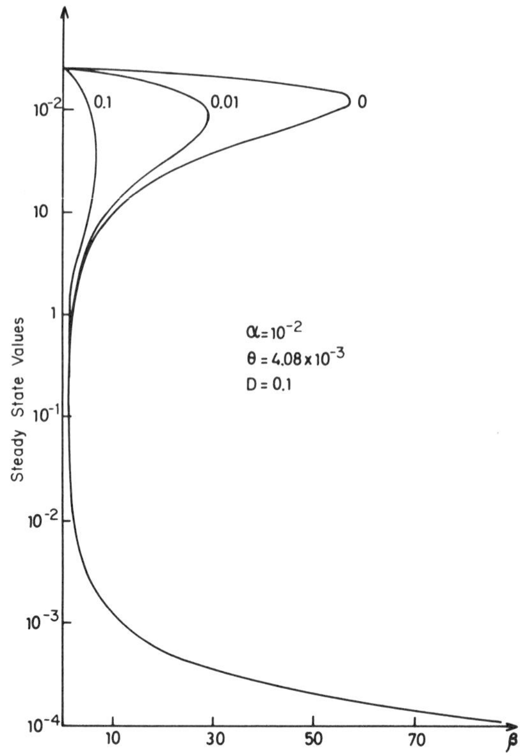

FIG. 2. Logarithmic plot of the steady-state solutions of Eq. (16) as a function of β. Each curve corresponds to a different value of γ, the parameters α, θ, and D being kept constant.

of view will be refined in Section VI, where we show that the influence of these parameters on behavior with respect to fluctuations is quite different.

On the other hand, it is interesting to see how γ is responsible for the accumulation of cytotoxic cells. Inside (ΔV) the population of cytotoxic cells is given by

$$\sigma(\Delta V) = \frac{\sigma_0(1 + \gamma x)}{1 + \gamma x_1} \tag{24}$$

It is simply proportional to the x population. Taking for the parameters the same values as in Fig. 2, considering that cytotoxic cells

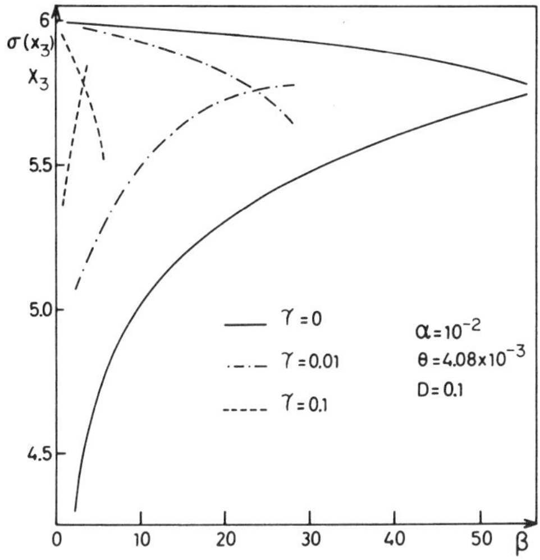

FIG. 3. Estimation of γ from the condition of equal malignant (X_3) and cytotoxic populations $\sigma(X_3)$ in the tumor state. The logarithm of the cellular populations is plotted vs. β.

represent 50% of all cells found in tumors and that the realistic values of β are likely to be smaller than 10, the value of γ may be guessed (in this matter the exact value of AN is of little importance). Indeed, in Fig. 3 we have plotted vs. β the tumor steady state solution (x_3) calculated with Eq. (23) and the cytotoxic population $\sigma(x_3)$ obtained by replacing x in Eq. (24) by x_3 and x_1 by the corresponding microcancer solution of Eq. (23). The intersections of these curves represent a percentage of 50% cytotoxic cells in the tumor state. We see that for $\gamma = 0$ and $\gamma = 0.01$, the values of β corresponding to this intersection are not plausible. The case $\gamma = 0.1$ is more compatible with our numerical discussion; it suggests that in reality the inequality $\gamma \gtrsim 0.1$ holds.

VI. CRITICAL FLUCTUATIONS AND THE MECHANISM OF ONSET OF TUMOR GROWTH

The relation between the instability or metastability of microcancer states and the onset of cancer growth raises the question of evaluating the size of the critical fluctuations able to trigger this phenomenon. The microscopic formulation of such a problem, which involves many degrees of freedom, presents great difficulties. Our approach will be based on the techniques of Markovian probability theory which in recent years have been extended with success to non-equilibrium situations in chemical systems McQuarrie, 1967; Nicolis and Babloyantz, 1969; Nicolis and Prigogine, 1971; Nicolis, 1972; Nitzan et al., 1974; Schlögl, 1972; McNeil and Walls, 1974; Matheson et al., 1975). An ansatz has been proposed describing fluctuations locally (Prigogine et al., 1975; Malek-Mansour and Nicolis, 1975). Our objective in this section will be primarily to illustrate some of the benefits gained by such an approach and the essential differences which may arise between the predictions of a purely kinetic description, as outlined above, and a stochastic description in which local fluctuations are taken into account. Our discussion will not be quantitative; the consideration of numerical values like those reported earlier is extremely time consuming with the computer and for that reason has not yet been done.

For the sake of clarity, let us first consider in general the problem of the spontaneous onset of a new regime and the idea which has lead to the local fluctuations theory considered here.

Suppose we have a system whose average state can be described in terms of macroscopic variable X (the extension to more than one variable is straightforward). The time evolution of this variable obeys a kinetic equation of the form (for simplicity let us momentarily neglect diffusion)

$$\frac{dX}{dt} = f(X) \tag{25}$$

where f(X) is a polynomial function of X. The effect of fluctuations does not appear in Eq. (25), which only refers to the average state of the system. In order to analyze the behavior of the fluctuations taking place around this average state we need a description giving the probability P(X, t) of having at time t the concentration or rather the number of particles X inside the system. A simple way to introduce such a description is by assuming that in the space of the numbers of particles (or number of cells), Eq. (25) defines a Markovian master equation of the type

$$\frac{dP(X, t)}{dt} = -\sum_r W(X \to X + r)P(X, t) + \sum_r W(X - r \to X)P(X - r, t) \qquad (26)$$

where $W(X \to X + r)$ represents the transition probability per unit time between states X and X + r. This transition probability is further assumed to be of the usual birth and death type. From Eq. (26) an equation for the time evolution of the first moment of the distribution P(X, t) can easily be derived. It is of the form

$$\frac{d\langle X \rangle}{dt} = \langle f(X) \rangle \qquad (27)$$

In a nonlinear system, it will in general differ from Eq. (25) by terms related to the mean square deviation or higher moments of P(X, t)

$$\frac{d\langle X \rangle}{dt} = f(\langle X \rangle) + 0\left[\langle (\sigma X)^2 \rangle\right] \qquad (28)$$

where

$$\langle (\sigma X)^2 \rangle = \sum_X (X - \langle X \rangle)^2 P(X, t) \qquad (29)$$

Comparing Eqs. (25) and (28), we see that the corrections to the deterministic description arise from the statistical deviations or fluctuations, around the average behavior as predicted by Eq. (25). In the case of the cancer problem these corrections cannot be neglected. The reasons for this are both experimental and theoretical. Indeed, experimentally the monoclonal origin of many tumors is well proved; this means that their onset seems related to some unique event taking place in a limited region of the tissue. This fact is also in agreement with the vanishingly small microcancer populations predicted by our numerical analysis [cf Eq. (18)]; even the addition of a single cancer cell would constitute a large fluctuation. From a theoretical point of view, we have shown that the microcancer state is likely to be unstable or metastable. This

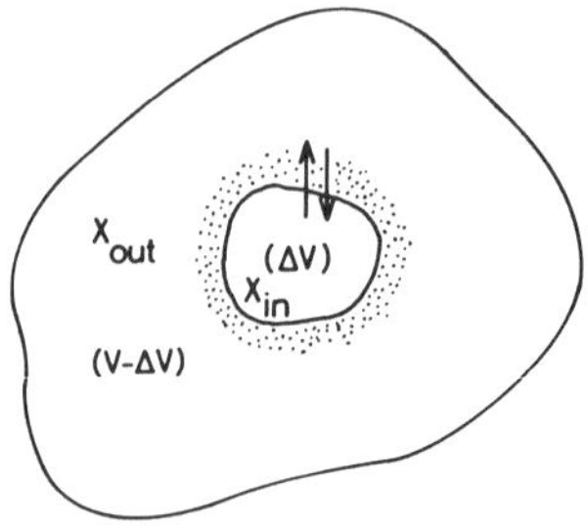

FIG. 4. The exchange of matter between (ΔV) and its local environment is illustrated, represented by the dotted area in $(V - \Delta V)$.

means that even if the correction terms, Eq. (29), are initially negligible in Eq. (28), they may grow in the course of time so that finally they will drive the average value $\langle X \rangle$ completely away from the unstable or metastable regime. The results of fluctuation theory within the framework of birth and death formalism have clarified the mechanism of such a fluctuation-driven evolution. The essential point to realize in this respect is that in order to build up a satisfactory description of fluctuations from a physical point of view, it is imperative to take into account explicitly their local character. This can be done with the help of a nonlinear master equation whose general properties shall first be considered.

As in Section V, we consider a small subvolume (ΔV) embedded in a surrounding "big" system $(V - \Delta V)$. It is assumed that (ΔV) and $(V - \Delta V)$ interact only through diffusion across their interface. We are only interested in the effect of this transport of matter on the stability properties of some reference state and thus neglect all other kinds of coupling (see Fig. 4).

The complete master equation for this system is of the form in Eq. (26). But, as it requires the specification of the value of X both in (ΔV) and in $(V - \Delta V)$, it involves twice as many stochastic variables. A way of eliminating this difficulty is to average this complete master equation which refers to the whole system, over the environment of (ΔV) (i.e., over $V - \Delta V$); this procedure can be justified as long as the size of (ΔV) is negligible compared with

(V - ΔV). This yields an equation for the time change of the probability P(X, t) of having "state" X inside (ΔV) which is of the form

$$\frac{dP(X, t)}{dt} = R_{(\Delta V)}[X, P(X, t)] + D\langle X\rangle[P(X - 1, t) - P(X, t)] + D[(X + 1)P(X + 1, t) - XP(X, t)] \tag{30}$$

with

$$\langle X\rangle = \sum_X XP(X, t) \tag{31}$$

and

$$D = \frac{\eta(T)}{\ell\ell_r} \tag{32}$$

The transport coefficient D describes the exchange of particles between (ΔV) and a layer surrounding (ΔV) of thickness ℓ_r (the mean free path of X) (Malek-Mansour and Nicolis, 1975). The function $\eta(T)$ depends on temperature and corresponds to Fick's diffusion coefficient; ℓ represents some characteristic parameter related to the size of (ΔV).

We see that three kinds of contributions enter the master equation (30) and determine the state of (ΔV). First, we have $R_{(\Delta V)}[X, P(X, t)]$, which is equal to the right hand side of Eq. (26) and stands for the chemical processes taking place inside (ΔV). Second, we have a diffusion term which describes the variation of P(X, t) due to the exchange of particles passing from (V - ΔV) to (ΔV); the transition probability of this process is simply proportional to the average $\langle X\rangle$ of (V - ΔV). Furthermore, as we want to assume that the entire system is macroscopically homogeneous (i.e., that there are *no local macroscopic gradients*), we had to impose the condition that the average values of X in (V - ΔV) and (ΔV) be equal. Third, we have a contribution coming from the motion of particles which pass from (ΔV) to (V - ΔV) and whose transition probability is proportional to the actual state of (ΔV). The main advantage of Eq. (30) as compared to the master equation for the entire system is obviously that it involves a reduced number of stochastic variables. This result, however, is obtained at the expense that we pass from a linear equation in the probabilities to one which is nonlinear.

From Eq. (30) we can easily obtain the kinetic equation describing the time volution of the moments of the distribution. For the first two moments $\langle X \rangle$ and $\langle X^2 \rangle$ we have the following interesting properties:

1. The equation for the time evolution of the first moment $\langle X \rangle$ is independent of D (as required by the condition of macroscopic homogeneity) and equal to Eq. (27).
2. The second moment obeys an equation of the form

$$\frac{d\langle X^2 \rangle}{dt} = \sum_X X^2 \; R[X, P(X, t)] + 2D[\langle X \rangle - \langle (\delta X)^2 \rangle] \qquad (33)$$

As we can see from Eqs. (28), (29), and (33), the evolution of the first moment $\langle X \rangle$ may be driven by the system's fluctuations even if $d\langle X \rangle/dt = 0$ initially, provided $d\langle X^2 \rangle/dt$ is not equal to zero simultaneously. Consequently, Eq. (33) tells us that if $\langle X \rangle$ is a steady-state solution of Eq. (27), such a fluctuation driven evolution is impossible in the limit $D \to \infty$, that is, for the volume elements (ΔV) of small size ($\ell \to 0$); the probability distribution is then necessarily Poisson with $\langle X \rangle$ as a mean value. The two most important implications of this result are: first, it demonstrates the compatibility of the description of fluctuations based on Eq. (30) with the *local equilibrium assumption* on which nonequilibrium thermodynamics has been developed (Glansdorff and Prigogine, 1971). Second, it shows that the *spontaneous* onset of an instability which drives a system away from some particular steady-state solution bears some similarity with a nucleation phenomenon. Indeed, if the size of the fluctuation is very small ($X \to 0$), D tends to infinity and the steady-state regime of Eq. (30) must necessarily correspond to the Poisson distribution having $\langle X \rangle$ as mean value. The stabilizing effect of the external world acting through diffusion damps the fluctuation and restores the average value of X existing in $(V - \Delta V)$. On the contrary, if the fluctuation is very large $(\ell \to \infty)$, the terms due to diffusion are negligible compared to the destabilizing contribution coming from the chemical processes going on in (ΔV). The fluctuation can grow and finally drive the average value of the entire system to a new state.

Let us now analyze this behavior more in detail in the case of the immune surveillance against cancer. The appropriate master equation involves three stochastic variables, referring to the cellular populations X, M_0, and M_1. It reads:

$$\frac{dP(X, M_0, M_1, t)}{dt} = R_{(\Delta V)}[X, M_0, M_1, t)]$$
$$+ \mu \left\langle \frac{M_0}{1 + KX} \right\rangle [P(X, M_0 - 1, M_1, t) - P(X, M_0, M_1, t)]$$
$$+ \frac{\mu}{1 + KX} [(M_0 + 1)P(X, M_0 + 1, M_1, t) - M_0 P(X, M_0, M_1, t)]$$
$$+ \mu \left\langle \frac{M_1}{1 + KX} \right\rangle [P(X, M_0, M_1 - 1, t) - P(X, M_0, M_1, t)]$$
$$+ \frac{\mu}{1 + KX} [(M_1 + 1)P(X, M_0, M_1 + 1, t) - M_1 P(X, M_0, M_1, t)] \quad (34)$$

Formally, Eq. (34) differs from Eq. (30) only by the coefficient multiplying the diffusion terms, which are due to the sticky barrier effect whereby malignant cells inhibit diffusion of the cytotoxic cells. As in our deterministic analysis, we shall reduce the number of variables of Eq. (34) by assuming that the M_0 and M_1 populations equilibrate rapidly with respect to X. This is done by obtaining from Eq. (34) the moment equations for M_0 and M_1 and using them as algebraic relations (quasi steady state) to express everything in terms of X (Lefever and Garay, 1977):

$$\frac{dP(X, t)}{dt} = \left\{\alpha + (X - 1)[1 - \theta(X - 1)]\right\}P(X - 1, t)$$
$$- \left[\alpha + X(1 - \theta X) + \beta \langle M_0 \rangle_X X\right]P(X, t)$$
$$+ \beta \langle M_0 \rangle_{X+1} (X + 1)P(X + 1, t) \quad (35)$$

with

$$\langle M_0 \rangle_X = \frac{(1 + KX)[(1 + KX)\langle (1 + KX)(1 + LX)\rangle + D(1 + K\langle X\rangle)]}{\langle (1 + LX)(1 + KX)\rangle (1 + K\langle X\rangle)[(1 + LX)(1 + KX) + D]}$$

and

$$\langle (1 + KX)(1 + LX)\rangle = \sum_{X=0}^{N} (1 + KX)(1 + LX)P(X, t)$$

The steady-state solution for P(X, t) is given by the recurrence

$$P(0) = 1$$

$$P(X) = \frac{\{\alpha + (X - 1)[1 - (X - 1)\theta]\}}{X\beta \langle M_0 \rangle_X} P(X - 1)$$

$$= \frac{\langle (1 + LX)(1 + KX)\rangle^X (1 + K\langle X\rangle)^X}{X!\beta^X}$$

$$\times \prod_{s=1}^{X} \frac{\{\alpha + (s - 1)[1 - (s - 1)\theta]\}[(1 + Ls)(1 + Ks) + D]}{(1 + Ks)[(1 + Ks)\langle (1 + KX)(1 + LX)\rangle + D(1 + K\langle X\rangle)]} \tag{36}$$

Let us first consider the homogeneous case where there is no cellular motion (D, $\gamma = 0$). Eq. (36) reduces to

$$P(X) = \frac{\alpha + (X - 1)[1 - \theta(X - 1)](1 + LX)}{X\beta} P(X - 1) \tag{37}$$

and the properties of the steady state distribution may be summmarized as follows.

1. Inside the domain defined by Eqs. (16) and (19), the distribution P(X) is bimodal; the maxima of the two peaks being located near $X_1 \simeq L^{-1}x_1$ and $X_3 \simeq L^{-1}x_3$, where x_1 and x_3 are the values of Eqs. (18) and (17). Outside this domain it is unimodal with a peak either at $X_1 (\beta > \beta_2)$, or at $X_3(\beta < \beta_1)$.
2. When the distribution is bimodal, the highest peak corresponds either to X_1 or X_3 according to whether $\beta > \beta_c$ or $\beta < \beta_c$. In the limit $N \to \infty$, each peak tends towards a δ-function and the ratio $P(X_1)/P(X_3)$ tends either to zero $(\beta < \beta_c)$ or to infinity $(\beta > \beta_c)$; only at $\beta = \beta_c$ do the two peaks have equal height.

3. As a consequence of (1) and (2), the first moment $\langle X \rangle$ of the distribution in Eq. (37) is a single-valued function of β. It tends either to $X_3(\beta < \beta_c)$ or to $X_1(\beta > \beta_c)$; the transition occurs at $\beta = \beta_c$ and its steepness increases with N (all other parameters being kept constant). In the limit $N \to \infty$, $\beta_c \to \infty$; as a result, the x_1 branch of steady states becomes entirely metastable ($\beta_2 \simeq 1/4\theta \to \infty$). The distribution in Eq. (35) can then no longer be normalized as we necessarily have $P(\infty) \to \infty$. This reflects the fact that for $N \to \infty$, the tissue always evolves in the course of time towards the tumor state. Thus in the homogeneous case, the stochastic analysis does not permit the existence of a stable steady-state distribution corresponding to a microcancer state. This is a direct consequence of the linearity of Eq. (26).

Remarkably, the effect of diffusion is to allow for a *multiplicity of steady-state solutions* in Eq. (36). Indeed it can be shown that in the interval $\beta_1 < \beta < \beta_c$ provided D is greater than some critical value D_c, there exists another steady-state distribution whose mean value corresponds to the metastable steady state. This value D_c furnishes a *lower bound* to the fluctuation size, below which the transition towards the tumor state is impossible. In Fig. 5, we have plotted D_c (dashed curve) as a function of β in the metastable domain of X_1. We notice that $D_c \to 0$ as $\beta \to \beta_c$, while on the contrary for $\beta \to \beta_1$, it tends to infinity. These results are similar to that reported earlier with a much simpler chemical system (Prigogine et al., 1975). Their interpretation is as follows: when $\beta \to \beta_1$, the size of critical fluctuations tends to zero. Consequently, as fluctuations of small size are very probable, near β_1, the probability that the transition between X_1 and X_3 takes place, tends to 1. We reach the point where any fluctuation induces the onset of cancer. Near β_c on the contrary, fluctuations of very large size would be required. Their probability of spontaneous occurrence being small, the lifetime of metastable states may be extremely long.

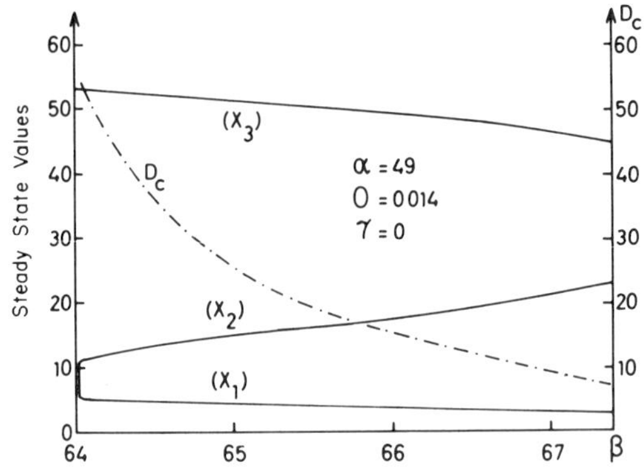

FIG. 5. Plot of steady-state values (full line) and of D_c in the metastable region as a function of β. An unrealistically large value of α has been considered simply for numerical convenience.

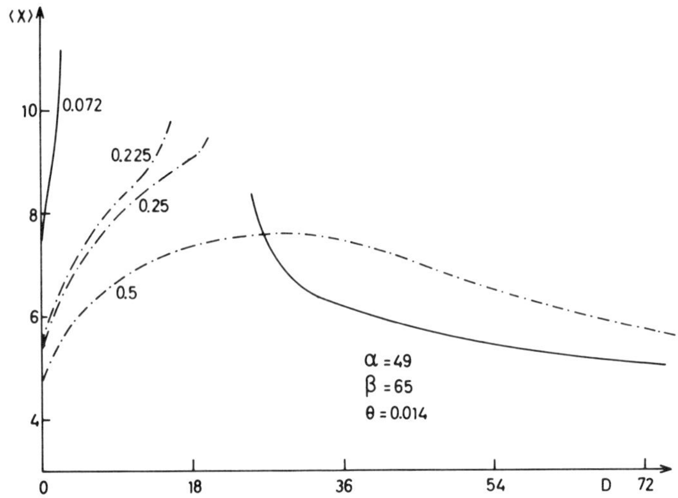

FIG. 6. Stochastic metastable solution ⟨X⟩ as a function of D. On the right side, the curves for various values of γ are overlapping over practically their entire domain of existence; therefore, only the curve corresponding to γ = 0.072 has been plotted (full line). The branch of steady-state values which appears on the left when γ increases is much more sensitive to the value of this parameter. For large values of γ ($\gamma \gtrsim 0.4$), a stable microcancer value of ⟨X⟩ exists with respect to fluctuations of any size.

In Fig. 6, we illustrate the effect of γ. The first moment $\langle X \rangle$ is plotted as a function of D, for various values of γ. The curves correspond to values of D for which a steady-state distribution with mean value $\langle X \rangle$ near the metastable branch exists. When this solution of Eq. (36) disappears, only the distribution whose mean lies near the tumor state remains. When $\gamma = 0$, in agreement with Fig. 5, this happens for small β values (below 0.072). However, as β increases, we find the remarkable result that a second branch of solutions appears on the side of the small β values. Thus in the case of the figure, there exists an interval for γ

$$0.072 \lesssim \gamma < 0.5$$

such that fluctuations of both large and small size are damped; the metastable state can only be destabilized by fluctuations of intermediate size. For larger values of γ no spontaneous fluctuation is able to cause the transition.

These results furnish a much clearer view of the relation between the parameters D and γ and metastability. In the analysis of Section V, the effect of increasing D or γ is rather similar: it reduces the domain of metastability. D in itself has no effect on the existence of a metastable region. Hence, we could say that the metastable region is defined through the existence of a finite value of D_c $(0 < D_c < \infty)$ beyond which the lifetime of the microcancer state becomes infinite. Spontaneous fluctuations are thus divided into two classes according to their size. The role of γ in the stochastic approach is to suppress completely the class of fluctuations which leads to a tumor invasion.

Up to now, we have treated D and N as independent parameters. This is, however, a convenience which limits the predictions of the stochastic analysis from a quantitative point of view. The density of cells for a given tissue is a constant, and the characteristic length ℓ should be related to N. In fact for a spherical volume element (ΔV), D is proportional to $N^{-2/3}$. In terms of N, the effect of D_c could also be reinterpreted in the following way: to D_c

corresponds a critical N_c, such that for $N < N_c$ the metastable branch is stable, thus has an infinite lifetime. When N is greater than N_c, there is no metastable solution of Eq. (36), thus an initial condition in its neighborhood has a finite lifetime. This lifetime, when N increases, first diminishes; however, there is a minimum to this decrease. Indeed, we know from the thermodynamic limit that such initial conditions will again exhibit an infinite lifetime when $N \to \infty$. The value of N for which the shortest lifetime is observed, could be viewed as some optimal nucleus of germination.

VII. CONCLUSION

It seemed to us that there existed a gap between the precise experimental data on tumor growth, the recent observations on the reaction between tumor and immune cells, and the interpretation of these data from the point of view of stability and fluctuation theory. The model presented here is an attempt to fill this gap: it furnishes in terms of a minimum number of parameters a physical interpretation of the phenomenon of immune surveillance against cancer and places it within the general class of behaviors and instabilities related to nonequilibrium. Our results also illustrate that not only is a theoretical description of cancer onset possible, but furthermore, to be entirely satisfactory, this description has to incorporate explicitly the effect of fluctuations which is usually neglected. The understanding of their mechanism of growth or damping is a key step towards the understanding of such biologically important notions as the threshold of instability of the microcancer population.

ACKNOWLEDGMENTS

We would like to thank Professors I. Prigogine, G. Nicolis, and J. Urbain for their interest in this work and the numerous discussions we had with them. We thank the Caisse Generale d'Epargne et de Retraite (CGER) whose financial support makes this research possible.

REFERENCES

Ames, B. N. (1973). Carcinogens are mutagens: their detection and classification. *Environ. Health Perspectives Exp. 6:* 115-118.

Baldwin, R. W. (1976). Role of immunosurveillance against chemically induced rat tumors. *Transplant. Rev. 28:* 62-74.

Baldwin, R. W. and Moore, M. (1968). Isolation of membrane associated tumour-specific antigens from rat hepatomas induced by aminoazo dye. *Nature 220:* 287-289.

Bernstein, I. D., Thor, D. E., Zbar, B., and Rapp, H. J. (1971). Tumor immunity: tumor suppression in vivo initiated by soluble products of specifically stimulated lymphocytes. *Science 173:* 729-731.

Bloom, B. R. and Bennett, B. (1966). Mechanism of a reaction in vitro associated with delayed type hypersensitivity. *Science 153:* 80-82.

Brunner, K. T., Mavel, J., Cerottini, J. C., and Chapuis, B. (1968). Quantitative assay of the lytic action of immune lymphoid cells on chromium-51-labelled allogeneic target cells in vitro; inhibition by isoantibody and by drugs. *Immunology 14:* 181-196.

Burnet, F. M. (1964). Immunological factors in the process of carcinogenesis. *Br. Med. Bull. 20:* 154-158.

Burnet, F. M. (1967). Immunological aspects of malignant disease. *Lancet i:* 1171-1174.

Burnet, F. M. (1971). Immunological surveillance in neoplasia. *Transplant. Rev. 7:* 3-25.

Cairns, J. (1975). The cancer problem. *Sc. Am. 233:* 64-78.

Calvin, M. (1975). Carcinogenesis. *Naturwissenschaften 62:* 405-413.

Cerottini, J. C. and Brunner, K. T. (1974). Cytotoxicite lymphocitaire antitumorale. *Adv. Immunol. 18:* 67-132.

Dumonde, D. C., Wolstencroft, R. A., Panayi, G. S., Matthew, M., Morley, J., and Howson, W. T. (1969). "Lymphokines;" nonantibody mediators of cellular immunity generated by lymphocyte activation. *Nature (London) 224:* 38-42.

Eccles, S. A. and Alexander, P. (1974). Immunologically-mediated restraint of latent tumour metastases. *Nature 257:* 52-53.

Ehrlich, P. (1957). Uber den Getzigenstand der Karzinomforschung. In *The Collected Papers of Paul Ehrlich*, vol. II, Pergamon, London, p. 550.

Evans, R. (1972). Macrophages in syngeneic animal tumours. *Transplantation 14:* 468-473.

Evans, R. and Alexander, P. (1970). Cooperation of immune lymphoid cells with macrophages in tumour immunity. *Nature 228:* 620-622.

Foley, E. J. (1953). Antigenic properties of methylcholanthrene-induced tumours in mice of the strain of origin. *Cancer Res. 13:* 835-842.

Friedman, J. M. and Fialkow, P. J. (1976). Cell marker studies of human tumorigenesis. *Transplant. Rev. 28:* 18-33.

Garay, R. and Lefever, R. (1977a). The immune barrier and the stability of microcancer states. To appear *C. R. Acad. Sci. Paris.*

Garay, R. and Lefever, R. (1977b). A kinetic approach to the immunology of cancer: stationary state properties of effector-target cell reactions. Submitted *J. Theor. Biol.*

Glansdorff, P. and Prigogine, I. (1971). *Thermodynamic Theory of Structure, Stability and Fluctuations.* Wiley-Interscience, New York.

Greaves, M. F., Falk, J. A., and Falk, R. E. (1975). A surface antigen marker for human monocytes. *Scand. J. Immunol. 4:* 555-562.

Habel, K. (1961). Resistance of polyoma virus immune animals to transplantized polyoma tumor. *Proc. Soc. Exp. Biol. N.Y. 106:* 722-725.

Haughton, G. and Whitmore, A. C. (1976). Genetics, the immune response and oncogenesis. *Transplant. Rev. 28:* 76-97.

Hellström, I. and Hellström, K. E. (1971). Colony inhibition and cytotoxicity assays. In *In Vitro Methods In Cell-Mediated Immunity* (B. R. Bloom and P. R. Glade, eds.). Academic, New York, p. 409.

Hellström, I. and Hellström, K. E. (1973). Some recent studies on cellular immunity to human melanomas. *Fed. Proc. 32:* 156-159.

Hellström, K. E. and Hellström, I. (1974). Lymphocyte-mediated cytotoxicity and blocking serum activity to tumour antigen. *Adv. Immunol. 18:* 209-277.

Henkart, P. and Blumenthal, R. (1975). Interaction of lymphocytes with lipid bilayer membranes: a model for lymphocyte-mediated lysis of target cells. *Proc. Nat. Acad. Sci. (USA) 72:* 2789-2793.

Hochova, B., Krejci, J., Pekarek, J., Svejcar, J., and Johanovsky, J. (1975). Further characterization of antigen-dependent migration inhibition factor in mice. *Immunology 29:* 231-236.

Huebner, R. J., Kelloff, G. J., Sarma, P. S., Lane, W. T., Gidden, R. V., Oroszlan, S., Meier, H., Myers, D. D., and Peters, R. L. (1970). Group-specific antigen expression during embryogenesis of the genome of the C-type RNA tumor virus: implication for ontogenesis and oncogenesis. *Proc. Nat. Acad. Sci. (USA) 67:* 366-376.

Lefever, R. and Garay, R. (1977). Cytotoxic cell diffusion and the behavior of the threshold for cancerization. To appear *C. R. Acad. Sci. Paris.*

Linder, D. and Gartler, S. M. (1965). Glucose-6-phosphate dehydrogenase mosaicism: utilization as a cell marker in the study of leiomyomas. *Science 150:* 67-69.

Lohmann-Matthes, M. L. and Fischer, H. (1973). T-cell cytotoxicity and amplification of the cytotoxic reaction by macrophages. *Transplant. Rev. 17:* 150-171.

McNeil, K. J. and Walls, D. F. (1974). Nonequilibrium phase transitions in chemical systems. *J. Stat. Phys. 10:* 439-448.

McQuarrie, D. (1967). Stochastic approach to chemical kinetics. In *Supplementary Review Series in Applied Probability* (J. Gani, ed.). Methuen, London, pp. 1-68.

Malek-Mansour, M. and Nicolis, G. (1975). A master equation description of local fluctuations. *J. Stat. Phys. 13:* 197-217.

Matheson, I., Walls, D. F., and Gardiner, C. W. (1975). Stochastic models of first order nonequilibrium phase transitions in chemical reactions. *J. Stat. Phys. 12:* 21-34.

Möller, G. and Möller, E. (1976). The concept of immunological surveillance against neoplasia. *Transplant. Rev. 28:* 3-16.

Moore, M., Lawrence, N., and Nisbet, N. W. (1975). Tumour inhibition mediated by BCG in immunosuppressed rats. *Int. J. Cancer 15:* 897-911.

Nicolis, G. (1972). Fluctuations around nonequilibrium states in open nonlinear systems. *J. Stat. Phys. 12:* 195-222.

Nicolis, G. and Babloyantz, A. (1969). Fluctuations in open systems. *J. Chem. Phys. 51:* 2632-2637.

Nicolis, G. and Prigogine, I. (1971). Fluctuations in nonequilibrium systems. *Proc. Nat. Acad. Sci. (USA) 68:* 2102-2107.

Nitzan, A., Ortoleva, P., Deutch, J., and Ross, J. (1974). Fluctuations and transitions at chemical instabilities: the analogy to phase transitions. *J. Chem. Phys. 61:* 1056-1074.

Pimm, M. V. and Baldwin, R. W. (1975). BCG immunotherapy of rat tumours in athymic nude mice. *Nature 254:* 77-78.

Plescia, O. J., Smith, A. H., and Grinwich, K. (1975). Subversion of immune system by tumor cells and role of prostaglandins. *Proc. Nat. Acad. Sci. (USA) 72:* 1848-1851.

Potter, M., Sklar, M. D., and Rowe, W. P. (1973). Rapid viral induction of plasmacytomas in pristane-primed BALB/c mice. *Science 182:* 592-594.

Prehn, R. T. (1970). Analysis of antigenic heterogeneity within individual 3-methylcholanthrene-induced mouse sarcomas. *J. Nat. Cancer Inst. 45:* 1039-1045.

Prehn, R. T. (1976). Do tumors grow because of the immune response of the host? *Transplant. Rev. 28:* 34-42.

Prehn, R. T. and Lappé, M.A. (1971). An immunostimulation theory of tumor development. *Transplant. Rev. 7:* 26-54.

Prehn, R. T. and Main, J. M. (1957). Immunity to methylcholanthrene-induced sarcomas. *J. Nat. Cancer Inst. 18:* 769-778.

Prigogine, I., Lefever, R., Turner, J., and Turner, J. (1975). Stochastic theory of metastable states and nucleation. *Phys. Lett. 51A:* 317-319.

Prigogine, I., Nicolis, G., Herman, R., and Lam, T. (1975). Structure, stability and complexity. *Cooperative Phenomena 2:* 103-109.

Rygaard, J. and Povlsen, C. O. (1976). The nude mouse versus the hypothesis of immunological surveillance. *Transplant. Rev. 28:* 43-61.

Salomon, J. C. (1975). La surveillance immunitaire. *La Recherche 58:* 640-655.

Schlögl, F. (1972). Chemical reaction models for nonequilibrium phase transitions. *Z. Physik 253:* 147-161.

Simpson-Herren, L. and Lloyd, H. H. (1970). Kinetic parameters of growth curves for experimental tumor systems. *Cancer Chemother. Rep., 1 54:* 143-179.

Sjögren, H. O., Hellström, I., and Klein, G. (1961). Resistance of polyoma virus immunized mice to transplantation of established polyoma tumor. *Exp. Cell. Res. 23:* 204-208.

Svejcar, J., Johanovsky, J., and Pekarek, J. (1967). Studies on the mechanism of delayed hypersensitivity in tissue cultures. XI. The influence of the substances released during the cultivation of lymph node cells from sensitized organisms with antigen on the migration activity of normal spleen cells. *Z. Immun. Forsch. 133:* 259-274.

Thomas, L. (1959). Reactions to homologous tissue antigens and relation to hypersensitivity. In *Cellular and Humoral Aspects of the Hypersensitive States* (H. S. Lawrence, ed.). Hoeber, New York, pp. 529-532.

Wagner, H., Harris, A. W., and Feldmann, M. (1972). Cell-mediated immune response in vitro. II. Role of thymus and thymus-derived lymphocytes. *Cell. Immunol. 4:* 39-50.

Weisbart, R. H., Isaacson, J., Bluestone, R., and Goldberg, L. S. (1975). Human polymorphonuclear leucocyte migration inhibitory factor. *Immunology 29:* 223-230.

Zilber, L. A. (1958). Specific tumor antigens. *Adv. Cancer Res. 5:* 291-329.

Chapter 18

THE INFILTRATION OF LYMPHOCYTES AND MACROPHAGES INTO A SITE OF INFECTION

Rutherford Aris

Department of Chemical Engineering
and Materials Science
University of Minnesota
Minneapolis, Minnesota

The two models put forward by Mackaness (1971) for the occlusion of a phagocyte infected by tubercle bacilli are set up in mathematical terms. Emphasis is on the basic strategy of mathematical modeling, and suggestions are made as to how the models might be discriminated and the progress of modeling continued.

I. INTRODUCTION

The purpose of this chapter is to consider carefully the process of setting up a mathematical model of an immunological problem. The value of mathematical modeling lies firstly in sharpening the analysis of the problem, secondly in establishing the degree of validity of the model by the correspondence of its consequences with observation, and thirdly in suggesting further lines of development. Mathematical models must be cultivated at different levels of sophistication if the greatest progress is to be made, for it is comparatively easy to set up a model of a biological process which is so complicated as to hold out little hope of any solution or, if by an exercise of mathematical virtuosity a solution is obtained, the model is found to have a solution so complex as to forbid any useful tie back into biological reality. Usually there is a process of rational simplification which must go on to achieve a model which is both soluble and interpretable. While the work of Polya (1945, 1954, 1962, 1965) has much to say to the art of problem solving, few applied mathematicians have addressed the general question of setting up the equations. The notable exception is the unusually fine text of Lin and Segel (1974), where the processes of modeling are described and illustrated by a problem in osmotically driven flow. Some aspects of the craft of modeling are considered explicitly by Aris (1976), but they are of course implicit in all sound work — a particularly beautiful example has recently been published by Fife (1976).

II. THE DYNAMICS OF CONSOLIDATION

The situation to be considered has been described by Mackaness (1971) in his discussion of cell-mediated immunity to infection. A phagocyte infected by tubercle bacilli will become consolitated by the accession of other monocytes. This involves the cooperative activity of these monocytes with committed lymphocytes, and Mackaness put forward two mechanisms which might account for the consolidation. The dramatis personae of the models are six:

1. An infected phagocyte located in the tissue
2. Monocytes circulating in an adjacent capillary loop
3. Committed lymphocytes also in the blood
4. Antigen produced by the infected phagocyte
5. A chemotactic factor
6. A migration inhibitor

The two scenarios proposed by Mackaness are as follows:

a. Monocyte (2) and committed lymphocyte (3) encounter one another in the bloodstream, with the latter sensitizing the former by the transfer of specific reactivity (i.e., 2 becomes 2* with the loss of 3).
b. In response to the antigen (4) released by the infected region of the tissue, the sensitized monocyte (2*) migrates through the cell wall to the infected site.
c. The migrating monocytes consolidate around the infection and seal it off.

alternatively:

α. The committed lymphocyte (3) migrates into the tissue.
β. It there reacts with the antigen (4) and releases a chemotactic factor (5) which attracts the monocytes (2).
γ. Having been attracted to the infected region (1), the consolidation takes place by a migration inhibitory factor (6).

The two mechanisms are sufficiently distinct that it might be hoped that modeling might lead to results that would allow them to be distinguished. They are shown schematically in Fig. 1.

III. THE GEOMETRY OF THE SITUATION

Clearly, the topography of the locus of infection will have to be vastly simplified and this in itself shows how mathematical models come in hierarchies. A fully three-dimensional idealization is shown in Fig. 2(III). The blood vessel is idealized to a vertical cylinder of radius r with the infected region a sphere of radius a whose center is a perpendicular distance d from the axis of the cylinder. This three-dimensional picture will obviously face considerable difficulty, since even the simplest problem of diffusion between a cylinder and sphere is a nontrivial one. To reduce the dimensions to two we can suppose either that the action takes place in a plane perpendicular to the axis of the cylinder and so involves diffusion in a plane between two circles as indicated in Fig. 2(IIa), or that the plane of of action should contain the axis of the cylinder. In the latter case the bloodstream might be held to occupy the left half-plane and diffusion be between a plane and a sphere as shown in Fig. 2(IIb). Finally, we recognize that in order to get started on a solution we may need to ignore geometrical similitude and consider the blood to be in the left half-plane and the infected area to be the half-plane to the right of the line $x = d$ [Fig. 2(I)]. The final stage is a reduction to one dimension which we recognize as possibly necessary to get a start on the solution, but certainly a dangerous divorcement from reality.

In honor of the original formulation, Z and K will denote the domains occupied by the blood and by the infected region, respectively. Their boundaries are ∂Z and ∂K, and will denote the intervening region of tissue.

If the process of occlusion is represented as a growth of the region K, we shall have the further complication of a moving boundary

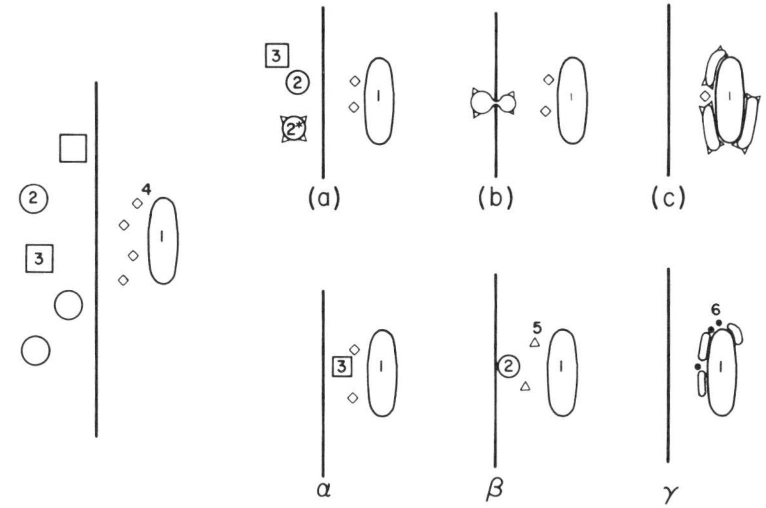

FIG. 1. The two scenarios: 1, tubercle; 2, monocyte; 2*, activated monocyte; 3, committed lymphocyte; 4, antigen; 5, chemotactic factor; 6, migration inhibitor (see text for details).

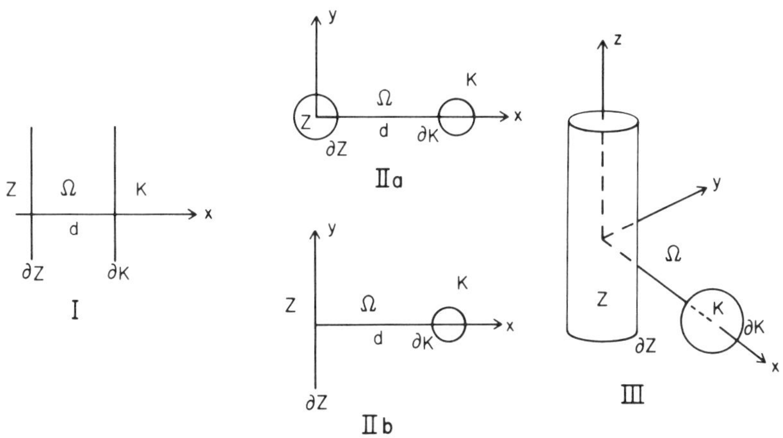

FIG. 2. The geometrical possibilities (see text for details).

problem. To avoid this we take the occlusion to be measured by the accumulation of monocytes at the boundary of the infected region.

IV. EQUATIONS FOR THE ANTIGEN

Since the equations for the antigen will be the same for both models, we may derive them first. We shall let c denote the concentrations, using the suffixes 1 through 6 to connote the different species as listed above. Within the tissue, the antigen diffuses with diffusion coefficient D_4 and reacts at rate R; the expression for this rate will depend on the model and must be specified later. For c_4, therefore,

$$\frac{\partial c_4}{\partial t} = D_4 \nabla^2 c_4 - R \qquad \text{in} \quad \Omega \tag{1}$$

Its generation at the site of infection is a function of the monocyte concentration there, and the rate decreases as $\hat{c}_2$ builds up, that is, as occlusion progresses. Thus with $\hat{c}_2$ denoting the occluded monocyte concentration

$$- D_4 \frac{\partial c_4}{\partial n} = G(\hat{c}_2) \qquad \text{on} \quad \partial K \tag{2}$$

One of the simpler forms for G would be

$$G(\hat{c}_2) = \begin{cases} a'(C_2 - \hat{c}_2)^{b'} & 0 \leqslant c_2 \leqslant C_2 \\ 0 & c_2 > C_2 \end{cases} \tag{3}$$

where C_2 is the completely occluded state. If the antigen is confined to the tissue

$$\frac{\partial c_4}{\partial n} = 0 \qquad \text{on} \quad \partial Z \tag{4}$$

V. THE FIRST MODEL

If the three-dimensional geometry of Fig. 2III obtains, the concentrations of monocyte (c_2), sensitized monocyte (c_2^*), and committed lymphocyte (c_3) would be specified far upstream as, say, $\bar{c}_{if}$. The concentrations of several species would then be functions of position, creating a problem of immense difficulty. Rather, we will have to assume the blood volume is well mixed in the neighborhood of the infection and that the flow is characterized by a residence time, θ. Then, if the process of sensitization is irreversible and depends on the transfer of a specific group (as Mackaness suggests), the concentrations of 2, 2*, and 3 in the region Z denoted by $\bar{c}_2$, c $\bar{c}_2^*$, and $\bar{c}_3$ are functions only of time and governed by

$$\frac{d\bar{c}_2}{dt} = \frac{1}{\theta}(\bar{c}_{2f} - \bar{c}_2) - k_+\bar{c}_2\bar{c}_3$$

$$\frac{d\bar{c}_2^*}{dt} = \frac{1}{\theta}(\bar{c}_{2f}^* - \bar{c}_2^*) + k_+\bar{c}_2\bar{c}_3 - Ah^*(\bar{c}_2^* - c_2^*) \tag{5}$$

$$\frac{d\bar{c}_3}{dt} = \frac{1}{\theta}(\bar{c}_{3f} - \bar{c}_3) - k_+\bar{c}_2\bar{c}_3$$

where c_2^* refers to the concentration just inside the tissue and A denotes a suitable averaging over the wall of the blood vessel. If the transfer of specific activity incapacitates the committed lymphocyte, there will be a loss in the active population of lymphocytes which is reflected in the last term of the last equation. A reversible sensitization would lead to a further set of terms, $k_-\bar{c}_2^*$, representing the decay of the sensitized monocyte. This is a possibility that should be investigated but which will not be pursued here. If h* is small and the initial values of the $\bar{c}_i$ are compatible with the feed $\bar{c}_{if}$ (cf Aris, 1965), then we have $\bar{c}_2 = \bar{c}_{2f} + \bar{c}_{2f}^* - \bar{c}_2^*$ and $\bar{c}_3 = \bar{c}_{3f} + \bar{c}_{2f}^* - \bar{c}_2^*$. Thus we can make do with only one of the equations in Eqs. (5) and

$$\frac{d\bar{c}_2^*}{dt} = Q(\bar{c}_2^*) = \frac{1}{\theta}(\bar{c}_{2f}^* - \bar{c}_2^*) + k_+(\bar{c}_{2f} + \bar{c}_{2f}^* - \bar{c}_2^*)$$

$$\times\ (\bar{c}_{3f} + \bar{c}_{2f}^* - \bar{c}_2^*) - Ah^*(\bar{c}_2^* - c_2^*) \tag{6}$$

the right side being quadratic in $\bar{c}_2^*$.

In the first model the antigen acts as an attractant for the sensitized monocytes. Hence their diffusion within the tissue is governed by

$$\frac{\partial c_2^*}{\partial t} = D_2^*\nabla[\nabla c_2^* - \chi^* c_2^* \nabla c_4] \qquad \text{in } \Omega \tag{7}$$

We do not distinguish between the monocytes before and after they may combine with the antigen, since this is not considered to have an effect on the occlusion. For this model the reaction rate for antigen in Eq. (1) is

$$R = kc_2^{*p}\ c_4^q \tag{8}$$

If the antigen is capable of affecting the permeability of the wall between the capillary and tissue

$$D_2^* \frac{\partial c_2^*}{\partial n} = h^*(c_4)(c_2^* - \bar{c}_2^*) \qquad \text{on } \partial Z \tag{9}$$

If the permeability is unaffected, h^* is a constant. On ∂K the monocytes build up and are fixed hence

$$D_2^* \frac{\partial c_2^*}{\partial n} = k_f c_2^* = \frac{\partial \hat{c}_2}{\partial t} \qquad \text{on } \partial K \tag{10}$$

Note that the normal derivative is always into the tissue and that the chemotactic term does not come into Eq. (9) on account of Eq. (4).

The initial conditions should be taken to correspond to the state just before the antigen is released and so would be

$$c_2^* = c_4 = 0 \qquad \text{in } \Omega \tag{11}$$

It seems natural to take the initial and feedstream conditions to be the same in the bloodstream, since encounters of lymphocyte and monocyte have been taking place upstream, and it is only the infection that disturbs the steady state. Thus

$$\bar{c}^*_{2f} = \bar{c}^*_2(0) = c^*_{2e} \qquad \bar{c}_{2f} = \bar{c}_2(0) = c_{2e} \qquad \bar{c}_{3f} = \bar{c}_3(0) = c_{3e} \tag{12}$$

where e denotes the undisturbed steady value. If the sensitization were reversible and terms $k_-\bar{c}^*_2$ were used in Eqs. (5), then we would have

$$\frac{c^*_{2e}}{c_{2e}c_{3e}} = K_e = \frac{k_+}{k_-} \tag{13}$$

VI. REDUCTION OF THE FIRST MODEL

The natural units of time and distances are θ and d, since the latter appears in all the geometries. For the concentrations of sensitized monocyte we can either work back from C_2, the concentration related to complete occlusion, or forward from $\bar{c}^*_{2f}$. The latter is preferable since different forms of Eq. (3) might be used. The reference concentration of antigen will be written as c_{4r} and chosen later to be as convenient as possible. Then by letting

$$\tau = \frac{t}{\theta} \qquad \xi = \frac{x}{d} \qquad \eta = \frac{y}{d} \qquad \zeta = \frac{z}{d}$$

$$u^*_2 = \frac{c^*_2}{\bar{c}^*_{2f}} \qquad \bar{u}^*_2 = \frac{\bar{c}^*_2}{\bar{c}^*_{2f}} \qquad \hat{u}_2 = \frac{\hat{c}_2 d}{\theta D^*_2 c^*_{2f}} \qquad u_4 = \frac{c_4}{c_{4r}} \tag{14}$$

$$\Delta^*_2 = \frac{D^*_2\theta}{d^2} \qquad \Delta_4 = \frac{D_4\theta}{d^2} \qquad \chi = \chi^* c_{4r}$$

$$\kappa = k\theta \bar{c}^{*p}_{2f}\, c^{q-1}_{4r} \qquad \kappa_f = \frac{k_f d}{D^*_2} \qquad \kappa_+ = k_+\theta \bar{c}^*_{2f}$$

$$\mu = \frac{D_4 c_{4r}}{dG(0)} \qquad \Gamma(\hat{u}_2) = \frac{G(\hat{c}_2)}{G(0)} \qquad U_2 = \frac{C_2 d}{\theta D^*_2 c^*_{2f}} \tag{15}$$

$$\lambda' = A\theta h^* \qquad \lambda = \frac{dh^*}{D^*_2} \qquad \alpha = 1 + \frac{\bar{c}_{2f}}{\bar{c}^*_{2f}} \qquad \beta = 1 + \frac{\bar{c}_{3f}}{\bar{c}^*_{2f}}$$

we have the equations

$$\frac{\partial u_4}{\partial \tau} = \Delta_4 \nabla^2 u_4 - \kappa\, u_2^{+p}\, u_4^q \qquad \text{in } \Omega \tag{16}$$

$$\mu \frac{\partial u_4}{\partial \nu} = \Gamma(\hat{u}_2) = 0 \qquad \text{on } \partial K \tag{17}$$

$$\frac{\partial u_4}{\partial \nu} = 0 \qquad \text{on } \partial Z \tag{18}$$

$$\frac{\partial u^*_2}{\partial \tau} = \Delta^*_2 \nabla[\nabla u^*_2 - \chi^*_2 \nabla u_4] \qquad \text{in } \Omega \tag{19}$$

$$\frac{\partial u^*_2}{\partial \nu} = \kappa_f u^*_2 = \frac{d\hat{u}_2}{d\tau} \qquad \text{on } \partial K \tag{20}$$

$$\frac{\partial u^*_2}{\partial \nu} = \lambda(u_4)(u^*_2 - \bar{u}^*_2) \qquad \text{on } \partial Z \tag{21}$$

$$\frac{d\bar{u}^*_2}{d\tau} = 1 - \bar{u}^*_2 + \kappa_+(\alpha - \bar{u}^*_2)(\beta - \bar{u}^*_2) - \lambda'(\bar{u}^*_2 - u^*_2) \tag{22}$$

It is convenient to choose c_{4r} to make $\mu = 1$, that is, $c_{4r} = dG(0)/D_4$, and then $\Gamma(0) = 1$. The alternative of choosing c_{4r} so that $\chi = 1$ is inferior if we wish to study the influence of chemotaxis.

These equations have to be integrated with the initial conditions $u_2^+ = u_4 = 0$, $\bar{u}^*_2 = 1$, and the occlusion is complete when $\hat{u}_2 = U_2$, say $\tau = T$. A simplified set of equations is obtained if κ_+ is very large for then Eq. (22) can be discarded and θ chosen to make κ or one of the Δ's equal to 1. The last term in Eq. (22) is the dimensionless averaged transfer to the tissue.

VII. THE SECOND MODEL

In the second scenario, it is the committed lymphocyte (3) that diffuses into the tissue and there reacts with the antigen (4) to produce the chemotactic factor (5). Thus

$$\frac{\partial c_3}{\partial t} = D_3 \nabla^2 c_3 - k' c_3 c_4 \tag{23}$$

$$\frac{\partial c_5}{\partial t} = D_5 \nabla^2 c_5 + k' c_3 c_4 \tag{24}$$

describe this process, while Eq. (1) becomes

$$\frac{\partial c_4}{\partial t} = D_4 \nabla^2 c_4 - k' c_3 c_4 \tag{25}$$

In place of the chemotactic influence of the antigen we have that of the factor (5) so that

$$\frac{\partial c_2}{\partial t} = D_2 \nabla [\nabla c_2 - \chi_2' c_2 \nabla c_5] \tag{26}$$

The lymphocyte and monocyte come from the bloodstream, where it will be assumed that they are maintained in spatially constant concentrations,

$$D_2 \frac{\partial c_2}{\partial n} = h_2 (c_2 - \bar{c}_2) \qquad \text{on} \quad \partial Z \tag{27}$$

$$D_3 \frac{\partial c_3}{\partial n} = h_3 (c_3 - \bar{c}_3) \qquad \text{on} \quad \partial Z \tag{28}$$

while the antigen and chemotactic factor are confined to the tissue

$$\frac{\partial c_4}{\partial n} = \frac{\partial c_5}{\partial n} = 0 \qquad \text{on} \quad \partial Z \tag{29}$$

The generation of antigen is again described by Eq. (20) and the process of occlusion by

$$\frac{d\hat{c}_2}{dt} = k_f' c_2 = D_2 \frac{\partial c_2}{\partial n} \qquad \text{on} \quad \partial K \tag{30}$$

If the immobilizing factor is considered, then D_2 or k_f could be made functions of c_6; however, this would only add to an already large set of equations.

VIII. REDUCTION OF THE SECOND MODEL

Retaining as many as possible of the dimensionless variables in Eq. (15), we have the same independent variables τ, ξ, η, and ζ but now

$$u_2 = \frac{c_2}{\bar{c}_2} \qquad u_3 = \frac{c_3}{\bar{c}_3} \qquad u_4 = \frac{c_4}{\bar{c}_{4r}} \qquad u_5 = \frac{c_5}{\bar{c}_{5r}}$$

$$\Delta_i = \frac{D_i\theta}{d^2} \qquad \chi_2 = \chi_2' c_{5r} \qquad \lambda_i = \frac{dh_i}{D_i} \tag{31}$$

$$\kappa_3 = k'\theta c_{4r} \qquad \kappa_4 = k'\theta\bar{c}_2 \qquad \kappa_5 = \frac{k'\theta\bar{c}_3 c_{4r}}{c_{5r}}$$

$$\frac{\partial u_2}{\partial \tau} = \Delta_2\nabla[\nabla u_2 - \chi_2 u_2 \nabla u_5] \tag{32}$$

$$\frac{\partial u_3}{\partial \tau} = \Delta_3\nabla^2 u_3 - \kappa_3 u_3 u_4 \tag{33}$$

$$\frac{\partial u_4}{\partial \tau} = \Delta_4\nabla^2 u_5 + \kappa_5 u_3 u_4 \tag{34}$$

$$\frac{\partial u_5}{\partial \tau} = \Delta_5\nabla^2 u_5 + \kappa_5 u_3 u_4 \tag{35}$$

By choosing c_{4r} as before we can take c_{5r} to make $\kappa_5 = 1$ and then

$$c_{4r} = \frac{dG(0)}{D_4} \qquad c_{5r} = \frac{k'\bar{c}_3\theta\ dG(0)}{D_4} \qquad \kappa_3 = \frac{k'\theta\ dG(0)}{D_4}$$

$$\kappa_4 = k'\theta\bar{c}_3 \tag{36}$$

As boundary conditions we have

$$\frac{\partial u_i}{\partial \nu} = \lambda_i(u_i - 1) \qquad \text{on } \partial Z \text{ with } \lambda_4 = \lambda_5 = 0 \tag{37}$$

while

$$\frac{d\hat{u}_2}{d\tau} = \frac{\partial u_2^*}{\partial \nu} = \kappa_f u_2^* \tag{38}$$

$$\frac{\partial u_3}{\partial \nu} = \frac{\partial u_5}{\partial \nu} = 0 \qquad \text{on} \quad \partial K \tag{39}$$

$$\frac{\partial u_4}{\partial \nu} + \Gamma(\hat{u}_2) = 0 \tag{40}$$

Again these equations are to be integrated with zero initial conditions and occlusion is complete when $\hat{u}_2 = U_2$.

IX. THE SIMPLEST FORM OF THE EQUATIONS

The equations take their simplest form in the plane geometry of Fig. 2I. We will compare these in their simplest form. For model I we assume equilibrium is maintained in the bloodstream, then: in Ω, $0 < \xi < 1$,

$$\frac{\partial u_2^*}{\partial \tau} = \Delta_2^* \frac{\partial^2 u_2^*}{\partial \xi^2} - \chi \, \Delta_2^* \left(u_2^* \frac{\partial^2 u_4}{\partial \xi^2} + \frac{\partial u_2^*}{\partial \xi} \frac{\partial u_4}{\partial \xi} \right) \tag{41}$$

$$\frac{\partial u_4}{\partial \tau} = \Delta_4 \frac{\partial^2 u_4}{\partial \xi^2} - \kappa \, u_2^{*p} \, u_4^q \tag{42}$$

on ∂K, $\xi = 1$,

$$\frac{\partial u_2^*}{\partial \xi} = \kappa_f u_2^* = \frac{d\hat{u}_2}{d\tau} \tag{43}$$

$$\frac{\partial u_4}{\partial \xi} + \Gamma(\hat{u}_2) = 0 \tag{44}$$

while on ∂Z, $\xi = 0$,

$$\frac{\partial u_2^*}{\partial \xi} + \lambda(1 - u_2^*) = 0 \tag{45}$$

$$\frac{\partial u_4}{\partial \xi} = 0 \tag{46}$$

The simplest form of $\Gamma(\hat{u}_2)$ is $(1 - \hat{u}_2)$. If p = 0 and q = 1, Eq. (42) can first be solved leaving Eq. (41) as a linear equation. The solutions to both of these will depend linearly on $\hat{u}_2(\tau)$ through the boundary conditions, Eqs. (43) and (44), the former providing an ordinary differential equation for this unknown function. With other values of p and q this method is not feasible.

In model II we cannot avoid nonlinear equations, for Eqs. (33) to (35) take the form

$$\frac{\partial u_i}{\partial \tau} = \Delta_i \frac{\partial^2 u_i}{\partial \xi^2} \pm \kappa_i u_3 u_4 \qquad i = 3, 4, 5 \tag{47}$$

Nor can the equations for u_3 and u_4 be solved first, for $\hat{u}_2$ appears in the boundary condition. For this model it seems best to proceed immediately to simultaneous numerical solution.

X. DISCUSSION

The equations of either model, even in their simplest forms, are not trivial to solve and recourse must be had to numerical methods almost from the start. The appropriate methods will be those of weighted residuals over finite elements (Strang and Fix, 1973) or of collocation (Finlayson, 1972). To discriminate between the models some feature of the solution which is readily testable must be isolated, and the characteristics of the way in which it depends on the parameters must be determined. Thus, experiments suggest a range of possible models which in turn suggest further experiments, and this leads to the discarding of some models and the refinement of others. Mackaness' experiments suggested the two possible models we have examined here. The measure by which the models are to be compared might well be T, the time for the tubercle to reach critical size and be occluded. Calculations are to be undertaken to see how this might depend on the parameters.

The parameters of the case can be divided into several classes according to the following table:

Class of parameter	Model I	Model II
Geometric	a/d, r/d	a/d, r/d
Kinetic	κ, κ_+, κ_-	κ_3, κ_4
Diffusion coefficients	Δ_2^*, Δ_4	Δ_2, Δ_3, Δ_4, Δ_5
Chemotactic	χ	χ_2
Transfer or permeability	λ, λ'	λ_2, λ_3
Occlusion	U_2, κ_f	U_2, κ_f
Blood	α, β	- -

Clearly, much more remains to be done with these models, but the principles of their construction are what has principally been at issue here. The continuation of this work is connected with a more general study of chemotaxis which is being pursued in cooperation with K. H. Keller.

APPENDIX: NOMENCLATURE

a	Radius of sphere representing infected region
a', b'	Constants in Eq. (3)
C_2	Concentration of c_2 for complete occlusion
c_i	Concentration of species i in tissue
$\hat{c}_2$	Concentration of monocyte at site of infection
c_2^*	Concentration of sensitized monocyte
$\bar{c}_i$	Concentration of species i in bloodstream
$\bar{c}_{if}$	Concentration of species i in bloodstream far from infected region
c_{ie}	Equilibrium concentrations in the sensitizing reaction
D_i	Diffusion coefficient of species i
d	Distance of infected region from bloodstream
G	Rate of generation of antigen at infected site
h	Permeability of vessel wall
i	Index for species (1, tubercle; 2, monocyte; 2*, sensitized monocyte; 3, committed lymphocyte; 4, antigen; 5, chemotactic factor; 6, migration inhibitor)

K	Spherical region representing the region of infection
K_e	Equilibrium constant for sensitizing reaction
k_f	Rate constant for occlusion, Eq. (10)
k_+, k_-	Forward and back rate constants for sensitization, Eq. (6)
k	Rate constant for antigen-monocyte reaction, Eq. (8)
k'	Rate constant for antigen-lymphocyte reaction, Eq. (23)
p, q	Orders in antigen-monocyte reaction
Q	Rate of change of $\bar{c}_2^*$, Eq. (6)
r	Radius of Z
R	Rate of reaction consuming antigen, Eq. (1)
T	Time for complete occlusion
t	Time
U_2	Dimensionless form of C_2, Eq. (15)
u_i	Dimensionless form of c_i, Eqs. (14) and (31)
x, y, z	Spatial coordinates
Z	Cylindrical region representing blood vessel
α, β	Parameters of bloodstream concentrations, Eq. (15)
Γ	Dimensionless form of G, Eq. (15)
Δ	Dimensionless diffusion coefficients, Eqs. (15) and (31)
∂K, ∂Z	Surfaces of K and Z
θ	Residence time in bloodstream
κ, κ_f, κ_+, κ_-	Dimensionless forms of k's, Eq. (15)
κ_3, κ_4, κ_5	Dimensionless rate constants, Eq. (31)
λ, λ', λ_i	Dimensionless permeabilities, Eqs. (15) and (31)
μ	Ephemeral parameter in Eqs. (15) and (17)
ξ, η, ζ	x/d, y/d, z/d, dimensionless coordinates
τ	t/θ
χ^*	Chemotactic factor in model I, Eq. (7)
χ	Dimensionless form of χ^*
χ_2'	Chemotactic factor in model II
χ_2	Dimensionless form of χ_2'
Ω	Tissue region

ACKNOWLEDGMENTS

The author is indebted to that most wide-ranging of mathematicians and stimulating of colleagues, Richard Bellman, for the opportunity to spend some time on these problems in the summer of 1973. The work was supported by the National Science Foundation (Grant No. GP 29049) and the Atomic Energy Commission [Contract No. AT(04-3)-113, Project 19].

REFERENCES

Aris, R. (1965). *Introduction to the Analysis of Chemical Reactors.* Prentice-Hall, Englewood Cliffs, New Jersey.

Aris, R. (1977). How to get the most out of an equation without actually solving it. *Chem. Eng. Educ. 10:* 114.

Fife, P. C. (1976). Pattern formation in reacting and diffusing systems. *J. Chem. Phys. 64:* 554.

Finlayson, B. A. (1972). *The Method of Weighted Residuals and Variational Principles.* Academic, New York.

Lin, C. C. and Segel, L. A. (1974). *Mathematics Applied to Deterministic Problems in the Natural Sciences.* Macmillan, New York.

Mackaness, G. B. (1971). Cell-mediated immunity to infection. In *Immunobiology* (R. A. Good and D. W. Fisher, eds.). Sinauer Assoc., Stamford, Connecticut.

Polya, G. (1945). *How to Solve It.* Princeton University Press, Princeton, New Jersey.

Polya, G. (1954). *Mathematics and Plausible Reasoning*, 2 vols. Princeton University Press, Princeton, New Jersey.

Polya, G. (1962 and 1965). *Mathematical Discovery*, 2 vols. Wiley, New York.

Strang, G. and Fix, G. J. (1973). *An Analysis of the Finite Element Method.* Prentice-Hall, Englewood Cliffs, New Jersey.

Wilkinson, P. G. (1974). *Chemotaxis and Inflammation.* Churchill-Livingstone, Edinburgh.

Part VII

LYMPHOCYTE NETWORK THEORY

Chapter 19

THE NETWORK IDEA AND THE IMMUNE RESPONSE

Peter H. Richter*

Department of Biochemical Kinetics
Max-Planck-Institut für Biophysikalische Chemie
Göttingen-Nikolausberg, Federal Republic of Germany

A network model of the immune response is presented which essentially rests on the simple axiom that an antigen specifically stimulates certain precommitted functional units which then act back on it in an aggressive manner. The network character is introduced via the specific antigenic properties of the functional units themselves. The unbalancing between cellular and molecular aspects as expressed

*Present affiliation: Department of Theoretical Chemistry, Massachusetts Institute of Technology, Cambridge, Massachusetts

in the dominant constitutive role of the lymphocytes is reflected in unequal sharing among T and B cells in regulation. The model ascribes fundamental significance to the low zone tolerance mode of response. The normal response, as well as high zone tolerance, are derived from it, on entering deeper and deeper into the system. In addition to these basic types of response, phenomena are reproduced which arise from heterogeneity in affinities, cross-reactivity among antigens, or T-cell impairment (Mitchison phenomenon, maturation, original antigenic sin, oscillatory behaviour, postrecovery overshoot). This leads to a straightforward understanding of self-nonself discrimination, and of its generation in early life. Allotype-mediated effects and the hapten-carrier dichotomy are examined in the light of the network concept, and finally, a number of relevant experiments are discussed.

I. INTRODUCTION

A growing body of experimental findings concerning the regulation of the immune response is lending more and more support to the network hypothesis as proposed and strongly advocated in recent years by Jerne (1972, 1974, 1976); for a review see Nisonoff and Bangasser (1975). The network concept is not meant to challenge the well-established precommitment axiom (Lefkovits, 1974) of Burnet's clonal selection theory (1957). Rather it attempts, on the basis of this axiom, to cope with the wealth of phenomena which seem to reflect more involved systemic potentialities than mere antigen-driven amplification of preexisting clones. Its most characteristic feature is to emphasize the importance of specific interrelations among different clones which allows intraclonal complexity to be relatively simple. The more conservative approaches, on the other hand, adhere to the implicit assumption that each antigenic specificity defines a little immune system of its own, uncoupled from the rest; accordingly they tend to invoke increasingly complex signaling and functioning on the cellular level (Bretscher and Cohn, 1970).

The evidence in favor of the network idea is twofold. First, there is the principal need to account for the phenomenon of idiotypy, that is, the specific antigenic nature of the antibodies themselves (Hopper and Nisonoff, 1971). The problem here is whether a population of lymphocytes that grows in response to an antigen can avoid being recognized and attacked like an external aggressor. From the point of view of strict self-nonself discrimination, one would be inclined to exclude any such internal excitation by postulating a mechanism which from the outset identifies and tolerates the idiotypes as self antigens. There is, however, a strong argument against this kind of evasion. The idiotypic diversity is generally believed to be of the same order of magnitude as the number of different antigen combining sites, or "paratopes." With 10^{20} antibody molecules, 10^{12} lymphocytes, and 10^{7} specificities for a human immune system (Jerne, 1972), we arrive at some 10^{10} molecules and 10^{2} cells per milliliter and specificity. These concentrations are one or two orders of magnitude lower than those typically needed to elicit any effect at all, namely low zone tolerance. We therefore conclude that in a virgin immune system the individual specificities are below threshold for effective recognition of their idiotypes. Only in the course of an immune response will an idiotype manifest itself, and when it does, it naturally induces a chain of idiotope-paratope interactions within the system. Although at first sight one may worry about the stability of such a situation, closer inspection reveals that it provides quite a powerful regulation scheme.

Accordingly, the main corroboration of the network concept comes from a considerable number of experiments on immune regulation. Various reviews are now available for orientation (Rowley et al., 1973; Nisonoff and Bangasser, 1975; Jerne, 1976), and a detailed discussion of several of the most pertinent results will be given below. The present state of affairs may be summarized as follows. Regulation is mainly a T-cell phenomenon; specificity can be mediated by at least three different agents: idiotypes, allotypes, and carrier determinants. As a rule, the same kind of agent can be employed for suppression or enhancement, depending on the circumstances. Thus antiidiotypic antibodies have been demonstrated to suppress (Cosenza and Köhler, 1972; Eichmann, 1974, 1975; Bangasser et al., 1975) or enhance (Eichmann and Rajewsky, 1975) the expression of a certain idiotype, by exerting some influence on the T-cell population. Likewise, antiallotypic antibodies have been used to induce suppressor T cells (Herzenberg et al., 1975) as well as T-cell help (Lees and Sinclair, 1975). Finally, carrier-primed T-cell suppression has recently been established by Tada et al. (1975), whereas carrier-induced helper T cells are an almost classical finding (reviewed by Katz and Benacerraf, 1972).

This remarkable plasticity of the T-cell system has been christened its "thymostat" character by Gershon (1974). To account for it, a network picture seems to be particularly appropriate, although it should perhaps not solely be woven out of idiotype specificities. Yet, in order to have a basis for further discussion we shall first elaborate a detailed model which centers on idiotope-paratope interactions (Richter, 1974, 1975), and which allows one to reproduce many characteristic observations. We shall then briefly comment on possible extensions of this model, to include the allotypic effects and the hapten-carrier problem. In addition, a number of crucial experiments will be selected for critically testing the theory. Here it will turn out that one of the strengths of the network concept is also its main shortcoming: its ability to reconcile what sometimes appear as contradictory alternatives (cf the analysis of tolerance induction by Weigle et al., 1975) is impaired by a concomitant vagueness in its predictive value. The only vindication for this could be that it reflects a true complexity of immunoregulation.

II. A NETWORK MODEL

The skeleton of a network based on paratope-idiotope interactions is depicted in Fig. 1. We adopt Jerne's terminology (1976) to denote by Ab-1 the antibodies produced against an antigen Ag, and by Ab-2 the antiidiotypic antibodies directed against Ab-1. The sequence

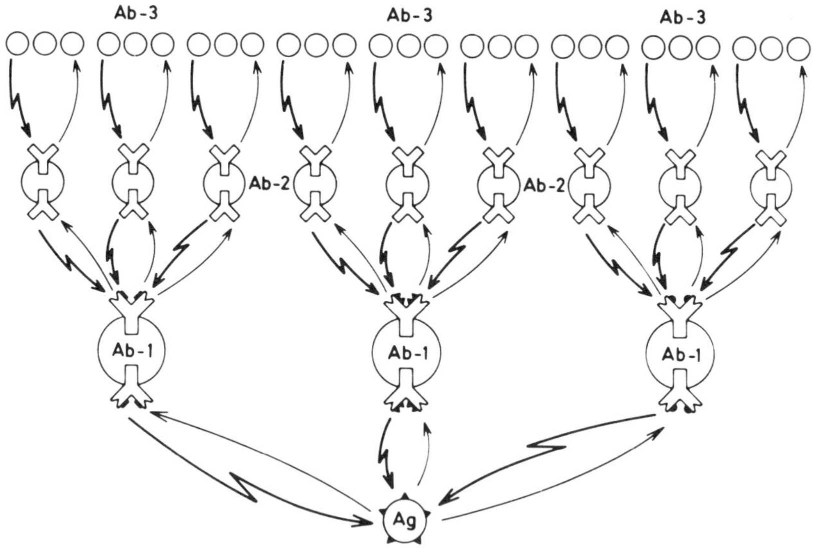

FIG. 1. Schematic view of the network based on idiotope-paratope interactions. Ab-i appears as an antigen to Ab-(i + 1) which it activates (arrow); the response is aggression (notched arrow). Inhibition and buffering are not indicated.

may be continued until at a certain level the whole system becomes involved; with an estimate of 25 different antibodies for a typical antigen, the Ab-5 population would exhaust 10^7 specificities. In the following, however, we shall never get beyond the Ab-4 level, so that it appears justified to disregard accidental double-membership of an antibody in the various Ab groups.

There are, however, theories by Hoffmann (1975, see also Chap. 20) and Köhler (1975) in which Ab-1 and Ab-3 are assumed to be identical, the network terminating on the Ab-2 level. Their basic postulate is a mirror-image relation between paratope and idiotope, with strict reciprocity of stimulatory or suppressive signaling. Appealing as it is at a first glance, this assumption probably cannot withstand closer inspection. X-Ray studies are now at hand (Poljak et al., 1973) which reveal how the hypervariable regions of the amino acid sequences are distributed around the antigen combining site, except for a small segment that lies somewhat apart. The paratypic specificity may be visualized as the interior of a well-defined groove into which the antigenic determinant must fit, whereas the idiotype should rather be conceived as a pattern of protruding side groups which in turn fit into the grooves of certain other antibodies. An antigen bound to the paratope may well inhibit the binding of an antiidiotypic antibody and vice versa. A functional identity, however, would require effective triggering of a protein regardless of the exact location of ligand binding, in marked contrast to the commonly observed high degree of precision. Our point of view will therefore be to assume functional separation as a starting point, and to consider incidental functional overlap as a possible second-order phenomenon. This seems to be in agreement with the difficulties encountered when trying to replace antigen by Ab-2 for induction of an adoptive secondary response (Eichmann and Rajewsky, 1975).

Before specifying the interactions in more detail, a note should be in order to further clarify the nature of the Ab-i populations (Fig. 1). They are not, in the first place, mere antibody molecules. Rather they are functional units which comprise everything that bears the specificity of these antibodies. The most important constituents are the lymphocytes, because it is their proliferation or destruction which decides upon the fate of a functional unit. The antibodies, being in their service perform a twofold role: they act as receptors on the lymphocyte surfaces, and as transmitters of specific interactions when in solution. We shall not go into a more refined description of the internal structure of a functional unit (Bell, 1970, 1971), because our emphasis is on the interclonal rather than on the intraclonal aspect.

The assumptions concerning the dominant interactions between functional units are derived from an elementary picture of the immune reaction: antigen stimulates its Ab-1 populations which in turn tend to eliminate the antigen. Thus there is activation in one direction, and suppression the other way around. In general, the paratopes of the Ab-i receptors take up a stimulatory signal from Ab-(i - 1) while their idiotopes render the i-lymphocyte vulnerable to attack from Ab-(i + 1). Conversely, in their role as transmitters the Ab-i antibodies stimulate the Ab-(i + 1) through their idiotopes whereas their paratopes mediate suppression of the Ab-(i - 1). Both types of processes may be complicated on the cellular and molecular levels, requiring a considerable unspecific subsidiary machinery like complement, macrophages, patch and cap formation, mitogens, etc. For our purposes, however, this is of marginal interest; it only enters the theory via the phenomenological parameters specifying growth and destruction characteristics.

It is well known that there is a pronounced division of labor within the immune system, in that B cells are responsible for the humoral, and T cells for the so-called cell-mediated immunity. In a given case the actual type of response depends on the nature of the antigen. Roughly speaking, molecular antigens usually elicit B-cell responses on the Ab-1 level whereas cellular antigens tend to require T-cell defense. Recalling now that the dominant representatives of a functional unit are its lymphocytes, we should all but expect that from the Ab-2 level onwards mainly T-cell populations are involved. Regulation would then very naturally be a T-cell phenomenon, with Ab-2 operating as suppressors and Ab-3 as helpers because they suppress the suppressors. A straightforward consequence of such a scheme would be that an impairment of the T-cell population, for example, by anti-Θ treatment, should first affect the helper function, whereas elimination of suppressor activity might be quite difficult to achieve.

In order to arrive at a reasonable first guess for the set of equations describing the system we have to make some additional remarks with respect to the interactions. The first is related to stability and concerns the relative strength of activation and suppression. It is by now familiar from various other fields of model building (Gierer and Meinhardt, 1972; Wilson and Cowan, 1973) that by and large the negative influences must be dominant for stability to be guaranteed. In our case it is certainly not unreasonable to assume that destruction of a lymphocyte is easier to bring about than proliferation. More precisely, we shall postulate that the threshold concentration for a suppressive agent to be operative is lower than the threshold for activation, and furthermore that destruction is a faster process than growth. These two requirements are important for preventing network explosion: an antigenic stimulus may propagate up several levels in the scheme of Fig. 1, but then suppression will inevitably set a limit.

A second remark is to introduce the mutual inhibition of stimulatory and suppressive activity. As noted above, the functional separation of paratope and idiotope, on a lymphocyte receptor, does not prevent their impeding each other. The actual amount of inhibition will strongly depend on the individual circumstances, and may be different for antibody-mediated and direct cell-cell interactions. Note that inhibition of stimulation by a suppressor cannot have a marked effect because the suppressive activity is stronger anyway. However, inhibition of suppression will turn out to be quite important for the induction of a normal response.

The last point on interactions takes some care of the separation into a cellular and a humoral aspect. When there are many Ab-i molecules in solution they will combine with Ab-(i - 1) and Ab-(i + 1) and thereby prevent their encountering the Ab-i lymphocytes. This effect will be referred to as buffering and is generally believed to operate, for example, in immune maturation.

Activation, suppression, their inhibition, and buffering are thus the essential ingredients of our model. It is now a routine matter to write down a corresponding set of equations. Although it is possible to laboriously derive such a set from a somewhat more detailed picture of cell triggering (Richter, 1974), an ad hoc formulation does just as well from our phenomenological point of view. The point of a mathematical theory at this stage cannot be to quantitatively reproduce nature, which is itself quite capricious. Rather it serves as a guide for our reasoning when things become intricate.

The rate equations will be given for a set of dimensionless variables s_i which denote the sizes of the Ab-i functional units, and may be understood as products of their concentrations and typical binding constants. The general form of these equations is

$$\frac{ds_i}{dt} = \frac{1}{\tau_b} f(s_{i-1}, s_i, s_{i+1})s_i - \frac{1}{\tau_d} g(s_{i-1}, s_i, s_{i+1})s_i \tag{1}$$

The first term describes growth, the second destruction. f and g are normalized to one so that τ_b and τ_d are the intrinsic birth and death time constants. Since stimulation comes from s_{i-1} we assume

$$f(s_{i-1}, s_i, s_{i+1}) = \frac{1}{1 + (B_i/s_{i-1})^m} \tag{2}$$

which is a typical threshold curve: there is no stimulation if $s_{i-1} \ll B_i$ and full triggering at high concentrations, $s_{i-1} \gg B_i$. The relative width of the threshold region is $\sim 1/m$, which identifies m as a cooperativity parameter. A large m, with a resulting switch like behavior of f, should be realistic for activation through patching and capping (Bell, 1975; DeLisi and Perelson, 1976), while direct cell-cell activation would probably imply a small m. The effectivity argument, however, strongly favors at least some degree of cooperativity, and $m = 5$ will be arbitrarily chosen to account for it. Analysis has shown that higher m does not modify the picture any more, whereas $m \lesssim 3$ makes triggering too easy at low concentrations (Tiedge, 1976).

The threshold position B_i depends on s_{i+1} via inhibition and s_i via buffering. This can be adequately represented by

$$B_i = B \frac{1 + s_{i+1}}{1 + \xi s_{i+1}} (1 + \eta s_i) \tag{3}$$

which takes into account that the intrinsic threshold B gets shifted towards higher concentrations because of inhibition $(1 + s_{i+1})$ and buffering $(1 + \eta s_i)$, and that inhibition is limited above $s_{i+1} \sim 1/\xi$. This can be interpreted as a reduction of the binding constant between i-paratopes and (i - 1)-idiotopes, due to the simultaneous binding of an (i + 1)-paratope to the i-idiotope.

The same kind of reasoning leads to the following suppression characteristics,

$$g = \frac{1}{1 + (D_i/s_{i+1})^n} \qquad D_i = D\,\frac{1 + s_{i-1}}{1 + \xi s_{i-1}}\,(1 + \eta s_i) \tag{4}$$

As mentioned above, the intrinsic threshold for destruction D should be lower than B. This may be rationalized by recalling that every single unit on the i'th level has to stand up against a whole set of functional units on the next level (see Fig. 1). We choose D/B = 0.1 throughout.

In order to have maximum transparency we shall use the same set of equations on all levels Ab-i. This can of course only be a first-order approximation to reality, but it does illustrate the capacity of straightforward network modeling, as will be seen in the next section. The actual choice of parameters is clearly of utmost importance for quantitative results. Qualitatively, however, the restrictions inferred by our above reasoning roughly determine the possible modes of behavior. Our standard set of parameters should therefore be quite representative:

$$B = 0.1 \qquad D = 0.01 \qquad \tau_b = 0.3 \qquad \tau_d = 0.1$$

$$m = n = 5 \qquad \xi = \eta = 0.01 \tag{5}$$

An intuition for the model may be gained from the phase diagram in Fig. 2. It shows the course of the thresholds on a s_{i+1}/s_{i-1}-plane, and the z direction gives $f/\tau_b - g/\tau_d$ which is the rate of change of log s_i. Given the concentrations s_{i+1} and s_{i-1}, the immediate fate of s_i may conveniently be derived from this diagram. The dominance of suppression is very perceptible.

Special consideration must be given to the antigen behavior which is most versatile in nature. For simplicity we shall disregard the possibility that the antigen itself may grow. Rather we confine ourselves to a naive model of Ab-1-mediated elimination, with some low cooperativity,

$$\dot{a} = -\frac{1}{\tau_a}\,\frac{1}{1 + (1/s_1)^2}\,a \tag{6}$$

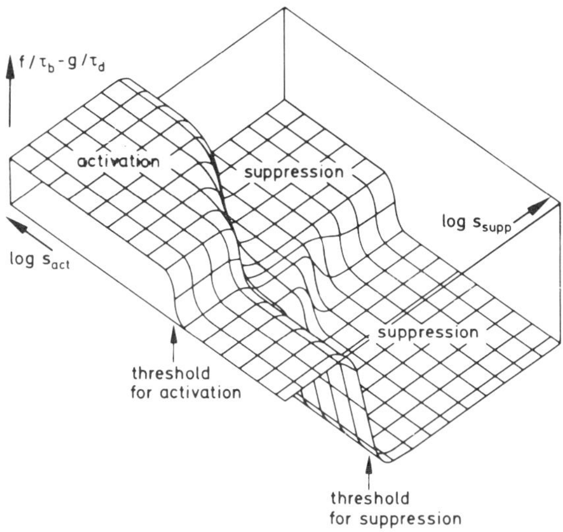

FIG. 2. Phase diagram showing the combined effects of activation and suppression upon a functional unit i. The z direction depicts the rate of change of log s_i. It is positive above the activation threshold, provided suppression is not too strong. The deflection of the threshold for suppression is due to the inhibitory influence of high enough activator concentration ($\xi = 10^{-2}$, $\eta = 0$).

It would be just as well to take an externally monitored a(t) curve and feed it into the above set of equations for the s_i, with a identified as s_0. This is because the antigen is usually kept under the experimenter's control. Here we can simulate an experiment by means of the decay time τ_a and the initial concentration a(0). A long time τ_a, for example, would sufficiently well represent a situation of repeated injection, as it is common for tolerance induction. The value of a(0) will be crucial for determining the mode of response.

III. THE BASIC MODES OF RESPONSE

Three main types of immune response can be derived from the above model, corresponding to low zone tolerance, normal response, and high zone tolerance. They will be discussed successively in the following, with low zone tolerance to play a particularly prominent role. Before entering an evaluation of the equations, however, we have to define the initial conditions. For the time being we want to consider a fully competent but virgin immune system, and since there is no a priori reason to discriminate between the functional units, we assume equal initial concentrations for the s_i. Their actual value, according to the introductory remarks, should be somewhat below the thresholds B and D, which leads us to take $s_i(0) = 10^{-3}$ for a reasonable guess. In terms of cell numbers, this may mean as little as some 10 cells/ml, so that whenever an s_i curve gets below 10^{-4}, we shall consider the respective functional unit as extinct.

A. Low Zone Tolerance (LZT)

From the point of view of absolute values of the antigen concentration, the lowest possible mode of response is tolerance induction (Dresser and Mitchison, 1968). The experimental procedure is to repeatedly challenge the animal with a low dose of the antigen. A subsequent standard dose will then fail to elicit a normal response.

Figure 3 shows how this phenomenon is described in the framework of our model. The repeated injections are simulated by a nearly constant antigen concentration. The antigen triggers Ab-1 which, after crossing the corresponding threshold, activates Ab-2. Because of its low amount the antigen is incapable of inhibiting the aggressive action of Ab-2 on Ab-1. Therefore Ab-1 becomes extinct, whereas Ab-2 is left on a moderately elevated level which is insufficient for stimulation of Ab-3.

In more familiar terms, suppressor T cells are activated against the idiotopes of the originally stimulated B cells, which thereupon disappear. This picture combines what is often presented as mutually exclusive explanations for tolerance, namely active suppression and clonal depletion. Furthermore, it gives a straightforward interpretation to the general saying that LZT is a "T cell phenomenon" (Chiller et al., 1971); taking T cells from a tolerant animal along with normal B cells, the existing suppressors will counteract every Ab-1 attempt to respond to antigenic challenge. On the other hand,

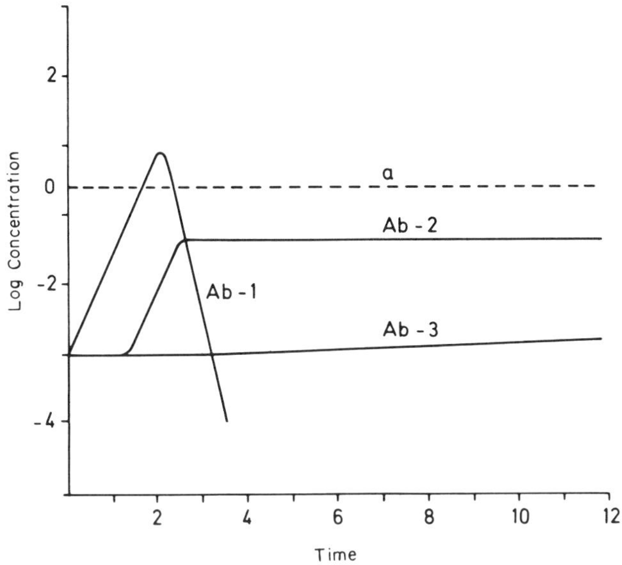

FIG. 3. Low zone tolerance. Ab-1 is stimulated and soon activates its own suppressors.

"tolerant B cells" together with normal T cells do not dispose of any primed suppressors, and newly synthesized competent B-cell precursors can normally respond to antigenic challenge. In this sense, the long-term memory for tolerance induction is clearly a T-cell matter.

B. Normal Response (NRP)

The standard procedure for immunization consists of two stages. First, a medium dose of antigen is applied to elicit a primary response. After a time, another challenge provokes a much more pronounced secondary response. Figure 4 shows how this is a natural consequence of our model. The primary response is a phase of severe internal conflict where the Ab-1 must overcome the aggression from Ab-2, with the help of Ab-3. The secondary response can take place after the suppressors Ab-2 have been eliminated, which renders the Ab-1 free for an unhindered response to the antigenic stimulus.

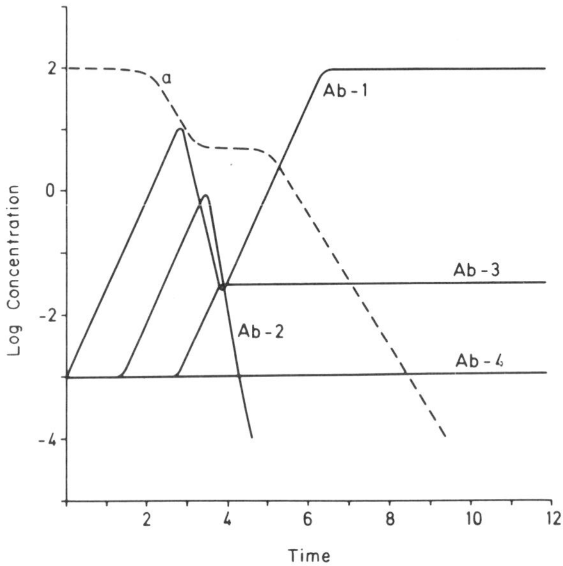

FIG. 4. Normal response. At higher antigen concentration, the suppressive action of Ab-2 on Ab-1 is delayed because of inhibition caused by the antigen. Helpers are thereby activated and eliminate the suppressors. This completes the primary response. Any antigen still present or applied afterwards leads to an unhampered secondary response.

The possibility for NRP to occur depends on the inhibition of suppression by larger amounts of the antigen. In this respect we formally agree with Jerne (1974) who visualizes the immune response as a break of a suppression-dominated steady state. The difference is that he thinks of suppression as already operating prior to antigenic stimulation, whereas here it is a consequence of Ab-2 induction after Ab-1 growth.

A similar line of formal agreement may be drawn to the Bretscher-Cohn two-signal theory (1970). They argue that for an adequate understanding of self-nonself discrimination, two signals must be assumed for effective Ab-1 triggering, the first of which is paralyzing and, moreover, part of the stimulatory signal. From our point of view, the mechanistic concept "signal" should be replaced by the operational term "mode," and then the reasoning becomes very similar. The funda-

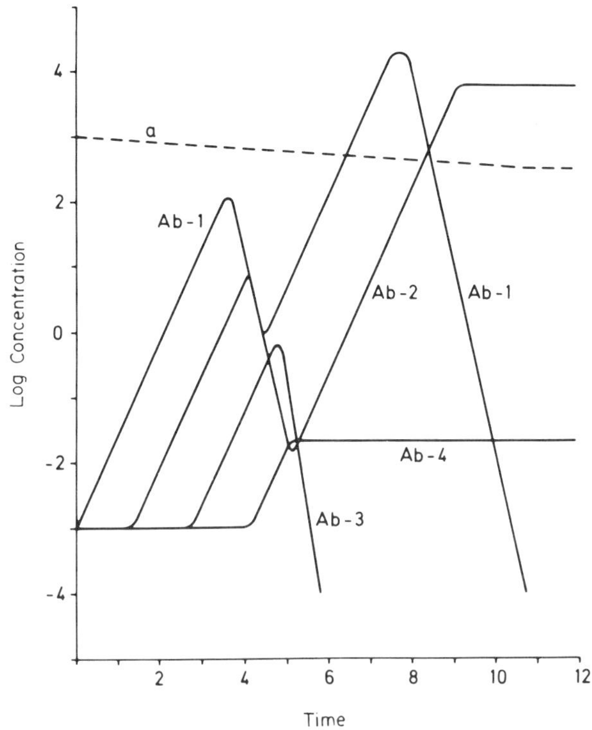

FIG. 5. High zone tolerance. Suppressors are pushed into a normal response. Ab-1 reaches a high intermediate level.

mental mode is LZT which means Ab-2 induction, with an obvious paralyzing effect. NRP requires a further step, namely Ab-3 induction, but it includes the first. The arguments in favor of a two-signal theory as listed by Cohn and Blomberg (1975) may therefore be translated into the language of the present model.

C. High Zone Tolerance (HZT)

The last type of response is presented in Fig. 5 and may be identified, though with some reservation, as high zone tolerance. As in LZT induction, the antigen is kept at an almost constant level through repeated injection, but this time the concentration is three or four orders of magnitude higher. The final result is again paralysis, with an intermediate phase of Ab-1 showing up. Following the sequence starting with Fig. 3 we would characterize HZT as LZT on the helper level Ab-3, or NRP on the suppressor level. This picture is straightforward but admittedly may be too simple. The very high concentrations involved surely give rise to marked second-order effects that have been neglected here.

There are no further modes beyond HZT, either in nature or in the model. The reason in the model is that inhibition has only a finite reach ($\xi = 10^{-2}$, not zero) so that suppression invariably takes over at a certain point. A more realistic argument might be that in the course of HZT the immune system is almost globally excited and therefore overall suppression dominant.

To sum up, three basic modes of response have been uncovered in the model which can be associated with the experimentally well-defined modes of LZT, NRP, and HZT. They may be characterized as LZT on the Ab-1, Ab-2 (suppressor), and Ab-3 (helper) levels, respectively. The simplicity of this sequence, and its derivation from one elementary set of equations, make it appear quite attractive from a theoretical point of view. There may, however, be more to it than merely aesthetics. Evolution could have followed a corresponding pathway, starting from a simple defense mechanism invented against the most common antigens, and possibly based on IgM effectors. A first limit was set up when the diverging system became a threat to self antigens. Suppressor T cells with their capacity of LZT induction were thus welcomed as a means of self-protection. The subsequent expansion of the T-cell population proceeded to the point where no further selective advantage could be gained. NRP obviously bears such an advantage, whereas HZT may not have much physiological relevance and for that reason be the last observed mode. As to the concomitant B-cell evolution, the invention of IgG may have facilitated the escape from Ab-2 suppression during the LZT phase: IgM-coated B cells could be better targets for suppressor T cells and thus be more efficiently eliminated than IgG-coated cells. The selection, during a primary response, against IgM-forming cells might reflect such a phylogenetic inheritance.

IV. FURTHER GENERAL OBSERVATIONS

A more detailed analysis of the three main modes of immune response reveals a number of accessory model characteristics which are in close correspondence to experimentally observed phenomena. They originate from certain particulars that have been left unconsidered so far: (a) there is not just one but a spectrum of affinities among each set of Ab-i populations; (b) the antigenic challenge may be more intricate, and relations between different antigens may play a role; (c) special treatment may affect the lymphocyte populations in various ways, with modified initial conditions arising.

To begin with, the representation of different affinities in our model is achieved by properly renormalizing the s_i. For example, if Ab-1 has an affinity χK towards the antigen, K being the typical binding constant used for all other relations, an adequate way to incorporate this into the set of equations (1) to (6) is to change B_1 and D_1,

$$B_1 = \frac{B}{\chi} \frac{1 + s_2}{1 + \xi s_2} (1 + \eta \chi s_1) \tag{7}$$

$$D_1 = D \frac{1 + \chi a}{1 + \xi \chi a} (1 + \eta s_1) \tag{8}$$

and to replace s_1 by χs_1 in Eq. (6). As a result, at low binding constants, $\chi \to 0$, the activation threshold for Ab-1 is effectively increased, and a given amount of antigen may no longer be sufficient to trigger Ab-1 production. Tiedge (1976) has discussed these complications in greater detail; here we review some consequences for LZT and NRP.

Because of the low antigen concentration, LZT at first affects the highest affinity antibodies only. The repeated injections, however, may well have a cumulative effect on the antigen so that Ab-1 populations with lower affinities become gradually activated and also undergo LZT elimination. A subsequent standard dose of antigen will only encounter very low affinity antibodies, and if they get triggered at all they will also run into extermination.

For a while, then, the induced suppressor T cells will be able to watch over any newly arising Ab-1, and thereby maintain tolerance. Their relatively low elevation above the average level, however, will soon fade away, and the memory get lost. This could be prevented by means of antigen being present (Dresser and Mitchison, 1968; Weigle, 1973): sporadically appearing Ab-1 would be enhanced and Ab-2 restimulated. This is an easy explanation of the well-known "Mitchison phenomenon" (Cohn and Blomberg, 1975), that tolerance induction depends on the antigen concentration whereas maintenance of tolerance does not.

In connection with the normal response, the main phenomenon to be discussed is immune maturation (reviewed by Siskind and Benacerraf, 1969). To simulate this in our model we assume two distinct Ab-1 populations, Ab-1(1) with an enhanced affinity χK towards the antigen, and Ab-1(2), which behaves like an average population. In addition to the modifications noted in Eqs. (7) and (8), there is a coupling between Ab-1(1) and Ab-1(2) due to the mutual buffering of stimulation: instead of $1 + \eta\chi s_{1(1)}$ in $B_{1(1)}$ and $1 + \eta s_{1(2)}$ in $B_{1(2)}$, both threshold expressions should contain the same buffering factor $1 + \eta(\chi s_{1(1)} + s_{1(2)})$. With these preparations, numerical integration yields Fig. 6. It is clearly seen how Ab-1(1) makes use of its initial advantage to depress the Ab-(2) response; the distribution among the different affinities changes to favor the higher ones.

A closely related explanation can be given to the phenomenon of the "original antigenic sin" (Webster, 1966; Fazekas de St. Groth and Webster, 1966). If somewhat lower affinity antibodies were included in the above discussion, they could be shown to end up in LZT suppression. Thus in the course of an immune response, the better responding Ab-1 populations tend to establish a pronounced individuality by outmatching their inferior competitors. This is an obvious threat to those populations which respond well to a cross-reacting antigen but poorly to the original one. When they get eliminated the only available responders to a challenge with the cross-reacting antigen are the originally stimulated Ab-1 populations, with high affinity to the original antigen, and low affinity to the challenging one.

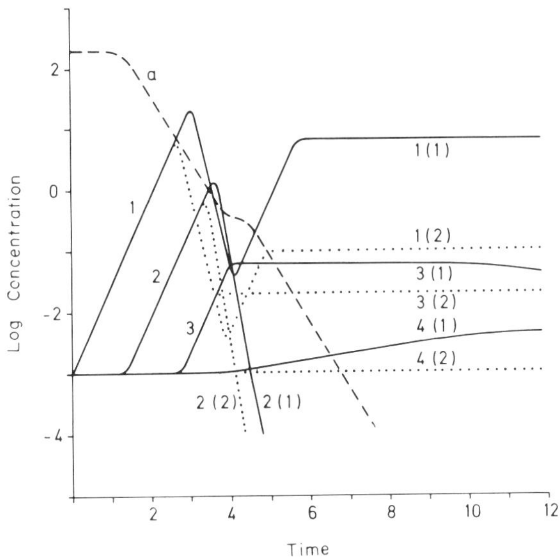

FIG. 6. Maturation in the immune response. The affinity of Ab-1(1) to the antigen a is 10-fold higher than the one of Ab-1(2) which is the same as all the other affinities used. Suppression of Ab-1(2) is less inhibited and therefore takes place earlier than of Ab-1(1). Buffering also disfavors Ab-1(2). The result here is that Ab-1(1) finally exceeds Ab-1(2) by a factor of 100.

Heterogeneity of the affinity between Ab-1 and its suppressors Ab-2 may account for another kind of phenomenon. Careful kinetic investigation of the immune response to a single persisting antigen frequently exhibits cyclical behavior in the concentration of Ab-1 (Weigle, 1975). There are usually two well-developed peaks, and the timing between them seems to be internally regulated. The explanation in the framework of our model is straightforward. In fact, Fig. 4 already discloses some tendency towards oscillations, which merely reflects the internal struggle for survival. A persisting antigen may give rise to cycling in the following way. In a first run, the Ab-1 reach only a moderate level before suffering from attack by their highest affinity suppressors. After elimination of these Ab-2, the Ab-1 start a next trial and attain a higher level than before. This may induce lower affinity suppressors which again reduce Ab-1, and another generation of helpers has to be awaited before Ab-1 may start its next expansion. Clearly, the time course of such cycling is a matter of internal regulation.

A great many experiments are done where the various subpopulations of lymphocytes are differentially affected, and several of them will be discussed in the following sections. At this point we only mention a few general predictions from our model that may have a bearing on a better understanding of the regulation system, and on the development of self-nonself discrimination during ontogeny. First of all, note that NRP leads further into T-cell participation than LZT does. Given an Ab-1 population, LZT requires only one more specific recognition, whereas NRP needs two. The reliability of LZT induction will therefore change in proportion to the total T-cell number [T], while NRP will depend on $[T]^2$. This implies that T-cell impairment will disfavor NRP to the benefit of the LZT mode. The general requirement for T-cell help in a normal response might be rationalized in such a way. The common means of T-cell depletion may be insufficient to put out of action every candidate for a suppressor cell in a given situation. (I disregard here the problem of thymus-independent antigens, lacking a safe knowledge of their specialities. Somehow they may protect their Ab-1 against the suppressive T-cell attack, under normal conditions. This would nicely go with the persisting IgM character of the responses.)

Figure 7 gives an example which simulates the effect of reduced T-cell number on the helper level. An antigenic challenge which normally induces NRP now leads to LZT. However, in this case the Ab-2 level has become high enough to also stimulate the Ab-3, which subsequently erases the memory for LZT. Recovery on the B-cell level could afterwards take advantage of the absence of suppressors and give rise to a postrecovery overshoot (Dresser and Mitchison, 1968, p. 164).

These considerations finally lead us to a simple hypothesis for the establishment of self-nonself discrimination in early life. During development of the immune system, the lymphocyte populations gradually expand. Under these conditions, the first mode of response

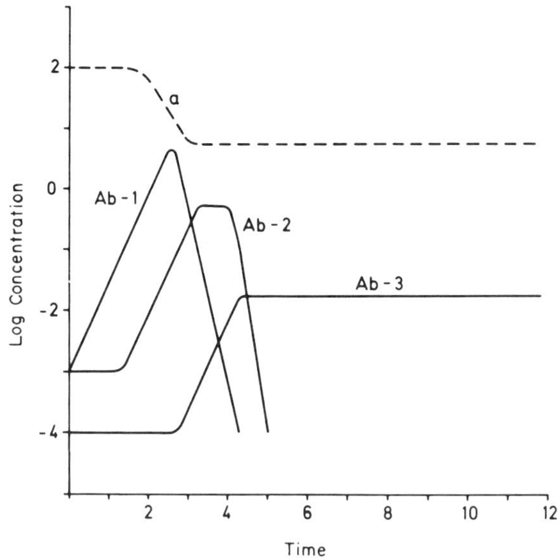

FIG. 7. Impairment of the T population. The availability of helpers is most severely reduced. Antigenic challenge that would normally yield a normal response now leads to low zone tolerance. In this particular case the suppressors still induce the residual helpers and thus get eliminated in the end. Tolerance is short-lived and after recovery may display overshoot characteristics.

to become operative is low zone tolerance, and for a while it will be the only one. The self antigens may cause some transient stimulus of Ab-1 populations, but suppressor cells will invariably arise to eliminate them. Occasionally, a helper population may happen to be already present, and drive the respective suppressor into death. But then there are other suppressors to take over, because of the system's built-in degeneracy. At the end of this period, a pattern of mildly elevated suppressor populations has been generated which protects against any anti-self directed Ab-1 production, and which is permanently stabilized by the presence of the self antigens, as in the Mitchison phenomenon.

This picture of ontogenetic unfolding corresponds well to Adam and Weiler's description (1976) of generation and limitation of antibody diversity. They also make use of antiidiotypic elimination as a main tool, but they do not attempt to explain self-nonself discrimination. The Bretscher-Cohn theory (1970), on the other hand, accounts for the maintenance of this discrimination but not for its ontogenesis.

V. POSSIBLE ROLES OF ALLOTYPES AND CARRIERS

As mentioned in the introduction, the idiotype-based network may not account for the totality of regulation phenomena that have been reported. We shall therefore briefly comment on the possibility of taking into consideration the marked effects associated with allotype and carrier interference. The main argument will be that allotype or carrier antigenicity may become operative on an Ab-i level and mask its comparatively weak idiotype antigenicity.

The work on allotype suppression induced by perinatal application of antiallotypic antibodies has recently been reviewed by Herzenberg et al. (1975). There seems to be no doubt that the suppressors are T lymphocytes directed against the allotype, that is, against a whole class containing many different idiotypes. We do not expect these suppressor cells to be distinct from the anti-idiotypic ones discussed so far because the nature of their respective targets is very similar. Under normal conditions, however, the allotype is present in much larger concentrations than any of the idiotypes, and during ontogeny it will induce tolerance like an ordinary self antigen. This means that it stimulates its suppressors. Now imagine that the number of allotype-bearing cells is severely reduced during that critical phase, for example, by means of anti-allotypic antibodies. Their stimulatory capacity is then reduced and they may become unable to drive the Ab-1 above threshold for Ab-2 triggering; rather they get eliminated first. Such a situation might be described as LZT on the zero'th level, and is a trivial case with external antigens. Here, however, it may achieve long-term persistence due to restimulation as in the Mitchison phenomenon: allotype-bearing cells continuously reappear, and it is a matter of balance between replenishment and elimination whether they finally overcome their suppressors. Accordingly, some species exhibit chronic allotype suppression, and some do not.

Allogeneic helper activity is also a well-established effect (Dutton, 1975; Schimpl and Wecker, 1975). In short, it is observed that an immune response which is impaired by T-cell depletion can be restored by allogeneic T cells, and they are superior for that purpose to syngeneic ones. Our interpretation is straightforward. T depletion is probably never complete; rather it favors suppressor dominance, with a tendency towards LZT induction. For NRP to recur, helpers are needed to suppress the suppressors. Syngeneic T cells can be used because of their potential antiidiotypic activity; however, allogeneic T cells attack via the allotype and should therefore be effective in much lower numbers. It has been observed that a T-cell replacing soluble factor (TRF) can substitute for the allogeneic cells, but this is of no particular interest for us since it concerns the internal organization of the functional units. A more pertinent finding is that TRF exerts an optimum effect some definite time after the antigenic challenge to the B cells. This might be related to the time needed for suppressor expansion during the response.

The carrier-hapten dichotomy is one of the fundamentals of immunology, and yet the very definition of carrier vs. hapten can only be given in operational terms. We do not want to question the practical usefulness of this distinction, but we should bear in mind that any particular antigenic determinant on a carrier molecule may be looked upon as a hapten, under appropriate circumstances. The most characteristic feature of a carrier is that it possesses many antigenic determinants, and of a variety of kinds.

The modification introduced in our standard network, when the antigen is a carrier or a carrier-linked hapten, lies in the relation between Ab-1 and Ab-2. The reason is that carrier determinants largely replace the receptor idiotypes in determining the antigenic character of the Ab-1 lymphocytes. Therefore, anticarrier-directed Ab-2 cells are expected to exert suppression upon the Ab-1 population.

The helper effect necessary for the induction of a normal response would then come from an anti-Ab-2 response on the Ab-3 level, as usual in our model.

This view of carrier priming markedly opposes the conventional picture, which assumes direct helper induction and associative signaling from the helpers towards the Ab-1 (Bretscher and Cohn, 1970). In our model, the anticarrier specificity is in the suppressor population whereas common thinking assigns it to the helper cells. A normal response should be characterized by the absence of any anticarrier T cells in the present network picture, although there may well be specificity with respect to the carrier because, after all, the carrier starts the weaving. By contrast, the usual two-signal theories predict the existence of anticarrier T cells in an NRP, without any experimental corroboration so far.

There is no difficulty in explaining numerous aspects of the carrier-hapten phenomenon, on the basis of our model. First of all, carrier-induced help is a typical T-cell matter in the sense that T-cell depletion tends to favor suppression. Next, the physical union of carrier and hapten is necessary for the hapten to profit from a previous carrier priming, for obvious reasons. And finally, overstimulation of help by means of higher doses of the carrier results in helper extinction and suppressor generation (Tada et al., 1975). A most interesting observation in this connection is that these suppressor T cells contain a molecule which can be absorbed with the carrier.

As a last point, we want to discuss the so-called "Weigle phenomenon" (Cohn and Blomberg, 1975), which is that breaking tolerance to an antigen α can be achieved with a cross-reacting antigen β in the absence of α, and once tolerance is lost, α can induce a secondary response. The simple idiotype-connected network does not account for this effect; the antigens used in these experiments, however, exhibit the typical characteristics of carrier molecules. Assume, therefore, that antigen α has determinants α_1 and α_2, and that β also possesses different antigenic sites β_1 and β_2. Let α_1 and β_1

cross-react, the others not. Tolerance to α means that there are anti-α T cells which suppress the anti-α B cells. Now let β challenge the system in the absence of α. The anti-β_1 B cells will undergo a normal primary response; the βs bound to their receptors will preferentially expose β_2 for T cell attack and not be harmed by the existing anti-α. The anti-β_2 B cells, on the other hand, suffer some suppression from the anti-α_1 T cells because they expose their cross-reacting determinant β_1. Thus there is a tendency towards production of antibodies against β_1, and once elicited they would soon give a secondary response to α challenge: the anti-β_1-bound α would expose α_2 and drive the anti-α_2 T cells into extermination. The presence of α during β challenge, however, would prevent anti-β_1 expression: the α would compete with β for anti-β_1 receptors and thereby render them vulnerable to anti-α_2 T-cell attack.

VI. SUPPORT FROM EXPERIMENTS

The evidence for suppressor T cells as a result of low zone tolerance induction is now quite convincing. As a typical experiment we mention the work of Kölsch et al. (1975) on LZT to phage fd in CBA mice. Transferable specific suppressor activity on the T-cell level has unambiguously been demonstrated. Furthermore, it has been concluded from the observations that suppressor T cells should have a lower triggering threshold than helper T cells, which is indeed an essential operational feature of our model. Finally, promotion of suppressor activity was found using hydrocortisone treatment, and resistance of suppressor T cells to radiation was found. This agrees well with our prediction that impairment of the T population should first affect helper function and thereby favor suppression. In their own model of LZT and NRP induction, Kölsch, Stumpf, and Weber come close to the picture presented here, except that they do not envisage helpers as being stimulated by the suppressors.

Antiidiotypic Ab-2 antibodies have recently been demonstrated to emerge during an immune response (Rodkey, 1974; Kluskens and

Köhler, 1974; McKearn et al., 1974), and they have been used as a tool for investigating regulation phenomena (Bangasser et al., 1975; Eichmann, 1975; Eichmann and Rajewsky, 1975).

The kinetics of Ab-2 appearance has been analyzed carefully by McKearn et al. (1974). Eight Lewis rats were immunized with 12 weekly intraperitoneal injections of 2×10^8 irradiated BN tumor cells, and sera were analyzed just before each renewed challenge. The total Ab-1 titer exhibited marked oscillatory behavior, with a first peak obviously originating from a lymphocyte species carrying the particular idiotype Id-1. The time course of Id-1 expression and the corresponding antiidiotypic Ab-2 level were also monitored. It was found that these Ab-2 appeared with a certain delay and that the Id-1 idiotypes concomitantly disappeared. This is in perfect agreement with the basic assumption underlying our theory that Ab-i stimulates Ab-(i + 1) and gets suppressed in turn. Recovery of the total Ab-1 titer is brought about by non-Id-1 bearing Ab-1 populations.

The effect of externally applied antiidiotypic antiserum on the expression of the idiotype, strongly depends on the experimental circumstances. We shall review here two examples where the tendency of the antiserum is to suppress the idiotype. Bangasser et al. (1975) treated normal A/J mice with a serum raised in rabbits which specifically acts against an idiotype of anti-p-azophenylarsonate (anti-Ar) antibodies, called CRI. Without any further manipulation, this anti-CRI treatment simply eliminates the CRI: adoptive transfer of 6×10^7 spleen cells to irradiated (700 R) recipients results in responses lacking CRI, whereas admixture of normal spleen cells restores the capacity for CRI responses because the normal cells contain this idiotype. The situation is different, however, when antigen is applied subsequent to the anti-CRI treatment, and prior to admixture of normal cells. In this case, the normal cells do not restore CRI expression. The investigators explain their observation in terms of competition for the antigen among the Ab-1 populations. From our point of view, an interpretation involving LZT induction seems to be more stringent. The anti-CRI serum severely hampers the CRI bearing lymphocytes in their response to the antigen. Therefore they effectively behave like low affinity responders, and in spite of a fair amount of antigen, do not surmount the LZT phase. Suppressor T cells should then be present which actively eliminate any CRI they encounter after adoptive transfer.

Corroboration of this expectation comes from Eichmann's experiments (1975) in which streptococcal Group A carbohydrate (A-CHO) is used as antigen, and guinea pig IgG_2 antiidiotypic antibody ($\bar{a}$Id2) is directed against the A5A idiotype of anti-A-CHO antibodies in A/J mice. The kinetics of A5A availability after $\bar{a}$Id2 application, and subsequent antigenic challenge, shows an interesting dose dependence. High doses of $\bar{a}$Id2 (5 μg idiotype binding capacity) rapidly diminish the A5A idiotype, but recovery is soon observed. A 50-fold lower dose, on the other hand, results in a slowly decreasing A5A level which remains chronically suppressed. Eichmann shows that suppressor T cells have been induced in this case, in contrast to the former. The rationalization is that the high dose immediately eliminates the A5A-bearing cells so that there is no opportunity for their triggering Ab-2. This situation therefore corresponds to the one elicited by anti-CRI treatment without antigenic challenge, in the experiment mentioned above. The suppressor induction in the low dose case should proceed similarly as suggested for the CRI suppressors.

Summarizing, we find good support from relevant experiments as far as the Ab-2 level is concerned. The techniques are just being developed for looking into the system in that detail, for example, by means of antiidiotypic antibodies. It will be much harder, accordingly, to go one step further and explore the Ab-3 level more directly.

VII. CONCLUSION

An attempt has been made, on the basis of a simple network model, to understand a variety of phenomena concerning regulation of the immune response. Underlying the whole reasoning was the asumption that regulation operates on the level of functional units defined via specificity. In a human, such a functional unit contains some 10^6 lymphocytes and 10^{14} antibody molecules on the average. We thus visualize the immune system as being organized on a distinctly higher level than its constituents. The internal structure of a functional unit is of course highly important for its very functioning, but for many purposes it may be quite sufficient, and even adequate, to know only a few phenomenological constants characterizing the interactions between these units.

To conclude, let us stress again that our model is conceived in a way which in principle allows for straightforward reconstruction of phylogenesis. The systematic sequence of modes may well reflect successive needs that came up during evolution, self-protection ranking at high priority. Our picture of the perinatal establishment of self-nonself discrimination would then very naturally fit into the general scheme that ontogeny reiterates phylogenetic acquisition. The question of germ-line fixation vs. somatic generation of individual diversity should also be reexamined in this context. If idiotypy is really at the heart of immunological regulation mechanisms, then at least this type of specificity should favorably be genetically preserved.

ACKNOWLEDGMENTS

I thank Prof. M. Eigen for his continued support. The numerical integrations were carried out by B. Morgeneyer whose expert assistance is gratefully acknowledged. Use has been made of the UNIVAC 1108 computer of the Ges. f. wiss. Datenverarbeitung, Göttingen.

REFERENCES

Adam, G. and Weiler, E. (1976). Lymphocyte population dynamics during ontogenetic generation of diversity. In *The Generation of Antibody Diversity* (A. J. Cunningham, ed.). Academic, London.

Bangasser, S. A., Kapsalis, A. A., Fraker, P. J., and Nisonoff, A. (1975). Competition for antigen by cell populations having receptors with the same specificity but of different idiotype. *J. Immunol. 114:* 610-614.

Bell, G. I. (1970). Mathematical model of clonal selection and antibody production. *J. Theor. Biol. 29:* 191-232.

Bell, G. I. (1971). Mathematical model of clonal selection and antibody production, II and III. *J. Theor. Biol. 33:* 339-398.

Bell, G. I. (1975). B lymphocyte activation and lattice formation. *Transplant. Rev. 23:* 23-36.

Bretscher, P. and Cohn, M. (1970). A theory of self-nonself discrimination. *Science 169:* 1042-1049.

Burnet, F. M. (1957). A modification of Jerne's theory of antibody production using the concept of clonal selection. *Austr. J. Sci. 20:* 67-68.

Chiller, J. M., Habicht, G. S., and Weigle, W. O. (1971). Kinetic differences in unresponsiveness of thymus and bone marrow cells. *Science 171:* 813-815.

Cohn, M. and Blomberg, B. (1975). The self-nonself discrimination: a one- or two-signal mechanism? *Scand. J. Immunol. 4:* 1-24.

Cosenza, H. and Köhler, H. (1972). Specific suppression of the antibody response by antibodies to receptors. *Proc. Nat. Acad. Sci. (USA) 69:* 2701-2705.

DeLisi, C. and Perelson, A. S. (1976). The kinetics of aggregation phenomena. I. Minimal models for patch formation on lymphocyte membranes. *J. Theor. Biol. 62:* 159-210.

Dresser, D. W. and Mitchison, N. A. (1968). The mechanism of immunological paralysis. *Adv. Immunol. 8:* 129-181.

Dutton, R. W. (1975). Separate signals for the initiation of proliferation and differentiation in the B cell response to antigen. *Transplant. Rev. 23:* 66-77.

Eichmann, K. (1974). Idiotype suppression. I. Influence of the dose and of the effector functions of anti-idiotypic antibody on the production of an idiotype. *Eur. J. Immunol. 4:* 296-302.

Eichmann, K. (1975). Idiotype suppression. II. Amplification of a suppressor T cell with anti-idiotypic activity. *Eur. J. Immunol. 5:* 511-517.

Eichmann, K. and Rajewsky, K. (1975). Induction of T and B cell immunity by anti-idiotypic antibody. *Eur. J. Immunol. 5:* 661-666.

Fazekas de St. Groth, S. and Webster, R. G. (1966). Disquisitions on original antigenic sin. *J. Exp. Med. 124:* 331-361.

Gershon, R. K. (1974). T cell regulation: the "second law of thymodynamics." In *The Immune System - Genes, Receptors, Signals* (E. E. Sercarz, A. R. Williamson, and C. F. Fox, eds.). Academic, New York, pp. 471-484.

Gierer, A. and Meinhardt, H. (1972). A theory of biological pattern formation. *Kybernetik 12:* 30-39.

Herzenberg, L. A., Okumura, K., and Metzler, C. M. (1975). Regulation of immunoglobulin and antibody production by allotype suppressor T cells in mice. *Transplant. Rev. 27:* 57-83.

Hoffmann, G. W. (1975). A theory of regulation and self-nonself discrimination in an immune network. *Eur. J. Immunol. 5:* 638-647.

Hopper, J. E. and Nisonoff, A. (1971). Individual antigenic specificity of immunoglobulins. *Adv. Immunol. 13:* 57-99.

Jerne, N. K. (1972). What precedes clonal selection? In *Ontogeny of Acquired Immunity.* CIBA Foundation Symposium 1971. Assoc. Scientific Publ., Amsterdam, pp. 1-15.

Jerne, N. K. (1974). Towards a network theory of the immune system. *Ann. Immunol. Inst. Pasteur 125C:* 373-389.

Jerne, N. K. (1976). The immune system. A web of V-domains. In *The Harvey Lectures,* Series 70. Academic, New York.

Katz, D. H. and Benacerraf, B. (1972). The regulatory influence of activated T cells on B cell responses to antigen. *Adv. Immunol. 15:* 1-94.

Kluskens, L. and Köhler, H. (1974). Regulation of immune response by autogenous antibody against receptor. *Proc. Nat. Acad. Sci. (USA) 71:* 5083-5087.

Köhler, H. (1975). The response to phosphorylcholine: dissecting an immune response. *Transplant. Rev. 27:* 24-56.

Kölsch, E., Stumpf, R., and Weber, G. (1975). Low zone tolerance and suppressor T cells. *Transplant. Rev. 26:* 56-86.

Lees, R. K. and Sinclair, N. R. S. (1975). Regulation of the immune response. IX. Resistance to antibody mediated immunosuppression induced by the presence of the allogeneic effect. *Cell. Immunol. 17:* 525-531.

Lefkovits, I. (1974). Precommitment in the immune system. *Curr. Topics Microbiol. Immunol. 65:* 21-58.

McKearn, T. J., Stuart, F. P., and Fitch, F. W. (1974). Anti-idiotypic antibody in rat transplantation immunity. I. Produciton of anti-idiotypic antibody in animals repeatedly immunized with alloantigens. *J. Immunol. 113:* 1876-1882.

Nisonoff, A. and Bangasser, S. A. (1975). Immunological suppression of idiotypic specificities. *Transplant. Rev. 27:* 100-134.

Poljak, R. J., Amzel, L. M., Avey, H. P., Chen, B. L., Phizackerley, R. P., and Saul, F. (1973). Three-dimensional structure of the Fab' fragment of a human immunoglobulin at 2.8 Å resolution. *Proc. Nat. Acad. Sci. (USA) 70:* 3305-3310.

Richter, P. H. (1974). *Die Phänomenologie der Immunantwort* (contribution to a competition of the Bavarian Academy of Sciences). Max-Planck-Institut für biophysikalische Chemie, Göttingen.

Richter, P. H. (1975). A network theory of the immune response. *Eur. J. Immunol. 5:* 350-354.

Rodkey, L. S. (1974). Studies of idiotypic antibodies. Production and characterization of autoantiidiotypic antisera. *J. Exp. Med. 139:* 712-720.

Rowley, D. A., Fitch, F. W., Stuart, F. P., Köhler, H., and Cosenza, H. (1973). Specific suppression of immune responses. *Science 181:* 1133-1141.

Schimpl, A. and Wecker, E. (1975). A third signal in B cell activation given by TRF. *Transplant. Rev. 23:* 176-188.

Siskind, G. W. and Benacerraf, B. (1969). Cell selection by antigen in the immune response. *Adv. Immunol. 10:* 1-50.

Tada, T., Taniguchi, M., and Takemori, T. (1975). Properties of primed suppressor T cells and their products. *Transplant. Rev. 26:* 106-129.

Tiedge, J. (1976). *Netzwerktheorie für Selektionsvorgänge in der Immunantwort.* Diplomarbeit, Marburg.

Webster, R. G. (1966). Original antigenic sin in ferrets: the response to sequential infections with influenza viruses. *J. Immunol. 97:* 177-183.

Weigle, W. O. (1973). Immunological unresponsiveness. *Adv. Immunol. 16:* 61-122.

Weigle, W. O. (1975). Cyclical production of antibody as a regulatory mechanism in the immune response. *Adv. Immunol. 21:* 87-111.

Weigle, W. O., Sieckmann, D. G., Doyle, M. V., and Chiller, J. M. (1975). Possible roles of suppressor cells in immunological tolerance. *Transplant. Rev. 26:* 186-205.

Wilson, H. R. and Cowan, J. D. (1973). A mathematical theory of the functional dynamics of cortical and thalamic nervous tissue. *Kybernetik 13:* 55-80.

Chapter 20

INCORPORATION OF A NONSPECIFIC T CELL DEPENDENT HELPER FACTOR INTO A NETWORK THEORY OF THE REGULATION OF THE IMMUNE RESPONSE

Geoffrey W. Hoffmann

Basel Institute for Immunology
Basel, Switzerland

Data concerning T cell dependent factors that influence humoral immune responses are reviewed. A simple way of incorporating a widely investigated nonspecific helper factor into a recently developed network theory of regulation is described. The extended model provides explanations for a number of well-characterized phenomena concerning the induction of unresponsiveness and of humoral immune responses. The phenomena discussed include immune responses to hapten-carrier conjugates, the adjuvant properties of "thymus-independent" antigens, high zone tolerance, and stimulation and suppression induced by anti-idiotypic antibodies.

I. INTRODUCTION

There are at least two basic theoretical propositions concerning the subject that most cellular immunologists would agree on. The first is that the clonal selection theory is correct, and the second is that almost everything else in cellular immunology is very complicated. For instance, Fig. 1 shows some of the components which, in addition to the antigen, are involved in the regulation of the production of antibodies by B cells.

Jerne has promoted the idea that the immune system may be viewed as a network, consisting of components that recognize each other specifically via idiotype-antiidiotype interactions (Jerne, 1972, 1973, 1974a,b, 1975). Similar ideas have been discussed in an article by Lindenmann (1973). The network hypothesis provides theoretical biologists with a difficult but fascinating problem. The challenge is to find simple models that can be shown to have the experimentally observed regulatory properties. The search for workable network models involves deciding which of the components in Fig. 1 are the most important, and just how they interact with each other. In view of the complexity of the problem, our only hope is to begin by simplifying it as much as possible by initially neglecting phenomena that we feel are probably of secondary importance. Whether or not such simplifications are justified can be judged only a posteriori, when we see whether the simplifications lead to a coherent scheme of regulation,

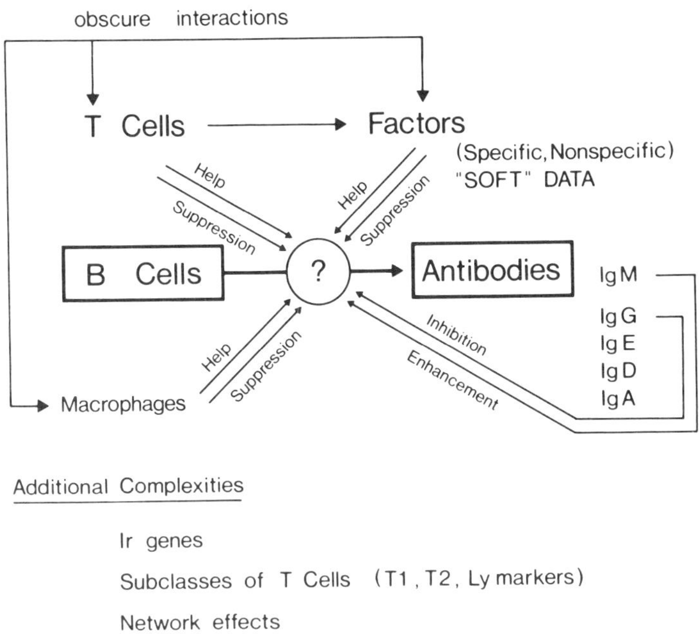

FIG. 1. Some of the components involved in the regulation of the production of antibodies by B cells.

providing explanations for phenomena that were not initially considered. Explicit models lead to testable predictions, and thus permit either refutation or substantiation of the postulates.

The purpose of this chapter is to show that much of the experimental data concerning the regulation of humoral immune responses may be integrated into a reasonably simple conceptual framework. I will describe an extended and slightly modified version of a recently published network theory of regulation (Hoffmann, 1975). The extension involves showing how a fairly extensively investigated nonspecific T cell dependent factor may be most simply incorporated into the model. For convenience, the model will be referred to as the plus-minus network theory.

Much of the experimental data available for model building may be roughly classified into the categories of molecular component data and system response data. Molecular component data include the

TABLE 1

Reported Properties of Some Antigen-specific Factors[a]

References	Factor	Size (MW)	Properties	Antigen	Genetic region	Comments
Nelson (1970)	"cytophilic antibody"	α_1 globulin	Arms MØ	Sheep RBC		Identical Factor in serum
Evans et al. (1972)	SMAF (specific MØ arming factor)	50,000-60,000	Arms MØ	Allogeneic cells		
Feldmann et al. (1972, 1973, 1974)	IgT	∿ 180,000	Cytophylic for MØ Helps, suppresses	KLH		Size determined from membrane extraction
Erb and Feldmann (1975) Erb et al. (1976)	"Genetically related MØ factor"	55,000 ± 3,000	Forms complex with antigen	KLH, TGAL	H2I	
Tada et al. (1975) Taniguchi et al. (1976)	Suppressor factor in vivo, in vitro	35,000-60,000	Carrier-specific. Enhances in one instance	Asc, KLH	H2I	
Taniguchi and Tada (1974)	Helper factor	100,000-200,000	Helps	Asc		Not found in the mouse (personal communication
Benacerraf et al. (1975)	GAT suppressor factor	∿ 45,000	Suppresses IgG	GAT	H2I	

Taussig and Munro (1974) Munro and Taussig (1975); and Taussig et al. (1976)	In vivo, helper factor	∼ 50,000	Helps IgM in vivo. Acts across species	TGAL	H2I	Binds to "purified B cells"
Zembala and Asherson (1974); Asherson and Zembala (1975)	TCP (T-cell product)	∼ 50,000	Suppresses contact sensitivity, arms macrophages	Picrylchloride		
Yu and Gordon (1973)	Helper factor	Nondialysable	Specific for particulate Ag	Sheep RBC Chicken RBC		
Amos and Lachmann (1970)	MIF (MØ inhibition factor)	35,000-55,000	Inhibits MØ migration in presence of antigen	PPD, β-lactoglobulin		

[a]MØ, macrophage; Asc, *Ascaris suum* extract; KLH, keyhole limpet hemocyanin; PPD, purified protein derivative

properties of various "factors" that have been reported to influence the production of antibodies by B cells. These data are essential for model building, but most are quite new and "soft," and there are disputes concerning the cellular sources of such factors, their molecular weights, whether or not they are antigen-specific, and so on. (See Table 1 for a brief review.) Thus, molecular component data provide important clues, but in view of the softness of some of the data, it is fortunate that they do not constitute the sole data base available to the model builder.

In addition, there is an extensive body of older, partly harder data concerning the way the *system as a whole* responds to various types of antigenic stimuli. Such data provide a means of testing the viability of any model, which may initially be conceived on the basis of soft data concerning the individual components.

In the following, I will review what I consider to be the most relevant molecular component data as of the time of writing (March, 1976). I will then formulate the extended model, and give a description of the events which, according to the model, are provoked by various types of antigenic stimulation. It will be seen that a reasonably simple set of interactions postulated on the basis of molecular component data exhibits much of the observed system response behavior.

The type of experiments that are required to test and quantify the model are discussed in the final section.

II. MOLECULAR COMPONENT DATA

A. Antigen-specific T-Cell Factors

Table 1 lists some of the reported properties of helper and suppressor factors for which the data indicate some antigenic specificity. The simplest hypothesis concerning antigen-specific T cell dependent factors that can accomodate an optimal amount of data, is that there is only one such factor, that it has a molecular weight of the order of 50,000, that it carries Ia (H2I region associated) antigenic determinants, and that it is cytophilic for nonspecific accessory cells (e.g., macrophages). These are the properties that were assigned to the antigen-specific factor in the plus-minus network theory (Hoffmann, 1975). On the basis of the molecular weight of the factor, it is furthermore postulated in the theory that the factor is monovalent. (Immunoglobulins with a molecular weight of about 150,000 are divalent.) This property of monovalency is important in the theory, which involves the cross-linking of receptors as a general mechanism for stimulating lymphoid cells. A monovalent factor could not cross-link receptors, whereas it could block receptors that are complementary to itself, and thus inhibit stimulation.

B. Nonspecific T Cell Dependent Factors That Provide B Cells with a "Second Signal"

Nonspecific helper factors have been generated by a number of procedures, as reviewed in Table 2. Some of the published data concerning these factors are also contradictory (unless there is a large number of such factors), but there is nevertheless widespread agreement concerning a number of points. Thus it is generally accepted that 24-hr mixed lymphocyte culture supernatants (MLC S/N) can provide B cells with the second (nonspecific) signal required for the in vitro formation of plaque-forming cells in response to sheep red blood cells (sheep RBC), and that a similar activity can be obtained by challenging appropriately primed T-cell suspensions with the antigen used for priming.

Some of the biochemical properties of these nonspecific factors are controversial. It was reported by Armerding et al. (1974) that a nonspecific helper factor, which they called allogeneic effect factor (AEF), prepared by in vivo sensitization to alloantigens, followed by in vitro incubation with the educating cell type, bears Ia determinants. The protocol for producing AEF is quite similar to that used by Munro and Taussig (1974) for producing specific factor, and since the activities had similar molecular weights, it seemed possible that it could have been the same factor. Waldmann et al. (1976) and Schimpl and Wecker (personal communication) have, however,

TABLE 2

Some Reported Properties of Non-specific "Second Signal" Factors for Activating B cells

A. Factors produced by uneducated cells

References	Factor production	Size (MW)	Antigen for assay	Optimal time of addition	Comments
Dutton (1975)	MLC S/N	Dialysable and 28,000	Sheep RBC	48 hours	
Schimpl and Wecker (1975)	MLC S/N	25,000-35,000	Sheep RBC	48 hours	Help IgM and IgG. No Ia determinants on factor (personal communication)
Britton (1972)	MLC S/N		Sheep RBC		
Sjöberg et al. (1972)	MLC S/N	Nondialyzable	Sheep RBC		MØ required for production
Feldmann and Basten (1972)	Allogeneic cells	Dialyzable	Various		
Schrader (1973)	Activated MØ S/N		FγG		Obtained also with MØ from nu/nu mice
Farrer (1975)	Human PBL[a]		Sheep RBC		Acts across species
Waldmann et al. (1976)	Con A stimulation of spleen cells[b]		Sheep RBC		Still produced after macrophage depletion, no Ia determinants detected.
Rubin et al. (1974)	Human lymphocyte	35,000	Sheep RBC		Acts across species

B. Factors produced by in vivo education with antigen followed by in vitro incubation with educating antigen

Gorczynski et al. (1972,1973)	F1 cells[c]	150,000-300,000	Sheep RBC	48 hours	Activity absorbed by antigen-stimulated cells
Vann and Galloway (1973)	F1 cells[c]		Sheep RBC		
Armerding and Katz (1974); Armerding et al. (1974, 1975)	F1 cells[c]	30,000-40,000	Sheep RBC, MØ-bound DNP-KLH, DNP-FγG[d]		β_2 microglobulin and Ia determinants reported present on factor
Rubin, MacDonald and Coons (1973)	Tetanus toxoid	75,000	Sheep RBC		
Waldmann and Munro (1975); Waldmann et al. (1975)	KLH	30,000-50,000	Sheep RBC	0 hours	Factor production enhanced by addition of MØ
Kishimoto and Ishizaka (1975a)	Ascaris, Ragweed	150,000	DNP-KLH	24 hours	Helps IgE response
Kishimoto et al. (1975a,1975)	Ascaris, Ragweed	20,000-40,000	DNP-KLH		Helps IgG, binds to anti-Ig activated B cells
Nakano and Braun (1967)	Chicken erythrocytes		Sheep RBC		In vivo activity
Watson (1973)	Sheep RBC, allogeneic cells	< 7000 15,000-40,000 and 150,000	Sheep RBC		T cells not required for production of the smaller factors

[a]Human peripheral blood lymphocytes [b]Concanavalin A = Con A.
[c]Parental thymus cells were sensitized in vivo to alloantigens on irradiated F1 cells, and then incubated with identical irradiated F1 cells.
[d]FγG = fowl gamma globulin.

been unable to find any evidence of Ia determinants on nonspecific helper factors. Furthermore, Waldmann et al. (1976) report a second distinguishing feature between nonspecific helper factor and specific T-cell factor. The latter binds to lentil lectin, whereas the former does not. The simplest reasonable interpretation at this point is, therefore, that both an antigen-specific and at least one nonspecific helper factor are directly involved in the regulation of B-cell responses. (The protocol used by Katz and Armerding and by Taussig and Munro and coworkers quite possibly leads to the production of a mixture of both nonspecific, non-Ia-bearing factors and specific, Ia-bearing T cell dependent factors.)

Schimpl and Wecker (1975) and Dutton (1975), who discovered nonspecific helper factors and have contributed much towards their characterization, have proposed that these factors are involved in the differentiation of B cells to antibody-secreting plasma cells. This hypothesis is based firstly on the finding that the factor is most effective if added to the cultures late, and secondly on the fact that B-cell proliferation can begin in the absence of this T-dependent help. But if the factor is nonspecific, how could it lead to the differentiation of only the relevant B cells? The answer is provided by an important finding of Gorczynski et al. (1973) and Kishimoto et al. (1975), who report that lymphoid cells stimulated by antigen or by antiimmunoglobulin can absorb out the activity of nonspecific factor. The simplest interpretation appears to be that the cross-linking of receptors on a B cell leads to the expression of a receptor for a T cell dependent nonspecific factor, which ensures that only antigen-stimulated B cells receive this "second signal."

The nonspecific helper factor seems to substitute for both T-cell and adherent cell functions in obtaining responses to particulate antigens, such as sheep RBC. Thus an anti-sheep RBC response may be obtained with cultures that include only thoracic duct lymphocytes from nude mice (a fairly pure B-cell source), nonspecific helper factor, and sheep RBC (I. Lefkovits and J. Sprent, personal communication).

We do not know what the sequence of events is that leads to the production of the nonspecific factor. Schimpl and Wecker (1975) call the nonspecific factor "T cell replacing factor," and it is usually thought of as being synthesized by T cells. The data suggest that both T cells and adherent cells (possibly monocytes or macrophages) are involved, but this by itself does not enable one to distinguish between an adherent cell-dependent T-cell factor and a T cell dependent adherent-cell factor. This difficulty is aggrevated by the fact that macrophages and monocytes, for instance, are heterogeneous in their adherence properties, and it is practically impossible to deplete completely a culture of some adherent-cell, functions, as has been demonstrated in detail by Rosenstreich and Rosenthal (1974).

III. THE BASIC POSTULATES OF THE PLUS-MINUS NETWORK THEORY AND THE INCORPORATION OF A NONSPECIFIC HELPER FACTOR

The plus-minus network theory has been developed (so far) in two stages. I will refer to the first published model (Hoffmann, 1975) as Mark I and the present extended version as Mark II. In the Mark I model only specific effects were considered; additional complications due to nonspecific mediators were not included.

A basic postulate of the plus-minus network theory is that stimulation involves the cross-linking of receptors for three cell types: T cells, B cells, and a nonspecific accessory cell that lacks endogeneous specific receptors (e.g., a macrophage). The requirement for cross-linking in the stimulation of B cells has been demonstrated by the elegant experiments of Kishimoto and Ishizaka (1975b). Evidence that the induction of an unresponsive state also involves cross-linking has been provided by Feldmann and Diener (1971, 1972). That nonspecific nonlymphoid cells can also be triggered by the cross-linking of receptors has been shown for basophils by Siraganian et al. (1975).

A lymphocyte that recognizes a given antigen is denoted as a "positive" cell (with respect to that antigen), and cells that are specific for determinants on the receptors of positive cells (anti-idiotypic cells) are called "negative" cells. As a first approximation, no fundamental distinction is made between an antigenic determinant on a V region, and the combining site of the V region [i.e., epitope and paratope in Jerne's terminology, (Jerne 1973, 1974a,b)]. This introduces an important symmetry into the system, which is a basic distinguishing feature of the plus-minus network theory from the only other network theory of regulation that has been precisely formulated (Richter, 1975).

The regulatory roles ascribed to the main components of the system in the Mark I model are as follows.

1. Cells are efficient antigens, and therefore cells with mutually complementary receptors (positive and negative cells) can stimulate each other to proliferate.

2. Specific monovalent T-cell factors cannot cross-link receptors, but can block receptors of a complementary specificity and therefore can inhibit the mutual stimulation of cells, and the stimulation of antigen-specific cells by the antigen.

3. Both antibodies and activated nonspecific accessory cells* (to be referred to here as A cells), armed with specific T-cell factors, eliminate (kill) cells of the complementary specificity.

4. Nonspecific accessory cells are postulated to be activated by the cross-linking of a receptor by antigen (and/or by other negative stimulators) in conjunction with antigen-specific T-cell factors. The specific T-cell factors are assumed to provide a link between the antigen and a receptor on the nonspecific accessory cell.

---

*In the original description of the Mark I model (Hoffmann, 1975), the nonspecific accessory cells were called "cytotoxic effector cells" and denoted by K. This was perhaps an unfortunate abbreviation, since "K cell" has been used in a different context in immunology. In this paper this cell will be denoted by A for "accessory cell," and it will be assigned an additional function.

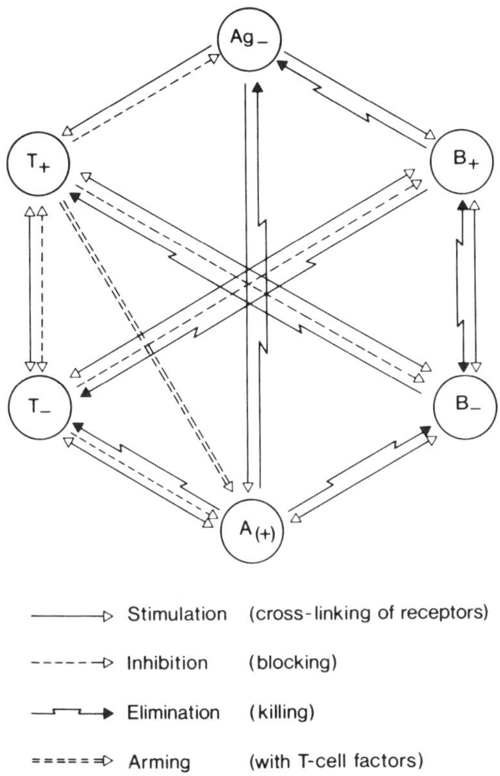

FIG. 2. The complete set of interactions invoked in the Mark I model of the plus-minus network theory. T_+ and B_+ denote antigen-specific T and B cells, T_- and B_- denote corresponding antiidiotypic cells and $A_{(+)}$ denotes a positively armed nonspecific accessory cell ("cytotoxic effector cell"). This apparently complex set of interactions is obtained by simply applying the basic postulates of the theory to a minimal set of cells.

The complete set of interactions of the Mark I model, including T, B, and A cells, is shown in Fig. 2. At first sight this set of interactions appears complicated. The details of such a figure are, however, obtained simply by applying the basic postulates of the model (which are not complicated) to a minimal set of cells. All these interactions need to be considered and mathematically simulated to ensure that any such model is self-consistent. The virgin, suppressed, and immune states are viewed in the theory as stable or quasi-stable states in a "species space," and the induction of either tolerance or immunity is interpreted as switching between these states. It is well known that antibody production by B cells is regulated primarily by T cells. I shall therefore begin by describing the virgin, suppressed, and immune states in terms of the levels of T_+ and T_-. These levels are illustrated in Fig. 3.

In the virgin state there is a subthreshold amount of mutual stimulation of T_+ and T_- cells. In the suppressed state there are elevated levels of both T_+ and T_- cells, and their mutual stimulation is limited by monovalent T-cell factors. Thus negative factors block positive receptors and positive factors block negative receptors. In the immune state there is an elevated level of positive cells, and a depressed level of negative cells. The negative populations are assumed to be relatively depleted in the immune state due to killing by positive antibodies and/or by positively armed A cells. A crude mathematical model of the set of interactions shown in Fig. 2 verified that they could lead to these stable states and to two modes of switching between states, namely the induction of an immune response, and the induction of low zone tolerance.

The working hypothesis concerning the nonspecific helper factor, that is now incorporated into the model is as follows.

5. A nonspecific factor is produced by activated nonspecific accessory cells (as reported by Schrader, 1973), and binds to an acceptor expressed on antigen-stimulated B cells (as described by Kishimoto et al., 1975), giving them a differentiation signal, and thus enabling them to become antibody-producing cells (as proposed by Schimpl and Wecker, 1975, and by Dutton, 1975).

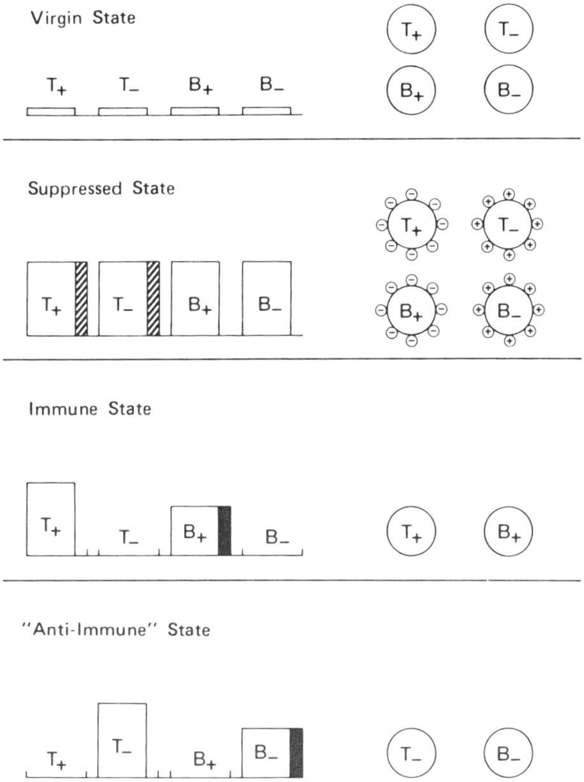

FIG. 3. Schematic representations of the virgin state (plus and minus both down), suppressed state (plus and minus both up), immune state (plus up and minus down), and a hypothetical "anti-immune state" (plus down and minus up). Shaded bars denote monovalent factors, solid bars antibodies.

The reason for making this postulate is that it seems to be the simplest possibility that is consistent with most of the molecular component data, and which furthermore (as described below) yields a set of interactions that has a considerable amount of the observed system response behavior. More complex models can be readily conceived and may correspond to reality. The present postulate, I should like to emphasize, seems merely to be the simplest possibility that provides explanations for a wide range of system response data, and therefore is worthy of consideration. The

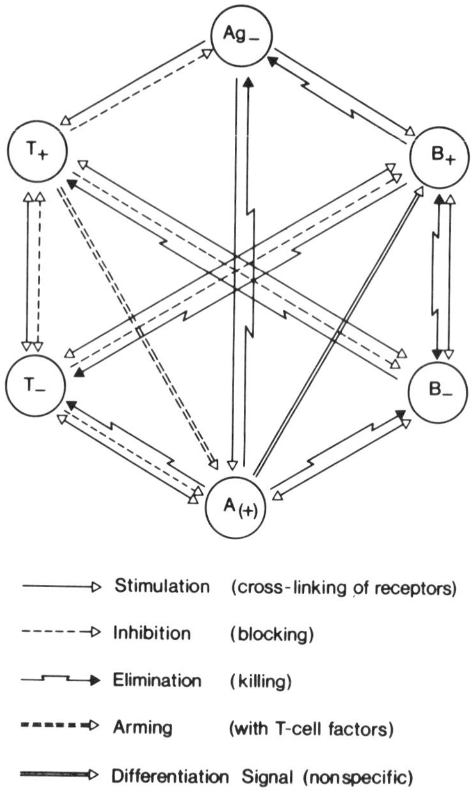

FIG. 4. The set of interactions of the Mark II model, obtained by addition of the nonspecific differentiation faction to the Mark I model. An immune response involves the stimulation of T_+ cells, leading to the arming of the A cell (or of the antigen), and thus facilitating A-cell activation by the antigen. Activated A cells produce nonspecific helper factor, which binds to a receptor expressed on antigen-stimulated B cell. This provides a differentiation signal for B cells to become antibody-forming cells. Positively armed A cells may also help inhibit the induction of the suppressed state by killing T_- and B_- cells.

complete set of interactions, including the nonspecific factor, are shown in Fig. 4, and will be referred to as the "Mark II model."

IV. SYSTEM RESPONSE DATA

A. The Immune Response

The induction of an immune response as envisioned in this extended model is actually quite simple and hardly radical. The antigen stimulates T_+ cells to secrete positive specific T-cell factors, which are cytophilic for the nonspecific A cell. The antigen cross-links the receptors on the A cell via these specific factors, activating the A cell, which then secretes nonspecific factor. The stimulation of the B cell by the antigen meanwhile leads to proliferation and the expression of a receptor for nonspecific factor. Thus, only antigen-stimulated cells receive this "second signal," which leads to the differentiation of such cells to antibody-producing cells.

As described in the Mark I model, nonspecific accessory cells armed with positive T-cell factors may help to prevent the induction of a suppressed state by killing T_- and B_- cells. The limited data currently available make it difficult to make quantitative estimates concerning the extent to which such A-cell mediated cytotoxicity may be important in the induction of a humoral immune response, since the effect is comparatively indirect. It is probably unimportant in inducing responses to so-called T-independent antigens (see below) but could be important in the induction of some T-dependent responses.

B. "T-Independent" Antigens

Some antigens with regularly repeating determinants are often referred to as "T-independent" antigens, since they give rise to antibody responses in the presence of very few or no T cells and adherent cells (Feldmann et al., 1975; Lee et al., 1976). Such antigens

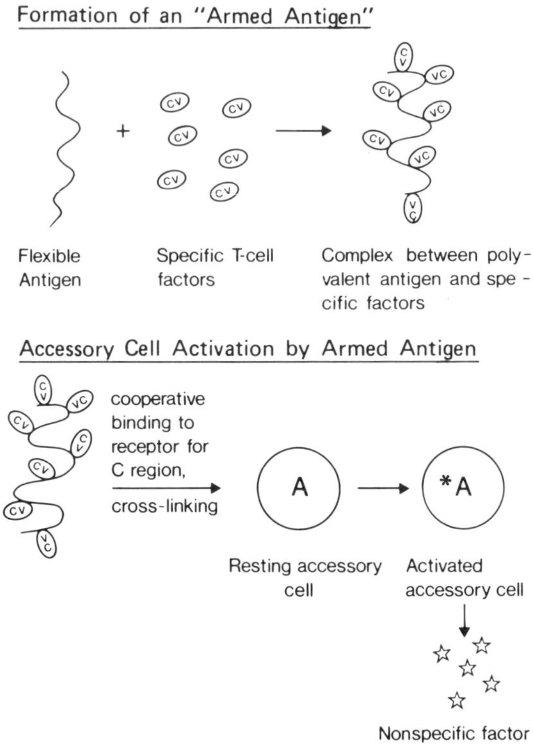

FIG. 5. An ultra-efficient mechanism for obtaining T-cell dependent nonspecific helper factors with T-independent antigens. A multivalent complex is formed between specific T-cell factors and the antigen, which typically has repeating determinants. The multivalent complex efficiently stimulates accessory cells to produce nonspecific helper factor. (C and V denote the constant and variable portions of the specific T-cell factors.)

would be ultraefficient in eliciting nonspecific factor production, as shown in Fig. 5. The antigen stimulates T_+ cells to produce antigen-specific factors, and this leads to the production of an "armed antigen." The repeating determinants of the armed antigen leads to multipoint cooperative binding to, and stimulation of, the nonspecific accessory cell. The model accounts for the early response and small clone size observed with T-independent antigens (Cosenza et al., 1975), since the expanding B-cell clones receive the differentiation signal early. It also accounts for the adjuvant properties of such polymeric antigens (Waldmann and Munro, 1975b). Some "T-independent" antigens presumably effectively stimulate excess nonspecific factor production, and thus provide less immunogenic antigens with nonspecific "help."

C. The Induction of the Suppressed State with Monomers

Soluble monomeric protein antigens that have been subjected to ultracentrifugation in order to eliminate any aggregates have been shown to be tolerogenic (Weigle, 1973). The injection of such an antigen leads to a different sequence of events, due to the fact that the antigen by itself is unable to cross-link receptors or can do so only comparatively inefficiently. For simplicity, we may think of an antigen as having two sides ("side 1" and "side 2"), each side having an antigenic determinant. T cells that are specific for side one and side two (T_{+1} and T_{+2} cells, respectively) could mutually stimulate each other, with the monomers acting as a bridge. Such mutual stimulation of T_{+1} and T_{+2} cells via the antigen would lead to the production of corresponding specific T-cell factors, and hence to the arming of the A cell. Since the antigen is inefficient in cross-linking the armed receptors of the A cell and thus activating it, there is very little nonspecific factor production. Under these circumstances, the positively armed A cell stimulates T_{-1} and T_{-2} cells, and hence the production of T_{-1} and T_{-2} factors. The A cell becomes armed with a mixture of T_+ and T_- factors, and may thus be thought of as a cellular catalyst, that is, a "reflector cell" which catalyzes the mutual stimulation of positive and negative cells. Such catalysis could account for the very rapid induction of unresponsiveness in the T-cell compartment that has been observed with such antigens (Chiller et al., 1971). It is noteworthy that heat-killed macrophages have been demonstrated to have suppressive properties (Ptak and Gershon, 1975). This phenomenon could be due to the catalytic action of the macrophage surface on specific plus-minus stimulation.

There is experimental evidence that has been interpreted as indicating that T cells are more sensitive to antigenic stimulation than B cells, (Mitchison, 1971). The B-cell function assayed in these experiments was antibody production, not proliferation. Thus the data do not exclude the possibility that B cells are just as sensitive as T cells to the first (proliferative) signal. If this is the case, there may be elevated levels of B_+ and B_- in the suppressed state, in addition to the elevated levels of T_+ and T_- (cf Fig. 3).

D. Low Zone Tolerance

The description of the events leading to the induction of low zone tolerance in the extended model is almost the same as in the Mark I model, and is analogous to the induction of unresponsiveness with monomers. The stimulation of positive cells leads to proliferation and/or the arming of A cells, which leads to the eventual stimulation of corresponding negative cells, thus leading to the suppressed state shown in Fig. 3. The low doses of antigen involved would mean that there is less activation of the A cells than is necessary for the production of sufficient nonspecific factor to permit differentiation to yield antibody-forming cells. Suppressor T cells have been shown to be responsible for low zone tolerance in at least two systems (Kölsch et al., 1975; Baker et al., 1974).

E. The Carrier Effect

A large fraction of experiments in cellular immunology involve hapten-carrier systems (reviewed by Katz and Benacerraf, 1972). Any postulated general model for regulation should therefore include a mechanism for this type of cooperation. The simplest way of doing so in the present model is illustrated in Fig. 6, and consists of a combination of antigen presentation and nonspecific factor production. Some of the main features of this model have been suggested before by Waldmann and Munor (1975b). Stimulation of the carrier-primed T cells by antigen leads to the arming of the A cell with carrier-

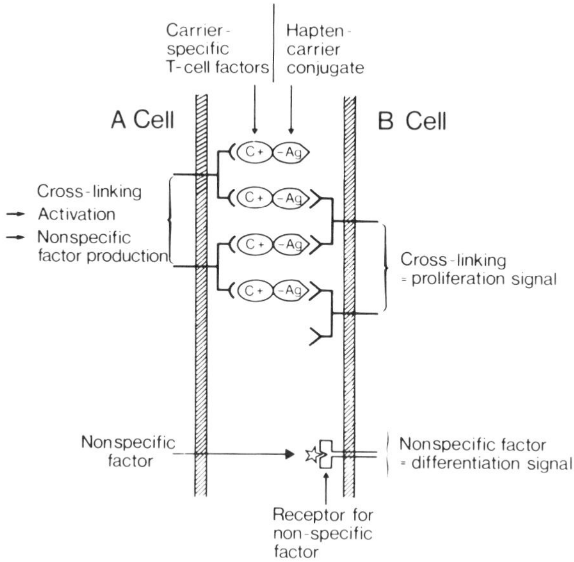

FIG. 6. The carrier effect is ascribed to a combination of antigen presentation and nonspecific factor production. Small soluble hapten-carrier conjugates (e.g., DNP-BSA) are bound to the A cell via carrier-specific T-cell factors. This provides the B cell with an immunogenic array of the hapten. Cross-linking of the receptors on the A cell activates it to produce nonspecific helper factor. Cross-linking of the immunoglobulin receptors on the B cell results in the expression of a receptor for nonspecific factor. (C and + denote the constant and carrier-specific variable parts of the specific T-cell factor, respectively; - denotes the carrier part of the antigen.)

specific T-cell factors. This provides a matrix of sites for the carrier to bind to the A cell, providing in turn a matrix of the hapten in immunogenic form, that is, a form that should be efficient in the cross-linking of receptors on a B cell. Stimulation of the A cell, meanwhile, by the cross-linking of the receptors, leads to the production of a nonspecific factor. The non-specific factor is cytophilic for the hapten-specific B cells, since due to the stimulation they have received, they express a receptor for nonspecific factor.

Nonspecific factor provides all the T-cell help that is required for in vitro B-cell responses to haptenated particulate antigens such as dinitrophenylated sheep RBC (Waldmann, 1975). This is interpreted as being due to the particulate antigen providing appropriate antigen presentation; only the differentiation signal is required in addition for B cells to become plaque forming cells. The same hapten, however, on a soluble protein carrier has generally been found to require carrier-primed T cells (and hence presumably the presence of specific T-cell factor) in order to evoke a B-cell response. This would be due to the requirement for efficient antigen presentation in this case. This model suggests that it may be possible to obtain a response to soluble antigens by using appropriately primed, adherent cell depleted T and B cells, nonspecific factor, and heat-killed adherent cells. Heat-killed A cells together with specific T-cell factor would then provide B cells with the required antigen presentation, while nonspecific factor would provide the differentiation signal.

F. High Zone Tolerance

The production of excessive amounts of specific T-cell factors by too much antigen would result in the inhibition of activation of A cells (Fig. 7). The binding sites on the A cell and the determinants on the antigen are blocked, thus inhibiting the required interaction. The stimulation of negative cells by the armed A cell is nevertheless unimpeded, leading to the induction of the suppressed state. The induction of unresponsiveness may be thought of as being due to too much help in one sense (too much specific T-cell factor) and not enough help in another sense (insufficient nonspecific factor). Both B cells and T cells are said to be "tolerant" under these circumstances (Weigle, 1973). This could be due to both B_+ and B_- populations being expanded, so that if they are transferred to a recipient with uneducated T cells, the suppressed state could be induced by the B_+ and B_- cells themselves.

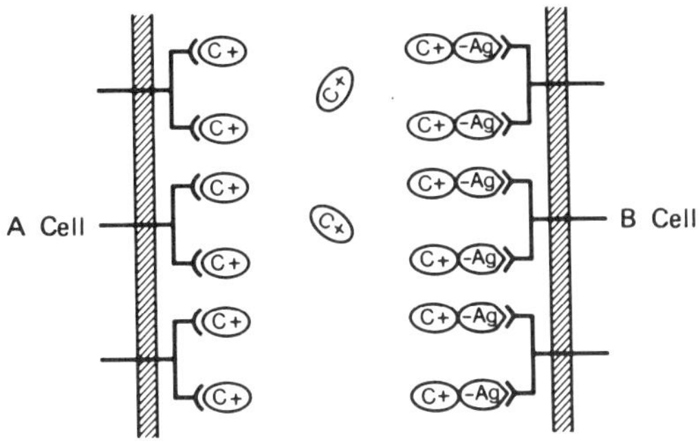

FIG. 7. Excess specific T-cell factor inhibits both the appropriate presentation of antigen to B cells (compare with Fig. 6) and also the activation of the A cell by the antigen. Positively armed A cells can nevertheless stimulate negative cells, leading to the suppressed state with elevated levels of both positive and negative populations. Too much specific help is thus seen to result in insufficient nonspecific help, and the induction of unresponsiveness.

This interpretation of the mechanism of high zone tolerance induction is consistent with the fact that it is readily induced by polymeric antigens, which would be expected to stimulate an excessive number of T cells, and by haptenic conjugates of such antigens (Howard, 1972; Feldmann et al., 1975; Coutinho and Möller, 1975). It is also consistent with the otherwise seemingly paradoxical finding that unresponsiveness is induced by lower doses of antigen and lower epitope densities on such antigens with primed cells than with normal cells (Klaus and Humphrey, 1975).

G. Idiotype Suppression

Administration of antiidiotype can lead to specific idiotype suppression (reviewed by Rowley et al., 1973; Nisonoff and Bangasser, 1975). Recent work by Eichmann (1975) shows that a suppressed state can be extremely stable. Eichmann transfers a small number of idiotype suppressor cells to a recipient mouse, and waits for several weeks until (according to the present model) T_+ and T_- cells have amplified each other up to yield the suppressed state. Multiple transfers of the suppressor cell can be performed, without any decrease in suppressive activity being observed. A prediction of the plus-minus network model, that suppressor cells carry Ia (Hoffmann, 1975) has been verified in that system (Hämmerling and Black, 1976).

It has been found by Nisonoff and Bangasser (1975) and by Cosenza and Augustin (personal communication) that idiotype-specific suppression can be transferred by B cells as well as by T cells. This is not incompatible with the Mark II plus-minus model. Expanded B_+ and B_- clones, which may exist in a suppressed animal, can also stimulate T_+ and T_- cells in a recipient to produce the suppressed state.

H. Stimulation with Antiidiotypic Antibody

Direct in vivo evidence for the bidirectional stimulation arrows of Figs. 2 and 4 has been obtained recently by Eichmann and Rajewsky (1975), who have demonstrated that both B cells and T cells in the mouse can be primed using antiidiotypic antibodies produced in the guinea pig (i.e., with heterologous antibodies). In their system, only priming (expansion of the B-cell clone) and not antibody production by the B cells is observed. This is explained in the present model by assuming that such antiidiotypic antibodies are not sufficiently potent cross-linkers to be able to activate enough A cells, and hence to provide enough of the nonspecific factor to permit differentiation to plaque forming cells.

The induction in vitro of a specific antibody response by antiidiotypic antibodies has been reported by Trenckner and Riblet (1975). They used mouse spleen cells and rabbit antiidiotypic antibodies, and demonstrated that a T-cell response to the (foreign) Fc portion of the rabbit antiidiotypic antibodies was necessary in order for the B-cell response to occur. Homologous antiidiotypic antibody was found to be ineffective in stimulating a response. This finding may be explained in the present model by assuming that carrier-specific T-cell factors are involved in efficiently presenting the antigen (here the antiidiotypic antibody) to B cells, and/or in the production of nonspecific factor by A cells. The model suggests that it may be possible to induce both priming and expression of a given idiotype using polymerized isologous antiidiotypic sera. Antiidiotypes have been raised using polymerized isologous idiotype together with adjuvant (Rodkey, 1974; Sakato and Eisen, 1975). The model suggests that the use of adjuvant may not be necessary in order to obtain such responses.

V. WHERE DO WE GO FROM HERE?

A basic aim of theoretical immunology is to understand the various types of immune response in terms of the physical characteristics of the antigen. With the present model a considerable range of system response data can be related to the cross-linking ability of the antigen. A number of qualitative predictions of the model have been mentioned (see the above sections on the carrier effect and stimulation with antiidiotype antibody).

Just which experiments should have the highest priority depends on the theoretical framework within which one operates. It is therefore useful, I think, for me to describe a line of investigation I consider to be extremely important for gaining an understanding of how the immune system functions as a network. The essence of the network consists in its dynamic properties. We would therefore like to measure as directly as possible, the *kinetics* of the system, in particular, the kinetics of what are believed to be its controlling elements. Thus we need to develop techniques that will enable us to monitor the levels of both specific and nonspecific factors, following antigenic stimulation.

Sensitive in vitro assays for characterizing the physical-chemical properties (e.g., binding constants) and the kinetics of production of specific T-cell factors have not yet been developed. One possibility would be to try to use them as haptens, to inhibit antibody-antigen reactions. This is assuming that, as postulated, they are monovalent.

Since the nonspecific helper factor works across species barriers (Farrer, 1975), it would seem to be worthwhile to purify it from larger animals, in quantities which are sufficient to prepare antibodies against it. The absolute level of this T-cell dependent "cooperating activity" could then be monitored directly following various forms of stimulation using a radioimmunoassay.

At the theoretical level, the elaboration of the basic plus-minus network model to include more cell types involves no principle difficulty. The elementary model shown in Fig. 4 may be readily generalized, with various types of effector cells being substituted for B_+ and B_-, and involving nonspecific factors for each class of effector cell. Distinct nonspecific helper factors for the IgG and IgE response have been reported (Kishimoto and Ishizaka, 1975a). The immune system could thus constitute the superposition of a number of such network systems.

A probably very important nonspecific factor is LAF (lymphocyte activating factor), the production of which has been ascribed to macrophages, and which seems to provide T cells with a second signal for proliferation (Gery, Gershon and Waksman, 1972; Gery and Waksman, 1972; Rosenstreich, Farrer and Dougherty, 1976). A simple way of incorporating it into the model would be to assume that it is produced and is received by antigen-stimulated cells in a way analogous to that proposed here for the nonspecific B-cell helper factor, possibly at lower levels of A-cell activation. Such a factor would introduce additional nonlinearities into a mathematical model of the system, and could have important consequences for its dynamic properties.

There is much more immune system phenomenology which will eventually have to be explained within the plus-minus network concept if it is to remain viable. The basic simplicity of the ideas, together with the successes that have already been achieved with the elementary plus-minus network model described here suggest, however, that the principles governing the regulation of the immune system may not be quite as complicated as the phenomenology sometimes seems to imply.

ACKNOWLEDGMENTS

The Basel Institute for Immunology continues to provide a stimulating and critical environment for the development of network theory. I thank Drs. H. Waldmann, I. Lefkovits, J. Sprent, H. Cosenza, and A. Augustin for the communication of experimental results prior to publication, and Professor N. K. Jerne for his continuing interest and encouragement. Ms. M.-C. Herzog provided excellent secretarial assistance.

REFERENCES

Amos, H. E. and Lachmann, P. J. (1970). The immunological specificity of a macrophage inhibition factor. *Immunology 18:* 269-278.

Armerding, D. and Katz, D. H. (1974). Activation of T and B lymphocytes in vitro. II. Biological and biochemical properties of an allogeneic effect factor (AEF) active in triggering specific B Lymphocytes. *J. Exp. Med. 140:* 19-37.

Armerding, D., Kubo, R. T., Grey, H. M., and Katz, D. H. (1975). Activation of T and B lymphocytes in vitro: Presence of β_2-microglobulin determinants on allogeneic effect factor. *Proc. Nat. Acad. Sci. (USA) 72:* 4577-4581.

Armerding, D., Sachs, D. H. and Katz, D. H. (1974). Activation of T and B lymphocytes in vitro. III. Presence of Ia determinants on allogeneic effect factor. *J. Exp. Med. 140:* 1717-1722.

Asherson, G. L. and Zembala, M. (1975). Inhibiting T cells. *Curr. Topics Microbiol. Immunol. 72:* 55-100.

Baker, P. J., Stashak, P. W., Amsbaugh, D. F., and Prescott, B. (1974). Regulation of the antibody response to Type III pneumococcal polysaccharide. IV. Role of suppressor T cells in the development of low-dose paralysis. *J. Immunol. 112:* 2020-2027.

Benacerraf, B., Kapp, J. A., Debre, P., Pierce, C. W., and de La Croix, F. (1975). The stimulation of specific suppressor T cells in genetic non-responder mice by linear random copolymers of L-amino acids. *Transplant. Rev. 26:* 21-38.

Britton, S. (1972). When allogeneic mouse spleen cells are mixed in vitro the T cells secrete a product which guides the maturation of B cells. *Scand. J. Immunol. 1:* 89-98.

Chiller, J. M., Habicht, G. S., and Weigle, W. O. (1971). Kinetic differences in unresponsiveness of thymus and bone marrow cells. *Science 171:* 813-815.

Coutinho, A. and Möller, G. (1975). Thymus-independent B cell induction and paralysis. *Adv. Immunol. 21:* 113-236.

Cosenza, H., Quintans, J., and Lefkovits, I. (1975). Antibody response to phosphorylcholine in vitro. I. Studies on the frequency of precursor cells, average clone size and cellular cooperation. *Eur. J. Immunol. 5:* 343-349.

Dutton, R. W. (1975). Separate signals for the initiation of proliferation and differentiation in the B cell response to antigen. *Transplant. Rev. 23:* 66-77.

Eichmann, K. (1975). Idiotype suppression. II. Amplification of a suppressor T cell with anti-idiotypic activity. *Eur. J. Immunol. 5:* 511-517.

Eichmann, K. and Rajewsky, K. (1975). Induction of T and B cell immunity by anti-idiotypic antibody. *Eur. J. Immunol. 5:* 661-666.

Erb, P. and Feldmann, M. (1975). The role of macrophages in the generation of T helper cells. III. Influence of macrophage-derived factors in helper cell induction. *Eur. J. Immunol. 5:* 759-766.

Erb, P., Feldmann, M., and Hogg, N. (1976). The role of macrophages in the generation of T-helper cells. IV. Nature of genetically related factor derived from macrophages incubated with soluble antigens. *Eur. J. Immunol. 6:* 365-372.

Evans, R., Grant, C. K., Cox, H., Steele, K., and Alexander, P. (1972). Thymus-derived lymphocytes produce an immunologically specific macrophage-arming factor. *J. Exp. Med. 136:* 1318-1322.

Farrer, J. J. (1975). The xenogeneic effect. I. Antigen and mitogen-stimulated human lymphocytes produce a nonantigen-specific factor which reconstitutes the antibody response of T cell-deficient mouse spleen cells. *J. Immunol. 115:* 1295-1300.

Feldmann, M. (1972). Cell interactions in the immune response in vitro. V. Specific collaboration via complexes of antigen and thymus-derived cell immunoglobulin. *J. Exp. Med. 136:* 737-760.

Feldmann, M. (1974). T cell suppression in vitro. II. Nature of specific suppressive factor. *Eur. J. Immunol. 4:* 667-674.

Feldmann, M. and Basten, A. (1972). Cell interactions in the immune response in vitro. IV. Comparison of the effects of antigen-specific and allogeneic thymus-derived cell factors. *J. Exp. Med. 136:* 722-736.

Feldmann, M., Basten, A., Boylston, A., Erb, P., Gorczynski, R., Greaves, M., Hogg, N., Kilburn, D., Kontiainen, S., Parker, D., Pepys, M., and Schrader, J. (1974). Interactions between T and B lymphocytes and accessory cells in antibody production. In *Progress in Immunology, II. 3.* (L. Brent and J. Holborow, eds.). North-Holland Publ. Company, Amsterdam, pp. 65-75.

Feldmann, M., Cone, R. E., and Marchalonis, J. J. (1973). Cell interactions in the immune response in vitro. VI. Mediation by T cell surface monomeric IgM. *Cell. Immunol. 9:* 1-11.

Feldmann, M. and Diener, E. (1971). Antibody-mediated suppression of the immune response in vitro. III. Low zone tolerance in vitro. *Immunology 21:* 387-404.

Feldmann, M. and Diener, E. (1972). Antibody-mediated suppression of the immune response in vitro. IV. The effect of antibody fragments. *J. Immunol. 108:* 93-101.

Feldmann, M., Howard, J. G., and Desaymard, C. (1975). Role of antigen structure in the discrimination between tolerance and immunity of B cells. *Transplant. Rev. 23:* 78-97.

Gery, I., Gershon, R. K., and Waksman, B. H. (1972). Potentiation of the T-lymphocyte response to mitogens. I. The responding cell. *J. Exp. Med. 136:* 128-142.

Gery, I. and Waksman, B. H. (1972). Potentiation of the T-lymphocyte response to mitogens. II. The cellular source of potentiating mediator(s). *J. Exp. Med. 136:* 143-155.

Gorczynski, R. M. (1972). Ph.D. thesis, University of Toronto, Toronto.

Gorczynski, R. M., Miller, R. G., and Phillips, R. A. (1973). Reconstitution of T cell-depleted spleen cell populations by factors derived from T cells. III. Mechanism of action of T cell-derived factors. *J. Immunol. 111:* 900-913.

Hämmerling, G. J., Black, S. J., Segal, S., and Eichmann, K. (1976). Cellular expression of Ia antigens and their possible role in immune reactions. *Proc. Tenth Leucocyte Culture Conference* (V. P. Eijsvoogel, D. Roos, and W. P. Zeijlmaker, eds.). Academic, New York.

Hoffmann, G. W. (1975). A theory of regulation and self-nonself discriminationin an immune network. *Eur. J. Immunol. 5:* 638-647.

Howard, J. G. (1972). Cellular events in the induction and loss of tolerance to pneumococcal polysaccharides. *Transplant. Rev. 8:* 50-75.

Jerne, N. K. (1972). What precedes clonal selection? In *Ontogeny of Acquired Immunity* (R. Porter and J. Knight, eds.). Ciba Foundation Symposium, New Series 5. Assoc. Scientific Publ., Amsterdam, pp. 1-15.

Jerne, N. K. (1973). The immune system. *Sci. Am. 229:* No. 1, 52-60.

Jerne, N. K. (1974a). Towards a network theory of the immune system. *Ann. Immunol. Inst. Pasteur 125C:* 373-389.

Jerne, N. K. (1974b). Clonal selection in a lymphocyte network. In *Cellular Selection and Regulation in the Immune Response* (G. M. Edelman, ed.). Raven, New York, pp. 39-48.

Jerne, N. K. (1975). The immune system - a web of V-domains. *The Harvey Lectures*, in press.

Katz, D. H. and Benacerraf, B. (1972). The regulatory influence of activated T cells on B cell responses to antigen. *Adv. Immunol. 15:* 1-94.

Kishimoto, T. and Ishizaka, K. (1975a). Immunologic and physiochemical properties of enhancing soluble factors for IgG and IgE antibody responses. *J. Immunol. 114:* 1177-1184.

Kishimoto, T. and Ishizaka, K. (1975b). Regulation of antibody response in vitro. IX. Induction of secondary anti-hapten IgG antibody response by antiimmunoglobulin enhancing soluble factor. *J. Immunol. 114:* 585-591.

Kishimoto, T., Miyake, T., Nishizawa, Y., Watanabe, T., and Yamamura, Y. (1975). Triggering mechanism of B lymphocytes. I. Effect of antiimmunoglobulin and enhancing soluble factor on differentiation and proliferation of B cells. *J. Immunol. 115:* 1179-1184.

Klaus, G. G. B. and Humphrey, J. H. (1975). B cell tolerance induced by polymeric antigens. I. Comparison of the dose and epitope density requirements for inactivation of primed and unprimed B cells in vivo. *Eur. J. Immunol. 5:* 361-365.

Kölsch, E., Stumpf, R., and Weber, G. (1975). Low zone tolerance and suppressor T cells. *Transplant. Rev. 26:* 56-86.

Lee, I-C., Shiozawa, C., Shaw, A., and Diener, E. (1976). Requirement for accessory cells in the antibody response to T cell-independent antigens in vitro. *Eur. J. Immunol. 6:* 63-68.

Lindenmann, J. (1973). Speculations on idiotypes and homobodies. *Ann. Immunol. Inst. Pasteur 124C:* 171-184.

Mitchison, N. A. (1971). The relative ability of T and B lymphocytes to see protein antigen. In *Cell Interactions and Receptor Antibodies in Immune Responses.* O. Mäkelä, A. Cross, and T. U. Kosunen, eds.). Academic, London and New York.

Munro, A. J. and Taussig, M. J. (1975). Two genes in the major histocompatibility complex control immune responses. *Nature 256:* 103-106.

Nakano, M. and Braun, W. (1967). Cell-released non-specific stimulators of antibody-forming spleen cell populations. *J. Immunol. 99:* 570-575.

Nelson, D. S. (1970). Studies on cytophilic antibodies. A mouse serum "antibody" having an affinity for macrophages and fast α-globulin mobility. *Austr. J. Exp. Biol. Med. Sci. 48:* 329-341.

Nisonoff, A. and Bangasser, S. A. (1975). Immunological suppression of idiotypic specificities. *Transplant. Rev. 27:* 100-134.

Ptak, W. and Gershon, R. K. (1975). Immunosuppression effected by macrophage surfaces. *J. Immunol. 115:* 1346-1350.

Richter, P. H. (1975). A network theory of the immune response. *Eur. J. Immunol. 5:* 350-354.

Rodkey, L. S. (1974). Studies of idiotypic antibodies. Production and characterization of autoanti-idiotypic antisera. *J. Exp. Med. 139:* 712-720.

Rosenstreich, D. L., Farrer, J. J., and Dougherty, S. (1976). Absolute macrophage dependency of T lymphocyte activation by mitogens. *J. Immunol. 116:* 876-880.

Rosenstreich, D. L. and Rosenthal, A. S. (1974). Peritoneal exudate lymphocyte. III. Dissociation of antigen-reactive lymphocytes from antigen-binding cells in a T lymphocyte enriched population in the guinea pig. *J. Immunol. 112:* 1085-1093.

Rowley, D. A., Fitch, F. W., Stuart, F. P., Köhler, H., and Cosenza, H. (1973). Specific suppression of immune responses. *Science 181:* 1133-1141.

Rubin, A. S., MacDonald, A. B., and Coons, A. H. (1973). Specific heterologous enhancement of immune responses. V. Isolation of a soluble enhancing factor from supernatants of specifically stimulated and allogeneically induced lymphoid cells. *J. Immunol. 111:* 1314-1325.

Rubin, A. S., MacDonald, A. B., and Coons, A. H. (1974). Specific heterologous enhancement of immune response. VI. Partial purification of a non-specific enhancing factor from supernates of allogeneically stimulated human lymphocyte cell lines. *J. Exp. Med. 139:* 439-444.

Sakato, N. and Eisen, H. N. (1975). Antibodies to idiotypes of isologous immunoglobulins. *J. Exp. Med. 141:* 1411-1426.

Schimpl, A. and Wecker, E. (1975). A third signal in B cell activation given by TRF. *Transplant. Rev. 23:* 176-188.

Schrader, J. W. (1973). Mechanism of activation of the bone marrow derived lymphocyte. III. A distinction between a macrophage-produced triggering signal and the amplifying effect on triggered B lymphocytes of allogeneic interactions. *J. Exp. Med. 138:* 1466-1480.

Sjöberg, O., Andersson, J., and Möller, G. (1972). Reconstitution of the antibody response in vitro of T cell deprived spleen cells by supernatants from spleen cell cultures. *J. Immunol. 109:* 1379-1385.

Siraganian, R. P., Hook, W. A., and Levine, B. B. (1975). Specific in vitro histamine release from basophils by bivalent haptens: evidence for activation by simple bridging of membrane bound antibody. *Immunochem. 12:* 149-157.

Tada, T., Taniguchi, M., and Takemori, T. (1975). Properties of primed suppressor T cells and their products. *Transplant. Rev. 26:* 106-129.

Taniguchi, M., Hayakawa, K., and Tada, T. (1976). Properties of antigen-specific suppressive T cell factor in the regulation of antibody response of the mouse. II. In vitro activity and evidence for the I region gene product. *J. Immunol. 116:* 542-548.

Taniguchi, M. and Tada, T. (1974). Regulation of homocytotropic antibody formation in the rat. X. IgT-like molecule for the induction of homocytotropic antibody response. *J. Immunol. 113:* 1757-1769.

Taussig, M. J. (1974). T cell factor which can replace T cells in vivo. *Nature 248:* 234-236.

Taussig, M. J., Munro, A. J., and Luzzati, A. L. (1976). I-region gene products in cell cooperation. In *The Roles of Products of the Histocompatibility Gene Complex in Immune Responses,* Brook Lodge Symposium (D. H. Katz and B. Benacerraf, eds.). Academic, New York, pp. 553-567.

Trenkner, E. and Riblet, R. (1975). Induction of antiphosphorylchloine antibody formation by anti-idiotypic antibodies. *J. Exp. Med. 142:* 1121-1132.

Vann, D. C. and Galloway, P. C. (1973). Stimulation of the in vitro responses to sheep red blood cells activated to histocompatibility antigens. *J. Immunol. 110:* 1542-1553.

Waldmann, H. (1975). T cell dependent mediator in the immune response. III. The role of non-specific factor (NSF) in the in vitro immune response. *Immunology 28:* 497-507.

Waldmann, H. and Munro, A. (1975a). B cell activation. *Transplant. Rev. 23:* 213-222.

Waldmann, H. and Munro, A. (1975b). The interrelationship of antigenic structure, thymus-independence and adjuvanticity. IV. A general model for B-cell induction. *Immunology 28:* 509-522.

Waldmann, H., Poulton, P., and Desaymard, C. (1976). Antigen-non-specific T-cell factor in B cell activation. Origin, biological properties and failure to show a relationship to H-2. *Immunology 30:* 723-733.

Watson, J. (1973). The role of humoral factors in the initiation of in vitro primary immune response. III. Characterization of factors that replace thymus-derived cells. *J. Immunol. 111:* 1301-1313.

Weigle, W. O. (1973). Immunological unresponsiveness. *Adv. Immunol. 16:* 61.

Yu, H. and Gordon, J. (1973). Helper function in antibody synthesis mediated by soluble factor(s). *Nature New Biology 214:* 20-21.

Zembala, M. and Asherson, G. L. (1974). T cell suppression of contact sensitivity in the mouse. II. The role of soluble suppressor factor and its interaction with macrophages. *Eur. J. Immunol. 4:* 799-804.

Chapter 21

THEORETICAL MODELS OF LYMPHOCYTE NETWORK INTERACTIONS IN ONTOGENETIC GENERATION OF ANTIBODY DIVERSITY

Gerold Adam

Fachbereich Biologie
Universität Konstanz
Konstanz, Federal Republic of Germany

Lymphocyte population dynamics in early ontogeny are described as governed by cell proliferation, random somatic expression of receptor specificities and antireceptor suppression. Two different models for these processes are formulated quantitatively using the following modes of suppression by antireceptor interaction: (a) clonal stabilization by inhibition of cell proliferation and differentiation into longliving cells, and (b) clonal elimination. These two models are applied to T-cell and B-cell branches of the lymphoid system, respectively, and compared with experimental data on that of the mouse.

I. INTRODUCTION

The lymphoid system of the adult mouse contains about 4×10^8 T-lymphocytes and about 2×10^8 B-lymphocytes, subpopulations of which can be identified by structural and functional properties. The total number of receptor specificities expressed by these cells may amount to up to about 10^6 or 10^7. The embryonic precursor cells for lymphoid cells are believed to arise from blood islands seen first on about day 7 of gestation in the yolk sac mesoderm of the mouse (Metcalf and Moore, 1971). Starting from these very limited cell numbers, multi-potent precursor cells then seed, proliferate, and mature in different body compartments and within 40 days of gestational and postnatal life give rise to the functional lymphoid system of the mouse.

These processes of ontogenetic formation of cellular subpopulations of the immune system have recently been the subject of considerable scientific interest. Their detailed analysis might contribute not only to a better understanding of cellular interactions in the functioning of the mature immune system but also represent a fairly lucid example of organ development and cellular differentiation in general.

In spite of the emergence of a host of solid experimental data on the ontogeny of the immune system, no quantitative theory for description of the population dynamics of the T- and B-cell branches and their subpopulations during embryonic and postnatal development has been given. Jerne (1971) has presented a very stimulating concept of somatic generation of immune recognition. According to this proposal, germ-line antibodies are specific for a subset of histocompatibility antigens of the species. Clones that produce antibodies directed against the animal's own antigens are eliminated by a process inducing self-tolerance. Only somatic variants with lesser affinity for self antigens are counterselected and after proliferation give rise to the lymphocyte populations of the immune system. One of the attractive features of this hypothesis is the coupling of generation of diversity with the induction of self tolerance. However, this model does not include the effects of antireceptor interactions between different clones of lymphocytes. Experimental work of recent years has brought abundant evidence that specific mutual recognition of immunoglobulin species or receptors may give rise to profound functional and regulatory effects. Jerne (1972, 1974, 1975) has put forward the "network hypothesis," which proposes that a web of idiotypic-antiidiotypic interactions regulates and stabilizes the immune system. Adam and Weiler (1976) made use of such network interactions among V domains in order to describe the generation of antibody diversity corresponding to a large set of different lymphocyte clones. Their model provided for increase of cell numbers by cellular proliferation, increase in the number of receptor specificities by random somatic expression of variants of receptor V domains and for limitation of number of cells *and* of number of receptor specificities by a process of clonal elimination after specific antireceptor recognition. A preliminary comparison with experimental results on B- and T-cell ontogeny could show that basic features of early ontogeny of the lymphoid system may be described by such a model.

In the following, a model of lymphocyte population dynamics is formulated quantitatively, which uses another mode of antireceptor suppression: clonal stabilization by arrest of cell division and differentiation into a longliving lymphocyte with concomitant alteration of migratory behavior leading to transit into other subcompartments of the animal's lymph system. For comparison, the clonal elimination model of antireceptor suppression is represented also. Thereafter, the theoretical results are applied to experimental data on early ontogeny of T- and B-cell populations of the lymphoid system of the mouse.

II. MODEL I: SUBPOPULATION WITH CLONAL STABILIZATION BY ANTIRECEPTOR INTERACTION

A. Definition of Theoretical Parameters

In the following, the term system refers to the lymphycyte subpopulation under consideration, which may reside in one or several compartments of the lymphoid system of the animal. An example might be the subpopulation of lymphocytes seeding, proliferating, and maturing in the thymus of the mouse from day 12 of gestation to the fourth week after birth.

The discussion will be based on Burnet's (1959) clonal selection theory by postulating that the system under consideration consists of clones of cells each having a unique individual antibody or receptor specificity which may be referred to as "clonotype." Each of these species of receptor molecules is characterized by its antibody-combining site (paratope) and by its set of determinants for antireceptor interactions. Operationally, the distinction of the idiotypic and the allotypic set of determinants for antireceptor interactions has been found useful. Although in principle both sets of determinants should be subject to the same general mechanism of antireceptor interaction, the concentration of a species of allotypic determinants may be expected to be much higher than that of an idiotypic species, so that under physiological conditions antiallotypic and antiidiotypic interactions are probably not equivalent. Generation of antibody diversity, almost by definition, should depend on mechanisms involving the idiotypic aspect of the receptors. As a first approximation, therefore, we shall neglect in the following the classification of receptors by allotype and leave the effects of antiallotypic regulation for a later more detailed analysis.

Thus, the diversity of the representative subpopulation of lymphocytes in the system will be described by the average number M of idiotypes and the average number M' of paratopes. These quantities represent the available repertoires of idiotypes and paratopes. Averages here and in the following are understood as averages over an ensemble of equivalent animals (the animal strain). We shall use further the concept of the potential repertoires of idiotypes and of paratopes (Jerne, 1972, 1974). The total number of idiotypes that is possible for the subpopulation of lymphocytes under consideration for the animal strain ("the potential repertoire of idiotypes") is denoted by P and may be considered much larger than the number of idiotypes present in a representative system at time t [the available repertoire M(t) of idiotypes]. Similarly, the total number of paratopes in the potential repertoire of paratopes of the animal strain is denoted by P' and may be considered much larger than the number M'(t) of paratopes in the system of time t. The logical sum of the sets P and P' may be termed "potential repertoire of clonotypes."

The total number of lymphocytes in the system is denoted as N; it is again an average as defined above for M and M'. It is the sum of the average number D of lymphoyctes which are able to divide and of the average number I of lymphoyctes, the proliferation of which is inhibited by specific antireceptor interaction:

$$N = D + I \tag{1}$$

Each of the D noninhibited cells may divide with a rate constant k_b or disappear by indiscriminate death with a rate constant k_d. Immigration to and emigration from the system is neglected. Similarly, change of N by discriminate removal of cells from the system, for instance by processes resulting from selective interactions with antigens, etc., will be neglected also.

Somatic variants may appear in the system in proportion to cell division. They are defined by expression of a V domain, taken at random from the potential repertoire of clonotypes, and by clonal propagation. For the purposes of this paper it is of secondary importance whether the potential repertoire of clonotypes has arisen phylogenetically (germ-line hypothesis) or represents the total extent of possible somatic mutations.

The rate constant of somatic expression of idiotypic variants is denoted by k_m, giving the number of new idiotypes arising per noninhibited lymphocyte and per unit time. Thus, the number of new idiotypes appearing in the system per unit time is $k_m D$.

The process of limitation of cell number *and* of idiotype number M in this model is defined as follows. Consider two clonotypes in the system that recognize each other, that is, exhibit specific antiidiotypic interaction. It is postulated that, depending on receptor accessibility and presentation of idiotypic determinants, there exists a range of interaction that will lead to or keep the cells of both clones suppressed, that is, proliferation-inhibited and differentiated into longliving cells. Thus, if one or both of the cell clones before the antiidiotypic encounter belonged to the class of proliferating cells, the antiidiotypic interaction will lead for one or both clones, respectively, to arrest of cell division and differentiation to longevity, which may imply expression of another set of surface antigens, change in migratory behavior, preferential homing to other compartments of the lymphoic system, etc. In the following, this process will be called "clonal stabilization" and is described by a rate constant k_s'. The range of intensity of antiidiotypic interaction which leads to clonal stabilization may well extend only up to a certain threshold above which the effect of antiidiotypic interaction is "clonal stimulation." Although clonal stimulation by antiidiotypic interaction appears to play an important role in the processes of regulation of an immune response to antigenic stimulus, it is not discussed further in the present context, which is devoted to the generation of antibody diversity independent of and temporally before antigenic challenge.

We have to evaluate the relative probability that such an antiidiotypic stabilization of clonotypes occurs in the system. In line with current thinking on paratope binding (Inman, 1974), we allow for a certain overlap of specificity of antiidiotypic interaction. Accordingly, every idiotype of the potential repertoire of idiotypes may be recognized on the average by ν paratopes of the potential repertoire of paratopes. Conversely, every paratope from the potential repertoire of paratopes in the average may recognize σ idiotypes of the potential repertoire of idiotypes. The averaging implied in ν and σ is over the idiotypes and paratopes of the potential repertoires P and P', respectively. Clearly, the following relation must hold

$$P\nu = P'\sigma \tag{2}$$

Corresponding to reality, we shall use in the following $P \approx P' >> 1$ and $M \approx M' >> 1$.

The clonotypes in the system are assumed to be taken at random from the potential repertoire. Then, the relative probability that a given idiotype in the system is recognized by one given paratope of the system is ν/P'. On the basis of Eq. (2), an alternative formulation is σ/P. Since the number of idiotypes per system is M, the number of M' of paratopes in the system is given by:

$$M' = \frac{MP'}{P} \tag{3}$$

The relative probability that the given idiotype is recognized by any one of the (many) paratopes of the system is proportional to their number and thus given by $M'\nu/P' = M\nu/P$.

B. Kinetic Equations

On the basis of the above argumentation the number of idiotypes may increase with the rate $k_m D$. Random death of individual cells, as described by the rate constant k_d, generally does not lead to extinction of clonotypes. Thus, the balance equation for M in this model reads

$$\frac{dM}{dt} = k_m D \tag{4}$$

Since antiidiotypic interaction only transfers clonotypes from the proliferating clones to the "stabilized" clones, the total number N of cells in the system changes in strict proportion to birth and random death of proliferating cells:

$$\frac{dN}{dt} = (k_b - k_d)\ D \tag{5}$$

To arrive at the balance equation for the proliferating cells, we observe that their number D increases with the rate $(k_b - k_d)D$. The rate of transfer of cells from the proliferating pool to the stabilized pool is proportional to k_s', to the relative probability $M\nu/P$ that a given idiotype is recognized by any one of the paratopes present in the system, and to the number of proliferating cells. Thus, the kinetic equation of D reads:

$$\frac{dD}{dt} = r_s D - k_s MD \tag{6}$$

where

$$r_s = k_b - k_d \tag{7}$$

$$k_s = \frac{k_s'\nu}{P} \tag{8}$$

Since the number I of cells belonging to "stabilized" clones can increase only by transfer of clones from the proliferating pool, the rate of which was evaluated above as $(k_s'\nu/P)MD$, we have:

$$\frac{dI}{dt} = k_s MD \tag{9}$$

The system of coupled differential Eqs. (4), (5), (6), and (9) can be integrated in closed form as follows.

From Eqs. (4) and (6) we obtain

$$\frac{dD}{dM} = \frac{r_s - k_s M}{k_m} \tag{10}$$

With the initial conditions

$$t = t_0 \qquad M = M_0 \qquad D = D_0 \tag{11}$$

the solution of Eq. (10) reads

$$D = D_0 + \frac{r_s}{k_m}(M - M_0) - \frac{k_s}{2k_m}(M^2 - M_0^2) \tag{12}$$

Equations (4) and (12) define a first-order differential equation in M:

$$\frac{dM}{dt} = k_m D_0 + r_s(M - M_0) - \frac{k_s}{2}(M^2 - M_0^2) \tag{13}$$

For t = 0: $M = M_0$, the integration of Eq. (13) yields

$$M = \frac{M_\infty + M_1 H_0 \exp[-G(t - t_0)]}{1 + H_0 \exp[-G(t - t_0)]} \tag{14}$$

Here, the following abbreviatons are used:

$$G = \left[r_s^2 + 2k_s\left(k_m D_0 - r_s M_0 + \frac{k_s M_0}{2}\right)\right]^{1/2} \tag{15}$$

$$M_\infty = \frac{r_s + G}{k_s} \tag{16}$$

$$M_1 = \frac{r_s - G}{k_s} \tag{17}$$

$$H_0 = \frac{M_\infty - M_0}{M_0 - M_1} \tag{18}$$

From Eqs. (4) and (5), we obtain

$$\frac{dN}{dM} = \frac{r_s}{k_m} \tag{19}$$

and with $t = t_0$: $M = M_0$, $N = N_0$:

$$N = N_0 + \frac{r_s}{k_m}(M - M_0) \tag{20}$$

Since I = N - D, we have from Eqs. (12) and (20):

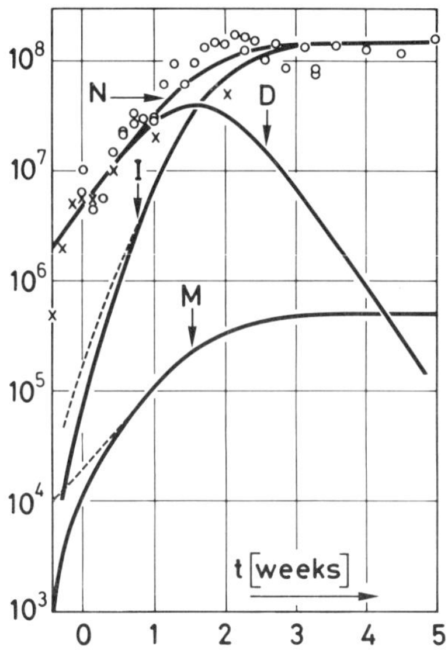

FIG. 1. Plot of total number of lymphocytes, N; number of proliferating lymphocytes, D; number of suppressed lymphocytes, I; and number of idiotypes M vs. time in weeks according to model I. Parameters used are: $r_s = 0.3$ day^{-1}, $k_m = 10^{-3}$ day^{-1}, $k_s = 1.2 \times 10^{-6}$ day^{-1}. Initial conditions are $t_0 = -3$ days, $N_0 = 2 \times 10^6$, $M_0 = 10^3$ (solid curve) or $M_0 = 10^4$ (broken curve). Experimental points refer to total number of lymphocytes in one lobe of mouse thymus vs. age: o is from Axelrad and van der Gaag (1962); x is from Ball (1963).

$$I = \frac{k_s}{2k_m}(M^2 - M_0^2) \tag{21}$$

Thus, if M is computed from Eqs. (14) through (18), the quantities N, D, and I may be computed from Eqs. (12), (20) and (21). In Fig. 1 are plotted the kinetics of M, N, D, and I as obtained by this procedure, using the parameters:

$$r_s = 0.3 \text{ d}^{-1} \qquad k_m = 10^{-3} \text{ d}^{-1} \qquad k_s = 1.2 \times 10^{-6} \text{ d}^{-1} \tag{22}$$

and the initial conditions

$$t_0 = -3 \text{ d} \qquad M_0 = 10^3 \qquad D_0 = N_0 = 2 \times 10^6 \tag{23}$$

This gives the full-drawn curve in Fig. 1.

With these numbers, the steady-state values read:

$$M_{\infty} = 5 \times 10^5 \qquad N_{\infty} = I_{\infty} = 1.5 \times 10^8 \qquad D_{\infty} = 0 \tag{24}$$

For a check of the effect of the initial conditions, we have used the above numbers except that $M_0 = 10^4$; this is shown as the broken curve in Fig. 1.

In a later section, model I will be compared with experimental data on thymic lymphocyte proliferation in early ontogeny of the mouse.

III. MODEL II: SUBPOPULATION WITH CLONAL ELIMINATION BY ANTIRECEPTOR INTERACTION

A. Definition of Theoretical Parameters

This model has been presented and compared preliminarily with experimental data on murine B- and T-cell populations in an earlier paper (Adam and Weiler, 1976). The basic approach is similar to the model developed above, except that antiidiotypic interaction in this case does not lead to clonal stabilization but to clonal elimination by processes such as suppression of cell proliferation and/or cell killing. In this model, no distinction is necessary between proliferating and stabilized cell clones. Thus, the two quantities M and N suffice for description of the system.

As before, the average number M of idiotypes increases by somatic expression of variants of V regions occurring in proportion to cell division which is proportional to the average number N of cells in the system. Therefore, the rate of increase of M is given by $k_m N$. However, the number of idiotypes decreases because of elimination of antiidiotypically interacting clones. If such a pair of antiidiotypically incompatible clones exist in the system, the rate constant of elimination is k_e'. The relative probability that one given idiotype in the system is recognized by existing paratopes in the system has been derived above as $\nu M/P$. Since each of the M existing idiotypes in the system is equivalent in being recognized, the rate of decrease of M per system and unit time by antiidiotypic elimination is $k_e'\nu M^2/P$.

B. Kinetic Equations

On the basis of the foregoing argumentation the kinetic equation for M reads

$$\frac{dM}{dt} = k_m N - k_e M^2 \tag{25}$$

where

$$k_e = \frac{k_e'\nu}{P} \tag{26}$$

Here again, we neglect immigration to and emigration from the system. The increase of N by random cell division is described by the rate constant k_b. Processes of decrease of N are those by indiscriminate death of cells with rate constant k_d and by antiidiotypic elimination of whole clones. The rate of clonal elimination was given before as $k_e M^2$. The average size of clones is

$$n = \frac{N}{M} \tag{27}$$

Thus, with each clone disappearing by antiidiotypic elimination, the number N decreases by $k_e M^2 n$. Using Eq. (27) the kinetic equation for N reads

$$\frac{dN}{dt} = r_e N - k_e MN \tag{28}$$

where

$$r_e = k_b - k_d \tag{29}$$

Steady state of the system is given by

$$M_\infty = \frac{r_e}{k_e} \tag{30}$$

$$N_\infty = \frac{r_e^2}{k_m k_e} = \frac{r_e n_\infty}{k_e} \tag{31}$$

$$n_\infty = \frac{N_\infty}{M_\infty} = \frac{r_e}{k_m} \tag{32}$$

The system of the two coupled first-order differential equations, Eqs. (25) and (28), has been solved numerically by a second-order Runge-Kutta method on a Hewlett-Packard calculator model 9830 using the following set of parameters

$$r_e = 0.7\ d^{-1} \qquad k_m = 0.035\ d^{-1} \qquad k_e = 7 \times 10^{-8}\ d^{-1} \tag{33}$$

and the initial conditions

$$t_0 = -3\ d \qquad M_0 = 100 \qquad N_0 = 10^4 \tag{34}$$

The results are given as the full curve in Fig. 2. In order to check the effect of the initial condition, we have also computed the cases $M_0 = 10$ and $M_0 = 1000$. The latter results are shown as the broken curves in Fig. 2 and demonstrate that differences of initial values M_0 fade away 3 to 4 days after t_0.

The above set of parameters Eq. (33) yields

$$N_\infty = 2 \times 10^8 \qquad M_\infty = 10^7 \qquad n_\infty = \frac{N_\infty}{M_\infty} = 20 \tag{35}$$

In a later section, these theoretical results are applied to experimental data on proliferation of virgin B cells in perinatal mouse.

IV. APPLICATION OF MODEL I TO LYMPHOCYTE PROLIFERATION IN THE THYMUS

A major part of lymphocyte proliferation in early ontogeny occurs in the thymus. Since the most detailed experimental data are available for the mouse, we shall restrict our discussion to this species except when stated otherwise.

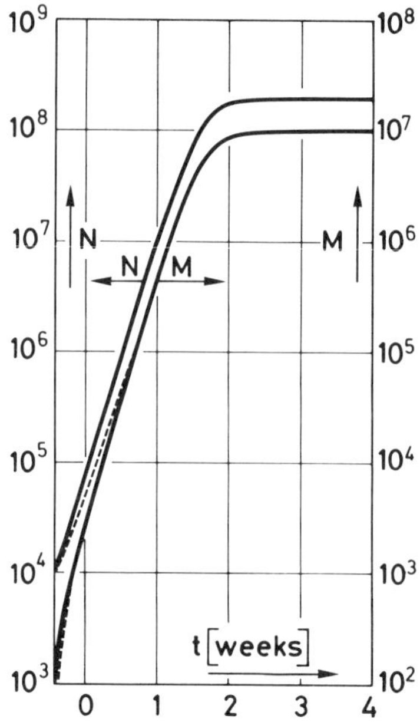

FIG. 2. Plot of lymphocyte number N (left ordinate) and number of idiotypes M (right ordinate) vs. time in weeks according to model II. Parameters used are: $r_e = 0.7\ \text{day}^{-1}$, $k_m = 0.035\ \text{day}^{-1}$, $k_e = 7 \times 10^{-8}\ \text{day}^{-1}$. Initial conditions are: $t_0 = -3$ day, $N_0 = 10^4$, $M_0 = 10^2$ (solid curve) and $M_0 = 10$ or 10^3 (broken curves).

At day 11 of murine gestation thymic precursor lymphocytes from the yolk sac and/or embryonic liver seed in the thymic anlage (Metcalf and Moore, 1971) and proliferate until at day 16 of gestation the number of thymic lymphocytes is about 10^6 (Ball, 1963). At that time, thymic lymphocytes begin to express TL-, Ly-, and Θ-alloantigens, which by day 18 of gestation are carried by about all of them (Owen and Raff, 1970; Goldschneider, 1974). At the same time, there is also a drastic increase in doubling time of thymic lymphocyte numbers (Ball, 1963). Thus, it appears that at day 16 of murine gestation the thymic microenvironment changes such that thymic precursor lymphocytes differentiate into thymocytes, which in turn may differentiate to functional T cells during the next weeks. Here and in the following thymocyte is defined as thymic lymphocyte after day

16 of gestation. We wish to apply model I to this thymocyte population up to the fourth week of postnatal life. This is a period with massive increase of thymocyte numbers. The predominant thymocyte cell types during this interval have been well characterized by different methods. These are small cortical lymphocytes ("type II") as well as medium-sized lymphocytes ("type IV") of high mitotic activity serving as precursors for the small lymphocytes of type II (Droege et al., 1974b). Analogous types of lymphocytes have been identified during early ontogeny in the chicken thymus (Droege et al., 1974a). The cortical small lymphocytes of type II presumably have suppressor function under physiological conditions (Droege et al., 1974b; Mosier and Johnson, 1975). At about the fourth week after birth, another type of small thymocyte appears ("type I") and is predominant at 6 months of age (Droege et al., 1974b). In the present paper we attempt to describe the thymocyte population dynamics only to about the fourth week of murine age.

Before applying our model to the proliferation interval specified above, we have to discuss the major approximations of the model. Certainly, the use of the proliferation parameter r_s is to be considered an approximation as it presumably comprises processes of asymmetric precursor cell division, proliferation of intermediates, and transit of these through maturation compartments. These processes are not elucidated fully (Bryant, 1972; Prothero and Tyler, 1975). In order to keep the number of theoretical parameters minimal, it appears justified at the present state of knowledge to use r_s as a lumped parameter. In the theoretical model, immigration to and emigration from the thymic compartment has been neglected. As the repopulation studies of Owen and Raff (1970) on embryonic thymus grafts have shown, immigration can indeed be considered minor as compared to proliferation. Emigration of lymphocytes from the thymus does occur in perinatal life. However, the extent of this emigration has yet to be determined in quantitative detail. For a rough estimate, we observe that up to 2 weeks of age the total number of T cells in the spleen (Spear et al., 1973; Sidman and Unanue, 1975a) and of lymphocytes in other lymphoid organs (Nossal and Pike,

1973; Friedberg and Weissman, 1974) remains less than about 10 or 15% of the number of thymocytes. Within an error limit of about this extent we may neglect emigration in the theoretical description.

Experimental data on thymocyte numbers during the time interval under consideration have been given by Axelrad and van der Gaag (1962) and Ball (1963) and are reproduced in Fig. 1. These data refer to one thymic lobe only. As Fig. 1 shows, this time course is well described by the theory, if one uses parameters and initial conditions as given in Eqs. (22) and (23). Since the choice $M_0 = 10^3$ is somewhat arbitrary, we have also given as the broken curve in Fig. 1, the result for $M_0 = 10^4$, showing that a change of M_0 by a factor of 10 affects appreciably the kinetics of M only to about the third day after birth. Of course, on the basis of the theory, the processes of proliferation and somatic expression of variants of V regions may be specified for the time interval *before* day 16 of gestation. Then M_0 and N_0 may be computed as arising from one or a few stem cells in the primitive blood islands after day 7 of gestation. The figure $M_0 \approx 10^3$ is entirely reasonable in this context.

According to the theoretical results shown in Fig. 1, the number of clonotypes in the thymic population, as described by M, rises to adult size in close proportion to the total number N of cells in the system. However, the number I of cells stabilized by antiidiotypic interaction rises to an asymptotic value with a certain delay and much steeper than N and M. Since the cells belonging to the stabilized clones are postulated to be differentiated into longliving cells exhibiting another set of surface antigens and a different migratory behavior, the rise of I should describe the maturation and peripherilization of early thymocytes to longliving and circulating T lymphocytes with suppressor function. The kinetics of I, as predicted by our model, parallels closely the relatively sudden appearance of T cells in the lymph nodes and in the spleen (Friedberg and Weissman, 1974; Spear et al., 1973; Sidman and Unanue, 1975a). Furthermore, the kinetics of I as predicted by the model reproduces closely the early postnatal appearance of reactivity of thymocytes to pokeweed mitogen or concanavalin A and in mixed lymphocyte reaction with allogeneic spleen cells (Mosier, 1974). The suppressing function of the early branch of thymocytes described by I is consistent with the predominance of suppressor activity observed in neonatal mice by Mosier and Johnson (1975).

Thus, the model of lymphocyte population dynamics with clonal stabilization by antiidiotypic interaction describes well basic features of the antigen-independent development of an early branch of thymic lymphocytes, with presumable suppressor function. It leads to an interesting pairwise clonal interconnection of the mature thymocytes, which might well be the prerequisite for subsequent mutual regulation by antiidiotypic interaction in the course of an immune response to antigenic perturbation.

The theoretical parameter r_s may be compared with the cell cycle time of $T_c \approx 8$ hr, as observed by Metcalf and Wiadrowski (1966). This number yields $k_b = 2.1\ d^{-1}$, which together with $r_s = 0.3\ d^{-1}$ implies a relatively high rate of random cell death during proliferation of D cells: $k_d = k_b - r_s = 1.8\ d^{-1}$. The "mutation rate" μ describing the expression of variants of V regions per cell divison may be estimated with these numbers as:

$$\mu = \frac{k_m}{k_b} = 4.76 \times 10^{-4} \qquad (36)$$

This number is not unusually high and, thus is compatible with a somatic mutation mechanism for generation of new variants.

The model in its present form does not describe the processes of appearance of "type I" small cortical lymphocytes at about 1 month of murine age and the gradual disappearance of the "type II" small cortical lymphocyte by about 6 months of age (Droege et al., 1974). Similarly, it does not describe the lymphocyte population dynamics in steady state of adult thymus, which is characterized by a high cell turnover (Metcalf and Wiadrowski, 1966) in contrast to a nonproliferating steady state of the theoretical model with $N = I = N_\infty$.

The latter deficiency probably is related to the neglect of stem cell immigration, which, according to the experiments of Owen and Raff (1970), seems to be a reasonable approximation up to about 3 weeks.

V. APPLICATION OF MODEL II TO PROLIFERATION IN THE B-CELL SYSTEM

According to recent results of different authors, the ontogenetic development of the B-cell branch of the immune system takes place multifocally (Nossal and Pike, 1973; Owen et al., 1975). According to this and other work (Spear et al., 1973; Friedman and Weissman, 1974; Sidman and Unanue, 1975a), spleen and liver are the major sites of perinatal lymphocyte proliferation in the murine B-cell line. Again, we restrict our discussion to experimental data on the mouse, except when stated otherwise. The number of immunoglobulin-positive (Ig^+) cells in these and other lymphoid organs rises essentially simultaneously during the first postnatal week and levels off thereafter. The main exception is bone marrow which develops later on at the expense of the lymphoid function of the early postnatal liver. The total number of Ig^+ cells in different compartments of the murine lymphoid system according to these studies is about 10^4 at day 16 of gestation when the first cellular Ig receptors are detected, rises to about 10^7 at 1 week of age, and reaches steady state with about 2×10^8 at 2 weeks of age. This expanding population of Ig-carrying cells may be considered as a branch of virgin, that is, antigenically unaffected, B cells. We wish to apply model II to this subpopulation which resides in several compartments of the lymphoid system. Very similar reservations as to the applicability of the theory with regard to the nature of r_e as a lumped parameter, and emigration and/or immigration may be discussed as in the application of model I to thymic proliferation. However, for the developing system of virgin B cells, an additional difficulty arises. Thymic proliferation occurs in a secluded compartment and can presumably be regarded as independent of interferences from the developing B-cell system. In contrast, B-cell proliferation occurs in a largely open compartment and in the presence of appreciable numbers of T lymphocytes. Since T-B cell interactions of different nature have been demonstrated in many physiological functions of the immune system, there is no a priori reason to expect that B-cell proliferation and maturation is independent of the T-cell system. On the other hand, the largely normal development of the B-cell branch in nude mice suggests that the diversification process of the virgin B cells, at least in its main features, is able to proceed independently of the mature T cells. Thus, we assume that the essentials of the ontogenetic development of the subpopulations of virgin B lymphocytes can be described in a first approximation by our model II, which disregards any regulative effect of T cells during this process. For the comparison of the model with the kinetics of Ig^+-cell populations reviewed above, we choose the parameters and initial conditions given in Eqs. (33) and (34). The resulting kinetic curves for N and M have been computed and shown as the solid curves in Fig. 2. Again the effect of a different choice of M_0 has been checked and is shown in Fig. 2 (broken curves) for $M_0 = 10$ and $M_0 = 10^3$. As in model I a change of M_0 by a factor of 10 is significant only up to about the third day after birth.

The theory describes well the kinetics of the B-cell population as experimentally determined by different authors (see references given above), that is, a doubling time of the cell number of about a day at the beginning and a leveling off of population growth during the second week after birth. Functional maturity of B lymphocytes during early ontogeny has been tested experimentally by T-cell independent antigens (Melchers et al., 1975; Mosier and Johnson, 1975) or by T-helper cell independent tests (Spear and Edelman, 1974; Rosenberg and Cunningham, 1975) and found to parallel closely the development of B-lymphocyte numbers. As shown in Fig. 2, this is well reproduced by the theoretical time course of the number M of idiotypes. Furthermore, the heterogeneity of antibody specificities has been studied experimentally and found severely restricted at about birth, but to achieve adult character by about 2 weeks of age

(Goidl and Siskind, 1974; Klinman and Press, 1975). Using the in vitro splenic focus technique combined with isoelectric focusing, the latter authors could give estimates for the number of clonotypes at different times during early ontogeny. From an analysis of the response to multiclonal determinants such as 2,4-dinitrophenyl, 2,4,6-trinitrophenyl, or fluorescein, they conclude that the adult mouse exhibits about 10^7 clonotypes, each expressed by 5 to 25 cells. In contrast, the neonatal mouse was estimated to express about 10^4 clonotypes, albeit with a higher number (200-400) of cells per clonotype. These specific experimental results on clonotype numbers agree well with the predictions of the theory (see Fig. 2). Even the larger clone size of neonatal B-cell population as compared to adult may be reproduced by the theory, if M_0 is smaller than $k_m N_0/r_e$.

Our model predicts the virgin B-cell population of the adult animal to be in continuous clonal flux: new clonotypes are continuously expressed and after a short lifetime eliminated by antiidiotypic interaction. Thus, the population of virgin B cells continuously scans through its potential repertoire of clonotypes. It is to be kept in mind that the model describes an antigen-independent diversification process. Antigenic stimulation may be thought of in effect removing the stimulated clone from the elimination mechanism. Some possible extensions of the model for description of antigenic disturbance of the virgin B-cell population, as well as questions regarding the size of the potential reservoires, the magnitudes of ν/P and of k_e' have been discussed elsewhere (Adam and Weiler, 1976). The magnitude chosen for the theoretical parameters r_e and k_m may be checked by some recent data pertaining to adult murine B lymphocytes. Osmond and Nossal (1974), among others, have shown for mice, and Strober (1975) for rat, that the subpopulation of virgin B lymphocytes is renewed continuously by rapid proliferation of stem cells as evidenced by a 90% [^{3}H]thymidine labeling after 2 days. This corresponds closely to our mean generation time of $T = 1/r_e = 1.4$ days. According to the results of Osmond and Nossal (1974), the newly divided stem cells enter a maturation compartment of about 1.5 to 2 days duration, which serves for synthesis and expression of Ig receptors. Thereafter, the cells are subject to imminent death by a mechanism which has not been detailed by experimental investigations. This life history of a virgin B lymphocyte is entirely compatible with our theoretical model II, which specifies cellular death as a consequence of clonal elimination by antiidiotypic interaction. The short life span of virgin B lymphocytes according to our model II, together with the longevity of matured thymocytes according to our model I, may give an explanation for the longstanding observation that in all lymphoid compartments except thymus, the tissues with the highest proportion of thymus-derived cells have the lowest percentage of short-lived cells (Parrot and de Sousa, 1971).

The relatively large magnitude of the parameter $k_m = 0.035\ \text{day}^{-1}$ as required by the theoretical model for description of the dynamics of virgin B cells is of considerable interest. In order to arrive at an estimate for the mutation rate μ in the virgin B-cell branch, we may use $r_e \leqslant k_b \leqslant 4\ \text{day}^{-1}$, the latter figure corresponding to a cellular generation time of 6 hr. These numbers, together with $k_m = 0.035\ \text{day}^{-1}$ give

$$0.01 \leqslant \mu = \frac{k_m}{k_b} \leqslant 0.05 \tag{37}$$

This means that one in 20 to 100 cell divisions leads to expression of a new clonotype. This is in good agreement with the recent observation in cloning experiments by Cunningham and Pilarski (1974) that variants of antibody specificity occur at a rate of one per 30 to 60 cell divisions.

VI. DISCUSSION

The application of our minimal models I and II to population dynamics and generation of antibody diversity in the early T cell line and the virgin B-cell line could show that the basic features of these processes occurring in early ontogeny of the mouse can be described in satisfactory agreement with the experimental data. In each of these models only three adjustable parameters are needed: r_s, k_m, and k_s (or r_e, k_m, and k_e).

Although the two modes of action of antiidiotypic recognition lead to very different consequences, they might be implemented by essentially the same cellular interaction mechanism. One may imagine that the essence of both modes is antiidiotypic interaction leading to suppression of cell division. The different outcome of this basic interaction may then be due to a different clone size and/or to a different rate constant for indiscriminate death of the cells from the suppressed clones of the two subpopulations of lymphocytes. A general cellular interaction mechanism of mutual suppression of cell proliferation obviously might be a basic feature of cell populations during organ formation of multicellular organisms. In the case of the lymphoid system, it suggests a generalization of the proposed theory to describe the processes of generation of tolerance and of self-tolerance. If the stem cells of the T-cell branch as well as of the B-cell branch are suppressed by suitable (e.g., subthreshold) interaction with self antigens or with passively administrated "tolerogenic" concentrations of foreign antigens, similar to the antiidiotypic suppression discussed above, their clonal expansion might be inhibited in a very early stage, so that the corresponding clones are eliminated by indiscriminate mechanisms of death of single cells. Nossal and Pike (1975) have described experiments with differentiating B lymphocytes from bone marrow, which suggest such a clonal elimination mechanism for generation of tolerance against hapten human gamma globulin. The cellular mechanism of suppression processes of this kind might involve ligand-induced inhibition of receptor reexpression (Sidman and Unanue, 1975b). In the case of the self antigens, this suppression might occur already in a stage of clonal sizes of one or a few cells at the very beginning of proliferation of precursor cells. Evidently, these processes can not be treated independently from the effects of immigration and emigration to or from the proliferation compartment, respectively. A pertinent modification of the theory is being investigated at present.

Furthermore, a more detailed treatment of the processes described by the lumped parameters r_s and r_e, as well as the consequences of maturation compartments in the cell cycle with the possibility of an oscillatory approach to steady state have been investigated (manuscript in preparation).

ACKNOWLEDGMENTS

I wish to thank Dipl.-Phys. M. Ernst for his help in some of the early numerical calculations. This work has been supported by grants for Deutsche Forschungsgemeinschaft to Sonderforschungsbereich "Biologische Grenzflächen und Spezifität" (SFB 138).

REFERENCES

Adam, G. and Weiler, E. (1976). Lymphocyte population dynamics during ontogenetic generation of diversity. In *The Generation of Antibody Diversity* (A. J. Cunningham, ed.). Academic, London.

Axelrad, A. A. and van der Gaag, H. C. (1962). Susceptibility to lymphoma induction by Gross' passage A virus in C3Hf/Bi mice of different ages: relation to thymic cell multiplication and differentiation. *J. Nat. Cancer Inst. 28:* 1065-1093.

Ball, W. D. (1963). A quantitative assessment of mouse thymus differentiation. *Exp. Cell Res. 31:* 82-88.

Bryant, B. J. (1972). Renewal and fate in the mammalian thymus: mechanisms and inferences of thymocytokinetics. *Eur. J. Immunol. 2:* 38-45.

Burnet, F. M. (1959). *The Clonal Selection Theory of Acquired Immunity.* Vanderbilt and Cambridge University Presses, Nashville, Tennessee and London.

Cunningham, A. J. and Pilarski, L. (1974). The generation of diversity within single clones of antibody-forming cells. In *The Immune System: Genes, Receptors, Signals* (E. E. Sercarz, A. R. Williamson, and C. F. Fox, eds.). Academic, New York, pp. 367-386.

Droege, W., Zucker, R., and Hannig, K. (1974a). Developmental changes in the cellular composition of the chicken thymus. *Cell. Immunol. 12:* 186-193.

Droege, W., Zucker, R., and Jauker, U. (1974b). Cellular composition of the mouse thymus: developmental changes and the effect of hydrocortisone. *Cell. Immunol. 12:* 173-185.

Friedberg, S. H. and Weissman, I. L. (1974). Lymphoid tissue architecture. II. Ontogeny of peripheral T and B cells in mice: evidence against Peyer's patches as the site of generation of B cells. *J. Immunol. 113:* 1477-1492.

Goidl, E. A. and Siskind, G. W. (1974). Ontogeny of B-lymphocyte function. I. Restricted heterogeneity of the antibody response of B-lymphocytes from neonatal and fetal mice. *J. Exp. Med. 140:* 1285-1302.

Goldschneider, I. (1974). Surface antigens and differentation of thymus-dependent lymphocytes. In *The Cell Surface in Development* (A. A. Moscona, ed.). John Wiley and Sons, New York, pp. 165-185.

Inman, J. K. (1974). Multispecificity of the antibody combining region and antibody diversity. In *The Immune System: Genes, Receptors, Signals* (E. E. Sercarz, A. R. Williamson, and C. F. Fox, eds.). Academic, New York, pp. 37-52.

Jerne, N. K. (1971). The somatic generation of immune recognition. *Eur. J. Immunol. 1:* 1-9.

Jerne, N. K. (1972). What precedes clonal selection? In *Ontogeny of Acquired Immunity, A Ciba Foundation Symposium.* Elsevier, Amsterdam, pp. 1-15.

Jerne, N. K. (1974). Toward a network theory of the immune system. *Ann. Immunol. Inst. Pasteur 125C:* 373-389.

Jerne, N. K. (1975). The immune system - a web of V-domains. In *The Harvey Lectures, Series 70.* Academic, New York.

Klinman, N. R. and Press, J. L. (1975). The B cell specificity repertoire: its relationship to definable subpopulations. *Transplant. Rev. 24:* 41-83.

Melchers, F., von Boehmer, H., and Phillips, R. A. (1975). B-lymphocyte subpopulations in the mouse. *Transplant. Rev. 25:* 26-58.

Metcalf, D. and Moore, M. A. S. (1971). *Haemopoietic Cells.* North Holland Publ. Company, Amsterdam, pp. 172-266.

Metcalf, D. and Wiadrowski, M. (1966). Autoradiographic analysis of lymphocyte proliferation in the thymus and in thymic lymphoma tissue. *Cancer Res. 26:* 483-491.

Mosier, D. E. (1974). Ontogeny of mouse lymphocyte function. I. Paradoxical effects of reactivity to allogeneic cells and phythaemagglutinin in BALB/c fetal thymocytes. *J. Immunol. 112:* 305-310.

Mosier, D. E. and Johnson, B. M. (1975). Ontogeny of mouse lymphocyte function. II. Development of the ability to produce antibody is modulated by T lymphocytes. *J. Exp. Med. 141:* 216-226.

Nossal, G. J. V. and Pike, B. L. (1973). Studies on the differentiation of B lymphocytes in the mouse. *Immunology 25:* 33-45.

Nossal, G. J. V. and Pike, B. L. (1975). Evidence for the clonal abortion theory of B-lymphocyte tolerance. *J. Exp. Med. 141:* 904-917.

Osmond, D. G. and Nossal, G. J. V. (1974). Differentiation of lymphocytes in mouse bone marrow. II. Kinetics of maturation and renewal of antiglobulin-binding cells studied by double labeling. *Cell. Immunol. 13:* 132-145.

Owen, J. J. T. and Raff, M. C. (1970). Studies on the differentiation of thymus-derived lymphocytes. *J. Exp. Med. 132:* 1216-1232.

Owen, J. J. T., Raff, M. C. and Cooper, M. D. (1975). Studies on the generation of B lymphocytes in the mouse embryo. *Eur. J. Immunol. 5:* 468-473.

Parrot, D. M. and de Sousa, M. (1971). Thymus-dependent and thymus-independent populations: origin, migratory patterns and life span. *Clin. Exp. Immunol. 8:* 663-684.

Prothero, J. W. and Tyler, R. W. (1975). A model of thymocyte proliferation. *J. Theor. Biol. 51:* 357-382.

Rosenberg, Y. J. and Cunningham, A. J. (1975). Ontogeny of antibody-forming cell line in mice. I. Kinetics of appearance of mature B cells. *Eur. J. Immunol. 5:* 444-447.

Sidman, C. L. and Unanue, E. R. (1975a). Development of B lymphocytes. I. Cell populations and critical event during ontogeny. *J. Immunol. 114:* 1730-1735.

Sidman, C. L. and Unanue, E. R. (1975b). Receptor-mediated inactivation of early B lymphocytes. *Nature 257:* 149-151.

Spear, P. G. and Edelman, G. M. (1974). Maturation of the humoral immune response in mice. *J. Exp. Med. 139:* 249-263.

Spear, P. G., Wang, A., Rutishauser, U. and Edelman, G. M. (1973). Characterization of splenic lymphoid cells in fetal and newborn mice. *J. Exp. Med. 138:* 557-573.

Strober, S. (1975). Immune function cell surface characteristics and maturation of B cell subpopulations. *Transplant. Rev. 24:* 84-112.

AUTHOR INDEX

Italic numbers give the page on which the complete reference is listed.

A

B

C

I

J

K

N

O

P

Q

R

S

T

Turner, J., 504,511,*518*

SUBJECT INDEX

The first page of a major discussion of a topic is indicated in italic numbers.